Chapter	Fig #	Video Titles
	20-86	Atypical large hypertrophied anal papilla
	20-87	Large tubular adenoma in distal rectum
	20-92	Rectal catheter transiently simulating a polyp at 3D (
	20-95	Squamous cell carcinoma of the anal canal detected
	20-100	Large tubulovillous adenoma involving the ileocecal
	20-102	Cecal tubulovillous adenoma superficially resemblin
	20-104	Inverted appendiceal stump manifesting as a polypo
	20-107	Mucocele of the appendix at 3D CTC
	20-112	Colonic leiomyoma detected at screening CTC
CH 21	21-1	CTC of CRC that was occlusive at OC
	21-2	Asymptomatic cancer detected at CTC screening
	21-3	22-mm malignant polyp in sigmoid colon
	21-7	Asymptomatic cancer in descending colon detected at screening CTC
	21-12	Colon cancer in patient with prior perforation at screening OC
	21-15	Occlusive cancer in transverse colon
	21-16	Cecal cancer at CTC following incomplete OC to the ascending colon
	21-19	Nonocclusive cancer detected at CTC screening
	21-24	Cecal lymphoma found at CTC following incomplete OC
	21-25	Squamous cell carcinoma of the anal canal detected at CTC screening
CH 22	22-2	Large colonic lipoma
	22-7	Rectal carcinoid tumor
	22-16	Colonic leiomyoma detected at screening CTC
	22-26	Mucocele of the appendix at 3D CTC
	22-48	Unsuspected endometriosis involving the sigmoid colon
	22-52	Extrinsic impression of the left kidney upon the descending colon
	22-56	Subtle impression from retrorectal cystic hamartoma
CH 23	23-1	Instructional video
	23-2	Mucosal coverage at one-way 3D fly-through with 90° FOV
	23-4	Comparison of 90°, 120°, and 150° field-of-view (FOV) angles for 3D fly-through
	23-5	Value of 120° versus 90° field-of-view (FOV) for polyp detection
	23-6	Sessile polyp and diverticulum in descending colon
	23-7	Pedunculated polyp on 3D perspective filet versus standard 3D endoluminal fly-through
	23-9	Rectal carpet lesion (villous adenoma with high-grade dysplasia)
	23-10	3D dynamic unfolded "band view" of CRC
	23-11	3D "band view" of small polyp behind a fold
	23-13	Unfolded cube display (3.5-cm tubulovillous adenoma)
		3D unfolded cube view of polyps in the ascending colon
CH 25	25-1	C-RADS C3 category for three 6-9 mm polyps
	25-4	Right-sided advanced adenoma in difficult location for OC detection
	25-9	Asymptomatic cancer in descending colon detected at screening CTC
	25-11	CRC near splenic flexure incorrectly localized to cecum at OC
	25-12	3.5-cm tubulovillous adenoma growing along fold
	25-13	8-cm rectal carpet lesion (villous adenoma)
CH 26	26-1	2-cm cecal adenoma missed at initial OC referral
	26-2	Polyp located at inner turn of flexure missed at initial OC
	26-4	Flat 14-mm right-sided polyp missed at initial OC
	26-10	Incorrect segmental localization of 7-mm adenoma at OC
CH 27	27-20	Ileal polyp (lymphangioma) incidentally detected at CTC screening
	27-20	Gastric polyp identified at CTC screening
CH 29	29-5	Instructional video

AUDIO VIDEO CLIPS

Video Titles

Instructional video

Coating of polyp surface with oral contrast at CTC

3D translucency rendering for soft tissue polyps versus tagged adherent stool

The utility of 3D translucency rendering in the presence of adherent tagged stool

3D translucency rendering to distinguish tagged stool from soft tissue polyps

Colonic leiomyoma detected at screening CTC

2D versus 3D polyp detection in advanced sigmoid diverticular disease

Primary 2D versus primary 3D polyp detection at CTC

Ileal polyp (lymphangioma) incidentally detected at CTC screening

CT Colonography

**PRINCIPLES AND PRACTICE
OF VIRTUAL COLONOSCOPY**

CT Colonography

PRINCIPLES AND PRACTICE OF VIRTUAL COLONOSCOPY

Perry J. Pickhardt, MD
Professor of Radiology
Abdominal Imaging Section
Department of Radiology
University of Wisconsin School of Medicine & Public Health
Madison, Wisconsin

David H. Kim, MD
Associate Professor of Radiology
Abdominal Imaging Section
Department of Radiology
University of Wisconsin School of Medicine & Public Health
Madison, Wisconsin

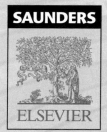

SAUNDERS

ELSEVIER

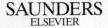

SAUNDERS
ELSEVIER

1600 John F. Kennedy Blvd.
Ste 1800
Philadelphia, PA 19103-2899

CT COLONOGRAPHY: PRINCIPLES AND PRACTICE
OF VIRTUAL COLONOSCOPY

ISBN: 978-1-4160-6168-7

Copyright © 2010 by Saunders, an imprint of Elsevier Inc.

Notice

Knowledge and best practice in this field are constantly changing. As new research and experience broaden our knowledge, changes in practice, treatment and drug therapy may become necessary or appropriate. Readers are advised to check the most current information provided (i) on procedures featured or (ii) by the manufacturer of each product to be administered, to verify the recommended dose or formula, the method and duration of administration, and contraindications. It is the responsibility of the practitioner, relying on their own experience and knowledge of the patient, to make diagnoses, to determine dosages and the best treatment for each individual patient, and to take all appropriate safety precautions. To the fullest extent of the law, neither the Publisher nor the Authors assume any liability for any injury and/or damage to persons or property arising out of or related to any use of the material contained in this book.

The Publisher

Library of Congress Cataloging-in-Publication Data

Pickhardt, Perry J.
  CT colonography : principles and practice of virtual colonoscopy /
Perry J. Pickhardt, David H. Kim.--1st ed.
     p. ; cm.
  Includes bibliographical references.
  ISBN 978-1-4160-6168-7
  1. Colon (Anatomy)--Tomography. I. Kim, David H. II. Title.
  [DNLM: 1. Colonography, Computed Tomographic--methods. 2. Colonic
Neoplasms--diagnosis. 3. Colonic Polyps--radiography. 4.
Colonoscopy--methods. 5. Colorectal Neoplasms--radiography. WI 520
P597c 2010]
  RC804.T65P53 2010
  616.99'43470754--dc22   2009008128

Acquisitions Editor: Rebecca Schmidt Gaertner
Developmental Editor: Martha Limbach
Design Direction: Ellen Zanolle

Printed in the United States of America

Last digit is the print number: 9 8 7 6 5 4 3 2 1

To my amazing wife, Bethney,
and my awesome boys, Silas & Henry,
for their unconditional love and support.
PJP

To Esther, my wife and best friend,
and my children, Mia and Jonathan:
You are the center of my life.
Also, to my parents for their guidance
and love over the years.
DHK

Preface

Since the introduction of cross-sectional abdominal imaging in the 1970s, there has been a steady stream of impressive advances in radiologic techniques. In particular, CT imaging has had a substantial impact on the diagnosis of intraabdominal disease in symptomatic patients. However, the role of abdominal imaging for the screen detection of asymptomatic disease has been quite limited. With the advent of CT colonography (CTC; also referred to as virtual colonoscopy) in the mid-1990s, a paradigm shift appears to be underway. Rarely has a technical innovation in medicine matched so beautifully with a medical need. Colorectal cancer is a prevalent and deadly disease. It represents a leading cause of cancer-related death throughout the industrialized world; however, it is largely preventable. The simple reason for this egregious disconnect is the disappointingly low rate of screening with the existing options. CTC has rapidly evolved to become a highly effective screening tool that has the potential to address this public health concern. In its current form, CTC is not only as sensitive as conventional (optical) colonoscopy for the detection of advanced neoplasia but is also a safer, more convenient, and more cost-effective alternative for screening. It has been extremely gratifying to take part in and to witness the impressive maturation of this technique. Although many key hurdles have been cleared, several important barriers to widespread implementation still remain, most of which are more political than clinical in nature. However, this test is simply too good to hold back for much longer. We look forward to the continuing progress and evolution of CTC, and also to the prospect of ever-decreasing mortality from colorectal cancer. This textbook represents our collective experience with this valuable radiologic technique. It is our hope that the pathway to clinical success with CTC will be made easier through this work.

PERRY J. PICKHARDT, MD

DAVID H. KIM, MD

Acknowledgments

This collective work would simply not have been possible without the invaluable contributions—both direct and indirect—of a number of other individuals who have also dedicated themselves to the advancement of CTC. First and foremost, Holly Casson, RN, BSN, deserves unparalleled recognition for her remarkable passion for patient advocacy with CTC screening. She has directly benefitted countless individuals during the past few years, counseling and convincing many to undergo screening and helping them make appropriate decisions. Her long hours and dedication to forwarding patient care have been absolutely vital to the success of our program. The other physician members of the CTC program at UW, including Andrew Taylor, MD; Louis Hinshaw, MD; and Tom Winter, MD, have been amazing colleagues. The success of the program is also directly related to their good judgment and clinical acumen. We sincerely thank the other team members—past and present—particularly Laura Misterek, RN, and Julie Rohrer, for their tireless efforts. We would also like to acknowledge the forward-thinking local insurance carriers (PPIC, Unity, GHC, and WPS) and the small core of primary care physicians in the Madison area who recognized early on the unique advantages of CTC screening for their patients. And finally, the academic CTC community—both in the United States and abroad—whose unselfish dedication for the greater good has resulted in the development of a superior screening examination that will undoubtedly impart a positive impact in the coming years.

PJP
DHK

Contents

Colorectal Polyps and Cancer

Colorectal Polyps: Overview and Classification

DAVID H. KIM, MD
PERRY J. PICKHARDT, MD

INTRODUCTION

Colorectal carcinoma (CRC) remains a major public health problem accounting for more than 150,000 new cancer diagnoses per year and resulting in more than 50,000 deaths.[1] Despite these grim statistics, this cancer holds a biology that is favorable to screening and prevention and a benign precursor lesion can be easily identified. This lesion is present in the colon for many years before transforming into cancer, and removal of this lesion effectively disrupts the pathway to cancer (Fig. 1-1). From 1998 to 2004, there has been a true decline in CRC incidence rates believed to be directly related to removal of these precancerous lesions at colonoscopy.[2]

The benign colorectal polyp is thus at the core of colorectal cancer screening (Fig. 1-2). As opposed to screening for other cancers such as breast or prostate, screening for CRC focuses not on early *cancer* detection to improve mortality but on the removal of a *benign precursor lesion* to prevent a future cancer. The detection of an early cancer is a secondary focus. The colorectal polyp has been used as this de facto target by optical colonoscopy (OC) screening where all detected polyps are removed to ensure the removal of the true

Progression to cancer

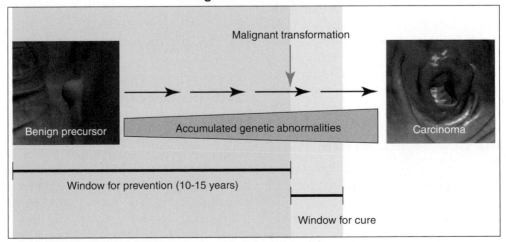

Figure 1-1 **Schematic pathway to cancer.** Screening for CRC is particularly effective because of the long time window *(blue pane)* in which to intervene before the target lesion transforms to cancer. Removal of this target effectively prevents a future cancer. Note that even after cancer conversion, there is a time window during which early detection may lead to a cure *(yellow pane)*.

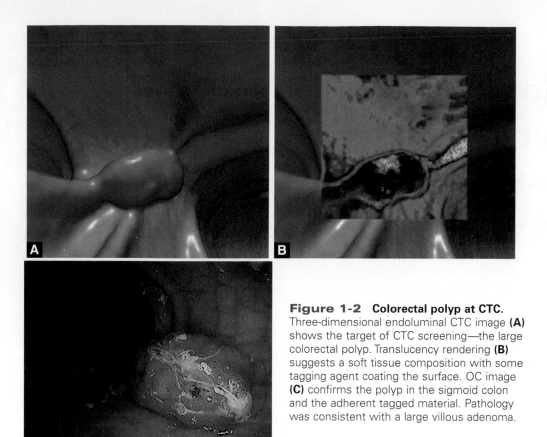

Figure 1-2 Colorectal polyp at CTC.
Three-dimensional endoluminal CTC image **(A)**
shows the target of CTC screening—the large
colorectal polyp. Translucency rendering **(B)**
suggests a soft tissue composition with some
tagging agent coating the surface. OC image
(C) confirms the polyp in the sigmoid colon
and the adherent tagged material. Pathology
was consistent with a large villous adenoma.

benign precursor. The polyp, however, represents an
inefficient surrogate and simply represents a morphologic descriptor for a focal soft tissue protrusion extending from the mucosa into the colonic lumen. It encompasses a variety of different lesions of differing histology
within the colon and rectum. Only a tiny fraction of
polyps removed have the correct histology and potential to accumulate the various genetic abnormalities to
transform into carcinoma. This chapter examines the
different histologic lesions that may present as a polyp
in the colon, highlighting the specific subtypes most
likely to progress to a future cancer. The rationale for
the application of a size criterion to create a more efficient target for screening at computed tomography
colonography (CTC) is explained.

HISTOLOGIC CLASSIFICATION OF POLYPS

Many individuals incorrectly use the terms colorectal
polyps and *adenomas* interchangeably. This practice
has led to confusion and many incorrect assumptions.
Adenomas are one histologic subtype of colorectal polyps. All polyps, however, are not adenomatous. Other
histologic subtypes include mucosal polyps, hyperplastic/
serrated polyps, juvenile polyps, and inflammatory polyps.

In addition, certain types of polyps can arise from layers
deeper than the mucosa, including lipomas, carcinoid
tumors, gastrointestinal stromal tumors (GIST), and
serosal lesions. Adenomas constitute approximately
half of colorectal polyps; hyperplastic and serrated lesions make up about one third or more; and mucosal
polyps make up approximately 10%.[3] The remaining
histologic subtypes constitute only a tiny percentage.
The histologic classification of polyps cannot be reliably determined by gross evaluation either at endoscopy
or at CTC; they require pathologic examination for
final diagnosis.

Adenomatous Polyps

The adenoma represents a benign *neoplastic* proliferation of epithelial origin. It is present throughout the
colorectum in equal proportion within the proximal
and distal colon.[4,5] The prevalence of adenomas in the
U.S. population ranges from 25% to 41% for asymptomatic individuals 50 years of age or older.[4,6,7] The
prevalence has a positive correlation with increasing
age (it significantly increases in patients older than age
60 years[8]) and is also higher in patients with a positive
family history of colorectal cancer and adenomas.[9] The
age distribution curves for adenomas generally parallel

those of colorectal cancer, where the cancer patients are several years older.[10]

Polyps of an adenomatous lineage hold the potential to transform into cancer, but the vast majority of adenomas never accumulate the necessary genetic abnormalities. For the small minority that do, it is estimated that this change from benign adenoma to cancer requires a protracted time period and may take 10 to 15 years.[11-13] This pathway accounts for the majority, or approximately 85%, of sporadic colorectal cancers and is termed the adenoma–carcinoma pathway (see Chapter 3). Until recently, the adenoma was considered the only precursor lesion with the potential for future transformation to carcinoma.

The three histologic classes of adenomas—tubular, tubulovillous, and villous—are based on the glandular architecture (Fig. 1-3). As a simplification, the architecture may demonstrate a crowded, branching glandular pattern, which is present in tubular adenomas; a more elongated, straight, finger-like frond pattern, which is present in villous adenomas; or a combination of both patterns, which is seen in tubulovillous adenomas. By convention, a tubular adenoma may contain up to 25% villous elements, a tubulovillous adenoma may contain 25% to 75% villous elements, and a villous adenoma may have at least 75% villous elements.[12] Tubular adenomas constitute the largest fraction, accounting for approximately 81% of adenomas, whereas tubulovillous adenomas make up 16% and villous adenomas constitute 3%.[14] The difference in future cancer risk is striking between *tubular* adenomas and adenomas with a significant villous component (e.g., tubulovillous and villous adenomas). In fact, considerable controversy arose in the mid-1900s regarding whether tubular adenomas held any malignant potential as opposed to "papillary" adenomas (the previous term describing tubulovillous or villous adenomas), which were considered a precancerous lesion.[15] It is now well established that large (10 mm or greater) tubular adenomas may progress onto cancer, whereas it is much less likely for smaller simple tubular adenomas to do so.[11,12]

The degree of adenoma dysplasia is probably a more important determinant of future cancer risk. It has been traditionally categorized into mild, moderate, and high grade. An adenoma is classified by the most advanced dysplastic focus present. By definition, all adenomas demonstrate at least a mild degree of dysplasia. The important distinction involves high-grade dysplasia (Fig. 1-4). Adenomas with high-grade dysplasia are at greatest risk for progression to cancer.[10,11,14] Conceptually, this makes sense. As adenomas acquire genetic mutations, they exhibit increasing degrees of cytotypic dysplasia prior to transforming to carcinoma. High-grade dysplasia represents the pathologic "bridge" to cancer.[14] It is important to be aware of some additional terms concerning this subject. *Carcinoma in situ* is a synonym for high-grade dysplasia; high-grade dysplasia, however, has become the preferred term. *Intramucosal carcinoma* represents carcinoma that has breached the basement membrane but does not extend beyond the lamina propria of the mucosa. Although a true carcinoma, it has no metastatic potential because no lym-

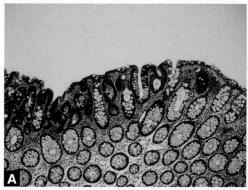
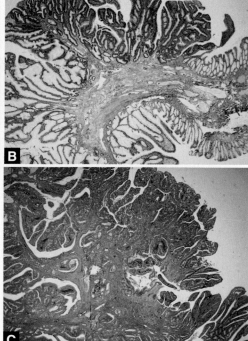

Figure 1-3 Histologic classes of adenomatous polyps. Photomicrograph **(A)** demonstrates a tubular adenoma. It is composed of branching tubules embedded in the lamina propria and thus presents as rounded structures in cut cross section. In contrast, photomicrograph **(B)** of a villous adenoma demonstrates the typical glandular architecture of long finger-like fronds that extend from the polyp surface to the muscularis mucosa. A tubulovillous adenoma **(C)** represents a combination of the two patterns. (Courtesy of Dr. Sara Zydowicz, University of Wisconsin.)

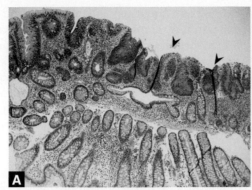
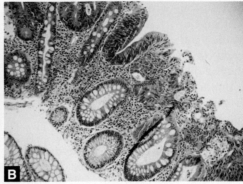

Figure 1-4 High-grade dysplasia (HGD). The bridge to cancer is through HGD. Photomicrograph at 10× magnification **(A)** shows a focus of HGD *(arrowheads)*. Note the difference from the other less dysplastic glands more inferior in the image. At 20× **(B)**, the HGD focus is characterized by pleomorphism of nuclei, more numerous and prominent nucleoli, increased nuclear–cytoplasmic ratio, and extreme glandular crowding. (Courtesy of Dr. Sara Zydowicz, University of Wisconsin.)

phatics are present at this level. *Invasive carcinoma* (with metastatic potential) is when cancer spreads past the muscularis mucosae into the submucosa. A *malignant polyp* is an adenoma with invasive carcinoma (i.e., a focus of cancer that has invaded past the muscularis mucosae). From a practical standpoint, it appears simply as a nondescript polyp at CTC or endoscopy (although typically large in size, ≥10 mm) as opposed to an annular or bulky carcinomatous mass.

Hyperplastic Polyps and Other Serrated Polyps

The hyperplastic polyp is a benign *non-neoplastic* growth characterized by a classic infolding of the crypt epithelium leading to a serrated ("sawtoothed") appearance in a longitudinal pathologic section (Fig. 1-5). No cytologic dysplasia is seen. The prevalence ranges from 10% to 35% of the population.[4,5] As opposed to adenomas, hyperplastic polyps hold no or weak correlation with advancing age.[16] Hyperplastic polyps are common, typically diminutive (≤5 mm), and sessile. They are pliable lesions that may flatten with colonic insufflation.[17] Traditionally, hyperplastic polyps have been considered innocuous lesions with no malignant potential. This view has changed considerably in recent years and is in a state of evolution. Although it is likely that the vast majority of these polyps indeed have no real malignant potential, a small minority can progress to carcinoma through a molecular pathway distinct from the adenoma–carcinoma sequence (see Chapter 3). A tiny number of hyperplastic polyps likely represent the previously unrecognized precursor of a newly described *serrated polyp pathway* that includes the sessile serrated "adenoma" (more aptly named a sessile serrated polyp or serrated polyp with abnormal proliferation), the traditional serrated adenoma, and the mixed hyperplastic/adenomatous polyp.[18,19] A small subset of these serrated polyps can progress to carcinoma

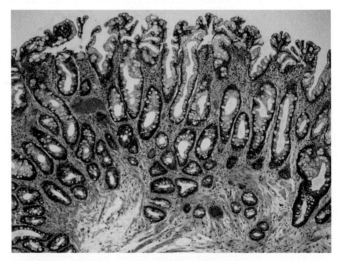

Figure 1-5 Histologic appearance of a hyperplastic polyp. Photomicrograph demonstrates the classic "sawtoothed" appearance of a hyperplastic polyp created by the infolding of the crypt epithelium seen in cut longitudinal section. Hyperplastic polyps are typically innocuous, but a tiny percentage may progress to cancer via the serrated polyp pathway. (Courtesy of Dr. Sara Zydowicz, University of Wisconsin.)

over an extended period (possibly 10 to 20 years).[20,21] It is hypothesized that these precursor lesions hold a higher distribution in the proximal colon[20] as opposed to the hyperplastic group as a whole, which is seen more commonly in the distal colon.[5]

The sessile serrated adenoma represents a hyperplastic variant, typically located in the right colon and large (≥10 mm). The nomenclature unfortunately causes much confusion. This lesion is not necessarily sessile in morphology and is not an adenoma. The term *sessile serrated adenoma* was selected to convey malignant potential of this benign lesion and to differentiate it from the previously described traditional serrated adenoma.[21] This lesion morphologically is similar to a large hyperplastic polyp and does not demonstrate cytologic dyplasia. Consequently, in the past this lesion has been underrecognized and likely was misclassified as a large hyperplastic polyp. It is estimated that 8% or more of large hyperplastic polyps have been misclassified and, in actuality, represent sessile serrated adenomas.[22] The sessile serrated adenoma resides in the serrated neoplastic pathway with the potential for malignant transformation, although controversy remains as to the specific level of risk.

The traditional serrated adenoma demonstrates the serrated architecture of hyperplastic polyps and the overlying dysplastic epithelium of adenomas.[18] Although originally considered a variant of adenomas, this lesion is now considered to reside in the serrated polyp–carcinoma pathway arising ultimately from a hyperplastic polyp. It is felt that this lesion represents a downstream lesion where there has been dysplastic progression of a hyperplastic precursor. In the same vein, the mixed hyperplastic/adenomatous polyp demonstrates discrete areas that resemble hyperplastic polyps and other areas that are adenomatous without a serrated architecture. This lesion is also felt to reside downstream in this molecular genetic pathway. The risk for progression of these lesions is not completely known. However, emerging evidence suggests a potential for malignant transformation similar to traditional adenomas.[23]

Other Histologic Polyps

The other histologic polyp subtypes arising from the mucosa include mucosal, juvenile, and inflammatory polyps. These polyps are benign in nature with no future malignant potential. *Mucosal polyps* are mamillary excrescences of normal mucosal epithelium. The vast majority are diminutive.[24] The *juvenile polyp* is a hamartomatous polyp most commonly seen in patients age 1 to 7 years old, although occasionally they are present in adults. They are usually solitary, pedunculated, and located in the rectosigmoid region. *Inflammatory polyps* are believed to be formed by local extrusion of mucosa as a result of peristaltic forces. A pale fibrinous cap may be seen at optical colonoscopy. It is important to remember that focal projections into the lumen creating polyps can arise from deeper layers. *Lipomas* are a common cause of submucosal polyp origin and may even appear pedunculated in some instances (see Chapter 22). Infrequent causes of submucosal polyps include *carcinoid tumors, hematogenous metastases, GIST,* and *serosal endometriomas.*

THE TARGET POLYP(S) OF COLORECTAL CANCER SCREENING

As discussed previously, the generic polyp has been used as the surrogate for the true precursor lesion of colorectal cancer screening. However, the generic colorec-

tal polyp represents an inefficient and dilute marker where the vast majority have no potential for malignant transformation. Only *adenomas* and *serrated lesions* represent the polyp subgroups that have the possibility for future transformation into cancer, and, even of this group, only a tiny fraction actually accumulate the specific genetic events to progress to cancer (Fig. 1-6). Consequently, it is these few select adenomas and serrated polyps encompassed by the concepts of the *advanced adenoma* and the *high-risk serrated polyp target,* respectively, that represent the true precursor lesions of colorectal cancer. These lesions should therefore represent the primary target polyps of colorectal screening. Unfortunately, these lesions cannot be reliably separated out from the larger population of polyps without histologic evaluation, although lesion size represents a useful surrogate.

The *advanced adenoma* defines those adenomas at high risk for cancer progression (Table 1-1). Criteria

Target versus polyp

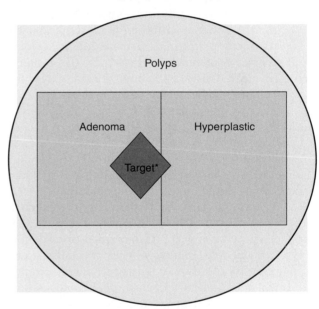

*Target group comprises advanced adenomas and high risk serrated lesions

Figure 1-6   Venn diagram of colorectal polyps. The relationship of the true target lesion of screening to the much larger population of all colorectal polyps is depicted in this Venn diagram. The true target lesion constitutes a tiny fraction of adenomas and hyperplastic lesions, with the majority of these target lesions deriving from an adenomatous lineage.

Table 1-1 ▪ Criteria for Advanced Adenomas

Any adenoma ≥10 mm in size
Harbors a significant villous component (>25%)*
Harbors high-grade dysplasia*

*Regardless of size.

include (1) an adenoma that is large (≥10 mm) and of any histologic subtype (tubular, tubulovillous, villous), (2) an adenoma of any size that contains a significant villous component (tubulovillous or villous histology), or (3) an adenoma of any size that harbors high-grade dyplasia. These factors have been shown to be markers for adenomas that are at increased risk for future progression to carcinoma.[10,25] It is important to remember that advanced adenomas constitute only a small percentage of all colorectal adenomas. A key defining characteristic of these lesions is their large size. In our experience, 90% to 95% of advanced adenomas are characterized by the size criterion and are 10 mm or larger.[26,27] Only a small minority of advanced adenomas are present in the subcentimeter size group, despite the overall preponderance of subcentimeter lesions. For the few small advanced adenomas, the vast majority are characterized by a villous component rather than by the presence of high-grade dysplasia.[26,27] Although both subtypes are lumped together in the definition of an advanced adenoma, the natural history of adenomas with a tubulovillous or villous component is likely different from an adenoma with high-grade dysplasia, with the former demonstrating a more prolonged course prior to cancer conversion.[12] High-grade dysplasia represents a closer histologic step toward carcinoma, whereas villous elements represent a glandular architectural change that is associated with a possible future transformation to carcinoma. Advanced adenomas are located throughout the colon with an approximately equal distribution proximally and distally.[27] They may demonstrate a variety of polyp morphologies including sessile, pedunculated, and flat appearances.

The *high-risk serrated polyp* represents the precursor lesion for the serrated polyp pathway. Increasing evidence suggests that the situation parallels the adenoma side.[23] As seen with adenomas, only a small subset of serrated lesions progress to carcinoma over an extended period. The vast majority of hyperplastic polyps never undergo a transformation to cancer—so much so that hyperplastic polyps have been historically thought not to harbor any malignant potential until recently. Molecular studies point to the likelihood that a tiny fraction of hyperplastic polyps do indeed represent the previously unrecognized precursor of dysplastic serrated lesions. Which of these polyps are the most likely to progress over time? There is gaining consensus that hyperplastic polyps that are 10 mm or greater and proximal in location appear to be more concerning, whereas the diminutive ones in the sigmoid and rectum are highly unlikely to progress, perhaps related to specific hyperplastic polyp subtypes and methylated state (see Chapter 3).[20,28] Multiplicity (greater than 20 in number) also appears to confer increased risk. Similarly, sessile serrated adenomas (which represent nondysplas-

tic serrated lesions with only some architectural changes and are often mistaken for large right-sided hyperplastic polyps) are at risk.[20] Other downstream serrated lesions including the traditional serrated adenoma and the mixed hyperplastic/adenomatous polyp likely have increased risk for future transformation as well. Traditional serrated adenomas have demonstrated similar cancer rates compared with conventional tubulovillous adenomas.[29] The reported prevalence of high-grade dysplasia and intramucosal carcinoma ranges from 4% to 16% in these lesions.[30-32] The time course for progression from a benign lesion to carcinoma in the serrated neoplasia pathway is unknown but is felt to be likely prolonged over many years, probably even longer than the classic adenoma–carcinoma sequence.

THE EFFICIENT TARGET LESION FOR CTC

Despite the knowledge that the true targets of screening are the advanced adenomas and high-risk serrated polyp, the inability to distinguish between these lesions from the larger population of all polyps at optical colonoscopy has led to the situation of the generic polyp (not otherwise specified) as the *de facto* target, and the strategy of universal polypectomy when screening is based on this modality. All polyps are removed to ensure the removal of the few true target lesions. Screening by CTC, however, presents an opportunity for alternative strategies to create a more efficient target for removal, in which select criteria can be used as a surrogate for advanced status. A strategy of selective polypectomy for high-risk lesions as identified by these criteria, with surveillance of patients with low-risk lesions, allows for more efficient identification of advanced adenomas and high-risk serrated polyps from the larger populations of polyps. High-risk lesions suitable for immediate polypectomy are defined by large size (≥10 mm) or multiplicity (three or more 6–9-mm polyps).[33] Patients with low-risk polyps may be placed in surveillance. Those polyps that demonstrate interval growth within surveillance more likely represent the few target lesions in the low-risk group and are then removed. The advantages of a more efficient target by such strategies include maintaining the numbers of advanced lesions while substantially decreasing the number of therapeutic interventions of little or no yield to decrease the procedural complication rate and conserve limited medical resources.

The benefits of a selective polypectomy strategy versus universal polypectomy are significant. In a comparison of the colorectal screening programs at the University of Wisconsin, there was no difference seen in the number of advanced neoplastic lesions between the CTC screening program and its OC counterpart (123 versus 121), whereas there was more than a fourfold decrease in the number of polypectomies (561 versus 2434) and a marked discrepancy in number of complications (zero versus seven perforations).[26] Chapter 2 examines the supporting evidence for using a more efficient polyp target and the selective polypectomy strategy in greater detail. Although selective polypectomy strategies are clearly beneficial at CTC, there is probably less benefit at primary OC screening because localization and assessment for interval growth may be difficult at colonoscopy. In addition, a polyp can be immediately removed once detected given the dual diagnostic and therapeutic nature of colonoscopy. Thus, for optical colonoscopy, one has breached the invasive threshold and can therefore make the case to "clear the colon."

SUMMARY

The colorectal polyp has traditionally represented the surrogate target of colorectal cancer screening programs. However, it is a dilute target where many polyps of little or no future malignant potential are removed to resect the few high-risk lesions. Of the various polyp histologies, only adenomatous and serrated lesions have the potential to undergo malignant transformation, and of these groups, ultimately only a few progress to cancer. These select polyps—the *advanced adenoma* and the *high-risk serrated polyp*—are the primary targets of CTC screening. A selective polypectomy strategy based on large size and multiplicity is at the core of this approach.

REFERENCES

1. Jemal A, Siegel R, Ward E, Murray T, Xu JQ, Thun MJ. Cancer statistics, 2007. CA Cancer J Clin. 2007;57(1):43-66.
2. Espey DK, Wu XC, Swan J, et al. Annual report to the nation on the status of cancer, 1975-2004, featuring cancer in American Indians and Alaska natives. Cancer. 2007;110(10):2119-2152.
3. Vatn MH, Stalsberg H. The prevalence of polyps of the large-intestine in Oslo—An autopsy study. Cancer. 1982;49(4):819-825.
4. Johnson DA, Gurney MS, Volpe RJ, et al. A prospective-study of the prevalence of colonic neoplasms in asymptomatic patients with an age-related risk. Am J Gastroenterol. 1990;85(8):969-974.
5. Disario JA, Foutch PG, Mai HD, Pardy K, Rao KM. Prevalence and malignant potential of colorectal polyps in asymptomatic, average-risk men. Am J Gastroenterol.1991;86(8):941-945.
6. Lieberman DA, Smith FW. Screening for colon malignancy with colonoscopy. Am J Gastroenterol.1991;86(8):946-951.
7. Lieberman DA, Weiss DG, Bond JH, et al. Use of colonoscopy to screen asymptomatic adults for colorectal cancer. N Engl J Med. 2000;343(3):162-168.
8. Arminski TC, McLean DW. Incidence and distribution of adenomatous polyps of the colon and rectum based on 1,000 autopsy examinations. Dis Colon Rectum. 1964;7:249-261.
9. Gaglia P, Atkin WS, Whitelaw S, et al. Variables associated with the risk of colorectal adenomas in asymptomatic patients with a family history of colorectal-cancer. Gut. 1995;36(3):385-390.
10. Morson BC. Evolution of cancer of colon and rectum. Cancer. 1974;34(3):845-849.
11. Muto T, Bussey HJR, Morson BC. Evolution of cancer of colon and rectum. Cancer. 1975;36(6):2251-2270.
12. Obrien MJ, Winawer SJ, Zauber AG, et al. The National Polyp Study—Patient and polyp characteristics associated with high-grade dysplasia in colorectal adenomas. Gastroenterology. 1990;98(2):371-379.
13. Kozuka S, Nogaki M, Ozeki T, Masumori S. Pre-malignancy of mucosal polyp in large-intestine .2. Estimation of periods required for malignant transformation of mucosal polyps. Dis Colon Rectum. 1975;18(6):494-500.
14. Konishi F, Morson BC. Pathology of colorectal adenomas—A colonoscopic survey. J Clin Pathol. 1982;35(8):830-841.
15. Castleman B, Krickstein HI. Do adenomatous polyps of the colon become malignant? N Engl J Med. 1962;267(10):469-475.
16. Morimoto LM, Newcomb PA, Ulrich CM, Bostick RM, Lais CJ, Potter JD. Risk factors for hyperplastic and adenomatous polyps: Evidence for malignant potential? Cancer Epidemiol Biomarkers Prev. 2002;11(10):1012-1018.
17. Waye JD, Bilotta JJ. Rectal hyperplastic polyps—Now you see them, now you don't—A differential point. Am J Gastroenterol.1990;85(12):1557-1559.
18. Jass JR, Biden KG, Cummings MC, et al. Characterisation of a subtype of colorectal cancer combining features of the suppressor and mild mutator pathways. J Clin Pathol. 1999;52(6):455-460.
19. Hawkins NJ, Bariol C, Ward RL. The serrated neoplasia pathway. Pathology. 2002;34(6):548-555.
20. O'Brien MJ. Hyperplastic and serrated polyps of the colorectum. Gastroenterol Clin N Am. 2007;36:947-968.
21. Snover DC, Jass JR, Fenoglio-Preiser C, Batts KP. Serrated polyps of the large intestine - A morphologic and molecular review of an evolving concept. Am J Clin Pathol. 2005;124(3):380-391.
22. Higuchi T, Sugihara K, Jass JR. Demographic and pathological characteristics of serrated polyps of colorectum. Histopathology. 2005;47(1):32-40.
23. Huang CS, O'Brien MJ, Yang S, Farraye FA. Hyperplastic polyps, serrated adenomas, and the serrated polyp neoplasia pathway. Am J Gastroenterol.2004;99(11):2242-2255.
24. Pickhardt PJ, Choi JR, Hwang I, Schindler WR. Nonadenomatous polyps at CT colonography: Prevalence, size distribution, and detection rates. Radiology. 2004;232(3):784-790.
25. Winawer SJ, Zauber AG. The advanced adenoma as the primary target of screening. Gastrointest Endosc Clin N Am. 2002;12(1):1-9.
26. Kim DH, Pickhardt PJ, Taylor AJ, et al. CT colonography versus colonoscopy for the detection of advanced neoplasia. N Engl J Med. 2007;357(14):1403-1412.
27. Kim DH, Pickhardt PJ, Taylor AJ. Characteristics of advanced adenomas detected at CT colonographic screening: Implications for appropriate polyp size thresholds for polypectomy versus surveillance. Am J Roentgenol. 2007;188(4):940-944.
28. Cunningham KS, Riddell RH. Serrated mucosal lesions of the colorectum. Curr Opin Gastroenterol. 2006;22(1):48-53.
29. Lazarus R, Junttila OE, Karttunen TJ, Makinen MJ. The risk of metachronous neoplasia in patients with serrated adenoma. Am J Clin Pathol. 2005;123(3):349-359.
30. Iwabuchi M, Sasano H, Hiwatashi N, et al. Serrated adenoma: A clinicopathological, DNA ploidy, and immunohistochemical study. Anticancer Res. 2000;20(2B):1141-1147.
31. Matsumoto T, Mizuno M, Shimizu M, Manabe T, Iida M, Fujishima M. Serrated adenoma of the colorectum: colonoscopic and histologic features. Gastrointest Endosc. 1999;49(6):736-742.
32. Rubio CA, Jaramillo E. Flat serrated adenomas of the colorectal mucosa. Jpn J Cancer Res. 1996;87(3):305-309.
33. Zalis ME, Barish MA, Choi JR, et al. CT colonography reporting and data system: A consensus proposal. Radiology. 2005;236(1):3-9.

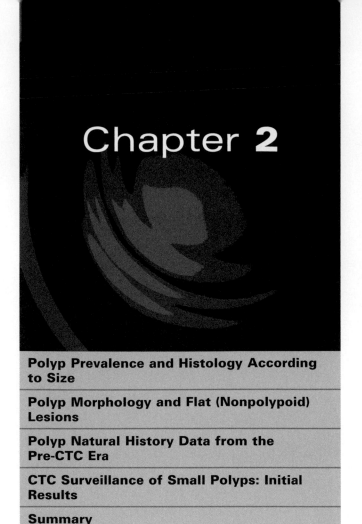

Chapter 2

Colorectal Polyps: Prevalence, Histology, Morphology, and Natural History

PERRY J. PICKHARDT, MD
DAVID H. KIM, MD

data based on actual screening cohorts now exist, which should replace this older teaching. This chapter will provide an update on a variety of key polyp topics to construct a proper framework for physicians who are interested in providing CTC screening as a clinical service.

INTRODUCTION

With convincing data confirming the excellent clinical performance, high safety profile, and superior cost-effectiveness of CT colonography (CTC) for colorectal cancer screening, the American Cancer Society officially endorsed this tool as a recommended screening test in March 2008.[1] With both clinical validation and acceptance by key medical societies secured, the final hurdle to widespread implementation of CTC screening—reimbursement by national third-party payers—now appears possible. With broader coverage and implementation for CTC screening on the horizon, involved physicians must be well versed in a number of key concepts with regard to colorectal polyps, including the expected screening prevalence, histologic characteristics, morphologic features, and existing evidence on natural history. These topics will generally not be covered adequately in CTC-specific reviews that focus more on technique or interpretation.[2] Furthermore, although some of these concepts may have been inculcated during residency or fellowship training, much of the "classic" data that have been passed down were based on high-risk or symptomatic cohorts. Unfortunately, these older statistics do not generalize to asymptomatic screening and may lead to inappropriate management decisions. Newer and more applicable

POLYP PREVALENCE AND HISTOLOGY ACCORDING TO SIZE

The need for rational evidence-based screening algorithms and surveillance guidelines based on polyp size is an important challenge facing large-scale implementation of CTC screening. Most experts agree that large polyps detected at CTC screening will generally warrant polypectomy, whereas immediate colonoscopy is not necessary for isolated diminutive polyps (≤5 mm).[3-11] Specifically with regard to diminutive lesions detected at CTC, an American Gastroenterological Association (AGA) future trends report from 2004 noted that "polyps ≤5 mm in size do not appear to be a compelling reason for colonoscopy and polypectomy."[11] Ransohoff added that "few clinicians would likely argue that colonoscopy is justified" for diminutive lesions, adding that "the overwhelming majority cannot possibly represent an important near-term health threat."[9] In an insightful editorial from 2001, Bond remarked that "a large volume of scientific data indicates that clinicians need to shift their attention away from simply finding and harvesting all diminutive colorectal adenomas toward strategies which allow the reliable detection of the much less common, but much more dangerous advanced adenoma."[3] Although a small number of gastroenterologists have suggested that colonoscopy referral might be considered for isolated CTC-detected diminutive lesions,[12] the real controversy regarding the clinical management of polyps detected at CTC clearly relates to the handling of small (6-9 mm) colorectal polyps.[1,4,10,11,13,14] To critically and objectively analyze this issue, we must strive to avoid the potential traps of protectionist "turf battles" and focus more on our current knowledge of the histology and, more importantly, our understanding of the behavior and natural history of small colorectal polyps in a screening population.

Because most polyps detected at primary optical colonoscopy (OC) screening are generally removed, polyp histology according to lesion size has been well established. However, one must keep in mind that the histology of resected polyps represents a static cross-sectional end point that does not provide any longitudinal information regarding clinical behavior or significance. Therefore, polyp histology alone does not describe its prior growth rate and it does not reliably predict what its future risk would have been if left in place. Furthermore, it is absolutely critical to ascertain whether the data are derived from asymptomatic screening populations or symptomatic high-risk cohorts because the rates of clinically important histology will greatly differ between these two groups. It is widely accepted that lesion size is undoubtedly the single most important determinant of clinical significance. Larger lesions are more often neoplastic, more frequently demonstrate advanced histology, and of course represent the vast majority of life-threatening cancers.

The ideal target for screening and prevention of colorectal cancer is the "advanced adenoma," which is defined as an adenoma that is large ($\geq$10 mm) and/or contains histologic findings of either high-grade dysplasia or a prominent villous component.[15] The serrated polyp pathway, which is distinct from the classic adenoma–carcinoma sequence, may account for about 15% of colorectal cancer cases.[16] Serrated adenomas less than 10 mm in size without significant dysplasia, which represent polyp entities along this pathway, should not be considered as histologically advanced lesions, but serrated adenomas that are large or exhibit dysplasia should be categorized as advanced.

In terms of prevalence data for colorectal polyps according to both size and relevant histology, a common pitfall is to quote the "classic" literature that is largely based on symptomatic, high-risk series.[17-19] Instead, one should realize the wealth of more recent data derived from a number of endoscopic screening trials[4,8,20-27] involving predominately healthy, asymptomatic cohorts including both men and women (Table 2-1). These modern studies, which are predominately OC trials but also include some combined CTC-OC studies, comprise more than 100,000 subjects and demonstrate some remarkably similar findings that should serve as our new reference point for screening in terms of expected polyp prevalence and histology according to lesion size.[2] Several other trials that either did not include a good gender mix or reported findings only in terms of proximal and distal disease were excluded from consideration but parallel the larger representative series.[2,28-30]

Table 2-1 ◘ Relevant Colorectal Polyp Data from Modern Screening Cohorts[2]

Variable	Typical Value	Reported Range	References
SCREENING PREVALENCE OF:			
All colorectal polyps $\geq$6 mm	14%	13-16%	4, 8, 23, 25, 27, 31
Small (6-9 mm) polyps	8%	8-9%	4, 8, 25, 27, 31
Large ($\geq$10 mm) polyps	6%	5-7%	4, 8, 25, 27, 31
Advanced neoplasia (any polyp size)	3-4%	3.3-6.9%*	4, 8, 21, 23, 26, 27
Small (6-9 mm) advanced adenomas	0.3%	0.17-0.46%	8, 25, 27
High-grade dysplasia in small polyps	0.05%	0.048-0.064%	8, 27
Invasive cancer in small polyps	0.01%	0-0.039%	4, 8, 21, 25, 27, 31
Rate of advanced histology in 6-9- mm adenomas	4%	2.7-5.3%†	8, 21, 25, 27
Rate of high-grade dysplasia in 6-9- mm adenomas	0.7%	0.5-0.8%	21, 27
Rate of invasive cancer in 6-9- mm adenomas	0.1%	0-0.49%	4, 8, 20, 21, 24, 25, 27, 31
Rate of invasive cancer in 1-2- cm adenomas	1%	0.5-2.4%	22, 25, 27

*Note: the rate increases to 7.1% in reference 27 if all small serrated adenomas are considered histologically advanced.
†Note: The rate increases to 6.6% in reference 27 if all small serrated adenomas are considered histologically advanced.

Although 35% to 50% of adults older than age 50 years may harbor at least one colorectal polyp,[4,8,23,25,27,31] the largest lesion will be diminutive in most cases. In fact, recent screening studies have demonstrated a remarkably narrow 13% to 16% prevalence range for polyps 6 mm and larger (Table 2-1), with a representative value of about 14% as an approximate average. The polyp prevalence at the 6-mm threshold is more reproducible than the prevalence for all polyps (i.e., including diminutive lesions) and is much more clinically relevant to CTC screening. The prevalence for large polyps is 5% to 6%, whereas about 8% will have a polyp in the 6- to 9-mm range (Table 2-1). As a general rule, approximately one third of diminutive lesions are adenomatous (almost exclusively tubular adenomas) and two thirds are nonadenomatous, predominately consisting of non-neoplastic mucosal tags and hyperplastic polyps.[4,32] Above the 6-mm size threshold, the ratio of adenomatous-to-nonadenomatous polyps reverses, with neoplastic lesions representing approximately two thirds of nondiminutive lesions.[4,31,32] It has been well established in the gastrointestinal literature that finding three or more adenomas at OC increases a patient's future risk for additional adenomas at surveillance,[33] but the risk related to multiple diminutive-only tubular adenomas is probably much lower. Therefore, CTC detection of at least one nondiminutive adenoma would presumably identify most patients at increased risk.

Because of the central importance of advanced adenomas for colorectal cancer prevention,[3,4,8,15,21] the overall and size-specific prevalence data for these lesions are critical considerations in determining appropriate screening strategies. The presence of high-grade dysplasia, previously termed "carcinoma in situ," is of particular interest because it is believed to be more clinically relevant than villous histology in terms of more imminent cancer transformation.[34,35] Of course, the prevalence of invasive cancer according to polyp size is also an important consideration. When recent data are analyzed in terms of important histology, it is again remarkable how closely the results agree with each other and how much they differ from the classic teaching. The overall prevalence of advanced adenomas in modern screening cohorts has ranged from 3.3% to 6.9% in most recent trials (Table 2-1), which is considerably lower than the prevalence values for groups at increased risk.

Although large adenomas comprise about 90%-95% of all advanced neoplasia,[21] approximately 4% of 6- to 9-mm adenomas will demonstrate advanced histology, with a reported range of 2.7% to 5.3%. By comparison, 10% of 5- to 10-mm adenomas were found to be advanced in a high-risk cohort.[36] Given the screening prevalence of 6- to 9-mm polyps of about 8% and a frequency of advanced histology in small adenomas of 4%, the overall screening prevalence of small advanced adenomas is approximately 0.3%, with a reported range of 0.17% to 0.56%. Fortunately, the presence of high-grade dysplasia in 6- to 9-mm adenomas is even more uncommon, with an overall prevalence of about 0.05%.

A commonly quoted historical figure for the cancer rate among small 6- to 9-mm adenomas is 0.9%.[11,17-19] However, when the recent large screening studies are tallied, the frequency of cancer dips to 0.1% or lower, ranging from 0% to 0.5%, with most reported cancers concentrated within one Korean series.[25] We have yet to encounter a subcentimeter invasive cancer in our combined CTC and OC experience, including more than 1000 6- to 9-mm polyps. Even for large 1- to 2-cm adenomas, the cancer rate appears to be only about 1% or less (Table 2-1), which is considerably lower than the commonly quoted historical range of 5% to 10%, which is again based on high-risk cohorts and not screening populations.[17,19] Given that about 30% to 40% of large polyps are nonadenomatous[4,31,32] and that some large lesions detected at CTC may be false-positive results,[31,37] the actual cancer risk for a 1- to 2-cm lesion detected at CTC is actually less than 1%, which is lower than the 1% to 2% frequency for significant complications at therapeutic OC referral.[38-41] This risk is also lower than the accepted 2% cancer rate for Breast Imaging Reporting and Data System 3 (BI-RADS) breast lesions at mammography, for which follow-up is recommended. The natural history data on 1- to 2-cm polyps from Stryker et al (discussed later) provide further evidence that even these relatively large lesions are predominately benign findings.

POLYP MORPHOLOGY AND FLAT (NONPOLYPOID) LESIONS

Polyps measuring ≤3 cm are generally divided into three major morphologic categories: sessile, pedunculated, and flat (Fig. 2-1). Invasive masses are generally bulky annular or semiannular tumors that comprise a morphologic category distinct from polyps. Sessile polyps have a relatively broad base of attachment, classically creating a "bowler hat" appearance, whereas pedunculated polyps have a defined head and stalk, which connects the lesion to the adjacent colonic surface. "Polypoid" lesions refer to both sessile and pedunculated polyps and account for the vast majority of cases, including most advanced adenomas and cancers.[8,21] Flat lesions represent a subset of sessile polyps that, as the name implies, have a "nonpolypoid" plaque-like morphology. A polyp height that is less than half its width has been commonly used as a morphologic descriptor,[42,43] but this definition is generally too forgiving and could include lesions that would be better labeled as sessile. For smaller flat polyps less than 3 cm in size, we have found that lesion elevation above the surrounding mucosal surface is typically 3 mm or less.[7] Categorization of large, superficially elevated lesions that are clearly flat in morphology

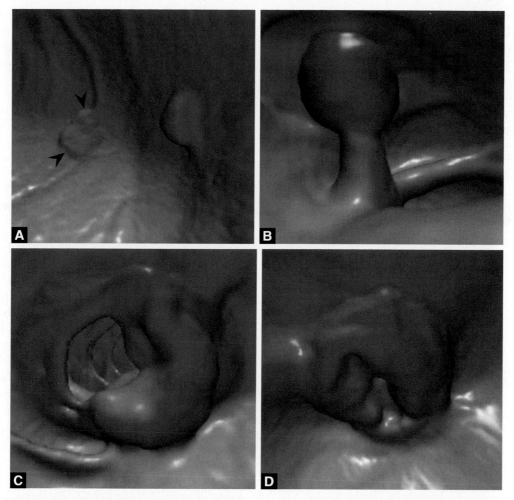

Figure 2-1   Morphology of colorectal polyps and masses. 3D endoluminal CTC image **(A)** shows a large sessile polyp adjacent to a large flat lesion *(arrowheads)*. Although the flat polyp is larger in linear size, it is less conspicuous and less voluminous than the sessile lesion. 3D endoluminal image from a second patient **(B)** shows a large pedunculated polyp. Images from two patients with invasive cancer demonstrate semiannular **(C)** and complete annular **(D)** morphology. The patient without circumferential involvement was asymptomatic, whereas the annular mass resulted in obstructive symptoms.

but that may exceed a maximal height of 3 mm is less uniform. The term "carpet lesion," also referred to as a laterally or superficially spreading tumor, best applies to this important subset of flat lesions that tend to be large in cross-sectional area (≥3 cm) but not bulky.[44]

Both the prevalence and clinical significance of flat (nonpolypoid) lesions have been the source of recent debate. Endoscopic detection of nonpolypoid lesions may be increased by the use of advanced endoscopic techniques such as chromoendoscopy and narrow band imaging. However, unlike the case for East Asia,[45] there is little evidence to suggest that small, flat, aggressive lesions represent a major problem in the U.S. screening population. Although a single-center Department of Veterans Affairs study[43] suggested that important nonpolypoid lesions may be more common in the United States than previously thought, closer inspection reveals that the conclusions are not supported by the findings.[46] First, a clear distinction must be made between the *rela-*

tively flat lesions primarily described in this study (defined as elevated lesions with a height less than half the diameter) and *completely flat* or *depressed lesions*. What has been widely overlooked is that the authors remarked that "completely flat lesions are exceedingly rare" and presumably were completely absent in this study. Furthermore, depressed lesions comprised less than 1% of all colorectal lesions (18 of 2770), only 4 of which were seen at screening. Therefore, nearly all nonpolypoid lesions from this study were elevated from the surrounding mucosa, which is a critical distinction that favors detection at both standard colonoscopy and CT colonography. In addition, the authors combined "carcinoma in situ," which is more appropriately termed "high-grade dysplasia," with invasive cancer. This is an unfortunate and misleading way to report histology, especially because the majority of nonpolypoid "cancers" in this study (11 of 15) were actually noninvasive advanced adenomas. The average size of advanced nonpolypoid lesions was relatively large (1.6 cm) and similar in size to their polypoid counterparts (1.9 cm), which also bodes well for detection at CTC. In contrast, data from the National Polyp Study showed that flat adenomas were actually *less* likely to harbor high-grade dysplasia compared with sessile or pedunculated adenomas.[47] In addition, patients with flat adenomas were not found to be at greater risk for advanced adenomas at subsequent surveillance colonoscopy. If aggressive flat lesions in this trial had somehow been missed, more incident cancers would have presumably developed over the course of longitudinal evaluation.[46,48] In fact, the relative frequency of flat adenomas in the National Polyp Study was similar to that reported when chromoendoscopic techniques are used.

Our own experience with 125 flat lesions measuring ≥6 mm detected at CTC screening has also demonstrated a nonaggressive picture.[49] Of 92 flat lesions less than 3 cm in size evaluated at subsequent OC, 23 (25.0%) were neoplastic, 5 (5.4%) were histologically advanced, and none were malignant. In comparison, polypoid lesions measuring less than 3 cm were much more likely to be neoplastic (60.3%; 363 of 602), histologically advanced (12.1%; 73 of 602), and malignant (0.5%; 3 of 602). None of the 9 flat lesions seen only at colonoscopy (i.e., CTC false negatives) were histologically advanced and only 2 were neoplastic (tubular adenomas). All 10 carpet lesions (i.e., laterally spreading tumors ≥3 cm in size) were neoplastic and 9 were histologically advanced. These findings indicate that flat lesions less than 3 cm in size are not a major concern compared with polypoid lesions of similar size and that large carpet lesions represent the subset of polyps with flat morphology of most interest.

Because flat lesions are generally less conspicuous than polypoid lesions, they tend to be more challenging to initially detect at CTC, as with OC. However, good sensitivity can be achieved with combined three-dimensional–two-dimensional (3D–2D) polyp detection, as shown in the Department of Defense CTC screening trial.[42] Both phantom and clinical studies have shown that 3D endoluminal evaluation improves the sensitivity for detecting flat lesions.[42,45,50] In our recent clinical experience, more large flat advanced adenomas were detected at primary CTC screening compared with primary OC screening, albeit they were uncommon in either arm.[8] It is interesting that histologically advanced or depressed small flat lesions appear to be exceedingly rare in our screening population. In fact, most flat lesions detected (Fig. 2-2) or missed (Fig. 2-3) at CTC are hyperplastic at pathologic examination.[32,51] The flat nature of many hyperplastic polyps at CTC likely results in part from their tendency to flatten out when the colonic lumen is well distended (Fig. 2-4).[52] In the Mayo Clinic experience, the great majority of occult polyps at CTC (i.e., missed lesions that could not be identified even retrospectively) were flat hyperplastic polyps ranging in size from 6 mm to

2.1 cm.[53] This mirrors our own clinical experience with occult lesions at CTC.[32,54] Given these collective findings, we believe that flat lesions remain a diagnostic challenge but do not represent a major drawback to widespread CTC screening.

Carpet lesions are an important subset of flat lesions that, despite their large surface area, can be relatively subtle on CTC because of the relative paucity of raised tissue. These lesions have a strong predilection for the rectum and cecum.[55] Despite their large linear size, they have a relatively low rate of malignancy but frequently demonstrate villous features, with or without high-grade dysplasia.[44,55] Although classic carpet lesions are less conspicuous than sessile or pedunculated polyps, they are nonetheless detectable at CTC in our experience as a result of fixed-fold distortion or edges with a rolled-up or polypoid appearance (Fig. 2-5). Optimal preparation and distention, and a hybrid 3D–2D detection strategy, allow for confident detection of carpet lesions. In some cases, endoscopic mucosal resection can serve as the definitive treatment, whereas others will require more aggressive surgery.[44]

POLYP NATURAL HISTORY DATA FROM THE PRE-CTC ERA

The natural history of small colorectal polyps has become a central issue of critical importance. One reason for this is that CTC is undoubtedly a highly efficacious and cost-effective approach to population screening when only large polyps (≥10 mm) necessitate referral for polypectomy.[5] If small (6-9 mm) polyps are deemed to carry a high enough risk to warrant therapeutic OC in all cases, the utility of CTC as an intermediate filter will be decreased somewhat, although it appears to remain useful.[4,6,8] To underscore the importance of this topic, the AGA issued a statement that "the need to define the natural history and biological significance of polyps smaller than a centimeter is central to refining colorectal cancer screening, irrespective of modality." Although our ongoing natural history study (discussed later) is, to our knowledge, the first to follow a substantial cohort of small 6- to 9-mm polyps using CTC as the surveillance tool, a number of older studies have followed small unresected polyps using other colorectal examinations, including endoscopy and barium enema. In fact, contrary to the prevailing general perception, a fair amount of data on polyp natural history already exists from these older longitudinal trials, which has somehow been forgotten over time. When considered together as a group, these longitudinal studies have repeatedly demonstrated the benign, indolent nature of unresected subcentimeter colorectal polyps. No study to date has ever shown that leaving 6- to 9-mm polyps in place is a harmful practice. It is instructive to briefly review these early trials, some of which are more than 40 years old.

In Norway, Hofstad et al performed serial colonoscopy on unresected subcentimeter polyps and found that only

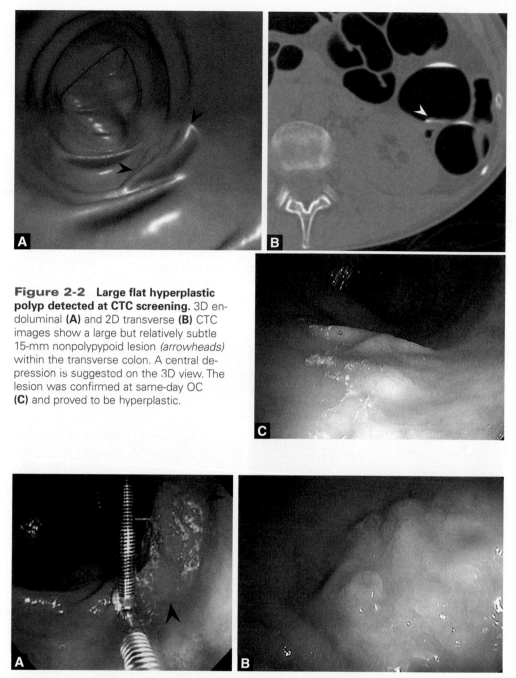

Figure 2-2   Large flat hyperplastic polyp detected at CTC screening. 3D endoluminal **(A)** and 2D transverse **(B)** CTC images show a large but relatively subtle 15-mm nonpolypypoid lesion *(arrowheads)* within the transverse colon. A central depression is suggested on the 3D view. The lesion was confirmed at same-day OC **(C)** and proved to be hyperplastic.

Figure 2-3   Large flat hyperplastic lesions missed at CTC screening. Large but subtle flat 2-cm hyperplastic lesion identified at OC **(A,** *arrowheads)* in the Department of Defense screening but not seen at CTC. Flat 5-cm hyperplastic lesion seen at the cecal base at OC in a second patient **(B)** but not called at CTC. Most large missed lesions at CTC are nonadenomatous and likely of no clinical significance. (A, from Pickhardt PJ, Choi JR, Hwang I, Schindler WR. Nonadenomatous polyps at CT colonography: Prevalence, size distribution, and detection rates. *Radiology.* 2004;232:784-790.)

1 (0.5%) of 189 lesions eclipsed the 10-mm threshold after a 1-year time interval.[56] At the 3-year follow-up mark, most polyps in this study remained stable or regressed in size, and there was an overall tendency to net regression among the "medium-sized" (5-9 mm) polyps.[57] The authors of this endoscopic trial concluded that following unresected 5- to 9-mm polyps for 3 years was a safe practice. Longitudinal studies using flexible sigmoid-oscopy have also demonstrated the stability of smaller polyps over time.[58-60] In one study that used serial sigmoidoscopy to follow polyps measuring up to 15 mm in size over a 3- to 5-year period, Knoernschild reported a significant increase in polyp size in only 4% of patients.[58] In a longitudinal study using barium enemas to follow colorectal polyps, Welin et al showed exceedingly slow growth rates by studying 375 unresected polyps over a

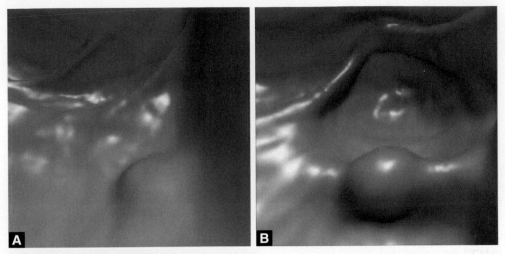

Figure 2-4 **Flattening of a hyperplastic polyp with increased luminal distention.** Supine **(A)** and prone **(B)** 3D endoluminal displays show a cecal hyperplastic polyp that has a relatively flat appearance on the well-distended supine view but a more sessile appearance on the prone view, where luminal distention is decreased (note the thickened appearance of the triangular fold surrounding the appendiceal orifice).

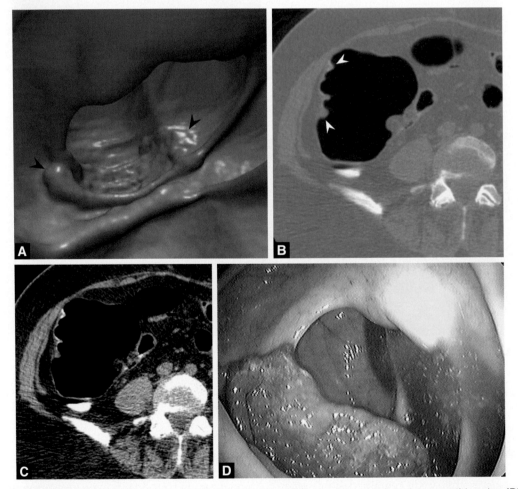

Figure 2-5 **Large cecal carpet lesion.** 3D endoluminal CTC image **(A)** and 2D transverse images with polyp **(B)** and soft tissue **(C)** windowing show a 6-cm area of mucosal irregularity and distorted fold thickening *(arrowheads)* opposite the ileocecal valve. This carpet lesion was confirmed at same-day OC **(D)** and proved to be a benign but histologically advanced tubulovillous adenoma with high-grade dysplasia.

mean interval of 30 months.[61] The high observed adenoma detection rates at surveillance in the National Polyp Study, in conjunction with the low observed colorectal cancer incidence, was felt to be explainable only by regression of adenomas.[62] Finally, in a classic barium enema study by Stryker et al,[63] the cumulative 5-year and 10-year risk of cancer related to large colorectal polyps ($\geq$1 cm) left in place was less than 3% and 10%, respectively. Although the authors concluded that their findings supported the practice of routine polypectomy for large lesions, it may come as a surprise to some how benign the behavior is for the great majority of these polyps, for which there is no debate on management.

CTC SURVEILLANCE OF SMALL POLYPS: INITIAL RESULTS

The longitudinal studies discussed previously that used endoscopic or barium enema techniques to follow unresected polyps are reassuring, but they have done surprisingly little to quell the current debate over the clinical management of small polyps detected at CTC screening.[12] Part of the problem is merely a lack of awareness that these studies even exist. However, issues beyond this simple fact reinforce the need for repeating a natural history trial using CTC as the instrument. For one, CTC provides superior polyp measurement capabilities compared with the other colorectal imaging examinations, including improved accuracy and reproducibility for linear size assessment.[64,65] Furthermore, CTC allows for polyp volume assessment, which greatly amplifies interval changes in polyp size compared with linear measurement (Fig. 2-6).[66] A secondary limitation of the prior polyp surveillance studies was that the sample sizes of some studies were underpowered to influence a change in practice. However, even without large-scale proof, the CT Colonography Reporting and Data System (C-RADS) consensus opinion from the Working Group on Virtual Colonoscopy felt that 3-year CTC surveillance for individuals

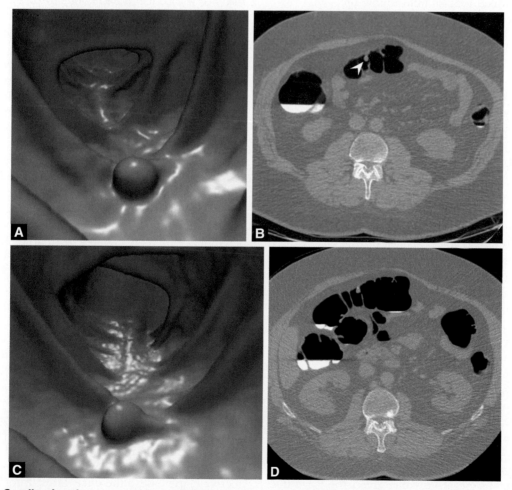

Figure 2-6 **Small polyp that was stable or slightly smaller in size at CTC surveillance.** 3D endoluminal **(A)** and 2D transverse **(B)** CTC images show a small sessile polyp in the transverse colon *(arrowhead)* that measured 7.8 mm in maximal linear dimension and 270 mm^3 in volume. Images from follow-up CTC performed 2 years later **(C** and **D)** show the same polyp, which now measured 7.6 mm in linear size and 230 mm^3 in volume. Although the changes in linear size and volume are not significant, note how the relative change in volume (15%) is amplified compared with the linear change (3%).

with one or two 6- to 9-mm polyps represented a reasonable clinical approach.[7]

To provide further evidence on the safety of short-term CTC surveillance for 6- to 9-mm polyps, and, it is hoped, to one day influence screening practice and policy, we undertook a prospective natural history study. This trial represents a collaborative effort between the University of Wisconsin (UW) and the National Naval Medical Center (NNMC) in Bethesda, MD. The precise protocol used at each center for polyp follow-up differs in a relatively small but meaningful way that provides even more complementary data. At UW, enrolled patients with a 6- to 9-mm polyp that has not measurably increased in size at 1 to 2 years after CTC follow-up are eligible for continued CTC surveillance (with an expanded interval out to 3-5 years). At NNMC, all patients undergo OC for polypectomy following CTC surveillance at 1 year. Therefore, the UW arm is relatively rich in polyp-years but lacks histologic data for most polyps that are stable or regressed, whereas the NNMC arm provides needed histologic data but loses the opportunity for continued longitudinal follow-up.

We presented the results of CTC surveillance for 128 small colorectal polyps from our initial 100 patients at the 2008 Annual Meeting of the Society of Gastrointestinal Radiologists.[67] A measurable change in linear polyp size was defined as an increase in diameter of 1 mm or greater. The average CTC follow-up interval was 1.4 years (range 362-1126 days), corresponding to 184 cumulative polyp-years of data. Of the 128 small polyps, 12 (9.4%) demonstrated interval growth, including 11 proven adenomas (1 polyp could not be retrieved at OC) in 9 patients but no cancers (Fig. 2-7). It is interesting to note that 5 of the adenomas that grew represented advanced lesions, which represent 4% of the 128 total polyps. Because this is the expected percentage of advanced lesions for the entire group of 6- to 9-mm polyps, this suggests that all advanced lesions were detectable by interval growth and removed. The remaining 116 polyps (90.6%) did not increase in size, including 73 polyps that were stable (Fig. 2-7), 9 that were measurably smaller, and 34 that were not seen at follow-up and had either completely regressed or represented a false positive at the initial examination. However, given that our positive predictive value for CTC-detected polyps ≥6 mm that go on to OC is more than 90%, it is highly likely that most of these lesions had truly regressed. None of the 128 6- to 9-mm polyps surpassed the 10-mm threshold at CTC follow-up. From the UW arm, 48 of the 128 polyps remain in extended CTC surveillance.

The mean growth rate for the entire polyp group was −1.41 mm/year—a negative value given the large fraction of lesions that regressed. The mean growth rate for proven adenomas and advanced adenomas was 0.40 mm/year and 1.43 mm/year, respectively. From these initial results, we concluded that short-term CTC surveillance appears to be a safe practice and can noninvasively identify the small subset of polyps (~10%) that are of potential clinical relevance, particularly the histologically advanced lesions. For the remaining 90% of cases, it is possible that unnecessary OC could be avoided. We are encouraged by these preliminary results but will continue our work to confirm these findings on a larger scale. We also plan to evaluate the role of polyp volume assessment for CTC follow-up (Fig. 2-8).

In addition to our ongoing longitudinal surveillance trial, we have looked at the theoretical cost effectiveness of immediate polypectomy versus 3-year CTC surveillance for small (6-9 mm) polyps detected at CTC screening.[14] Without any intervention, we estimated that the 5-year CRC death rate for patients with unresected 6- to 9-mm polyps was 0.08%, which already represents a sevenfold decrease from the 0.56% 5-year CRC death in the general screening population, the majority of whom do not harbor polyps. Therefore, for patients with 6- to 9-mm polyps detected at CTC screening, the exclusion of large polyps (≥10 mm) already confers a very low CRC risk. For the concentrated cohort with a small polyp, the death rate was further reduced to 0.03% with the CTC surveillance strategy and 0.02% with immediate colonoscopy referral. However, for each additional cancer-related death prevented with immediate polypectomy versus CTC follow-up, 10,000 additional colonoscopy referrals would be needed, resulting in 10 perforations and an exorbitant incremental cost-effectiveness ratio of $372,853. We concluded that the high costs, additional complications, and relatively low incremental yield associated with immediate polypectomy of 6- to 9-mm polyps support the practice of 3-year CTC surveillance, which allows for selective noninvasive identification of small polyps at risk. In addition to the management of small polyps, we have explored other economic aspects of CTC screening, which are covered in Chapter 10.

SUMMARY

As the medical community readies itself for large-scale CTC screening, we believe it is prudent to update and review several key concepts regarding colorectal polyps, which are generally not covered in works focusing on CTC technique and interpretation. With the advent of noninvasive colorectal screening tests such as CTC, strict adherence to a "leave no polyp behind" approach makes little sense on either clinical or economic grounds, let alone from a patient safety standpoint. At the very least, we must be open to novel approaches to colorectal screening beyond OC that can safely and effectively increase adherence rates. Simply because all cancers presumably arise from smaller benign polyps does not imply that all small lesions are therefore dangerous and worthy of resection. Although universal polyp harvesting may work at some level in terms of primary OC

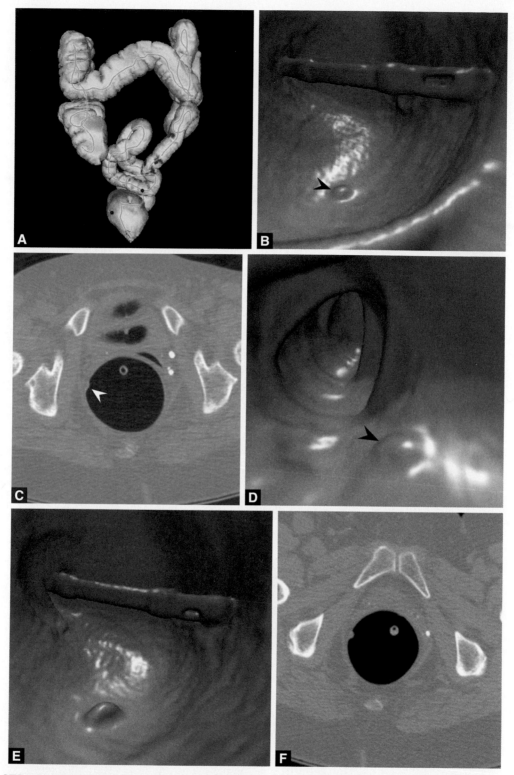

Figure 2-7   **CTC surveillance of small unresected polyps can demonstrate behavior and predict histology.** 3D colon map **(A)** shows the location of two small polyps detected at CTC screening *(red dots)*. 3D endoluminal **(B)** and 2D transverse **(C)** CTC images show a 6-mm rectal polyp *(arrowheads)*. A relatively flat 6-mm polyp in the sigmoid colon was also detected **(D,** *arrowhead)*. Matched images **(E-G)** from follow-up CTC performed 2 years later show interval growth of the rectal polyp to 8 mm **(E** and **(F)** and no change in the flat sigmoid lesion **(G).**

Illustration continued on following page

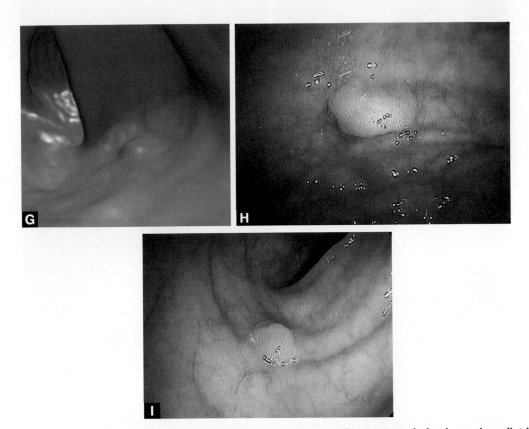

Figure 2-7 (Continued)   **CTC surveillance of small unresected polyps can demonstrate behavior and predict histology.** Matched images **(E-G)** from follow-up CTC performed 2 years later show interval growth of the rectal polyp to 8 mm **(E** and **(F)** and no change in the flat sigmoid lesion **(G)**. Given the demonstrable growth in the rectal polyp, the patient was referred to OC for polypectomy. The growing rectal lesion **(H)** proved to be neoplastic (tubular adenoma), whereas the stable sigmoid lesion **(I)** proved to be a hyperplastic polyp.

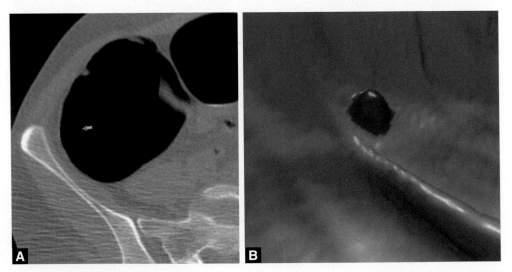

Figure 2-8   **Polyp volume assessment at CTC.** 2D transverse **(A)** and 3D endoluminal **(B)** CTC images from a patient undergoing surveillance for a small polyp *(arrow)* show the segmentation application for volume measurement. On some systems, such as the Viatronix V3D, this is an automated tool that can be further adjusted by the user to refine the polyp border determination.

screening, where the invasive barrier has already been breached, this represents an ineffective strategy for the safer and less expensive noninvasive tests that provide a filter between polyp detection and invasive therapy. Furthermore, it is important to move beyond the engrained older literature regarding polyp prevalence and histology that was derived from high-risk and/or symptomatic co-

horts. A bevy of data from modern screening cohorts can now replace this old information. It is also important to understand the current concepts and existing data surrounding nonpolypoid lesions and the natural history of small colorectal polyps. It is our hope that this overview of key polyp concepts can provide a solid foundation for those interested in providing quality CTC screening.

REFERENCES

1. Levin B, Lieberman DA, McFarland B, et al. Screening and surveillance for the early detection of colorectal cancer and adenomatous polyps, 2008: A joint guideline from the American Cancer Society, the US Multi-Society Task Force on Colorectal Cancer, and the American College of Radiology. *CA Cancer J Clin.* 2008;58(3):130-160.

2. Pickhardt PJ, Kim DH. Colorectal cancer screening with CT colonography: Key concepts regarding polyp prevalence, histology, morhpology, and natural history. *Am J Roentgenol.* 2009 (in press).

3. Bond JH. Clinical relevance of the small colorectal polyp. *Endoscopy.* 2001;33(5):454-457.

4. Pickhardt PJ, Choi JR, Hwang I, et al. Computed tomographic virtual colonoscopy to screen for colorectal neoplasia in asymptomatic adults. *New Engl J Med.* 2003;349(23):2191-2200.

5. Pickhardt PJ, Hassan C, Laghi A, et al. Small and diminutive polyps detected at screening CT colonography: A decision analysis for referral to colonoscopy. *Am J Roentgenol.* 2008;190(1):136-144.

6. Pickhardt PJ, Hassan C, Laghi A, Zullo A, Kim DH, Morini S. Cost-effectiveness of colorectal cancer screening with computed tomography colonography—The impact of not reporting diminutive lesions. *Cancer.* 2007;109(11):2213-2221.

7. Zalis ME, Barish MA, Choi JR, et al. CT colonography reporting and data system: A consensus proposal. *Radiology.* 2005;236(1):3-9.

8. Kim DH, Pickhardt PJ, Taylor AJ, et al. CT colonography versus colonoscopy for the detection of advanced neoplasia. *New Engl J Med.* 2007;357(14):1403-1412.

9. Ransohoff DF. Colonoscopy is justified for any polyp discovered during computed tomographic colonography—CON: Immediate colonoscopy is not necessary in patients who have polyps smaller than 1 cm on computed tomographic colonography. *Am J Gastroenterol.* 2005;100(9):1905-1917.

10. Rockey DC, Barish M, Brill JV, et al. Standards for gastroenterologists for performing and interpreting diagnostic computed tomographic colonography. *Gastroenterology.* 2007;133(3):1005-1024.

11. Van Dam J, Cotton P, Johnson CD, et al. AGA future trends report: CT colonography. *Gastroenterology.* 2004;127(3):970-984.

12. Rex DK. Colonoscopy is justified for any polyp discovered during computed tomographic colonography—PRO: Patients with polyps smaller than 1 cm on computed tomographic colonography should be offered colonoscopy and polypectomy. *Am J Gastroenterol.* 2005;100(9):1903-1905.

13. Pickhardt PJ. CT colonography (virtual colonoscopy) for primary colorectal screening: challenges facing clinical implementation. *Abdominal Imag.* 2005;30(1):1-4.

14. Pickhardt PJ, Hassan C, Laghi A, et al. Clinical management of small (6- to 9-mm) polyps detected at screening CT colonography: A cost-effectiveness analysis. *Am J Roentgenol.* 2008;191(5):1509-1516.

15. Winawer SJ, Zauber AG. The advanced adenoma as the primary target of screening. *Gastrointest Endosc Clin N Am.* 2002;12(1):1-9, v.

16. O'Brien MJ. Hyperplastic and serrated polyps of the colorectum. *Gastroenterol Clin North Am.* 2007;36(4):947-968.

17. Muto T, Bussey HJR, Morson BC. Evolution of cancer of colon and rectum. *Cancer.* 1975;36(6):2251-2270.

18. Matek W, Guggenmoosholzmann I, Demling L. Follow-up of patients with colorectal adenomas. *Endoscopy.* 1985;17(5):175-181.

19. Shinya H, Wolff WI. Morphology, anatomic distribution and cancer potential of colonic polyps. *Ann Surg.* 1979;190(6):679-683.

20. Church JM. Clinical significance of small colorectal polyps. *Dis Colon Rectum.* 2004;47(4):481-485.

21. Kim DH, Pickhardt PJ, Taylor AJ. Characteristics of advanced adenomas detected at CT colonographic screening: Implications for appropriate polyp size thresholds for polypectomy versus surveillance. *Am J Roentgenol.* 2007;188(4):940-944.

22. Odom SR, Duffy SD, Barone JE, Ghevariya V, McClane SJ. The rate of adenocarcinoma in endoscopically removed colorectal polyps. *Am Surg.* 2005;71(12):1024-1026.

23. Regula J, Rupinski M, Kraszewska E, et al. Colonoscopy in colorectal-cancer screening for detection of advanced neoplasia. *New Engl J Med.* 2006;355(18):1863-1872.

24. Sprung D. Prevalence of adenocarcinoma in small adenomas. *Am J Gastroenterol.* 2006;101:S199.

25. Yoo TW, Park DI, Kim YH, et al. Clinical significance of small colorectal adenoma less than 10mm: The KASID study. *Hepatogastroenterol.* 2007;54(74):418-421.

26. Barclay RL, Vicari JJ, Doughty AS, Johanson JF, Greenlaw RL. Colonoscopic withdrawal times and adenoma detection during screening colonoscopy. *New Engl J Med.* 2006;355(24):2533-2541.

27. Lieberman D, Moravec M, Holub J, Michaels L, Eisen G. Polyp size and advanced histology in patients undergoing colonoscopy screening: Implications for CT colonography. *Gastroenterology.* 2008;135(4)1100-1105.

28. Schoenfeld P, Cash B, Flood A, et al. Colonoscopic screening of average-risk women for colorectal neoplasia. *New Engl J Med.* 2005;352(20):2061-2068.

29. Imperiale TF, Wagner DR, Lin CY, Larkin GN, Rogge JD, Ransohoff DF. Risk of advanced proximal neoplasms in asymptomatic adults according to the distal colorectal findings. *New Engl J Med.* 2000;343(3):169-174.

30. Lieberman DA, Weiss DG, Bond JH, et al. Use of colonoscopy to screen asymptomatic adults for colorectal cancer. *New Engl J Med.* 2000;343(3):162-168.

31. Johnson CD, Chen MH, Toledano AY, et al. Accuracy of CT colonography for detection of large adenomas and cancers. *New Engl J Med.* 2008;359(12):1207-1217.

32. Pickhardt PJ, Choi JR, Hwang I, Schindler WR. Nonadenomatous polyps at CT colonography: Prevalence, size distribution, and detection rates. *Radiology.* 2004;232(3):784-790.

33. Winawer SJ, Zauber AG, Fletcher RH, et al. Guidelines for colonoscopy surveillance after polypectomy: A consensus update by the US Multi-Society Task Force on Colorectal Cancer and the American Cancer Society. *Gastroenterology.* 2006;130(6):1872-1885.

34. O'Brien MJ, Winawer SJ, Zauber AG, et al. The National Polyp Study—Patient and polyp characteristics associated with high-grade dysplasia in colorectal adenomas. *Gastroenterology.* 1990;98(2):371-379.

35. West AB, Mitsuhashi T. Cancer or high-grade dysplasia? The present status of the application of the terms in colonic polyps. *J Clin Gastroenterol.* 2005;39(1):4-6.

36. Butterly LF, Chase MP, Pohl H, Fiarman GS. Prevalence of clinically important histology in small adenomas. *Clin Gastroenterol Hepatol.* 2006;4(3):343-348.

37. Pickhardt PJ, Taylor AJ, Kim DH, Reichelderfer M, Gopal DV, Pfau PR. Screening for colorectal neoplasia with CT colonography: Initial experience from the 1st year of coverage by third-party payers. *Radiology.* 2006;241(2):417-425.

38. Waye JD, Lewis BS, Yessayan S. Colonoscopy—A prospective report of complications. *J Clin Gastroenterol.* 1992;15(4):347-351.

39. Silvis SE, Nebel O, Rogers G, Sugawa C, Mandelstam P. Endoscopic complications—Results of 1974 American Society for Gastrointestinal Endoscopy Survey. *JAMA.* 1976;235(9):928-930.

40. Levin TR. Complications of colonoscopy. *Ann Intern Med.* 2007;147(3):213-214.

41. Fruhmorgen P, Demling L. Complications of diagnostic and therapeutic colonoscopy in the Federal Republic of Germany—Results of an inquiry. *Endoscopy.* 1979;11(2):146-150.

42. Pickhardt PJ, Nugent PA, Choi JR, Schindler WR. Flat colorectal lesions in asymptomatic adults: Implications for screening with CT virtual colonoscopy. *Am J Roentgenol.* 2004;183(5):1343-1347.

43. Soetikno RM, Kaltenbach T, Rouse RV, et al. Prevalence of nonpolypoid (flat and depressed) colorectal neoplasms in asymptomatic and symptomatic adults. *JAMA.* 2008;299(9):1027-1035.

44. Tanaka S, Haruma K, Oka S, et al. Clinicopathologic features and endoscopic treatment of superficially spreading colorectal neoplasms larger than 20 mm. *Gastrointestinal Endosc.* 2001;54(1):62-66.

45. Park SH, Lee SS, Choi EK, et al. Flat colorectal neoplasms: Definition, importance, and visualization on CT colonography. *Am J Roentgenol.* 2007;188(4):953-959.

46. Pickhardt PJ, Levin B, Bond JH. Screening for nonpolypoid colorectal neoplasms. *JAMA.* 2008;299(23):2743; author reply 2744.

47. O'Brien M J, Winawer SJ, Zauber AG, et al. Flat adenomas in the National Polyp Study: Is there increased risk for high-grade dysplasia initially or during surveillance? *Clin Gastroenterol Hepatol.* 2004;2(10):905-911.

48. Pickhardt PJ. High-magnification chromoscopic colonoscopy: Caution needs to be exercised before changing screening policy—Reply. *Am J Roentgenol.* 2006;186(2):577-578.

49. Robbins J, Pickhardt PJ, Kim DH. Flat (nonpolypoid) lesions detected at CT colonography. Maui, HI: Annual Meeting for the Society of Gastrointestinal Radiologists; 2009.

50. Mang TG, Schaefer-Prokop C, Maier A, Schober E, Lechner G, Prokop M. Detectability of small and flat polyps in MDCT Colonography using 2D and 3D imaging tools: Results from a phantom study. *Am J Roentgenol.* 2005;185(6):1582-1589.

51. Fidler JL, Johnson CD, MacCarty RL, Welch TJ, Hara AK, Harmsen WS. Detection of flat lesions in the colon with CT colonography. *Abdominal Imag.* 2002;27(3):292-300.

52. Waye JD, Bilotta JJ. Rectal hyperplastic polyps—Now you see them, now you don't—A differential point. *Am J Gastroenterol.* 1990;85(12):1557-1559.

53. MacCarty RL, Johnson CD, Fletcher JG, Wilson LA. Occult colorectal polyps on CT colonography: Implications for surveillance. *Am J Roentgenol.* 2006;186(5):1380-1383.

54. Cornett D, Barancin C, Roeder B, et al. Findings on optical colonoscopy after positive CT colonography exam. *Am J Gastroenterol.* 2008;103(8):2068-2074.

55. Rubesin S, Saul S, Laufer I, Levine M. Carpet lesions of the colon. *Radiographics.* 1985;5(4):537-552.

56. Hofstad B, Vatn M, Larsen S, Osnes M. Growth of colorectal polyps—Recovery and evaluation of unresected polyps of less than 10 mm, 1 year after detection. *Scand J Gastroenterol.* 1994;29(7):640-645.

57. Hofstad B, Vatn MH, Andersen SN, et al. Growth of colorectal polyps: Redetection and evaluation of unresected polyps for a period of three years. *Gut.* 1996;39(3):449-456.

58. Knoernschild HE. Growth rate and malignant potential of colonic polyps: Early results. *Surg Forum.* 1963;14:137-138.

59. Hoff G, Foerster A, Vatn MH, Sauar J, Larsen S. Epidemiology of polyps in the rectum and colon—Recovery and evaluation of unresected polyps 2 years after detection. *Scand J Gastroenterol.* 1986;21(7):853-862.

60. Bersentes K, Fennerty B, Sampliner RE, Garewal HS. Lack of spontaneous regression of tubular adenomas in two years of follow-up. *Am J Gastroenterol.* 1997;92(7):1117-1120.

61. Welin S, Youker J, Spratt JS, Jr. The rates and patterns of growth of 375 tumors of the large intestine and rectum observed serially by double contrast enema study (Malmoe technique). *Am J Roentgenol Radium Ther Nucl Med.* 1963;90:673-687.

62. Loeve F, Boer R, Zauber AG, et al. National Polyp Study Data: Evidence for regression of adenomas. *Int J Cancer.* 2004;111(4):633-639.

63. Stryker SJ, Wolff BG, Culp CE, Libbe SD, Ilstrup DM, Maccarty RL. Natural history of untreated colonic polyps. *Gastroenterology.* 1987;93(5):1009-1013.

64. Pickhardt PJ, Lee AD, McFarland EG, Taylor AJ. Linear polyp measurement at CT colonography: In vitro and in vivo comparison of two-dimensional and three-dimensional displays. *Radiology.* 2005;236(3):872-878.

65. Park SH, Choi EK, Lee SS, et al. Polyp measurement reliability, accuracy, and discrepancy: Optical colonoscopy versus CT colonography with pig colonic specimens. *Radiology.* 2007;244(1):157-164.

66. Pickhardt PJ, Lehman VT, Winter TC, Taylor AJ. Polyp volume versus linear size measurements at CT colonography: Implications for noninvasive surveillance of unresected colorectal lesions. *Am J Roentgenol.* 2006;186(6):1605-1610.

67. Pickhardt PJ, Kim DH, Cash BD, Lee AD. The natural history of small polyps at CT colonography. Rancho Mirage, CA: Annual Meeting for the Society of Gastrointestinal Radiologists; 2008.

Colorectal Cancer: Pathogenesis and Risk Factors

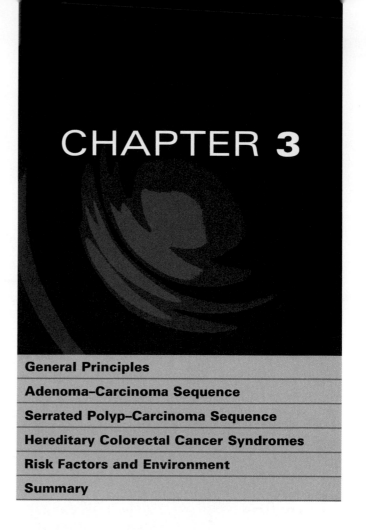

DAVID H. KIM, MD
PERRY J. PICKHARDT, MD

CHAPTER 3

INTRODUCTION

Since Lockhart-Mummery and Duke's original description in 1928,[1] it has been recognized that colorectal cancer (CRC) arises from a benign precursor. This has been refined over the subsequent decades where cancers were seen to arise specifically from an adenoma. The rapid accumulation of knowledge from molecular genetics in recent years has further defined this pathway, identifying the specific genetic abnormalities promoting this conversion. In addition, it has become evident that alternative pathways and other histologic precursors exist. Recently, a second pathway has been defined, accounting for 15% of sporadic cancers arising not from a colorectal adenoma but through serrated lesions ultimately derived from a hyperplastic polyp. This chapter delineates these pathways and highlights the factors that are associated with increased risk for colorectal cancer.

GENERAL PRINCIPLES

Colorectal carcinoma does not arise as a de novo lesion. Instead, it transforms from a defined benign precursor (Fig. 3-1). Multiple specific genetic abnormalities are acquired within this lesion over time, ultimately leading to the loss of regulated growth. The time period is extended over many years, and only a tiny percentage of these precursor lesions actually undergo complete trans-

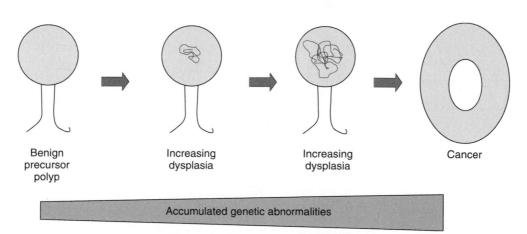

Figure 3-1 Colorectal carcinogenesis. The transformation of benign polyp target to cancer is a multistep process characterized by accumulation of genetic abnormalities that ultimately lead to dysregulated growth. The bridge to cancer is through increasing dysplasia as a result of these genetic changes. The time course of these changes is measured over many years.

formation to cancer. The vast majority remain benign and, over time, remain stable in size or regress. Contrary to past dogma, it is now recognized that colorectal carcinoma is a heterogenous disease with multiple precursor lesions and several different underlying genetic pathways. Most sporadic cancers arise from the adenomatous polyp, whereas a small fraction arise from a newly recognized precursor derived from the hyperplastic polyp. The molecular pathway of the *adenoma–carcinoma sequence* is termed the "suppressor" or "chromosomal instability" pathway and is characterized by loss or inactivation of large portions of chromosomes, whereas the *serrated polyp–carcinoma sequence* is termed the "mutator" pathway and is largely characterized by microsatellite instability where there are variations in areas of small microsatellite repeats within the chromosome as a result of uncorrected replication errors. A second minor pathway within the serrated polyp–carcinoma sequence is characterized by low microsatellite instability (MSI-low) cancers. The study of familial conditions such as familial adenomatous polyposis and hereditary nonpolyposis colorectal cancer, and a rare condition termed hyperplastic polyposis, have been instrumental in elucidating both the adenomatous and serrated polyp pathways.

ADENOMA–CARCINOMA SEQUENCE

The majority of sporadic cancers arise through this classically described pathway where the precursor lesion is the colorectal adenoma. It is estimated that 85% of sporadic colorectal cancers arise from this route.[2] The progression from adenoma to carcinoma is a prolonged one, typically requiring 8 to 10 years.[3,4] A number of specific genetic mutations are accumulated along the way, resulting in a multistage carcinogenesis. Histologi-

cally, the adenoma becomes increasingly dysplastic. Resultant high-grade dysplasia is felt to represent the extreme end of these histologic changes just short of invasive carcinoma and is a likely intermediary to cancer.[5,6] Carcinoma in situ is synonymous with high-grade dysplasia, but high-grade dysplasia is the preferred term.[6] Ultimately, only a small fraction of adenomas undergo the complete transition to cancer. The adenomas most likely to undergo progression to carcinoma are the advanced adenomas (see Chapter 1). Specifically, these are large adenomas (≥10 mm), regardless of glandular architecture; adenomas with a significant villous component (tubulovillous or villous histology) of any size; or adenomas with high-grade dysplasia of any size. Many aspects of this transition and of the natural history of adenomas in general are not completely known. However, cross-sectional observational studies and a few longitudinal studies suggest that adenomas typically grow to a fairly large size prior to the conversion to carcinoma.[3,7-11] In true screening populations, the prevalence of carcinoma in subcentimeter polyps is extremely low in comparison with polyps greater than 10 mm.[11-13] In our University of Wisconsin (UW) series, 18 invasive cancers were seen in an asymptomatic screening population of approximately 6,000 patients.[10] Of these cancers, 15 of 18 were greater than 2 cm in size, 3 were 1 to 2 cm, and none were present in the subcentimeter group. Studies also suggest that the time course from an advanced adenoma (or the high-risk polyp) to carcinoma is extended over several years.[14]

Originally defined by Vogelstein and colleagues,[15] the elucidation of the molecular pathway of the adenoma–carcinoma sequence has greatly increased our understanding of colorectal cancer pathogenesis (Fig. 3-2). The conversion from normal colonic mucosa to a benign adenoma to an invasive carcinoma involves a number of genetic mutations resulting in both the inactivation of

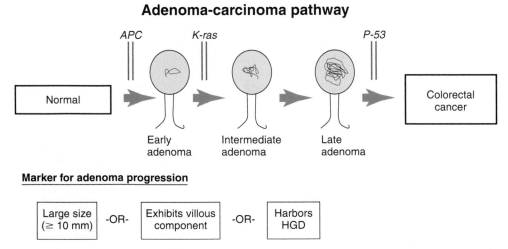

Figure 3-2 Adenoma–carcinoma sequence. Schematic of adenoma progression shows a multistep process involving several genes. Loss of the *APC* gene results in the initiation of an adenoma. *K-ras* abnormalities occur early in the life cycle of an adenoma, whereas loss of *p53* occurs late and results in the transformation to cancer. The markers for adenomas most likely to progress to cancer are listed here.

tumor suppression genes and activation of various oncogenes that promote tumor growth. Three main gene loci have been identified, including *APC* (adenomatous polyposis coli), *K-ras* (Kirsten-ras), and *p53* genes. In addition, alterations in the *DCC* (deleted in colon cancer) gene occur and may play a role in metastatic behavior. This pathway has been termed the chromosomal instability pattern because of the characteristic events of chromosomal truncation or loss of large portions of the chromosomes as a result of these mutations. Much of this pathway has been worked out from the study of patients with familial adenomatous polyposis (FAP) syndrome. The following description is a simplified overview of the complex genetic alterations that take place.

The first step of this pathway involves the *APC* gene, which is located on the long arm of chromosome 5 (5q). This is a tumor suppressor gene, and loss of this gene results in the initiation of an adenoma. The *APC* gene has thus been considered the gatekeeper of colorectal carcinogenesis.[16] For this tumor suppressor gene to be inactivated, both allelic copies within the same cell must be lost (from chromosome truncation or inactivated through mutation). One functioning *APC* copy within the cell prevents adenoma formation. When both copies are lost, this event is referred to as loss of heterozygosity (LOH), resulting in aneuploidy. This is the case for sporadic colorectal cancer, in which both copies are initially present in each cell and both copies are subsequently inactivated, initiating the formation of an adenoma. For the FAP syndrome, only a single functioning allele is present in each cell because a germline mutation has resulted in loss of one copy. Thus, it requires only one genetic event to form an adenoma and it is statistically much more likely that an adenoma will arise in patients with FAP. This is evident clinically because these patients typically have hundreds of adenomas carpeting their colon by the third decade. The *APC* gene encodes for a protein that plays a role in several cellular processes, including cell proliferation, differentiation, migration, and apoptosis.[2] One significant interaction involves β-catenin. The APC protein can form a complex with other proteins to bind β-catenin. When β-catenin is bound, it can be phosphorylated and down-regulated. If the APC protein is not functional, β-catenin is not down-regulated and may migrate from the cytoplasm to the nucleus, where it can up-regulate target genes and initiate adenoma formation.[17,18]

The next genetic step in this pathway involves the *K-ras* proto-oncogene. Mutation leading to *K-ras* activation is felt to occur during the early to intermediate stage of the life of an adenoma. This gene encodes for a GTP binding protein and confers a growth advantage in the setting of pre-existing *APC* inactivation by permitting continued signal transduction across the cell membrane.[19]

Loss of the *DCC* gene is thought to occur late in the life of an adenoma. It is located on the long arm of chromosome 18 and encodes for a neural cell adhesion molecule receptor. Loss of the DCC protein correlates with a poor prognosis and may be involved in CRC invasion and metastasis.[20]

The final gene alteration involves *p53* located on the short arm of chromosome 17 (17p).[2,21] *p53* allows for either G1 cell cycle arrest to allow the cell to repair the genetic damage or help to initiate apoptosis (i.e., cell death) if the damage is too extensive. Loss of *p53* results in the loss of the cell's ability to correct the previous damage and completes the transition from adenoma to carcinoma. The resultant carcinomas have been termed microsatellite instability stable (MSI-S) cancers—a concept to be discussed in the next section.

SERRATED POLYP–CARCINOMA SEQUENCE

The newly recognized serrated polyp–carcinoma pathway accounts for approximately 15% of sporadic colorectal cancers.[2,22,23] Many of the concepts are in evolution, and the following is a simplified version. The putative precursor lesion is likely the hyperplastic polyp, which has long been considered a non-neoplastic lesion without any malignant potential. The transition to cancer is over many years. As with the adenoma in the adenoma-carcinoma pathway, only a tiny percentage of hyperplastic polyps will progress to cancer. The progression is from a hyperplastic polyp to an intermediary hyperplastic polyp with architectural disorganization ("sessile serrated adenoma") or through the intermediaries of a traditional serrated adenoma or a mixed hyperplastic/adenomatous polyp (Fig. 3-3). With increasing number of genetic events, these serrated polyps become increasingly dysplastic and may ultimately progress to carcinoma.[23] The majority of resultant carcinomas demonstrate microsatellite instability and are termed MSI-H tumors (i.e., "microsatellite instability high" cancers). A minority of cancers from this pathway are MSI low or stable. Microsatellite instability refers to mutations with resultant variability of length of repeating short nucleotide sequences, or "microsatellites." This phenomenon is related to inactivation of DNA repair genes such as *hMLH1* or *MGMT*. DNA mismatch repair (MMR) genes allow for correction of errors introduced into the genome during replication from slippage of the DNA polymerase on the template strand.[24] Although most errors are of little significance in noncoding regions, mutations introduced into genes regulating cell growth can ultimately result in the progression of a serrated lesion to cancer.

Two molecular pathogenic pathways have been described in the serrated polyp–carcinoma sequence.[22] The major pathway accounting for 75% of these cancers results in MSI-H carcinomas, whereas the minor pathway results in MSI-L or MSI-S cancers. In the major pathway, a defining genetic marker is activation of the *BRAF* on-

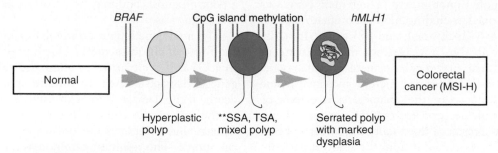

Serrated polyp-carcinoma pathway*

*Major pathway (MSI-H). Minor pathway leading to MSI-L or MSI-S tumors not shown.

**Histologic subtypes along the
serrated polyp pathway: SSA—sessile
serrated adenoma; TSA—traditional
serrated adenoma; Mixed polyp—mixed
hyperplastic/adenomatous polyp

Figure 3-3 Serrated polyp–carcinoma sequence. Schematic of hyperplastic polyp progression to cancer. The major molecular driver is CpG island methylation, which is a nonrandom methylation event typically in promoter regions that silences genes. Ultimately, genes regulating growth are affected leading to cancer transformation.

cogene. Mutations in *BRAF* have been highly correlated with a serrated histologic appearance.[25] This oncogene encodes a kinase that is normally activated by *RAS* and resides in the RAS-RAF-MEK-ERK signaling pathway.[26] This signal network is integral to a number of cell processes, including cell proliferation, differentiation, survival, and apoptosis. It is hypothesized that *BRAF* oncogene activation results in adaptive responses from the cell including induction of cell senescence to prevent cell transformation.[27] Loss of these adaptive responses by way of silencing of various growth regulator genes may then result in initiation down the serrated polyp pathway to cancer. In the BRAF serrated polyp pathway, the molecular process felt to drive this process is CpG island methylation (CIM).[28] CpG island methylation is an epigenetic event in which a gene is silenced or inactivated by the binding of methyl groups to recurrent cytosine–guanine dinucleotide sequences, typically in a gene's promoter region. It is termed an epigenetic event distinct from a mutational event because the underlying genetic sequence is not altered. However, as with mutation, it can be transmitted to progeny but theoretically is reversible. Thus, characteristic of lesions along the BRAF pathway is a CIMP (CpG island methylator phenotype) high status. Another feature involves MSI-H carcinomas. Microsatellite instability is felt to be a late occurrence in this pathway resulting from the methylation and silencing of a DNA mismatch repair gene, typically *hMLH1* (Fig. 3-3).[23,29]

The minor molecular pathway of the serrated polyp–carcinoma sequence is estimated to account for 25% of the cancers along this sequence.[22] Here, the defining genetic marker is *K-ras*. Like *BRAF*, *K-ras* also transcribes a protein in the signaling RAS-RAF-MEK-ERK

pathway.[26] Activation of this pathway may result in similar adaptive responses as described in the previous paragraph. In distinction to *BRAF*, *K-ras* serrated lesions demonstrate low levels of CIM, which preferentially targets different genes such as *MGMT*. Cancers arising from this pathway are typically MSI-low or MSI-stable. There may be overlap of molecular features with the classically described suppressor pathway.[30]

HEREDITARY COLORECTAL CANCER SYNDROMES

Hereditary colorectal cancer syndromes account for 5% to 10% of all colorectal cancers.[31] For the afflicted individual, this obviously represents the ultimate risk factor for future cancer development and the absolute risk of a future cancer is markedly increased over baseline. Studies of these individuals and families have greatly increased our knowledge of the molecular pathogenesis of sporadic colorectal cancers in addition to knowledge about these specific disorders. From the standpoint of a practitioner engaged in CRC screening, it is important to be familiar with these entities and how they fit in within the realm of colorectal cancer. Once discovered, genetic testing and counseling for the individual and family members is mandatory. As a general rule, patients with such syndromes are best evaluated by endoscopic means rather than by computed tomography colonography (CTC), although an alternating strategy of colonoscopy and CTC may become useful for some in the future.

The classic hereditary colorectal cancer syndrome is FAP (Fig. 3-4). It is inherited in an autosomal dominant fashion with high penetrance. FAP involves a germline mutation of the *APC* gene leading to only a

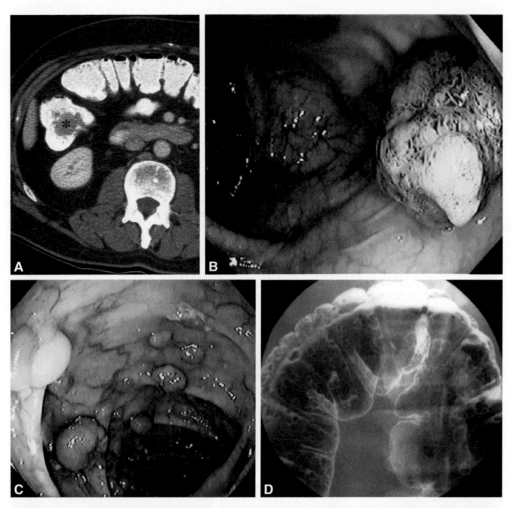

Figure 3-4   Familial adenomatous polyposis (FAP). Contrast-enhanced CT **(A)** shows a dominant polyp in the ascending colon *(asterisk)*. Multiple soft tissue polyps are identified elsewhere on CT throughout a contrast-filled colon (not shown). OC **(B and C)** confirms the dominant adenoma and other multiple adenomas in this patient with FAP. Barium enema spot view **(D)** in a different patient demonstrates multiple polyps from FAP carpeting the hepatic flexure. Note that neither BE nor CTC is typically indicated in the evaluation of patients with FAP. (A-C from Pickhardt PJ. Differential diagnosis of polypoid lesions seen at CT colonography [Virtual colonoscopy]. *Radiographics.* 2004;24:1535-1559.)

single copy of this allele in all somatic cells. Consequently, the likelihood of adenoma formation is markedly increased where loss of this second copy initiates the formation of an adenoma. Afflicted individuals often have hundreds of adenomas carpeting their colon by their 20s or 30s. The risk for adenoma progression to cancer for each adenoma is no different than that of a sporadic cancer situation, but the sheer increased numbers of adenomas markedly increase overall risk. A colorectal cancer is inevitable in these individuals unless a colectomy is performed. It is estimated that despite intensive screening and surveillance programs, approximately 25% of patients with FAP present with colorectal cancer at the time of colectomy.[32] CTC currently does not yet play role in the management of these patients, although an alternating surveillance strategy with colonoscopy could be considered.

Patients with FAP often develop gastric and small bowel polyps. The gastric polyps are typically fundic gland polyps (Fig. 3-5). Although typically considered innocuous in the sporadic setting, they are considered at risk in this patient population because of the underlying APC mutation. Gastric adenomas represent a minority of these polyps, typically located in the antrum. A significant increase in gastric carcinoma has not been seen in the U.S.-based FAP population. More concerning is the development of duodenal adenomas, particularly in the periampullary region (Fig. 3-6). Duodenal adenocarcinoma is the leading cause of death for those patients who successfully undergo colectomy. Overall, there is an estimated lifetime risk of 4% to 12%.[33,34] Adenomas are seen in the jejunum and ileum, but malignant transformation appears to be rare.

Because the germline mutations affect all somatic cells, tumors have been described throughout the body in addi-

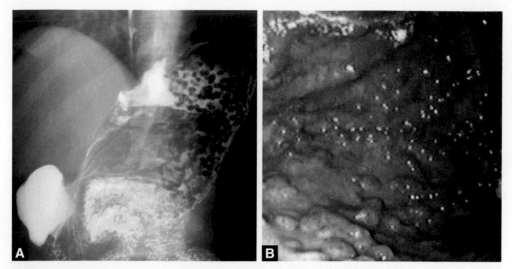

Figure 3-5 **Fundic gland polyposis in FAP.** Upper gastrointestinal **(A)** and esophagogastroduodenoscopy (EGD; **B**) images show innumerable benign fundic gland polyps in two different patients.

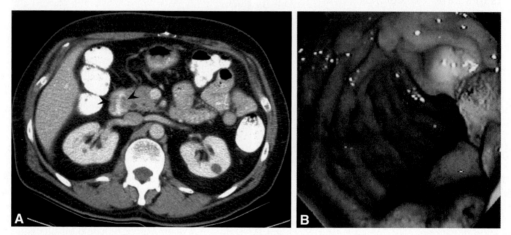

Figure 3-6 **Duodenal adenomas in FAP.** Contrast-enhanced CT **(A)** shows irregular wall duodenal wall thickening *(arrowhead)*, which correlates with multiple large sessile adenomas at EGD **(B)**.

tion to the gastrointestinal tract. These include neoplasms of the thyroid, biliary tree, liver, and adrenal glands.[35-38] Approximately one third of patients with FAP develop intraabdominal desmoid tumors (fibromatosis).[39,40] This complication can be lethal as a result of intestinal obstruction or vascular occlusion. The tumors tend to recur after surgical resection and unfortunately are not typically responsive to either radiation or chemotherapy.

With the understanding of the molecular underpinnings of this disease, many related but separate syndromes are now considered under the umbrella of FAP. For example, Gardner's syndrome of intestinal polyposis and benign osseous lesions (e.g., osteomas of the mandible) is a variable manifestation of mutations within the *APC* gene. Turcot's syndrome of colonic polyposis and central nervous tumors is another FAP variant.[41] The colonic phenotype ranges from very few adenomas to thousands. Finally, hereditary flat adenoma syndrome

characterized by adenomas of a flat morphology, typically few in number and proximal in location, has been renamed *attenuated FAP*. As a result of germline mutations at the ends of the *APC* gene of all somatic cells,[42] these individuals are susceptible to extracolonic tumors as in classic FAP. The colorectal cancers in attenuated FAP typically present at an older age (approximately age 55 years) than in classic FAP.

Hereditary nonpolyposis colorectal cancer (HNPCC) is the second major familial hereditary cancer syndrome (Fig. 3-7). It is an autosomal dominant condition with high penetrance. It involves a germline mutation of a DNA mismatch repair gene (typically *hMLH1* or *hMSH2*) and leads to a MSI-high cancer in most cases.[31] Study of afflicted patients and those with hyperplastic polyposis has helped to elucidate the newly described serrated polyp–carcinoma sequence and molecular pathways (see previous section). Previously,

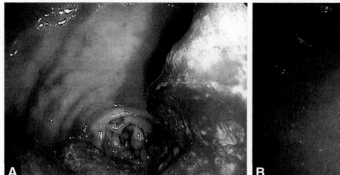
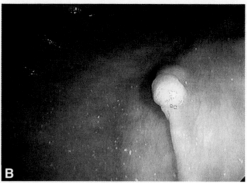

Figure 3-7   HNPCC. A 47-year-old man who met Amsterdam criteria for HNPCC. Colonoscopic images show a hemicircumferential sigmoid cancer **(A)** and 5-mm tubular adenoma **(B)** in the ascending colon. As a general rule, CTC should not be in the evaluation pathway for patients with HNPCC. (Courtesy of Dr. Deepak Gopal, University of Wisconsin.)

HNPCC was called Lynch syndrome and was classified into two types. Patients with Lynch I demonstrated only colonic tumors, whereas those with Lynch II demonstrated tumors in addition to colonic lesions, including those of endometrial, ovarian, gastrointestinal, hepatobiliary, pancreatic, central nervous system, and urologic origin (the "cancer family syndrome"). HNPCC encompasses both previous subtypes in which mutations in a particular mismatch repair gene correlate with a different propensity for a given tumor.

Clinically, patients with HNPCC present with colonic adenocarcinoma at a younger age. The mean age of presentation is 45 years (approximately 30 years earlier than the average risk population).[43] The lifetime risk is markedly increased when afflicted individuals hold a greater than 80% risk of developing a colon cancer as opposed to the lifetime risk held by an individual at an average of 5%.[44,45] The colon cancers tend to be proximal in location, and 70% are distributed proximal to the splenic flexure.[31] Histologically, the cancers are more often poorly differentiated, with mucoid and signet-cell features.[46,47] Infiltrating lymphocytes within the tumor and aggregates surrounding the cancer can be seen. It is interesting that survival stage for stage for a given HNPCC cancer is improved over the typical adenocarcinoma. One study demonstrated a 65% 5-year survival rate for HNPCC tumors versus 44% in patients with sporadic colorectal cancers.[48] Despite the moniker of hereditary *nonpolyposis* colorectal cancer, patients with this condition do present with polyps. The prevailing theory suggests that there is an accelerated carcinogenesis of these benign precursors with quicker transformation to cancer (2 to 3 years).[46,49] This is in distinction to sporadic colorectal cancers (without a germline mutation in a DNA mismatch repair gene) arising from the serrated polyp pathway in which the time course is felt to be elongated over many years between benign precursor to cancer.

Various criteria have been used to identify patients with HNPCC. The most widely used are the Amsterdam

I and II criteria (although they are somewhat restrictive, leading to underdiagnosis), whereas the more sensitive Bethesda criteria are helpful to suggest which patients should undergo MSI typing of the tumor to suggest HNPCC (Tables 3-1 and 3-2).[50-52]

Table 3-1 ▫ Amsterdam Criteria*

- ≥3 relatives with proven CRC, one of whom is a first-degree relative of the other two
- CRC involving at least two generations
- ≥1 CRC diagnosed before age of 50 years

*FAP must be excluded.
From Vasen HF, Mecklin JP, Khan PM, Lynch HT. *Dis Colon Rectum*. 1991;34:424-425.

Table 3-2 ▫ Bethesda Guidelines for MSI Testing

- Individuals with cancer in families that meet the Amsterdam criteria
- Individuals with two HNPCC-related cancers, including synchronous and metachronous colorectal cancers or associated extracolonic cancers*
- Individuals with colorectal cancer and a first-degree relative with colorectal cancer and/or HNPCC-related extracolonic cancer and/or a colorectal adenoma; one of the cancers diagnosed at age <45 years, and the adenoma diagnosed at age <40 years
- Individuals with colorectal cancer or endometrial cancer diagnosed at age <45 years
- Individuals with right-sided colorectal cancer with an undifferentiated pattern (solid/cribriform) on histopathology diagnosed at age <45 years†
- Individuals with signet ring cell type colorectal cancer diagnosed at age <45 years
- Individual with adenomas diagnosed at age <40 years‡

*Endometrial, ovarian, gastric, hepatobiliary, or small bowel cancer or transitional cell carcinoma of the renal pelvis or ureter.
†Solid/cribriform defined as poorly differentiated or undifferentiated carcinoma composed of irregular, solid sheets of large eosinophilic cells and containing small glandlike spaces.
‡Composed of >50% signet ring cells.
From Rodriguez-Bigas MA, Boland CR, Hamilton SR, et al. *J Natl Cancer Inst.* 1997;89:1758-1762.

RISK FACTORS AND ENVIRONMENT

The average lifetime risk for development of colorectal cancer is 5%.[45] Of colorectal cancers, 90% occur after the age of 50 years. Factors that increase risk over the baseline of increasing age include a family or personal history for CRC or adenomatous polyps, a personal history of inflammatory bowel disease, and a personal history of a polyposis syndrome such as FAP or HNPCC. It is estimated that approximately 30% of the population harbors one of these risk factors, leaving 70% of individuals at average risk.[53] Dietary and environmental factors are also postulated to potentially play a role in altering the possibility of developing a colorectal cancer.

A *family history* of CRC or adenomatous polyps is defined as an individual with a first-degree relative (parent, sibling, child) with a CRC or adenoma diagnosed before the age of 60 years or two or more first-degree relatives diagnosed at any age. Meta-analyses have shown an approximately twofold increase of relative risk with a positive family history in a first-degree relative.[54] This risk may increase to fourfold with multiple first-degree relatives with CRC or CRC diagnosed at a young age (<45 years) in a first-degree relative. A *personal history* for CRC also increases risk. Such individuals are at risk for synchronous or metachronous cancers. Synchronous cancers have been seen in 3% of individuals.[55]

Individuals with longstanding inflammatory bowel disease are at increased risk for development of CRC. The risk increases with increased duration and severity of the inflamed colon.[56,57] As discussed in the previous section, hereditary colorectal cancer syndromes markedly increase risk. Nearly all patients with FAP succumb to CRC without a prophylactic colectomy and the lifetime risk for patients with HNPCC has been estimated to increase to 80%.[44]

Diet and environment presumably have an impact on the incidence of CRC, as illustrated by the difference in colorectal cancer rates seen in Japanese individuals living in Japan from those who have migrated to Hawaii. However, specific elements within the diet or environment as a modifier of risk are difficult to ascertain. Epidemiologic observational studies often have many confounding variables, and prospective prevention clinical trials often alter associated behaviors in addition to the primary dietary intervention. Although initially suggestive of protective effects, dietary fiber does not appear to decrease risk.[58] Some fruits and vegetables may be somewhat protective, although the association is variable.[59,60] Antioxidants such as beta-carotene, vitamin C, and vitamin E appear not to reduce risk.[61] Dietary fat from red meat appears to increase risk.[62] Nonsteroid antiinflammatory agents, selenium, calcium, and folate supplementation may confer protective effects against adenomas and colon cancer.[63-66] Lifestyle may have an impact because obesity and increased alcohol intake both increase risk for future CRC.[66,67] Smoking has a weaker association. It is interesting to note that smoking has no correlation with risk for increasing adenoma prevalence, although there is a positive correlation for hyperplastic polyps, which may account for the discrepant studies related to smoking and increased cancer risk.[67] Cancers through the serrated polyp pathway may be affected by smoking, whereas cancers through the adenoma–carcinoma sequence may not.

SUMMARY

Colorectal cancer is a heterogenous disease with several molecular pathways from a benign precursor lesion to cancer. The major pathway involves the adenoma–carcinoma sequence, whereas a minority of lesions follow the newly described serrated polyp pathway. In addition to the classically described benign target of the adenoma, a small fraction of hyperplastic polyps are thought to potentially transform to cancer. All pathways take many years and multiple genetic events. The majority of colorectal cancers are sporadic in nature, but 5% to 10% of CRC cases are related to a hereditary polyposis syndrome. FAP and HNPCC have been instrumental in increasing the understanding of the genetic underpinnings of this cancer.

REFERENCES

1. Lockhart-Mummery J, Dukes C. The precancerous changes in the rectum and colon. *Surg Gynecol Obstet.* 1928;46:591-596.
2. Robbins DH, Itzkowitz SH. The molecular and genetic basis of colon cancer. *Med Clin North Am.* 2002;86(6):1467-1495.
3. Muto T, Bussey HJR, Morson BC. Evolution of cancer of colon and rectum. *Cancer.* 1975;36(6):2251-2270.
4. Winawer SJ, Zauber A, Diaz B. The National Polyp Study—Temporal sequence of evolving colorectal cancer from the normal colon. *Gastrointestinal Endosc.* 1987;33(2):167.
5. Konishi F, Morson BC. Pathology of colorectal adenomas—A colonoscopic survey. *J Clin Pathol.* 1982;35(8):830-841.
6. Obrien MJ, Winawer SJ, Zauber AG, et al. The National Polyp Study—Patient and polyp characteristics associated with high-grade dysplasia in colorectal adenomas. *Gastroenterology.* 1990;98(2):371-379.
7. Hofstad B, Vatn MH, Andersen SN, et al. Growth of colorectal polyps: Redetection and evaluation of unresected polyps for a period of three years. *Gut.* 1996;39(3):449-456.
8. Morson BC. Evolution of cancer of colon and rectum. *Cancer.* 1974;34(3):845-849.
9. Kim DH, Pickhardt PJ, Taylor AJ. Characteristics of advanced adenomas detected at CT colonographic screening: Implications for appropriate polyp size thresholds for polypectomy versus surveillance. *Am J Roentgenol.* 2007;188(4):940-944.
10. Kim DH, Pickhardt PJ, Taylor AJ, et al. CT colonography versus colonoscopy for the detection of advanced neoplasia. *N Engl J Med.* 2007;357(14):1403-1412.
11. Stryker SJ, Wolff BG, Culp CE, Libbe SD, Ilstrup DM, Maccarty RL. Natural history of untreated colonic polyps. *Gastroenterology.* 1987;93(5):1009-1013.

12. Lieberman D, Moravec M, Holub J, Michaels L, Eisen G. Polyp size and advanced histology in patients undergoing colonoscopy screening: Implications for CT colonography. *Gastroenterology.* 2008;135(4):1100-1105.

13. Odom SR, Duffy SD, Barone JE, Ghevariya V, McClane SJ. The rate of adenocarcinoma in endoscopically removed colorectal polyps. *Am Surg.* 2005;71(12):1024-1026.

14. Kozuka S, Nogaki M, Ozeki T, Masumori S. Pre-malignancy of mucosal polyp in large-intestine. 2. Estimation of periods required for malignant transformation of mucosal polyps. *Dis Colon Rectum.* 1975;18(6):494-500.

15. Vogelstein B, Fearon ER, Hamilton SR, et al. Genetic alterations during colorectal-tumor development. *N Engl J Med.* 1988;319(9):525-532.

16. Kinzler KW, Vogelstein B. Lessons from hereditary colorectal cancer. *Cell.* 1996;87(2):159-170.

17. Korinek V, Barker N, Morin PJ, et al. Constitutive transcriptional activation by a beta-catenin-Tcf complex in APC(-/-) colon carcinoma. *Science.* 1997;275(5307):1784-1787.

18. Rubinfeld B, Souza B, Albert I, et al. Association of the Apc gene-product with beta-catenin. *Science.* 1993;262(5140):1731-1734.

19. Yashiro M, Carethers JM, Laghi L, et al. Genetic pathways in the evolution of morphologically distinct colorectal neoplasms. *Cancer Res.* 2001;61(6):2676-2683.

20. Shibata D, Reale MA, Lavin P, et al. The DCC protein and prognosis in colorectal cancer. *N Engl J Med.* 1996;335(23):1727-1732.

21. Fearon ER, Vogelstein B. A genetic model for colorectal tumorigenesis. *Cell.* 1990;61(5):759-767.

22. Jass JR. Classification of colorectal cancer based on correlation of clinical, morphological and molecular features. *Histopathology.* 2007;50(1):113-130.

23. O'Brien MJ. Hyperplastic and serrated polyps of the colorectum. *Gastroenterol Clin N Am.* 2007;36:947-968.

24. Shibata D, Peinado MA, Ionov Y, Malkhosyan S, Perucho M. Genomic instability in repeated sequences is an early somatic event in colorectal tumorigenesis that persists after transformation. *Nat Genet.* 1994;6(3):273-281.

25. Tateyama H, Li WX, Takahashi E, Miura Y, Sugiura H, Eimoto T. Apoptosis index and apoptosis-related antigen expression in serrated adenoma of the colorectum—The saw-toothed structure may be related to inhibition of apoptosis. *Am J Surg Pathol.* 2002;26(2):249-256.

26. Kolch W. Meaningful relationships: The regulation of the Ras/Raf/MEK/ERK pathway by protein interactions. *Biochem J.* 2000;351:289-305.

27. Minoo P, Jass JR. Senescence and serration: A new twist to an old tale. *J Pathol.* 2006;210(2):137-140.

28. Jass JR, Iino H, Ruszkiewicz A, et al. Neoplastic progression occurs through mutator pathways in hyperplastic polyposis of the colorectum. *Gut.* 2000;47(1):43-49.

29. Thibodeau SN, French AJ, Cunningham JM, et al. Microsatellite instability in colorectal cancer: Different mutator phenotypes and the principal involvement of hMLH1. *Cancer Res.* 1998;58(8):1713-1718.

30. Jass JR, Baker K, Zlobec I, et al. Advanced colorectal polyps with the molecular and morphological features of serrated polyps and adenomas: Concept of a "fusion" pathway to colorectal cancer. *Histopathology.* 2006;49(2):121-131.

31. Lynch HT, de la Chapelle A. Genomic medicine—Hereditary colorectal cancer. *N Engl J Med.* 2003;348(10):919-932.

32. Jang YS, Steinhagen RM, Heimann TM. Colorectal cancer in familial adenomatous polyposis. *Dis Colon Rectum.* 1997;40:312-316.

33. Bjork J, Akerbrant H, Iselius L, et al. Periampullary adenomas and adenocarcinomas in familial adenomatous polyposis: Cumulative risks and APC gene mutations. *Gastroenterology.* 2001;121(5):1127-1135.

34. Debinski HS, Spigelman AD, Hatfield A, Williams CB, Phillips RKS. Upper intestinal surveillance in familial adenomatous polyposis. *Eur J Cancer.* 1995;31A(7-8):1149-1153.

35. Garber JE, Li FP, Kingston JE, et al. Hepatoblastoma and familial adenomatous polyposis. *J Natl Cancer Inst.* 1988;80(20):1626-1628.

36. Lesher AR, Castronuovo JJ, Filippone AL. Hepatoblastoma in a patient with familial polyposis coli. *Surgery.* 1989;105(5):668-670.

37. Plail RO, Bussey HJR, Glazer G, Thomson JPS. Adenomatous polyposis—An association with carcinoma of the thyroid. *Br J Surg.* 1987;74(5):377-380.

38. Walsh N, Qizilbash A, Banerjee R, Waugh GA. Biliary neoplasia in Gardner's syndrome. *Arch Pathol Lab Med.* 1987;111(1):76-77.

39. Gurbuz AK, Giardiello FM, Petersen GM, et al. Desmoid tumors in familial adenomatous polyposis. *Gut.* 1994;35(3):377-381.

40. Jones IT, Jagelman DG, Fazio VW, Lavery IC, Weakley FL, McGannon E. Desmoid tumors in familial polyposis coli. *Ann Surg.* 1986;204(1):94-97.

41. Hamilton SR, Liu B, Parsons RE, et al. The molecular basis of Turcot's syndrome. *N Engl J Med.* 1995;332(13):839-847.

42. Spirio L, Olschwang S, Groden J, et al. Alleles of the Apc gene—An attenuated form of familial polyposis. *Cell.* 1993;75(5):951-957.

43. Lynch HT, de la Chapelle A. Genetic susceptibility to non-polyposis colorectal cancer. *J Med Genet.* 1999;36(11):801-818.

44. Vasen HF, Wijnen JT, Menko FH, et al. Cancer risk in families with hereditary nonpolyposis colorectal cancer diagnosed by mutation analysis. *Gastroenterology.* 1996;110(4):1020-1027.

45. Jemal A, Siegel R, Ward E, Murray T, Xu JQ, Thun MJ. Cancer statistics, 2007. *CA Cancer J Clin.* 2007;57(1):43-66.

46. Jass JR, Stewart SM. Evolution of Hereditary Nonpolyposis Colorectal-Cancer. *Gut.* 1992;33(6):783-786.

47. Messerini L, Vitelli F, DeVitis LR, et al. Microsatellite instability in sporadic mucinous colorectal carcinomas: Relationship to clinico-pathological variables. *J Pathol.* 1997;182(4):380-384.

48. Sankila R, Aaltonen LA, Jarvinen HJ, Mecklin JP. Better survival rates in patients with MLH1-associated hereditary colorectal cancer. *Gastroenterology.* 1996;110(3):682-687.

49. Vasen HFA, Nagengast FM, Meera Khan P. Interval cancers in hereditary non-polyposis colorectal cancer (Lynch syndrome). *Lancet.* 1995;345(8958):1183-1184.

50. Vasen HF, Mecklin JP, Khan PM, Lynch HT. The International Collaborative Group on Hereditary Non-Polyposis Colorectal Cancer (ICG-HNPCC). *Dis Colon Rectum.* 1991;34(5):424-425.

51. Vasen HFA, Watson P, Mecklin J-P, Lynch HT. New clinical criteria for hereditary nonpolyposis colorectal cancer (HNPCC, Lynch syndrome) proposed by the International Collaborative Group on HNPCC. *Gastroenterology.* 1999;116(6):1453-1456.

52. Rodriguez-Bigas MA, Boland CR, Hamilton SR, et al. A National Cancer Institute Workshop on Hereditary Nonpolyposis Colorectal Cancer Syndrome: Meeting highlights and Bethesda guidelines. *J Natl Cancer Inst.* 1997;89(23):1758-1762.

53. Winawer SJ, Fletcher RH, Miller L, et al. Colorectal cancer screening: Clinical guidelines and rationale. *Gastroenterology.* 1997;112(2):594-642.

54. Johns LE, Houlston RS. A systematic review and meta-analysis of familial colorectal cancer risk. *Am J Gastroenterol.* 2001;96(10):2992-3003.

55. Passman MA, Pommier RF, Vetto JT. Synchronous colon primaries have the same prognosis as solitary colon cancers. *Dis Colon Rectum.* 1996;39(3):329-334.

56. Eaden JA, Abrams KR, Mayberry JF. The risk of colorectal cancer in ulcerative colitis: A meta-analysis. (Statistical data included). *Gut.* 2001;48(4):526.

57. Rutter M, Saunders B, Wilkinson K, et al. Severity of inflammation is a risk factor for colorectal neoplasia in ulcerative colitis. *Gastroenterology.* 2004;126(2):451-459.

58. Fuchs CS, Giovannucci EL, Colditz GA, et al. Dietary fiber and the risk of colorectal cancer and adenoma in women. *N Engl J Med.* 1999;340(3):169-176.

59. Michels KB, Edward G, Joshipura KJ, et al. Prospective study of fruit and vegetable consumption and incidence of colon and rectal cancers. *J Natl Cancer Inst.* 2000;92(21):1740-1752.

60. Graham S, Dayal H, Swanson M, Mittelman A, Wilkinson G. Diet in epidemiology of cancer of colon and rectum. *J Natl Cancer Inst.* 1978;61(3):709-714.

61. Greenberg ER, Baron JA, Tosteson TD, et al. A clinical trial of antioxidant vitamins to prevent colorectal adenoma. *N Engl J Med.* 1994;331(3):141-147.

62. Willett WC, Stampfer MJ, Colditz GA, Rosner BA, Speizer FE. Relation of meat, fat, and fiber intake to the risk of colon cancer in a prospective study among women. *N Engl J Med.* 1990;323(24): 1664-1672.

63. Thun MJ, Namboodiri MM, Heath CW. Aspirin Use and Reduced Risk of Fatal Colon Cancer. *N Engl J Med.* 1991;325(23): 1593-1596.

64. Reid ME, Duffield-Lillico AJ, Sunga A, Fakih M, Alberts DS, Marshall JR. Selenium supplementation and colorectal adenomas: An analysis of the nutritional prevention of cancer trial. *Int J Cancer.* 2006;118(7):1777-1781.

65. Baron JA, Cole BF, Sandler RS, et al. A randomized trial of aspirin to prevent colorectal adenomas. *N Engl J Med.* 2003;348(10):891-899.

66. Giovannucci E, Rimm EB, Ascherio A, Stampfer MJ, Colditz GA, Willett WC. Alcohol, low-methionine low-folate diets, and risk of colon-cancer in men. *J Natl Cancer Inst.* 1995;87(4): 265-273.

67. Morimoto LM, Newcomb PA, Ulrich CM, Bostick RM, Lais CJ, Potter JD. Risk factors for hyperplastic and adenomatous polyps: Evidence for malignant potential? *Cancer Epidemiol Biomarkers Prev.* 2002;11(10):1012-1018.

Colorectal Cancer: Staging, Treatment, and Prognosis

DAVID H. KIM, MD
PERRY J. PICKHARDT, MD

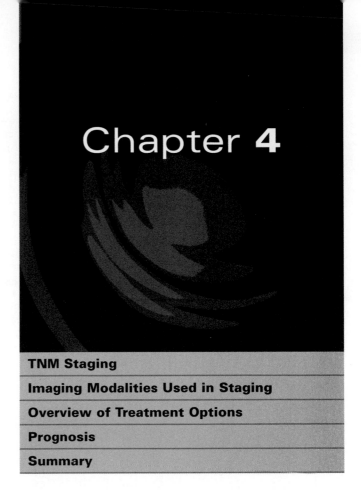

Chapter 4

TNM Staging

Imaging Modalities Used in Staging

Overview of Treatment Options

Prognosis

Summary

INTRODUCTION

Colorectal carcinoma accounts for approximately 52,000 deaths per year in the United States. The 5-year survival rates range from 10% to 90% depending on the anatomic extent of the disease and other prognostic factors.[1] In addition to the reference standard of pathologic staging, various imaging modalities are used in the determination of clinical stage. Treatment ranges from surgical resection alone to surgical resection with chemotherapy and/or radiation to systemic chemotherapy for metastatic disease. Metastectomy of isolated lesions, particularly those that are hepatic in location, can be beneficial. This chapter outlines the predominant staging system for colorectal cancer, the various modalities used, the treatment options, and prognostic factors.

TNM STAGING

The pattern of spread of a colorectal cancer typically follows a fairly predictable route. After conversion to malignancy, the cancer grows from the mucosa to involve deeper layers of the bowel wall. Once past the muscularis mucosae, there is the potential for spread through lymphatics with subsequent regional lymph node involvement. At this point, there is also the potential for involvement of the venous system, leading to metastatic lesions in the liver via the portomesenteric venous circulation. There may be subsequent hematogenous spread to the lungs. Specifically for rectal carcinoma, pulmonary metastases may preferentially occur as a result of systemic venous drainage from the hemorrhoidal veins to the inferior vena cava to the lungs.[2] Extension of the mass past the serosa of the bowel wall can lead to peritoneal involvement. Staging of anatomic extent of disease is a key determinant in the future prognosis of an individual with colorectal carcinoma. For example, depth of cancer inva-

sion within the colonic wall and number of involved regional lymph nodes are both key independent factors that help to determine prognosis.[3,4]

The predominant staging classification for colorectal carcinoma is the TNM (tumor-node-metastasis) system by the American Joint Committee on Cancer (AJCC) and the International Union Against Cancer (UICC).[5] To a large extent, it has replaced the older Dukes classification system and subsequent modifications for rectal and colon cancers. This system is based on evaluation of the primary tumor, of the regional lymph nodes, and of distant metastatic spread for the purpose of predicting prognosis (Tables 4-1 and 4-2). These individual subcategories evaluating the tumor, nodes, and metastases are then combined into larger, more encompassing stages ranging from Stage I to Stage IV. Each stage is grouped to form a homogenous collection of patients with respect to future survival. For example, patients with Stage I disease have much higher 5-year survival rates in comparison with patients with Stage IV disease. With the sixth edition of the AJCC staging system, Stages II and III were further subdivided into subgroups to increase the homogeneity of patient prognosis within each subgroup. Stage II was divided into Stage IIa (T3N0M0) and Stage IIb (T4N0M0), whereas Stage III was divided into Stage IIIa (T1/2N1M0), Stage IIIb (T3/4N1M0), and Stage IIIc (TanyN2M0). By providing prognostic survival information based on standardized categories, the TNM classification schema allows for the accurate evaluation of various therapeutic interventions

Table 4-1 ◘ Colorectal Cancer Staging*

Category	Subgroup	Definition
Primary tumor (T)	Tx	Primary tumor cannot be assessed
	T0	No evidence of primary tumor
	Tis	Intraepithelial or intramucosal carcinoma
	T1	Tumor invades the submucosa
	T2	Tumor invades the muscularis propria
	T3	Tumor invades through the muscularis propria into the subserosa or into nonperitonealized pericolic tissue
	T4	Tumor directly invades other organs or structures and/or perforates visceral peritoneum
Regional lymph node metastases (N)	Nx	Regional lymph nodes cannot be assessed
	N0	No regional lymph node metastases
	N1	Metastases to 1-3 regional lymph nodes
	N2	Metastases to 4 or more regional lymph nodes
Distant metastases (M)	Mx	Presence of distant metastases cannot be assessed
	M0	No distant metastases
	M1	Distant metastases present

*From Greene FL, Page DL, Morrow M, et al, eds. *AJCC cancer staging manual.* 6th ed. New York: Springer; 2002.

Table 4-2 ◘ Colorectal Cancer Staging*

Stage	T	N	M
0	Tis	N0	M0
I	T1 or T2	N0	M0
IIa	T3	N0	M0
IIb	T4	N0	M0
IIIa	T1 or T2	N1	M0
IIIb	T3 or T4	N1	M0
IIIc	Any T	N2	M0
IV	Any T	Any N	M1

*From Greene FL, Page DL, Morrow M, et al, eds. *AJCC cancer staging manual.* 6th ed. New York: Springer; 2002.

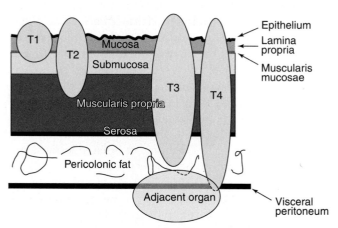

Figure 4-1 Schematic of T status. Diagrammatic representation of T classifications of wall layer involvement. One key differential point from an imaging perspective is the distinction between T2 and T3 lesions, which can be difficult for any modality.

having an impact on this disease. Clinical trials would not be possible without such a construct. In addition, it allows for the assessment of nonanatomic prognostic factors at specific anatomic stages. Ultimately, it helps to direct the appropriate therapeutic regimen for a given patient and to define the expected outcome.

For the primary tumor, there are four categories of T classification in the TNM system (Fig. 4-1). A T1 lesion extends from the mucosa past the muscularis mucosae into the submucosa. A T2 lesion extends into but is limited by the muscularis propria. A T3 lesion invades through the muscularis propria into the bowel serosa or nonperitonealized pericolic tissue. A T4 lesion invades other organs or structures and/or perforates the visceral peritoneum.

For regional lymph nodes, N-positive status is divided into the categories of N1 and N2. With N1 status there are one to three cancer-involved regional lymph nodes, and with N2 status, a patient has four of more regional lymph nodes. Determining positivity of a lymph node can be problematic at clinical staging (see later) as a result of micrometastases, which do not significantly enlarge the lymph nodes. Even at pathologic staging, ac-

curate lymph node status may be difficult to achieve because of sampling issues, as suggested by observations from studies such as from Goldstein et al.[6] Here, an analysis of patients with T3 tumors (n = 2427) demonstrated a survival difference based on the number of analyzed lymph nodes in which recovery of ≤7 lymph nodes had a 5-year survival of 62.2%, whereas those with ≥17 lymph nodes sampled had a survival of 75.8%. Studies such as this suggest that understaging related to sampling is an issue. Current recommendations from the AJCC include sampling at least 12 lymph nodes to decrease false-negative lymph status.[5]

The M status is a binary decision as to whether distant metastatic disease is present (M1) or not (M0). Solitary metastatic implants may be amenable to surgical and interventional options, as discussed later.

IMAGING MODALITIES USED IN STAGING

The TNM classification involves a determination of both clinical stage (cTNM) and pathologic stage (pTNM). The clinical stage is undertaken before treatment and includes the use of various imaging modalities, whereas the pathologic stage is completed after surgical intervention. Several imaging modalities are used to help determine the clinical stage, including computed tomography (CT), magnetic resonance imaging (MR), and endoscopic ultrasound (EUS). The main aims of imaging include the following: (1) assessment for distant disease in the abdomen or pelvis, typically undertaken by CT, and (2) local tumor staging (in the case of rectal carcinoma) to assess for need of neoadjuvant chemoradiation therapy. For local tumor evaluation, the primary imaging modality has been EUS, although MR has shown increasing utility in this regard.

Imaging Determination of Distant Disease

CT is the main imaging modality to assess for distant disease in most institutions (Fig. 4-2). It is typically undertaken with both intravenous and oral contrast.

CT is well suited to assess the liver and other areas in the abdomen and pelvis for metastatic lesions. Even back in the mid-1990s accuracies for hepatic metastatic disease of 85% were reported.[7] Given the significant advances in CT technology over the past decade leading to multislice acquisition of thin images during rapid administration of contrast boluses, the capabilities of CT for distant metastatic detection within the liver have improved considerably. However, accuracy of regional and distant adenopathy remains difficult. It is important to note that the determination of pathologic involvement of lymph nodes based predominantly on size may miss some involved lymph nodes. When lymph nodes become rounded or demonstrate a necrotic center, neoplastic involvement can be suspected even when the lymph node does not meet size criteria.

Another imaging option for distant metastatic evaluation includes MR. This modality is also sensitive for distant metastases to the liver. Newer sequences and protocols have allowed for more complete evaluations of the entire abdomen and pelvis. Whereas areas such as the small bowel mesentery and retroperitoneum were previously sometimes difficult to assess with MR, these are now well seen with current volume breath-held three-dimensional (3D) series. Overall, however,

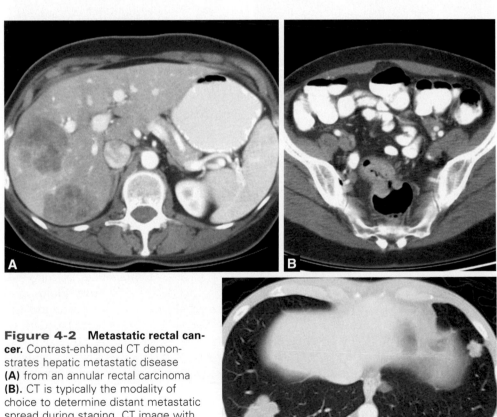

Figure 4-2 Metastatic rectal cancer. Contrast-enhanced CT demonstrates hepatic metastatic disease **(A)** from an annular rectal carcinoma **(B)**. CT is typically the modality of choice to determine distant metastatic spread during staging. CT image with lung windows **(C)** from a different patient demonstrates pulmonary metastases from a rectal cancer.

MR is typically less available and demonstrates more variability in examination quality between patients and institutions. Finally, positron emission tomography (PET) may be helpful and is used increasingly by some institutions to aid in staging for distant metastatic disease.

Imaging Determination of Bowel Wall and Local Lymph Node Involvement

Clinical staging involving depth of local wall invasion and of local lymph node involvement is particularly important in the case of rectal cancer because it determines the need for neoadjuvant (preoperative) therapy. The traditional mainstay of imaging evaluation involves endoscopic ultrasound. EUS allows for depiction of the various layers of the bowel wall, which present as alternating hyperechoic and hypoechoic concentric bands. A cancer appears as a hypoechoic mass, which disrupts the various involved layers of the bowel wall (Fig. 4-3). Of the available imaging modalities, EUS and MR provide better assessment of the level of wall involvement than CT does.[8] EUS accuracy in T stage assessment is about mid-80%.[9] The central issue at EUS is similar to the other imaging modalities and concerns the distinction between a T2 lesion (contained by the muscularis propria) and a T3 lesion (spread beyond the muscularis propria) or, in other words, differentiating between Stage I and Stage II disease where treatment options may differ (see following section). Unfortunately, this is an area of difficulty, and the T2 category corresponds to the lowest accuracy for EUS.[9] Peritumoral inflammatory stranding can lead to overstaging a T2 lesion to a T3 lesion where

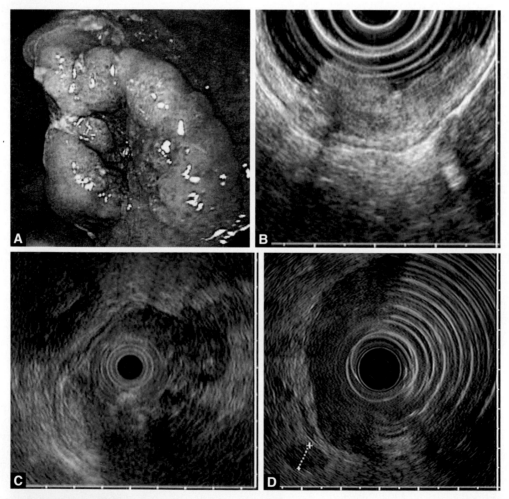

Figure 4-3 **Local staging by EUS.** Optical colonoscopy image **(A)** shows a lobulated mass in the rectum. EUS **(B)** demonstrates that the cancer is limited to the mucosa and submucosa with an intact muscularis propria seen as the outer hypoechoic stripe (T2 lesion). EUS image **(C)** in another patient demonstrates extension beyond the muscularis propria consistent with a T3 lesion. EUS in a third patient **(D)** also shows a T3 lesion with tumor extension into the perirectal fat. In addition, an involved rounded perirectal lymph node is seen *(calipers)*.

the inflammation is falsely interpreted as tumor spread beyond the muscularis propria. Conversely, microscopic infiltration in a T3 lesion would be nonapparent at conventional imaging, leading to an understaged T2 lesion.

Another area of relative weakness for EUS, and the other imaging modalities, concerns regional lymph node involvement. Sensitivities range around 60% with specificities at mid-70%s for all imaging modalities.[8] Size as a surrogate for tumor involvement is suboptimal related to the potential for micrometastases. Positive lymph nodes may not enlarge past the 1-cm threshold because of this phenomenon. In fact, it has been demonstrated that approximately 50% of lymph node metastases in rectal cancer are ≤5 mm in size.[10] Decreasing the size threshold to 5 mm increases sensitivity, as does the use of morphologic features such as a rounded appearance to the nodes. On the other hand, lymph nodes can enlarge past the 1-cm threshold as a result of reactive inflammatory etiologies and not because of tumor, leading to false overstaging. In addition, the depth of transducer range for EUS is overall limited where all regional lymph nodes may not be able to be evaluated.

Additional limitations of EUS include the potential inability to pass a stenotic lesion for evaluation and the inability to depict the mesorectal fascia well. Thus, the relationship of the tumor to this fascia cannot be made accurately, which represents a prognostic factor for rectal carcinoma that is gaining in importance.[11]

MR is also effectively used for local clinical staging. In the past, EUS has been considered the more accurate method. With the advancements in underlying hardware, sequence development, and surface coils, the capability of MR has significantly increased. The pelvic phased array coil is supplanting the endorectal coil for MR, demonstrating excellent signal-to-noise. Bianchi and colleagues compared EUS with MR with comparable results. MR with a phased array coil held an accuracy of 71% compared with EUS at 70%.[12] As with EUS, micrometastases to lymph nodes decrease the accuracy of MR assessment for lymph node involvement. Perhaps the major advantages that MR holds over EUS are the ability to visualize the mesorectal fascia for rectal cancer and the ability to visualize more distant nodes and other structures for metastatic involvement (Fig. 4-4).[13]

CT lacks the tissue contrast to clearly visualize the various layers of the bowel wall. Although it does well to characterize advanced disease with invasion into adjacent structures, it cannot differentiate between different categories of lesser extent disease. It holds the poorest accuracy for T status compared with EUS and MR.[14] Potentially, CT colonography (CTC) may improve this accuracy. CTC with colonic distention, thin collimation, and use of intravenous contrast has demonstrated improved results over the past reported standard CT results in early studies (Fig. 4-5).[15] Nodal involvement assessments by CT and CTC are similar to EUS and MR. This is not surprising, as stated previously, because all modalities use similar size and morphologic criteria to make this assessment. One situation in which CTC is clearly helpful is in the assessment of synchronous polyps and cancers proximal to a distal cancer. In cases where optical colonoscopy cannot pass a stenotic cancer, CTC allows evaluation of these proximal areas (Fig. 4-6).[16]

It is important to note that besides initial clinical staging, imaging plays an ongoing role in the evaluation for recurrent disease. Again, the role is predominantly related to evaluating for the presence of distant metastatic disease. Evaluation of the resection site with cross-sectional imaging techniques can be difficult because of postsurgical changes and postradiation changes (in those patients who received such therapy), in which gross interval progression of soft tissue is needed to make the

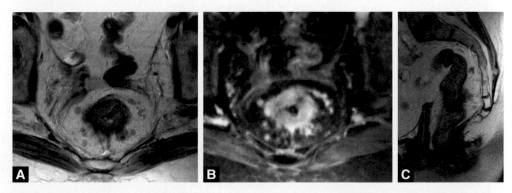

Figure 4-4   Local staging by MR. T2-weighted **(A)** and postcontrast, fat-suppressed T1-weighted **(B)** MR images show an annular T3 rectal cancer with gross extension past the muscularis propria. Several rounded perirectal lymph nodes are seen. Sagittal T2-weighted MR image **(C)** demonstrates posterior extension of tumor into the perirectal fat.

Illustration continued on following page

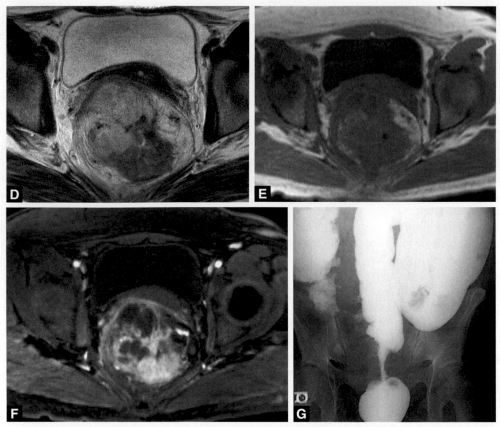

Figure 4-4 (Continued) **Local staging by MR.** T2-weighted **(D)**; precontrast T1-weighted **(E)**; and postcontrast, fat-suppressed T1-weighted **(F)** MR images in a second patient show a large rectal T4 cancer with multifocal involvement of the mesorectal fascia. Hypaque enema **(G)** demonstrates the classic "apple core" appearance at fluoroscopy. (Courtesy of Dr. Christine O. Menias, Washington University.)

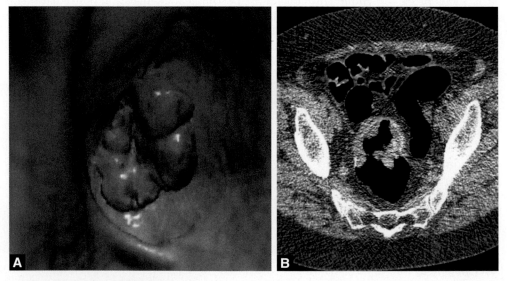

Figure 4-5 **Cancer evaluation at CTC.** 3D endoluminal image **(A)** shows a lobulated annular rectal cancer. Two-dimensional transverse CTC image **(B)** demonstrates circumferential soft tissue thickening. The CO_2 distention allows improved evaluation of the tumor, although the individual layers of the wall cannot be resolved. The lack of convex borders suggests a T2 lesion.

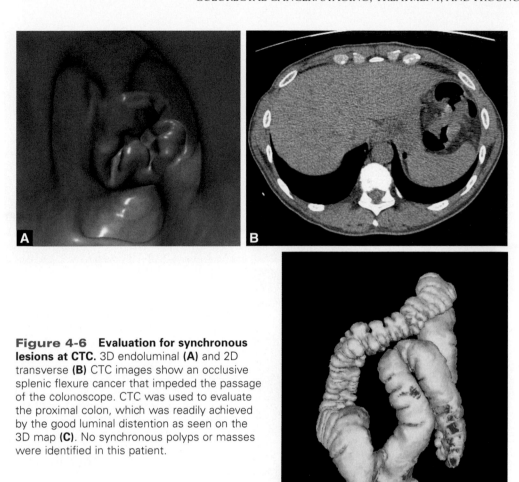

Figure 4-6 **Evaluation for synchronous lesions at CTC.** 3D endoluminal **(A)** and 2D transverse **(B)** CTC images show an occlusive splenic flexure cancer that impeded the passage of the colonoscope. CTC was used to evaluate the proximal colon, which was readily achieved by the good luminal distention as seen on the 3D map **(C)**. No synchronous polyps or masses were identified in this patient.

determination of recurrent disease. Modalities such as positron emission tomography (PET) can be helpful in this regard (Fig. 4-7).

OVERVIEW OF TREATMENT OPTIONS

Specific treatment regimens are continuously evolving and being modified, including refinement of the approach to various TNM subgroups. However, several general themes have held constant. First, the imaging approach and treatment of colon and rectal cancers differ in several regards as a result of the location of rectal cancers in which the bony constraints of the pelvis affect surgical access, leading to difficulty in negative margin control and increased recurrence rates. Second, surgical resection for cure is sufficient for localized disease, whereas chemotherapy is needed in addition to surgery for more advanced local disease when cure is the focus. Third, radiation has not shown to increase survival but is useful for local control for rectal carcinomas. It is not typically used for colon cancers unless the cancer holds a low location pelvic and is adherent to pelvic structures. Fourth, in metastatic disease, chemotherapy regimens can lengthen survival for the patient. Procedures directed at the removal or ablation of isolated/limited hepatic and pulmonary metastatic lesion(s) may also increase survival intervals.

Surgical resection alone is the treatment of choice for Stage I (T1/2N0M0) rectal and colon cancers and for Stage II (T3/4N0M0) colon cancer. For rectal cancer, the concept of the mesorectum and the tumor relationship to this structure has shown to correlate with future local recurrence and survival.[17] Total mesorectal excision (TME) has proved effective in reducing local recurrence rates.[18] Traditionally, resection was accomplished by means of an open procedure for both colon and rectal cancers. The curative surgical resection should include the primary tumor and sampling of at least 12 regional lymph nodes to pathologically stage the nodal status of the patient.[5] During the procedure, the entire abdominal cavity should be inspected for metastatic lesions. Biopsies of suspicious lesions should be performed. In recent years, laparoscopic tech-

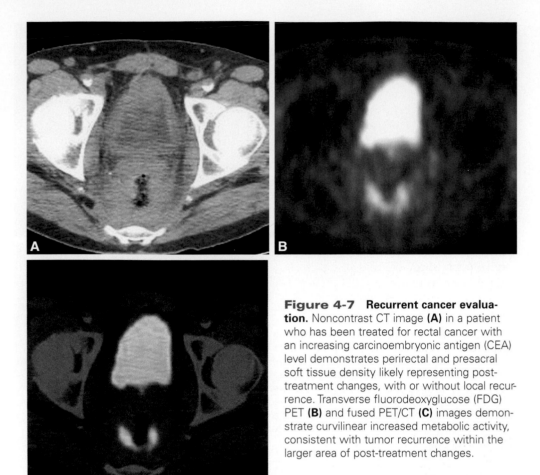

Figure 4-7 Recurrent cancer evaluation. Noncontrast CT image **(A)** in a patient who has been treated for rectal cancer with an increasing carcinoembryonic antigen (CEA) level demonstrates perirectal and presacral soft tissue density likely representing post-treatment changes, with or without local recurrence. Transverse fluorodeoxyglucose (FDG) PET **(B)** and fused PET/CT **(C)** images demonstrate curvilinear increased metabolic activity, consistent with tumor recurrence within the larger area of post-treatment changes.

niques have increasingly been used. A large randomized trial with experienced surgeons has demonstrated equivalency between the two approaches for colon cancer.[19]

The addition of chemotherapy to surgical resection improves survival rates for more advanced local disease. For colon cancers, adjuvant (postoperative) chemotherapy is given routinely for Stage III disease (TanyN1/2M0). A large trial of nearly 1300 patients conducted by the Eastern Cooperative Oncology Group (ECOG) demonstrated that adjuvant therapy could substantially decrease local recurrence and risk of death versus surgery alone.[20,21] It is controversial whether Stage II colon cancer (T3/4N0M0) benefits from adjuvant therapy. No survival advantage has been conclusively demonstrated in subset analysis of the majority of various trials, leading to the opinion against routine administration of adjuvant therapy in this group.[22] It has been proposed, however, to add such therapy for those Stage II colon cancers with unfavorable factors such as poor histology, colonic perforation/obstruction, or lymphovascular invasion.[22] Radiation typically does not play a role in colon cancer unless the tumor is low in the pelvis and adherent to pelvic structures. In that case, radiation may be helpful in decreasing local recurrences and related symptomatology.

For rectal cancers, both chemotherapy and radiation are given for Stage II (T3/4N0M0) and Stage III (TanyN1/2M0), in addition to surgical resection. Chemotherapy is given with the intent of increasing survival interval, whereas radiation is given with the intent of decreasing local recurrences. Neoadjuvant (preoperative) administration of chemoradiation is currently favored, whereas in the past, adjuvant (postoperative) therapy was undertaken. Evidence to support this approach was provided by Sauer et al.,[23] who demonstrated equivalency between the two approaches in terms of overall survival but improved local control and decreased toxicity with the neoadjuvant approach. The advantages of a neoadjuvant approach include potentially downstaging the tumor to a resectable state, increasing the possibility of preserving sphincter control and decreasing local recurrence rates. It is important to realize that neoadjuvant administration demands accurate clinical staging with imaging as opposed to the adjuvant situation where pathologic stage determines the need for chemoradiation. Given the known difficulties with the distinction between T2 and T3 status with imaging including EUS, some contend that a substantial percentage may be overstaged and thus treated unnecessarily by this approach. Evidence supports this;

Sauer et al. demonstrated that 18% of patients in the adjuvant therapy arm of their study actually were overstaged at resection. Presumably, a similar percentage would exist in the neoadjuvant arm.[23]

In the metastatic setting, the overall 5-year survival is poor at 10%.[1] Chemotherapy has been shown to increase survival intervals. Various regimens have increased the median survival of a patient with metastatic disease from less than 1 year to approximately 2 years with multiagent therapy. In addition, for isolated metastatic disease to the liver and lungs, surgical resection or ablative procedures have proved effective at increasing survival. For appropriate hepatic metastatic lesions, surgical resection has resulted in up to a 40% 5-year survival rate in some series.[24] The role of neoadjuvant or adjuvant chemotherapy in this situation is not firmly established. Minimally invasive image-guided techniques such as radiofrequency ablation (RFA) have shown similar promising results (Fig. 4-8).[25] Such methods have the advantage of quicker patient recovery and the ability to repeat treatment with recurrences because larger areas of normal liver are spared in

comparison with formal surgical resections. Other techniques that are potentially helpful in hepatic metastatic disease include hepatic arterial infusion chemotherapy to increase drug dose levels to the metastatic lesions and selective internal radiation therapy with yttrium-90 microspheres to increase radiation dose to a metastasis. Along similar principles, resection (and ablative therapies) may be helpful for isolated pulmonary metastases.[26]

PROGNOSIS

The TNM classification system groups various combinations of the primary tumor, regional lymph nodes, and distant metastatic disease into larger stages, which portend prognosis. As the stage progresses, survival rates generally decrease. Key anatomic features that correlate with prognosis include extent of cancer involvement of the bowel wall and number of affected regional lymph nodes. In addition, the presence of venous and lymphatic invasion has been identified as independent poor prognostic factors where it is theorized that this allows the

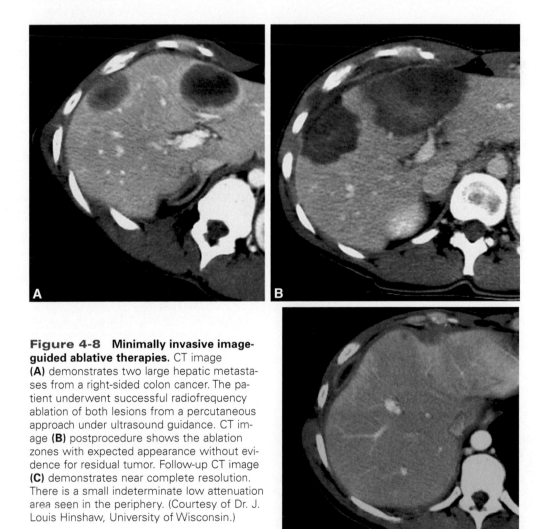

Figure 4-8   Minimally invasive image-guided ablative therapies. CT image **(A)** demonstrates two large hepatic metastases from a right-sided colon cancer. The patient underwent successful radiofrequency ablation of both lesions from a percutaneous approach under ultrasound guidance. CT image **(B)** postprocedure shows the ablation zones with expected appearance without evidence for residual tumor. Follow-up CT image **(C)** demonstrates near complete resolution. There is a small indeterminate low attenuation area seen in the periphery. (Courtesy of Dr. J. Louis Hinshaw, University of Wisconsin.)

implant of micrometastases.[27] A number of factors are not accounted for in the TNM system. However, this classification allows for assessment of impact of these various factors for a given anatomic extent or stage of disease. Morphologic features such as tumor budding and tumor border configuration have been shown to confer a worse prognosis.[28,29] Histology and grade have demonstrated prognostic value. Cells with signet ring histology portend a much worse prognosis than a standard adenocarcinoma stage for stage, with the exception of Stage I disease.[30] Although not recommended for routine examination, molecular mutation analysis such as loss of heterozygosity 18q and TP53 may be helpful to stratify prognosis. Immunohistochemical protein profiling has yet to be established.[31]

O'Connell and colleagues reported on the 5-year survival rates for colon cancer (excluding rectal) for the period January 1991 to December 2000 for patients in the SEER (Surveillance, Epidemiology, and End Results) national cancer registry.[30] The overall 5-year survival was 65.2%. From Stage I to IV, the rate was 93.2%, 82.5%, 59.5%, and 8.1%, respectively. Stage II and Stage III were also broken down into subcategories as outlined by the revised sixth edition staging system (see Table 4-2). Here, the 5-year survival rates for patients with Stage IIIa were significantly better than that of Stage IIb (83.4% versus 72.2%, respectively), leading the authors to suggest that this potentially reflected that patients with Stage III disease generally receive chemotherapy, whereas patients with Stage II disease do not.

SUMMARY

Colorectal cancer currently is a significant cause of cancer mortality, with 5-year survival ranging from 10% to 90%.[1] The TNM classification system, based on the anatomic extent of disease, creates groups of homogenous CRC populations to allow for important prognostic information. It allows the assessment of nonanatomic prognostic factors for a given stage and the assessment of various therapeutic options. Increasingly, imaging is being used in the determination of stage.

REFERENCES

1. Jemal A, Siegel R, Ward E, Murray T, Xu JQ, Thun MJ. Cancer statistics, 2007. CA Cancer J Clin. 2007;57(1):43-66.
2. Kirke R, Rajesh A, Verma R, Bankart MJG. Rectal cancer: Incidence of pulmonary metastases on thoracic CT and correlation with T staging. J Comput Assist Tomogr. 2007;31(4):569-571.
3. Adjuvant therapy of colon cancer—Results of a prospectively randomized trial. Gastrointestinal Tumor Study Group. N Engl J Med. 1984;310(12):737-743.
4. Wolmark N, Fisher ER, Wieand HS, Fisher B. The relationship of depth of penetration and tumor size to the number of positive nodes in Dukes C colorectal cancer. Cancer. 1984;53(12):2707-2712.
5. Compton CC, Greene FL. The staging of colorectal cancer: 2004 and beyond. CA Cancer J Clin. 2004;54(6):295-308.
6. Goldstein NS. Lymph node recoveries from 2427 pT3 colorectal resection specimens spanning 45 years—Recommendations for a minimum number of recovered lymph nodes based on predictive probabilities. Am J Surg Pathol. 2002;26(2):179-189.
7. Zerhouni EA, Rutter C, Hamilton SR, et al. CT and MR imaging in the staging of colorectal carcinoma: Report of the radiology diagnostic oncology group II. Radiology. 1996;200(2):443-451.
8. Bipat S, Glas AS, Slors FJM, Zwinderman AH, Bossuyt PMM, Stoker J. Rectal cancer: Local staging and assessment of lymph node involvement with endoluminal US, CT, and MR imaging—A meta-analysis. Radiology. 2004;232(3):773-783.
9. Savides TJ, Master SS. EUS in rectal cancer. Gastrointest Endosc. 2002;56(4):S12-S18.
10. Kotanagi H, Fukuoka T, Shibata Y, et al. The size of regional lymph nodes does not correlate with the presence or absence of metastasis in lymph nodes in rectal cancer. J Surg Oncol. 1993;54(4):252-254.
11. Nagtegaal ID, Marijnen CAA, Kranenbarg EK, van de Velde CJH, van Krieken J. Circumferential margin involvement is still an important predictor of local recurrence in rectal carcinoma—Not one millimeter but two millimeters is the limit. Am J Surg Pathol. 2002;26(3):350-357.
12. Bianchi PP, Ceriani C, Rottoli M, et al. Endoscopic ultrasonography and magnetic resonance in preoperative staging of rectal cancer: Comparison with histologic findings. J Gastrointest Surg. 2005;9(9):1222-1227.
13. Beets-Tan RGH, Beets GL, Vliegen RFA, et al. Accuracy of magnetic resonance imaging in prediction of tumour-free resection margin in rectal cancer surgery. Lancet. 2001;357(9255):497-504.
14. Kwok H, Bissett IP, Hill GL. Preoperative staging of rectal cancer. Intl J Colorectal Dis. 2000;15(1):9-20.
15. Chung DJ, Huh KC, Choi WJ, Kim JK. CT colonography using 16-MDCT in the evaluation of colorectal cancer. Am J Roentgenol. 2005;184(1):98-103.
16. Kim DH, Pickhardt PJ, Hoff G, Kay CL. Computed tomographic colonography for colorectal screening. Endoscopy. 2007;39(6):545-549.
17. Adam IJ, Mohamdee MO, Martin IG, et al. Role of circumferential margin involvement in the local recurrence of rectal cancer. Lancet. 1994;344(8924):707-711.
18. Soreide O, Norstein J. Local recurrence after operative treatment of rectal carcinoma: A strategy for change. J Am Coll Surg. 1997;184(1):84-92.
19. Guillou PJ, Quirke P, Thorpe H, et al. Short-term endpoints of conventional versus laparoscopic-assisted surgery in patients with colorectal cancer (MRC CLASICC trial): multicentre, randomised controlled trial. Lancet. 2005;365(9472):1718-1726.
20. Moertel CG, Fleming TR, Macdonald JS, et al. Levamisole and fluorouracil for adjuvant therapy of resected colon carcinoma. N Engl J Med. 1990;322(6):352-358.
21. Moertel CG, Fleming TR, Macdonald JS, et al. Fluorouracil plus levamisole as effective adjuvant therapy after resection of Stage III colon carcinoma—A Final Report. Ann Intern Med. 1995;122(5):321-326.
22. Benson AB, Schrag D, Somerfield MR, et al. American Society of Clinical Oncology recommendations on adjuvant chemotherapy for stage II colon cancer. J Clin Oncol. 2004;22(16):3408-3419.
23. Sauer R, Becker H, Hohenberger W, et al. Preoperative versus postoperative chemoradiotherapy for rectal cancer. N Engl J Med. 2004;351(17):1731-1740.

24. Fong Y, Fortner J, Sun RL, Brennan MF, Blumgart LH. Clinical score for predicting recurrence after hepatic resection for metastatic colorectal cancer—Analysis of 1001 consecutive cases. *Ann Surg.* 1999;230(3):309-318.

25. Solbiati L, Livraghi T, Goldberg SN, et al. Percutaneous radiofrequency ablation of hepatic metastases from colorectal cancer: Long-term results in 117 patients. *Radiology.* 2001;221(1):159-166.

26. Rotolo N, De Monte L, Imperatori A, Dominioni L. Pulmonary resections of single metastases from colorectal cancer. *Surg Oncol (Oxford).* 2007;16:S141-S144.

27. Compton CC, Fielding LP, Burgart LJ, et al. Prognostic factors in colorectal cancer - College of American Pathologists Consensus Statement 1999. *Arch Pathol Lab Med.* 2000;124(7):979-994.

28. Ueno H, Mochizuki H, Hashiguchi Y, et al. Risk factors for an adverse outcome in early invasive colorectal carcinoma. *Gastroenterology.* 2004;127(2):385-394.

29. Kanazawa H, Mitomi H, Nishiyama Y, et al. Tumour budding at invasive margins and outcome in colorectal cancer. *Colorectal Dis.* 2008;10(1):41-47.

30. O'Connell JB, Maggard MA, Ko CY. Colon cancer survival rates with the new American Joint Committee on cancer sixth edition staging. *J Natl Cancer Inst.* 2004;96(19):1420-1425.

31. Zlobec I, Lugli A. Prognostic and predictive factors in colorectal cancer. *J Clin Pathol.* 2008;61(5):561-569.

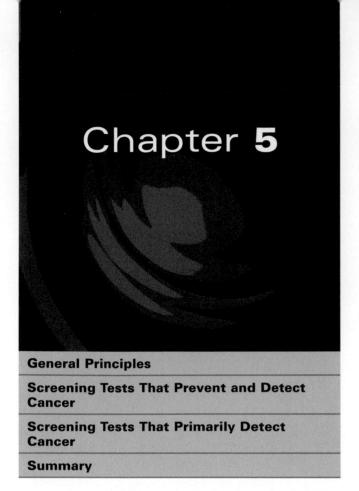

Chapter 5

Colorectal Cancer Screening: Rationale and Available Options

PERRY J. PICKHARDT, MD
DAVID H. KIM, MD

General Principles

Screening Tests That Prevent and Detect Cancer

Screening Tests That Primarily Detect Cancer

Summary

GENERAL PRINCIPLES

The basic rationale behind screening for colorectal cancer (CRC) is that this deadly disease is not only treatable with early detection, but, perhaps more importantly, it is also largely preventable through detection and removal of the precursor lesion: the advanced adenoma. This unique opportunity for prevention sets CRC apart from the screening efforts directed toward breast cancer and lung cancer, where the main target of screening is the cancer itself. For this reason, CRC screening is generally a cost-effective endeavor. The evidence that screening of average-risk lesions can reduce CRC mortality is compelling. The main challenge for CRC screening, however, lies not in proving its worth from either a clinical or economic standpoint. Rather, the predominant challenge is simply getting individuals tested because the majority of average-risk adults older than age 50 years have not engaged in any type of screening. Although some have argued that too many screening options lead to confusion that could have an overall negative impact on compliance rates, most believe that variations in test availability and patient preferences favor providing a menu of acceptable options.

The joint 2008 screening guidelines released by the American Cancer Society (ACS),[1] in conjunction with the American College of Radiology (ACR) and the U.S. Multi-Society Task Force on CRC (representing the three major U.S. gastroenterology societies: the American Gastroenterological Association, American College of Gastroenterology, and American Society for Gastrointestinal Endoscopy), represent a landmark effort for several reasons. For one, this marks the first time that the radiology and gastroenterology groups have formally come together with the ACS to issue joint guidelines. Second, these guidelines appropriately stress that CRC prevention should be considered the primary goal of screening. To underscore this message, the various screening tests are now divided into tests that serve to both prevent and detect CRC versus tests that primarily serve to simply detect the cancer itself (Table 5-1). In the past, all acceptable options were lumped together in a single list of recommended tests. Third, computed tomography colonography (CTC) has made the list of recommended tests for the first time and stands alongside optical colonoscopy (OC) as the tests that are best suited to both prevent and detect CRC.

The remainder of this chapter will review the salient features of the various acceptable screening options, including the relative advantages and disadvantages of each test. The discussion for CTC will be abbreviated because this information is provided elsewhere throughout this book. In the end, the best test for a given patient is the one that he or she is actually willing to undergo—provided that the test is done well.

SCREENING TESTS THAT PREVENT AND DETECT CANCER

Tests that detect both precancerous polyps and cancer include flexible sigmoidoscopy (FS), OC, double contrast barium enema (DCBE), and CTC. It was the strong opinion of the expert panel that convened for the recent ACS guidelines that CRC *prevention* should be the primary goal

Table 5-1 ▫ Acceptable Testing Options for Primary CRC Screening for Asymptomatic Adults Aged 50 Years and Older According to the 2008 American Cancer Society Guidelines

TESTS THAT DETECT ADENOMATOUS POLYPS AND CANCER

Flexible sigmoidoscopy (FS) every 5 years, or

Optical colonoscopy (OC) every 10 years, or

Double contrast barium enema (DCBE) every 5 years, or

CT colonography (CTC) every 5 years

TESTS THAT PRIMARILY DETECT CANCER

Annual guaiac-based fecal occult blood test (gFOBT) with high test sensitivity for cancer, or

Annual fecal immunochemical test (FIT) with high test sensitivity for cancer, or

Stool DNA test (sDNA) with high sensitivity for cancer, interval uncertain

Adapted with permission from Levin B, Lieberman DA, McFarland B, et al. Screening and surveillance for the early detection of colorectal cancer and adenomatous polyps, 2008: A joint guideline from the American Cancer Society, the US Multi-Society Task Force on Colorectal Cancer, and the American College of Radiology. *CA Cancer J Clin.* 2008;58(3):130-160.

of screening. Therefore, structural examinations that are designed to detect both early cancer and precancerous polyps should be encouraged if resources are available. Unlike the case of fecal occult blood testing (FOBT), there are no large randomized controlled trials confirming that these studies reduce mortality from CRC through routine screening. However, it is widely accepted that any test capable of detecting cancer as well as or better than FOBT will be beneficial, especially if the test can also detect precancerous advanced adenomas.[1]

OC, CTC, and DCBE all provide for full structural examination, whereas FS allows for only partial structural evaluation. Furthermore, detection of a large polyp or mass at CTC, DCBE, or FS will generally require subsequent OC for definitive therapy. For a variety of reasons discussed later, OC and CTC are likely to be the two predominate CRC screening tests going forward, assuming that widespread third-party reimbursement for the latter is imminent.

Flexible Sigmoidoscopy

Flexible sigmoidoscopy (FS) is an endoscopic procedure that examines the distal colon and rectum, typically to the level of the splenic flexure. FS can be performed alone every 5 years, or in combination with a sensitive fecal blood test performed annually. FS is usually performed without sedation and with a more limited bowel preparation than OC. As such, it can be performed in office-based settings and even by nonphysician providers, assuming that adequate training has been received.[2] FS

has been shown to significantly reduce mortality from distal CRC in two high-quality case-control studies[3,4] and has demonstrated a decrease in CRC incidence compared with unscreened control groups in a small randomized trial[5] and a case-control study.[6] A number of prospective randomized controlled trials are ongoing, with results expected in the near future. Additional evidence supporting the effectiveness of FS derives from OC studies, which can be used as a surrogate for FS. Studies have shown that FS may be up to 70% as sensitive as OC for detection of advanced adenomas and cancers.[7,8] However, there may be important differences in the prevalence of distal and proximal advanced neoplasms lesions based on age, gender, and ethnicity, which carry important implications for screening with FS.

The main advantages of FS are that it can be performed following a simple enema preparation, without sedation, by a variety of examiners. However, oral bowel preparation yields superior cleansing over enemas and may be favored by patients.[9] Furthermore, the lack of sedation is perceived by some as an overall disadvantage because of greater periprocedural discomfort compared with OC, which also has a negative impact on compliance with future screening.[10] Considerable variation between examiners has been shown for both depth of scope insertion and for adenoma detection,[11,12] which may reduce the overall effectiveness of FS screening. Scope insertion beyond 40 cm is considered one measure of study quality, but it does not guarantee adequate polyp detection. The major limitations of FS compared with OC are that it does not examine the entire colon and that full OC is often required when left-sided polyps are found. The ACS guidelines recommend that most patients who have adenomas discovered at FS should undergo OC evaluation. If biopsies are not obtained at FS, an alternative strategy is to refer all patients with one or more polyps greater than 5 mm to OC.[1,13] Perforation is a feared complication of FS but is much less frequently encountered compared with OC (fewer than 1 case per 20,000 examinations).[14] The appropriate screening interval following negative FS is debatable, but 5 years remains the standard recommendation, largely because of concerns about examination quality and completeness.

The incremental benefit of primary OC screening versus FS screening is less than one might expect, in part because proximal advanced adenomas may be found at OC in patients referred for small distal adenomas or nondiminutive polyps. Given the higher direct medical costs and indirect costs of OC, and the higher risk of complications with OC, the magnitude of this incremental benefit carries important policy implications.[15] As with DCBE, FS use in the United States has been steadily decreasing as a result of both low reimbursement and a shortage of adequately trained examiners. However, some pockets of relatively high FS use do remain.

Optical Colonoscopy

Since Medicare initiated reimbursement for screening optical colonoscopy in 2001, the volume of procedures has greatly increased. An estimated 14 million procedures were performed in 2003.[16] Like FS, OC allows for direct mucosal inspection, but it has the added benefit of covering the entire colon. The modern colonoscope is more advanced than a standard sigmoidoscope and is capable of air insufflation, irrigation, suction, and passage of biopsy forceps and polypectomy snares. Patients must undergo full oral bowel preparation, including a liquid diet 1 day or more before the examination, followed by either an oral lavage solution (polyethylene glycol) or saline laxatives (sodium phosphate). Although not always absolutely required, intravenous sedation and pain control are standard to avoid the discomfort of this invasive examination.

As noted previously, there are no prospective randomized controlled OC trials demonstrating a reduction in incidence or mortality from CRC. However, because OC is the final common pathway for less invasive screening tests, the ultimate benefit of CRC prevention results from polypectomy at OC. Strong indirect evidence lies in the National Polyp Study, where the incidence of CRC after clearing colonoscopy was reduced by 76% to 90% compared with three historical control populations.[17] Although not all subsequent trials were this convincing, the overall data support the conclusion that OC screening can have a significant impact on CRC incidence and, by extension, CRC mortality. The actual magnitude of the protective impact remains uncertain.

OC clearly represents the therapeutic gold standard for colorectal evaluation, but it has a number of important limitations as a primary screening tool. Chief among these are that OC represents the most invasive and most expensive initial screening test. OC complications can be severe and life threatening. Perforation and bleeding are feared complications that occur more often, but not exclusively, with polypectomy. Perforation at screening OC occurs in approximately 1 in 500 to 1000 cases (0.1%-0.2%).[15,18-20] In addition, significant cardiopulmonary complications, such as cardiac arrhythmias, hypotension, and oxygen desaturation, are usually related to sedation. Cardiopulmonary complications account for approximately one half of all adverse events at OC.[21] Other OC-related complications that may lead to hospitalization or surgery include splenic rupture and postpolypectomy syndromes.[22] Serious complications that affect patients without significant polyps could have been avoided by initial screening with a less invasive option. OC represents an expensive and limited resource. The charge for OC at our institution is three to five times the charge for CTC. Even when OC and CTC costs are assumed to be similar, CTC has been shown to be a more cost-effective option for primary screening.[23] When un-suspected extracolonic findings such as aneurysms and other cancers are considered, CTC screening appears to dominate OC, being both more clinically efficacious and cost effective.[24]

Beyond complications and cost issues, there are a number of other limitations to OC screening. Postprocedural recovery time and a chaperone for transportation are required, even for negative cases. A number of surveys indicate that many adults would prefer less invasive screening options.[25-28] Bowel preparation is required, which is a barrier for all the structural examinations. The OC miss rate for large adenomas and CRC is often overlooked but has been shown to be about 12% and 5%, respectively.[29-32] Formal quality assurance programs for OC do not exist, and the current reimbursement system does not reward careful examination or prevent premature follow-up studies.[33] Inappropriate use of surveillance OC following polypectomy has been well documented,[33,34] leading to further refinements in postpolypectomy follow-up recommendations.[35] Revised guideline recommendations continue to expand the interval between follow-up OC examinations in patients with low-risk adenomas.

The appropriate interval between negative OC screening examinations is uncertain because of lack of long-term follow-up data. Currently, a 10-year interval is considered an acceptable option for average-risk adults beginning at age 50 years. Providing adults with a choice between primary OC and primary CTC screening has the potential to substantially increase compliance and affect CRC incidence and mortality because personal preferences usually will favor one test over the other.

Double Contrast Barium Enema

The double contrast barium enema, also referred to as an air-contrast barium enema, evaluates the entire colon by coating the mucosal surface with high-density barium and distending the lumen with air introduced through a flexible rectal catheter. Multiple spot radiographs are then acquired during fluoroscopic evaluation, followed by overhead conventional radiographs. Again, complete bowel preparation is essential for an optimal examination. Sedation is not used, and the procedure typically lasts about 20 to 40 minutes. Patients generally experience mild to moderate discomfort during and after the procedure. The DCBE was first adopted as a recognized CRC screening option by the ACS in 1997 and continues to be included on the recently updated guidelines.[1] The DCBE was designated as a covered Medicare benefit in 1997.

There have been no randomized controlled or case control trials evaluating the efficacy of DCBE as a primary screening modality. Unfortunately, the existing studies that have attempted to evaluate DCBE performance have been severely limited by study design and are predominantly retrospective in nature.[36,37] Most studies evaluating cancer detection by DCBE have shown a high sensitivity, generally 85% or greater.[31,38-41] DCBE performance for polyp detection is less established. Studies involving asymptomatic individuals with a history of prior adenoma removal have demonstrated a sensitivity of approximately 50% for large adenomas.[42,43]

Potential benefits of DCBE screening are that it is relatively safe, provides full structural evaluation of the colon, and generally detects the majority of significant colorectal neoplasms. Bowel perforation is a rare event, with a rate of about 1 in 25,000 cases.[44] As with CTC, DCBE has proved useful for patients in whom OC is either incomplete or contraindicated. Limitations of DCBE include the prep requirement, periprocedural discomfort, and lack of therapeutic capability. As with CTC, detected polyps ≥6 mm in size should be considered for OC referral. Additional limitations of DCBE include the operator dependence, labor-intensive nature, low reimbursement rate, and declining expertise as a result of decreased volumes and lack of proper training. Although DCBE (every 5 years) remains an acceptable option for primary screening in places where CTC and other screening resources are limited, it is unlikely to continue as a viable option for much longer.

Computed Tomography Colonography

Discussion of CT colonography (CTC) will be kept brief herein because the technique, performance characteristics, limitations, benefits, and cost issues are covered extensively elsewhere throughout this book. According to the recent guideline recommendations, CTC (every 5 years) is now recognized as an acceptable screening option by the ACS, the ACR, and the major GI societies.[1] In our experience at the University of Wisconsin, CTC has proved to be a better, faster, safer, and cheaper primary CRC screening tool compared with OC.[19,45] At the very least, CTC has proved beyond any reasonable doubt that it belongs on the list of front-line recommended screening options. Now that CTC screening has been clinically validated, the challenges that remain relate more to the practical issues of widespread implementation. Currently, the single greatest barrier for CTC screening is the lack of third-party reimbursement at the national level. Assuming that insurance coverage is secured in the relatively near future, another major challenge that remains relates to adequate training of enough radiologists. A number of dedicated CTC training programs exist, but an increased capacity for training even larger numbers of radiologists will be needed. With regard to multidetector CT (MDCT) capacity, it appears that this may not be a major issue.[46] Alongside existing parallel OC screening, the institution of CTC screening will provide a highly complementary test that can substantially increase compliance for CRC screening.[19,45] If

executed properly, this symbiotic relationship has the potential to render CRC a minor contributor to cancer-related deaths.

SCREENING TESTS THAT PRIMARILY DETECT CANCER

Some patients will be reluctant, unable, or unfit to undergo some of the structural colorectal examinations described earlier as an initial screening test. Common barriers to the structural examinations include the need for bowel preparation, increased invasiveness, and inability to perform the test at home. In comparison, collection of fecal samples for blood or DNA testing can be performed at home, without bowel preparation or the potential for complications. However, providers and patients need to be aware of the limitations that these noninvasive stool tests all have in common. First, these tests generally do not provide for adequate CRC prevention because they are insensitive for benign adenomas. Although the revised ACS guidelines include some of these fecal tests as acceptable screening options (Table 5-1), the preference for structural tests that are capable of cancer prevention through detection and removal of advanced adenomas is repeatedly emphasized. In addition, these fecal tests must be repeated at more frequent intervals. If the test is positive, OC will then be indicated, so the patient must be potentially willing or able to undergo this more invasive test. If the patient is either not willing to undergo fecal testing at regular intervals or is not willing to undergo subsequent OC, these noninvasive fecal-based tests should not be performed.

Stool-based screening tests are designed to detect either occult blood or DNA alterations that suggest cancer development. The fecal occult blood tests include guaiac-based tests (gFOBT) and fecal immunohistochemical tests (FIT). FIT processing generally requires being sent off to a clinical laboratory, whereas gFOBT can be processed in either the physician's office or a clinical laboratory. Blood in the stool is a nonspecific finding but may originate from CRC or even some large adenomatous polyps. However, most benign polyps do not bleed, and bleeding from more advanced neoplasia may be intermittent, which may require repeated testing. A positive gFOBT or FIT result generally requires diagnostic workup with OC to evaluate for the possibility of CRC. There are many other causes of blood in the stool beyond colorectal neoplasia.

Guaiac-Based Fecal Occult Blood Tests

gFOBT is the most common stool blood test in use for CRC screening and is the only one for which there is direct evidence of efficacy. Three large, prospective randomized controlled trials have demonstrated significant reductions in CRC mortality of 15% to 33%.[47-49] However, a number of factors regarding specimen collection and handling can affect the accuracy of gFOBT; they are beyond the scope of this chapter but are described elsewhere.[1] The reported sensitivity of a single application of gFOBT for CRC has varied from as low as 9% to as high as 79.4%.[50-53] Specificity for CRC has ranged from 86.7% to 97.7%. Therefore, collection of three samples is important because test sensitivity improves with each additional stool sample.[54] Program sensitivity, which represents the outcome of repeat annual testing, is considerably higher than one-time application, but the systems to ensure regular testing often are not in place. The current ACS guidelines include annual screening with gFOBT as an acceptable option but stress that only versions with a proven high sensitivity for CRC (e.g., Hemoccult SENSA) should be used. Any positive test should be followed up with OC. Screening with gFOBT in the office setting following digital rectal examination is not recommended.

Fecal Immunochemical Tests

FIT for occult blood became commercially available in the United States in the 1980s, but implementation was slowed by its higher costs compared with gFOBT. However, recent increases in Medicare reimbursement have led to wider use of FIT.[53] FIT is more specific than gFOBT for human blood and has a number of other technical advantages over gFOBT, which are beyond the scope of this chapter.[1] In addition, sample collection for some variants of FIT are less demanding than gFOBT. The diagnostic accuracy of FITs has been evaluated in comparison with high-sensitivity gFOBT. Based on data from six separate studies, the ACS guidelines concluded that neither test is clearly superior to the other.[1] No FIT has been tested in a randomized controlled trial with an end point of reduction in CRC mortality. The benefits and limitations of FIT are similar to that for gFOBT. As with high-sensitivity gFOBT, the ACS guidelines include annual screening with FIT as an acceptable CRC screening option, with the same caveats that apply to gFOBT.

Stool DNA Tests

Stool DNA (sDNA) testing applies the knowledge gained from studying DNA alterations in the adenoma–carcinoma sequence of colorectal carcinogenesis. This relatively new method of CRC screening shows some promise but requires much additional research before possibly reaching its full potential. This testing method relies on the notion that neoplastic cells in colorectal tumors that contain altered DNA are continuously shed into the lumen and passed in feces. Because no single gene mutation is ubiquitous in all colorectal neoplasms, a multitarget stool assay is required to achieve adequate sensitivity. Most of the published evidence to date in-volves the PreGen-Plus assay (version 1.0), which consists of a multiple marker panel that searches for point mutations in the K-ras oncogene, contains a probe for BAT-26 (a marker of microsatellite instability), and a marker for DNA integrity assay (DIA). Version 1.1 of this assay, which is commercially available, includes this same marker panel but incorporates several technical advances related to processing and specimen preservation.[1] Unlike the gFOBT and FIT, this sDNA test generally requires the entire stool sample. Specialized kits have been designed to make specimen collection and mailing a more straightforward process.

A number of studies have been published on the sensitivity and specificity of stool DNA testing for CRC.[1] Test sensitivity for CRC in these studies has ranged from 52% to 91%, with specificity ranging from 93% to 97%. Lower sensitivity in some of these studies has been attributed to a number of specimen handling issues, which presumably will be addressed by subsequent version of the tests. Using version 1.0 of the PreGen-Plus assay, detection of advanced adenomas, the primary target for CRC screening and prevention, was only 15% in one large study of more than 2507 average-risk adults.[52] Sensitivity for CRC detection in this study was 52%, compared with only 13% for the nonrehydrated Hemoccult II FOBT. Newer-version assays with better DNA stabilization and simplified genetic analyses may be more sensitive than version 1.0 for advanced adenoma detection but currently still fall short of the structural screening tests.[55,56] As such, there is room for improvement to clearly distinguish sDNA from current high-sensitivity gFOBT and FIT, which all fall well short of CRC prevention and merely serve to detect CRC. Furthermore, the implications of a positive sDNA test result followed by a negative structural examination are unknown but may require more frequent followup and cause significant anxiety in patients. Based on the recent accumulation of evidence, the ACS guidelines concluded that sDNA is an acceptable option for CRC screening but that the interval between negative examinations is currently uncertain.

SUMMARY

The cumulative evidence in support of screening average-risk individuals older than 50 years of age for the purposes of detecting and preventing CRC is compelling. A number of screening options are acceptable, some of which can both detect and prevent CRC and others that primarily just detect CRC. Testing options that provide CRC prevention through detection of advanced adenomas need to be emphasized to reap the greatest benefit. No CRC screening test is perfect, and each option has certain advantages and disadvantages. In our opinion, full structural examination by either virtual or optical colonoscopy represents the two best options for the general screening population. However, in the end, the best test for a given individual is the one that is done well *and* that he or she is actually willing to undergo. Issues of patient preference, quality assurance, and cost effectiveness were not covered in depth in this chapter but are obviously important considerations. Better definition of the optimal target lesion is needed, but this will likely differ among the various testing options. Ongoing natural history studies will help to refine the optimal target lesion, particularly for CTC. The very fact that CRC remains the second-leading cause of cancer deaths in the United States, despite being largely preventable, shows just how far we have to go in promoting CRC screening.

REFERENCES

1. Levin B, Lieberman DA, McFarland B, et al. Screening and surveillance for the early detection of colorectal cancer and adenomatous polyps, 2008: A joint guideline from the American Cancer Society, the US Multi-Society Task Force on Colorectal Cancer, and the American College of Radiology. *CA Cancer J Clin.* 2008;58(3):130-160.

2. Levin TR, Farraye FA, Schoen RE, et al. Quality in the technical performance of screening flexible sigmoidoscopy: Recommendations of an international multi-society task group. *Gut.* 2005;54(6):807-813.

3. Newcomb PA, Norfleet RG, Storer BE, Surawicz TS, Marcus PM. Screening sigmoidoscopy and colorectal-cancer mortality. *J Natl Cancer Inst.* 1992;84(20):1572-1575.

4. Selby JV, Friedman GD, Quesenberry CP, Weiss NS. A case control study of screening sigmoidoscopy and mortality from colorectal cancer. *N Engl J Med.* 1992;326(10):653-657.

5. Thiis-Evensen E, Hoff GS, Sauar J, Langmark F, Majak BM, Vatn MH. Population-based surveillance by colonoscopy: Effect on the incidence of colorectal cancer—Telemark Polyp Study I. *Scand J Gastroenterol.* 1999;34(4):414-420.

6. Newcomb PA, Storer BE, Morimoto LM, Templeton A, Potter JD. Long-term efficacy of sigmoidoscopy in the reduction of colorectal cancer incidence. *J Natl Cancer Inst.* 2003;95(8):622-625.

7. Imperiale TF, Wagner DR, Lin CY, Larkin GN, Rogge JD, Ransohoff DF. Risk of advanced proximal neoplasms in asymptomatic adults according to the distal colorectal findings. *N Engl J Med.* 2000;343 (3):169-174.

8. Lieberman DA, Weiss DG, Bond JH, et al. Use of colonoscopy to screen asymptomatic adults for colorectal cancer. *N Engl J Med.* 2000;343(3):162-168.

9. Bini EJ, Unger JS, Rieber JM, Rosenberg J, Trujillo K, Weinshel EH. Prospective, randomized, single-blind comparison of two preparations for screening flexible sigmoidoscopy. *Gastroenterol Endosc.* 2000;52(2):218-222.

10. Zubarik R, Ganguly E, Benway D, Ferrentino N, Moses P, Vecchio J. Procedure-related abdominal discomfort in patients undergoing colorectal comparison screening: A comparison of colonoscopy and flexible sigmoidoscopy. *Am J Gastroenterol.* 2002;97(12):3056-3061.

11. Atkin W, Rogers P, Cardwell C, et al. Wide variation in adenoma detection rates at screening flexible sigmoidoscopy. *Gastroenterology.* 2004;126(5):1247-1256.

12. Pinsky PF, Schoen RE, Weissfeld JL, et al. Variability in flexible sigmoidoscopy performance among examiners in a screening trial. *Clin Gastroenterol Hepatol.* 2005;3(8):792-797.

13. Schoen RE, Weissfeld JL, Pinsky PF, Riley T. Yield of advanced adenoma and cancer based on polyp size detected at screening flexible sigmoidoscopy. *Gastroenterology.* 2006;131(6):1683-1689.

14. Levin TR, Conell C, Shapiro JA, Chazan SG, Nadel MR, Selby JV. Complications of screening flexible sigmoidoscopy. *Gastroenterology.* 2002;123(6):1786-1792.

15. Levin TR, Zhao W, Conell C, et al. Complications of colonoscopy in an integrated health care delivery system. *Ann Intern Med.* 2006;145(12):880-886.

16. Seeff LC, Richards TB, Shapiro JA, et al. How many endoscopies are performed for colorectal cancer screening? Results from CDC's survey of endoscopic capacity. *Gastroenterology.* 2004;127(6):1670-1677.

17. Winawer SJ, Zauber AG, Ho MN, et al. Prevention of colorectal cancer by colonoscopic polypectomy. *N Engl J Med.* 1993;329(27): 1977-1981.

18. Iqbal CW, Cullinane DC, Schiller HJ, Sawyer MD, Zietlow SP, Farley DR. Surgical management and outcomes of 165 colonoscopic perforations from a single institution. *Arch Surg.* 2008;143(7):701-706.

19. Kim DH, Pickhardt PJ, Taylor AJ, et al. CT colonography versus colonoscopy for the detection of advanced neoplasia. *N Engl J Med.* 2007;357(14):1403-1412.

20. Gatto NM, Frucht H, Sundararajan V, Jacobson JS, Grann VR, Neugut AI. Risk of perforation after colonoscopy and sigmoidoscopy: A population-based study. *J Natl Cancer Inst.* 2003;95(3):230-236.

21. Rex DK, Bond JH, Winawer S, et al. Quality in the technical performance of colonoscopy and the continuous quality improvement process for colonoscopy: Recommendations of the US Multi-Society Task Force on Colorectal Cancer. *Am J Gastroenterol.* 2002;97(6):1296-1308.

22. Kim DH, Pickhardt PJ, Taylor AJ, Menias CO. Imaging evaluation of complications at optical colonoscopy. *Curr Probl Diagn Radiol.* 2008;37(4):165-177.

23. Pickhardt PJ, Hassan C, Laghi A, Zullo A, Kim DH, Morini S. Cost-effectiveness of colorectal cancer screening with computed tomography colonography—The impact of not reporting diminutive lesions. *Cancer.* 2007;109(11):2213-2221.

24. Hassan C, Pickhardt P, Laghi A, et al. Computed tomographic colonography to screen for colorectal cancer, extracolonic cancer, and aortic aneurysm. *Arch Intern Med.* 2008;168(7):696-705.

25. Leard LE, Savides TJ, Ganiats TG. Patient preferences for colorectal cancer screening. *J Fam Pract.* 1997;45(3):211-228.

26. Ling BS, Moskowitz MA, Wachs D, Pearson B, Schroy PC. Attitudes toward colorectal cancer screening tests—A survey of patients and physicians. *J Gen Intern Med.* 2001;16(12):822-830.

27. Schroy PC, Lal S, Glick JT, Robinson PA, Zamor P, Heeren TC. Patient preferences for colorectal cancer screening: How does stool DNA testing fare? *Am J Manag Care.* 2007;13(7):393-400.

28. Gluecker TM, Johnson CD, Harmsen WS, et al. Colorectal cancer screening with CT colonography, colonoscopy, and double-contrast barium enema examination: Prospective assessment of patient perceptions and preferences. *Radiology.* 2003;227(2):378-384.

29. Bressler B, Paszat LF, Vinden C, Li C, He JS, Rabeneck L. Colonoscopic miss rates for right-sided colon cancer: A population-based analysis. *Gastroenterology.* 2004;127(2):452-456.

30. Pickhardt PJ, Nugent PA, Mysliwiec PA, Choi JR, Schindler WR. Location of adenomas missed by optical colonoscopy. *Ann Intern Med.* 2004;141(5):352-359.

31. Rex DK, Rahmani EY, Haseman JH, Lemmel GT, Kaster S, Buckley JS. Relative sensitivity of colonoscopy and barium enema for detection of colorectal cancer in clinical practice. *Gastroenterology.* 1997;112(1):17-23.

32. Heresbach D, Barrioz T, Lapalus MG, et al. Miss rate for colorectal neoplastic polyps: A prospective multicenter study of back-to-back video colonoscopies. *Endoscopy.* 2008;40(4):284-290.

33. Mysliwiec PA, Brown ML, Klabunde CN, Ransohoff DF. Are physicians doing too much colonoscopy? A national survey of colorectal surveillance after polypectomy. *Ann Intern Med.* 2004;141(4):264-271.

34. Boolchand V, Olds G, Singh J, Singh P, Chak A, Cooper GS. Colorectal screening after polypectomy: A national survey study of primary care physicians. *Ann Intern Med.* 2006;145(9):654-659.

35. Winawer SJ, Zauber AG, Fletcher RH, et al. Guidelines for colonoscopy surveillance after polypectomy: A consensus update by the US Multi-Society Task Force on Colorectal Cancer and the American Cancer Society. *Gastroenterology.* 2006;130(6):1872-1885.

36. Glick S. Opinion—Double-contrast barium enema for colorectal cancer screening: A review of the issues and a comparison with other screening alternatives. *Am J Roentgenol.* 2000;174(6):1529-1537.

37. De Zwart IM, Griffioen G, Shaw MPC, Lamers C, De Roos A. Barium enema and endoscopy for the detection of colorectal neoplasia: Sensitivity, specificity, complications and its determinants. *Clin Radiol.* 2001;56(5):401-409.

38. Tawn DJ, Squire CJ, Mohammed MA, Adam EJ. National audit of the sensitivity of double-contrast barium enema for colorectal carcinoma, using control charts—For the Royal College of Radiologists Clinical Radiology Audit Sub-Committee. *Clin Radiol.* 2005;60(5):558-564.

39. Johnson CD, Carlson HC, Taylor WF, Weiland LP. Barium enemas of carcinoma of the colon—Sensitivity of double-contrast and single-contrast studies. *Am J Roentgenol.* 1983;140(6):1143-1149.

40. Fork FT, Lindstrom C, Ekelund G. Double contrast examination in carcinoma of the colon and rectum—A prospective clinical-series. *Acta Radiologica Diagn.* 1983;24(3):177-188.

41. Kelvin FM, Gardiner R, Vas W, Stevenson GW. Colorectal carcinoma missed on double contrast barium enema study—A problem in perception. *Am J Roentgenol.* 1981;137(2):307-313.

42. Winawer SJ, Stewart ET, Zauber AG, et al. A comparison of colonoscopy and double-contrast barium enema for surveillance after polypectomy. *N Engl J Med.* 2000;342(24):1766-1772.

43. Williams CB, Macrae FA, Bartram CI. A prospective-study of diagnostic methods in adenoma follow-up. *Endoscopy.* 1982;14(3):74-78.

44. Blakeborough A, Sheridan MB, Chapman AH. Complications of barium enema examinations: A survey of UK consultant radiologists 1992 to 1994. *Clin Radiol.* 1997;52(2):142-148.

45. Pickhardt PJ, Taylor AJ, Kim DH, Reichelderfer M, Gopal DV, Pfau PR. Screening for colorectal neoplasia with CT colonography: Initial experience from the 1st year of coverage by third-party payers. *Radiology.* 2006;241(2):417-425.

46. Pickhardt PJ, Hassan C, Laghi A, et al. Is there sufficient MDCT capacity to provide colorectal cancer screening with CT colonography for the US population? *Am J Roentgenol.* 2008;190(4):1044-1049.

47. Mandel JS, Church TR, Bond JH, et al. The effect of fecal occult-blood screening on the incidence of colorectal cancer. *N Engl J Med.* 2000;343(22):1603-1607.

48. Hardcastle JD, Chamberlain JO, Robinson MHE, et al. Randomised controlled trial of faecal-occult-blood screening for colorectal cancer. *Lancet.* 1996;348(9040):1472-1477.

49. Kronborg O, Fenger C, Olsen J, Jorgensen OD, Sondergaard O. Randomised study of screening for colorectal cancer with faecal-occult-blood test. *Lancet.* 1996;348(9040):1467-1471.

50. Allison JE, Sakoda LC, Levin TR, et al. Screening for colorectal neoplasms with new fecal occult blood tests: Update on performance characteristics. *J Natl Cancer Inst.* 2007;99:1462-1470.

51. Allison JE, Tekawa IS, Ransom LJ, Adrain AL. A comparison of fecal occult-blood tests for colorectal-cancer screening. *N Engl J Med.* 1996;334(3):155-159.

52. Imperiale TF, Ransohoff DF, Itzkowitz SH, Turnbull BA, Ross ME. Fecal DNA versus fecal occult blood for colorectal-cancer screening in an average-risk population. *N Engl J Med.* 2004;351(26):2704-2714.

53. Collins JF, Lieberman DA, Durbin TE, Weiss DG, Veterans Affairs Cooperative Study #380 Group. Accuracy of screening for fecal occult blood on a single stool sample obtained by digital rectal examination: A comparison with recommended sampling practice. *Ann Intern Med.* 2005;142(2):81-85.

54. Lieberman DA, Weiss DG, Bond JH, et al. Use of colonoscopy to screen asymptomatic adults for colorectal cancer. *N Engl J Med.* 2000;343(3):162-168.

55. Itzkowitz SH, Jandorf L, Brand R, et al. Improved fecal DNA test for colorectal cancer screening. *Clin Gastroenterol Hepatol.* 2007;5(1):111-117.

56. Ahlquist DA, Sargent DJ, Loprinzi CL, et al. Stool DNA and occult blood testing for screen detection of colorectal neoplasia. *Ann Intern Med.* 2008;149(7):441-450, W81.

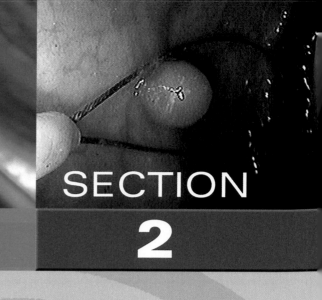

General Aspects of CT Colonography

CT Colonography: An Introduction and Historical Overview

PERRY J. PICKHARDT, MD

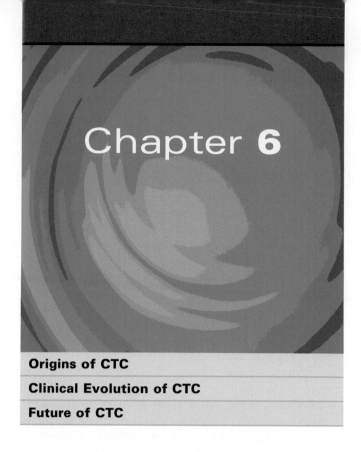

Chapter 6

Origins of CTC

Clinical Evolution of CTC

Future of CTC

INTRODUCTION

Computed tomography colonography (CTC), also referred to as virtual colonoscopy (VC), is a minimally invasive imaging examination of the large intestine. Simply put, CTC represents a modified CT examination in a patient who has undergone some form of bowel preparation and colonic distention, in which the images are then interpreted using advanced two-dimensional (2D) and three-dimensional (3D) display techniques. Since its introduction in the mid 1990s, there have been continuous advancements in both CTC technique and the advanced visualization software for interpretation. This chapter will review the origins of CTC as a natural extension of abdominal CT imaging; discuss the evolution of CTC through the clinical phases of feasibility, validation, and implementation; and briefly consider the future prospects for this examination.

ORIGINS OF CTC

Although Vining and Gelfand are appropriately credited as the first to demonstrate a 3D endoluminal fly-through of the colon using CT (i.e., "virtual colonoscopy") in 1994,[1] some of the basic groundwork for CTC technique was laid down earlier.[2] By the late 1980s, it was becoming clear that CT might be useful not only for evaluating patients with surgically proven colorectal carcinoma (CRC), but also potentially for preoperative assessment of CRC and perhaps even for patients with only suspected tumors.[2,3] The potential advantages for a cross-sectional imaging technique such as CT over the barium enema may now seem obvious in

retrospect. However, one must keep in mind that this was still the prehelical CT era, where conventional "step-and-shoot" studies took a considerable amount of time and typically generated 10-mm–thick sections. Nonetheless, in 1988, Balthazar et al. reported on the utility of a conventional CT technique that presaged subsequent CTC evaluation years later, including the use of both colonic air distention (pneumocolon) and positive oral contrast opacification.[2] In fact, this group showed that the sensitivity for detecting CRC was 95% when air distention was used, versus a sensitivity of 68% when no such attempts were made. The 95% sensitivity for CRC detection using colonic distention was similar to that reported in a meta-analysis for CTC nearly two decades later.[4] Overall, the barium enema actually outperformed CT for detecting CRC in this study, reflecting both the fluoroscopic expertise and nascent CT techniques in place at that time. Of course, this situation would not last much longer.

In revisiting the brief editorial by Vining on CTC published in *Radiology* in 1996,[5] he demonstrated impressive foresight in broaching the many potential hurdles and controversies facing this promising new examination. Included in his discussion were the topics of 2D versus 3D evaluation, colonic distention, oral contrast tagging, flat lesions, coding and reimbursement issues, standardized reporting, and appropriate clinical indications, all of which would indeed become core issues and many of which are in evolution today. By 1996 small clinical series using CTC technique began to appear.[6,7] The term "CT colography" was applied in some early works, but this term soon gave way to the more familiar terms of CT colonography and virtual colonoscopy, which both remain widely in use today.

The introduction of spiral CT in the early 1990s provided for more rapid image acquisition and volumetric data, which made detection of colorectal polyps and invasive CRC masses a feasible task. Multidetector CT (MDCT) soon allowed for even greater coverage and thinner sections within a single breath hold, which further improved the ability to render and detect polyps.[8] Once the four detector-row scanners were available, CTC imaging protocols were adopted that remain diagnostically adequate to this day.[9,10] At this point, MDCT scanner capability was no longer a major focus for continued CTC improvements, although some incremental gains were still apparent up to 16 detector-row scanners.

With the rapidly advancing MDCT technology that promptly met and surpassed the relatively forgiving imaging needs of CTC, the obvious weak link in the chain for performing time-efficient 3D endoluminal VC was the processing speed and ability of the computer software programs. By report, more than 8 hours of processing time was required to generate the first 3D endoluminal VC fly-through.[11] Although expected improvements in computer processing performance no doubt followed, the initial concept of "virtual colonoscopy" as a simulated virtual-reality colonoscopic examination gave way to a primary 2D evaluation, which is more properly termed "CT colonography" and not at all deserving of the VC moniker. As such, most CTC software platforms were initially based on a primary 2D paradigm and it would be nearly a decade before primary 3D evaluation began to make a mainstream return. Even Vining himself seemed resigned to a 2D approach, stating in a 2005 publication that "most practitioners of VC today agree that 2D review of CT images at a workstation is sufficient for lesion detection and that 3D imaging can be reserved for problem solving."[11] This ingrained 2D sentiment was also evident in a survey of 25 leading CTC experts that was published in the *American Journal of Roentgenology* in 2005,[12] where only one respondent felt that primary 3D review was necessary (more on this individual in the next section).

CLINICAL EVOLUTION OF CTC

Once the basic tenets of CTC were established and the various components of the examination were available, the next logical step was to begin clinical evaluation of this new diagnostic tool. We will consider the evolution of screening CTC in three sequential phases: a "feasibility phase" where early testing in high-prevalence cohorts provided the necessary proof of concept; a "validation phase," where testing in low-prevalence cohorts sought to prove its value for screening; and an "implementation phase," where proven techniques were applied in the clinical realm beyond the artificial setting of a clinical trial. In terms of testing, one fact that has repeatedly and unavoidably penalized CTC assessment is that optical colonoscopy (OC) is far from an infallible reference standard.[13] Even when painstaking steps are instituted to ameliorate the situation, particularly through the use of segmental unblinding of CTC findings at OC, there will still be problems with lesion matching. The most notable discrepancies are the OC false-negative results that are incorrectly registered as CTC false-positive results. Poor localization of OC findings can also lead to a CTC true positive finding being incorrectly labeled as both a CTC false-negative and false-positive result. Even more bias and uncertainty may be introduced if the endoscopist is either not blinded to the CTC results or if the CTC results are never revealed. Therefore, it is useful to remember that clinical trials using an OC reference standard will generally underestimate CTC accuracy. In addition, clinical validation trials that do not use segmental unblinding unfortunately position OC as the sole but fallible reference standard.[14]

Feasibility Phase

Beyond the earliest clinical reports on CTC performance noted previously, a number of single-center CTC trials were published between 1997 and mid-2003 that ranged in size from about 50 to 300 patients.[8,15-23] Common themes among nearly all of these trials were that polyp-rich high-risk and/or symptomatic cohorts were evaluated, single-detector MDCT was generally used, oral contrast tagging was rarely applied, a primary 2D polyp search was used, and segmental unblinding of CTC findings at OC was generally not used. Nonetheless, these early clinical trials provided the necessary proof of concept that CTC was a feasible technique and could detect large colorectal polyps with reasonably good sensitivity (70%-100%) and specificity (90%-100%). Noteworthy high-profile publications among this group include a study involving 100 subjects by Fenlon et al. in *The New England Journal of Medicine* in 1999 and a study involving 300 subjects by Yee et al. in *Radiology* in 2001.[15,20] Also during this time period, several clinical studies demonstrated the utility of CTC following incomplete OC,[24-27] which was important because this became the first widely accepted clinical indication for diagnostic CTC. With regard to screening CTC, however, the battle was still far from over.

Validation Phase

Once the feasibility trials in high-prevalence cohorts had demonstrated the necessary proof of concept to move forward, the next step was to assess the performance characteristics of CTC in a low-prevalence setting, preferably a true asymptomatic screening cohort. Although CTC occupies several useful niches for various diagnostic indications, the true "holy grail" for clinical CTC is asymptomatic screening. However, because significant polyps at screening are somewhat akin to a "needle in a haystack" of normal findings, the screening population represents a most difficult challenge. It should not really come as any surprise that there were more than a few bumps along the road to validation for screening CTC. The initial attempts in larger cohorts were not true asymptomatic average-risk adults but supposedly represented "the next best thing": relatively low-prevalence cohorts. However, the specific reason for having a low prevalence of polyps in a given study population turns out to be an important factor.

Using 500 subjects as an arbitrary threshold for a "large" study cohort, the first large low-prevalence CTC trial was published in late 2003 by Johnson et al. from the Mayo Clinic, evaluating a high-risk cohort of 703 adults.[28] Like the feasibility studies before it, this single-center trial used primary 2D for polyp detection and did not use oral contrast tagging or segmental unblinding. It is important to note that the reason that this high-risk cohort had a low prevalence of disease (5% of subjects had large polyps) was primarily because three fourths of patients were undergoing postpolypectomy surveillance, a fact that often goes unnoticed. However, this is an important distinction because polyps that were either missed at initial OC, or were partially resected and regrew, would presumably be harder to detect than a first-time evaluation.[29] A technical limitation in the trial by Johnson et al. was the use of an arbitrary low-volume cutoff of carbon dioxide for initial scanning, without active replacement, which likely lead to suboptimal distention in many cases. After all of these factors are taken into account, it is little wonder that the pooled sensitivity for large polyps was less than 50%. Specificity was generally greater than 95%, but this is of little consolation with such a low sensitivity. Clearly, there was room for improvement.

The next two large CTC trials evaluating low-prevalence cohorts were multicenter efforts led by two well-intentioned gastroenterologists, Drs. Cotton and Rockey, involving 600 and 614 subjects, respectively.[30,31] As with the Mayo Clinic study, neither of these trials evaluated a true screening cohort, and both used a primary 2D polyp search without oral contrast tagging. Additional issues that likely had a negative impact on CTC performance in these trials included use of suboptimal CTC software, low numbers of cases per participating center, and lack of performance feedback for learning. It should be made clear that although the studies by Cotton et al.[30] and Rockey et al.[31] were published after the Department of Defense (DoD) trial by Pickhardt et al.,[10] both trials began well before the DoD trial and therefore should be placed earlier on the CTC timeline. The performance in these two CTC trials closely mirrored the disappointing findings of Johnson et al., with a by-

patient sensitivity for large polyps of 55% to 59% and a by-patient specificity of 96%. If these three studies (i.e., Johnson et al., Cotton et al., and Rockey et al.) had actually all been published in chronological order before the DoD trial, it is conceivable that the screening CTC movement would have been effectively dead in the water. Fortunately, that is not how things played out.

Before discussing the specific methodology and results of the DoD multicenter screening trial, a little more background may be helpful to set the stage. When I first became involved in CTC in 2001, I was serving as an active-duty medical officer at the National Naval Medical Center in Bethesda, MD. A potential opportunity for funding arose to conduct a clinical trial evaluating CTC in a true screening cohort. Up to that time, only high-risk and/or symptomatic cohorts had been evaluated, as discussed earlier. Quite frankly, as I surveyed the existing landscape at that time, I was doubtful that CTC would prove effective for screening. Like everyone else, I started out as a primary 2D reader and was pessimistic that this approach could achieve adequate sensitivity in a true screening cohort. Nonetheless, I was prepared to forge ahead and began to assess several CTC software systems that were available. Fortunately, this is where serendipity struck and, as is often the case with a chance medical discovery on a prepared individual,[32] changed the future course of CTC screening. As I evaluated a variety of CTC software systems, it became clear that one system, from a small company I had not heard of previously—Viatronix—was fundamentally different in its ability for 3D polyp detection.[33] Not only was the volume rendering superior to the other systems available at the time (Fig. 6-1), but, more importantly, the navigational ease of the Viatronix V3D system allowed for an effective and time-efficient primary 3D evaluation.[33,34] Polyps that were missed on the usual primary 2D evaluation were generally obvious on the 3D fly-through, eventually prompting my colleagues and me to favor the latter for initial lesion detection. The ultimate choice for which CTC software system to use in the DoD trial became patently obvious (of note, none of the investigators had any financial relationship with Viatronix before or during the trial). The rest, as they say, is history.

In addition to instituting a novel primary 3D approach to polyp detection, the DoD trial was also the first large study to use oral contrast tagging. In our opinion, these two innovations allowed us to succeed, even in the face of "training-related adversity." Compared with the radiologists involved in the subsequent American College of Radiology Imaging Network (ACRIN) CTC trial, the radiologists involved in the DoD trial were woefully undertrained and inexperienced. We had no formal training and no set of proven cases to practice with, and some of us had read only 25 or fewer studies prior to commencing the trial. According to the "steep learning curve" theory for CTC training, we had

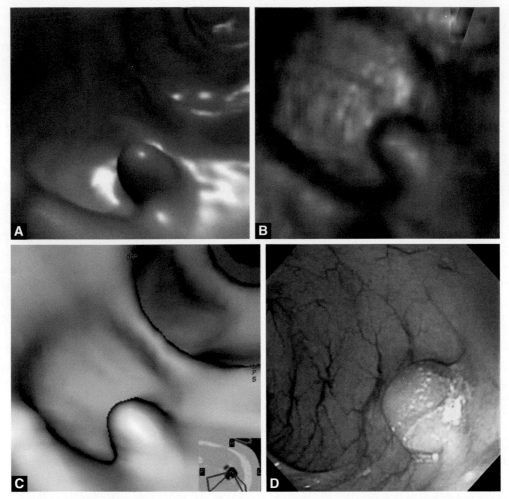

Figure 6-1 **Comparison of the quality of 3D endoluminal volume rendering on different CTC software systems around the time of initiation of the Department of Defense screening trial.** Matched 3D endoluminal displays using the same dataset show an 8-mm tubular adenoma on Viatronix V3D, version 1.2 **(A)**; Vital Images Vitrea 2, version 3.1 **(B)**; and General Electric Navigator, Advantage Workstation, version 4.0 **(C)**. Although substantial differences in volumetric rendering are apparent, even bigger differences in navigational abilities were present, which made effective and time-efficient primary 3D evaluation feasible only with the Viatronix V3D system. The endoscopic appearance of the polyp is shown in **D.** (From Pickhardt PJ. Three-dimensional endoluminal CT colonography (virtual colonoscopy): Comparison of three commercially available systems. *Am J Roentgenol.* 2003;181:1599-1606.)

every reason to fail. Fortunately, our chosen methodology and software prevented that from happening. Even with stringent inclusion and exclusion criteria to ensure an asymptomatic, predominately average-risk screening cohort, we still managed to achieve a 94% by-patient sensitivity for large adenomas, with a reasonable specificity of 96%.[10] Through the use of segmental unblinding, we were able to show that the miss rate for large adenomas was higher for the purported "gold standard" (OC) than for CTC. At the 6-mm threshold, the by-patient CTC sensitivity for adenomas was a respectable 89%, but specificity suffered at 80%. As discussed later, technical improvements in the years since the DoD trial have greatly improved CTC performance down to the 6-mm threshold. To apply the final blow to primary 2D evaluation for screen detection of polyps, we later showed that the 2D sensitivity of trained experts reading the naval subset of CTC cases from the DoD trial closely resembled the 2D polyp detection performance from the Cotton and Rockey trials.[35]

With the publication of the DoD trial in December 2003, our methodology for CTC screening with the Viatronix V3D system was clinically validated, leading to the first Food and Drug Administration approval of any such device for the purpose of screening. At this point, the other CTC systems and methodologies had either failed or remained largely unproven in the screening realm. More recently, however, other CTC studies and clinical experiences have provided additional and broader validation for screening.[14,36,37] The reasonably good sensitivity achieved in the ACRIN trial may help to validate the predominate CTC system used (Vital Image's Vitrea), but the low specificity and positive predictive value have raised some concerns.[14]

Implementation Phase

With a proven and published CTC screening methodology in hand,[10] I left the Navy in late 2003 and headed back home to Madison, WI, intent on implementing this newly validated screening tool at the University of Wisconsin. In February 2004 I met with the medical directors of the major local medical care organizations. After making the case for why screening CTC (with our proven methodology) deserved to be a covered benefit for patients under their plan as much as OC did, the medical director of one forward-thinking organization (Physician's Plus Insurance Corporation [PPIC]) saw the light. It is interesting that less than 1 day after the news hit that PPIC was to be the first third-party payer in the United States to reimburse for CTC screening, the other major payers at the meeting immediately acquiesced in a domino-like fashion. In April 2004 the CTC program at the University of Wisconsin embarked on the first reimbursed screening program, thus initiating the implementation phase. Of course, small-scale but much more diffuse implementation of diagnostic CTC, predominately for incomplete OC, was occurring simultaneously throughout the world. Incomplete OC and other diagnostic indications represent an important component of CTC practice but make up a relatively small percentage of the total volume once screening is instituted. Therefore, the evolution of screening CTC is emphasized herein.

The clinical results to date of the University of Wisconsin CTC program are detailed in Chapter 30. The results for our screening program have remained remarkably stable year by year through the initial 5,000 CTC subjects, although several staff radiologists have been added to the rotation and many more body-imaging fellows have cycled through the program.[38,39] The overall test positive rate at the 6-mm and 10-mm polyp size thresholds have held steady at about 13% and 5%, respectively. Early on, we noticed that the positive predictive value for CTC abnormalities, which we prefer to call the concordance rate between CTC and OC, was much higher than that seen in the DoD screening trial. More than 90% of the time, a correlate was found at OC for lesions called at CTC, compared with a positive predictive value of less than 60% in the DoD trial. In comparison, the positive predictive value for adenomas in the ACRIN trial was only 23% at the 10-mm threshold. Our results were gratifying and almost certainly related to the notable improvements in technique, including the preparation, distention, and CTC software. However, unlike the artificial trial setting, only positive CTC cases are considered for OC referral. Therefore, one could raise the question of whether we were simply calling only obvious lesions and perhaps missing more subtle ones to achieve such a high CTC–OC concordance rate. This question was the impetus behind the work that lead to our second CTC paper in *The New England Journal of Medicine*,[38] which was published in 2007 and is discussed in the next paragraph.

Because we have had parallel CTC and OC screening programs in place at the University of Wisconsin since 2004, we had a unique opportunity to compare the diagnostic yield of each method. We compared the results from more than 6000 individuals who either underwent primary CTC screening (n = 3120) or primary OC screening (n = 3163). The two cohorts were drawn from the same general population and were closely matched in terms of age and gender mix. There was a slight increase in positive family history within the OC cohort. The primary outcome measure was the detection and removal of advanced neoplasia, which represents the primary target of colorectal prevention and screening. Although only 8% of individuals in the CTC arm underwent OC (compared with a 100% OC utilization rate in the OC arm), the same number of advanced neoplasms were detected and removed (123 for CTC, 121 for OC). The test positive rates for both CTC and OC were similar at the 6-mm (12.9% and 13.4%) and 10-mm (5.3% and 4.2%) thresholds, respectively. When diminutive lesions are considered a positive test result at OC, the positive rate increases to 37.6%, despite the fact that only 3 diminutive advanced adenomas were found in the OC arm. Overall, only 4 (0.2%) of 2006 diminutive polyps were advanced adenomas. No subcentimeter cancers were found in either arm. One striking finding in this study was the difference in CRC detection, with 14 cancers found at primary CTC but only 4 found at primary OC, which raises the concern for potential missed cancers at OC.[40] To demonstrate the efficiency of CTC screening compared with OC, only 561 total polyps were removed in the CTC arm, compared with 2434 polypectomies in the OC arm. Furthermore, 167 of 561 polyps removed in the CTC cohort were diminutive lesions incidental to the CTC-detected polyps. Finally, to demonstrate the safety of CTC relative to OC, there were no significant complications in the entire CTC cohort but seven perforations (0.2%) among the 3163 individuals undergoing primary OC screening, in addition to other complications. This study demonstrated that, in actual clinical practice, CTC screening is just as effective as primary OC screening (perhaps even more effective) but is also clearly more efficient and less risky.

Besides the CTC program at the University of Wisconsin, the only other medical centers routinely performing actual CTC screening beyond a clinical trial to any significant degree have been the military hospitals that were involved in the DoD trial—namely, the National Naval Medical Center in Bethesda, MD and the Walter Reed Army Medical Center in Washington, DC. In particular, the Bethesda Naval Hospital has demonstrated the success of their clinical screening program, in addition to ongoing research projects.[36] Included in their investigations is the ongoing collaboration with the University of Wisconsin that is focused on the natural history of small (6-9 mm) polyps (see Chapter 2). With more widespread third-party coverage for CTC screening, the number of centers performing this examination and the overall screening volume will no doubt increase. The rate at which such broad implementation for CTC screening occurs will depend on many inter-related factors. For practices that are considering instituting a CTC program, careful planning will avoid the many predictable pitfalls (see Chapters 8 and 20).[41,42]

FUTURE OF CTC

As of the time of this writing, the future of CTC for both diagnostic indications and asymptomatic screening appears bright. Compared with optical colonoscopy, CTC offers a less invasive, more cost-effective, and more clinically effective method for population screening. Assuming widespread reimbursement for CTC screening by third-party payers transpires in the near future, the volume of studies performed in the United States should increase exponentially. Additional issues that will continue to play out as the field matures include the natural history and management of small (6-9 mm) polyps, the role of computer-aided detection, proper management of extracolonic findings, patient acceptance and compliance issues, polyp volume assessment, time intervals for follow-up and postpolypectomy surveillance, CTC interpretation by nonradiologists, the emergence of competing novel colorectal screening tests, and so on. Future chapters explores these issues and more in greater detail.

REFERENCES

1. Vining DJ, Gelfand DW, Bechtold RE, Sharling ES, Grishaw EK, Shifrin RY. Technical feasibility of colon imaging with helical CT and virtual reality (abstr). *Am J Roentgenol.* 1994; 162:104.
2. Balthazar EJ, Megibow AJ, Hulnick D, Naidich DP. Carcinoma of the colon—Detection and preoperative staging by CT. *Am J Roentgenol.* 1988;150(2):301-306.
3. Balthazar EJ. CT of the gastrointestinal tract—Principles and interpretation. *Am J Roentgenol.* 1991;156(1):23-32.
4. Halligan S, Altman DG, Taylor SA, et al. CT colonography in the detection of colorectal polyps and cancer: Systematic review meta-analysis and proposed minimum data set for study level reporting. *Radiology.* 2006;238(3):893-904.
5. Vining DJ. Virtual endoscopy: Is it reality? *Radiology.* 1996;200(1):30-31.
6. Vining DJ, Teigen EL, Stelts D, Vanderwerken B, Kopecky KK, Rex D. Experience with virtual colonoscopy in 20 patients. *Radiology.* 1995;197:514.
7. Lees WR, Amin Z, Boulos P. Spiral CT pneumocolon for suspected colonic neoplasm: Is virtual colonoscopy helpful? *Radiology.* 1996;201:1047.
8. Hara AK, Johnson CD, MacCarty RL, Welch TJ, McCollough CH, Harmen WS. CT colonography: Single-versus multi-detector row imaging. *Radiology.* 2001;219(2):461-465.
9. Levin B, Lieberman DA, McFarland B, et al. Screening and surveillance for the early detection of colorectal cancer and adenomatous polyps, 2008: A joint guideline from the American Cancer Society, the US Multi-Society Task Force on Colorectal Cancer, and the American College of Radiology. *CA Cancer J Clin.* 2008;58(3):130-160.
10. Pickhardt PJ, Choi JR, Hwang I, et al. Computed tomographic virtual colonoscopy to screen for colorectal neoplasia in asymptomatic adults. *N Engl J Med.* 2003;349(23):2191-2200.
11. Vining DJ. Virtual colonoscopy: The inside story. In: Dachman A, ed. *Fundamentals of virtual colonoscopy.* New York: Springer; 2005:1-3.
12. Barish MA, Soto JA, Ferrucci JT. Consensus on current clinical practice of virtual colonoscopy. *Am J Roentgenol.* 2005;184(3):786-792.
13. Pickhardt PJ, Nugent PA, Mysliwiec PA, Choi JR, Schindler WR. Location of adenomas missed by optical colonoscopy. *Ann Intern Med.* 2004;141(5):352-359.
14. Johnson CD, Chen MH, Toledano AY, et al. Accuracy of CT colonography for detection of large adenomas and cancers. *N Engl J Med.* 2008;359(12):1207-1217.
15. Fenlon HM, Nunes DP, Schroy PC, Barish MA, Clarke PD, Ferrucci JT. A comparison of virtual and conventional colonoscopy for the detection of colorectal polyps. *N Engl J Med.* 1999;341(20):1496-1503.
16. Fletcher JG, Johnson CD, Welch TJ, et al. Optimization of CT colonography technique: Prospective trial in 180 patients. *Radiology.* 2000;216(3):704-711.
17. Hara AK, Johnson CD, Reed JE, et al. Detection of colorectal polyps with CT colography: Initial assessment of sensitivity and specificity. *Radiology.* 1997;205(1):59-65.
18. Morrin MM, Farrell RJ, Kruskal JB, Reynolds K, McGee JB, Raptopoulos V. Utility of intravenously administered contrast material at CT colonography. *Radiology.* 2000;217(3):765-771.
19. Pineau BC, Paskett ED, Chen GJ, et al. Virtual colonoscopy using oral contrast compared with colonoscopy for the detection of patients with colorectal polyps. *Gastroenterology.* 2003;125(2):304-310.
20. Yee J, Akerkar GA, Hung RK, Steinauer-Gebauer AM, Wall SD, McQuaid KR. Colorectal neoplasia: Performance characteristics of CT colonography for detection in 300 patients. *Radiology.* 2001;219(3):685-692.
21. Rex DK, Vining D, Kopecky KK. An initial experience with screening for colon polyps using spiral CT with and without CT colography (virtual colonoscopy). *Gastrointest Endosc.* 1999;50(3):309-313.
22. McFarland EG, Pilgram TK, Brink JA, et al. CT colonography: Multiobserver diagnostic performance. *Radiology.* 2002;225(2):380-390.
23. Lefere PA, Gryspeerdt SS, Dewyspelaere J, Baekelandt M, Van Holsbeeck BG. Dietary fecal tagging as a cleansing method before CT colonography: Initial results polyp detection and patient acceptance. *Radiology.* 2002;224(2):393-403.
24. Fenlon HM, McAneny DB, Nunes DP, Clarke PD, Ferrucci JT. Occlusive colon carcinoma: Virtual colonoscopy in the preoperative evaluation of the proximal colon. *Radiology.* 1999;210(2):423-428.
25. Macari M, Berman P, Dicker M, Milano A, Megibow AJ. Usefulness of CT colonography in patients with incomplete colonoscopy. *Am J Roentgenol.* 1999;173(3):561-564.
26. Morrin MM, Kruskal JB, Farrell RJ, Goldberg SN, McGee JB, Raptopoulos V. Endoluminal CT colonography after an incomplete endoscopic colonoscopy. *Am J Roentgenol.* 1999;172(4):913-918.
27. Neri E, Giusti P, Battolla L, et al. Colorectal cancer: Role of CT colonography in preoperative evaluation after incomplete colonoscopy. *Radiology.* 2002;223(3):615-619.

28. Johnson CD, Harmsen WS, Wilson LA, et al. Prospective blinded evaluation of computed tomographic colonography for screen detection of colorectal polyps. *Gastroenterology.* 2003;125(2):311-19.

29. MacCarty RL, Johnson CD, Fletcher JG, Wilson LA. Occult colorectal polyps on CT colonography: Implications for surveillance. *Am J Roentgenol.* 2006;186(5):1380-1383.

30. Cotton PB, Durkalski VL, Benoit PC, et al. Computed tomographic colonography (virtual colonoscopy)—A multicenter comparison with standard colonoscopy for detection of colorectal neoplasia. *JAMA.* 2004;291(14):1713-1719.

31. Rockey DC, Poulson E, Niedzwiecki D, et al. Analysis of air contrast barium enema, computed tomographic colonography, and colonoscopy: Prospective comparison. *Lancet.* 2005;365(9456):305-311.

32. Meyers MA. *Happy accidents: Serendipity in modern medical breakthroughs.* New York: Arcade Publishing; 2007.

33. Pickhardt PJ. Three-dimensional endoluminal CT colonography (virtual colonoscopy): Comparison of three commercially available systems. *Am J Roentgenol.* 2003;181(6):1599-1606.

34. Pickhardt PJ. Differential diagnosis of polypoid lesions seen at CT colonography (virtual colonoscopy)—Author's response. *Radiographics.* 2004;24(6):1558-1559.

35. Pickhardt PJ, Lee AD, Taylor AJ, et al. Primary 2D versus primary 3D polyp detection at screening CT colonography. *Am J Roentgenol.* 2007;189(6):1451-1456.

36. Cash BD, Kim C, Jensen D, et al. Accuracy of computed tomographic colonography for colorectal cancer screening in asymptomatic individuals. *Gastroenterology.* 2007;132(4):A92.

37. Graser A, Stieber P, Nagel D, et al. Comparison of CT colonography, colonoscopy, sigmoidoscopy and faecal occult blood tests for the detection of advanced adenoma in an average risk population. *Gut.* 2009;58(2):241-248.

38. Kim DH, Pickhardt PJ, Taylor AJ, et al. CT colonography versus colonoscopy for the detection of advanced neoplasia. *N Engl J Med.* 2007;357(14):1403-1412.

39. Pickhardt PJ, Taylor AJ, Kim DH, Reichelderfer M, Gopal DV, Pfau PR. Screening for colorectal neoplasia with CT colonography: Initial experience from the 1st year of coverage by third-party payers. *Radiology.* 2006;241(2):417-425.

40. Kim DH, Pickhardt PJ. CT colonography versus colonoscopy for the detection of advanced neoplasia—Reply. *N Engl J Med.* 2008;358(1):90.

41. Pickhardt PJ. Screening CT colonography: How I do it. *Am J Roentgenol.* 2007;189(2):290-298.

42. Pickhardt PJ, Taylor AJ, Johnson GL, et al. Building a CT colonography program: Necessary ingredients for reimbursement and clinical success. *Radiology.* 2005;235(1):17-20.

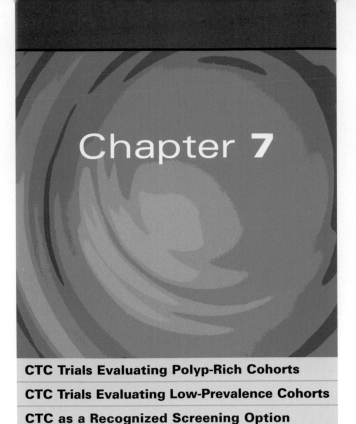

Chapter 7

Clinical Validation of CTC Performance

DAVID H. KIM, MD
PERRY J. PICKHARDT, MD

INTRODUCTION

CT colonography (CTC) has evolved from an experimental research tool with limited clinical application to a validated colorectal examination that is now poised for mainstream implementation. The road to widespread clinical acceptance, however, has not been entirely smooth, largely as a result of an unfortunate combination of poorly understood trial results and professional politics. In this chapter, we provide an overview of the performance results from the various CTC clinical trials. When faced with the task of critiquing these trials, one critical distinction that needs to be made up front is whether the study population represents an enriched high-prevalence cohort or a low-prevalence cohort. This distinction is particularly important if one is attempting to extrapolate the results to asymptomatic screening, for which only the results obtained from low-prevalence cohorts should be considered. The obvious tradeoff in study design is that low-prevalence trials generally require large study populations to include adequate numbers of positive cases. The smaller trials evaluating polyp-rich cohorts were nonetheless important as feasibility studies that provided the "proof of concept" for CTC.

CTC TRIALS EVALUATING POLYP-RICH COHORTS

In the years following the initial stunning display of nascent CTC technology at the Society of Gastrointestinal Radiology annual meeting in 1994, a handful of studies regarding CTC performance were published in the literature. They represented single institution experiences with CTC typically in polyp-enriched cohorts where there was increased risk for carcinoma.[1-5] They used the basic techniques for that time, including cathartic preparation without tagging agents, manual room air colonic distention, 3- to 5-mm collimation, and a primary two-dimensional (2D) interpretative approach. Despite the limitations from these older techniques, many studies demonstrated excellent polyp detection sensitivities, presumably related to the application of CTC in a polyp-rich setting. It is important to realize that performance in this situation can and does often result in artificially inflated sensitivities. However, these studies were a necessary and important step in demonstrating the feasibility of CTC in the detection of colorectal polyps. Two notable studies included the Boston University series by Fenlon et al. published in *The New England Journal of Medicine*[3] and the San Francisco Veterans Administration (VA) experience by Yee et al. published in *Radiology*.[4]

Fenlon and colleagues prospectively enrolled 100 high-risk individuals (60 men and 40 women) over a 2-year period. Patients underwent both CT colonography and optical colonoscopy (OC), with the latter serving as the reference standard where segmental unblinding was not used. At the 10-mm threshold, the sensitivity for polyps at CTC was 91% (20 of 22 polyps). The sensitivity decreased to 82% for small (6-9 mm) polyps and to 67% for diminutive polyps. All cancers (3 of 3) were detected at CTC. The results led investigators to conclude that CTC and conventional colonoscopy had a similar efficacy for the detection of polyps 6 mm or more in size for high-risk populations. On the heels of this study, Yee et al.[4] published positive results of a larger cohort of 300 patients. These were high-risk patients within the Veterans Administration system. Typical of a VA population, the cohort was largely male

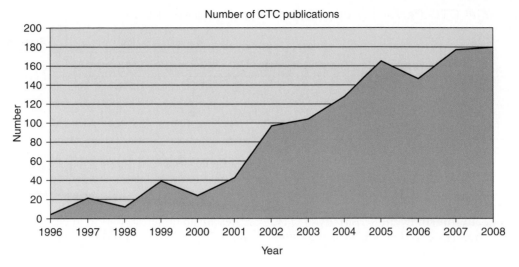

Figure 7-1   Graph of CTC publications over the last 12 years. Note the substantial increase in the number of publications beginning in the late 1990s. These studies have helped to advance the technique and interpretation of CTC.

(291 male, 9 female). All patients underwent both examinations where the CTC was performed 2 to 3 hours prior to colonoscopy. Segmental unblinding at colonoscopy was again not undertaken. At the 10-mm threshold, the sensitivity was 90% (74 of 82 polyps), which dropped to 80% for small polyps (6-9 mm). CTC detected all 8 carcinomas within this group. When examining polyps of adenomatous histology only, the sensitivity increased to 94% at the 10-mm size threshold and 82% for small polyps. This observation has been seen in other studies where the sensitivities of adenoma detection for a given size threshold are increased over polyps in general. The prevailing theory is that the pliable nature of hyperplastic and mucosal polyps allows flattening during colonic insufflation and thus decreases detection. The overall specificity in the Yee et al.[4] study was 72%. The results of these two studies conducted during the late 1990s and early 2000s helped to establish the feasibility of CTC as a viable modality to detect colorectal polyps, at least in polyp-rich cohorts.

Also during this time period, studies evaluating technical development and optimization were beginning to be published (Fig. 7-1). In the context of changing technique, an increasing number of studies demonstrated positive CTC performance (typically applied to higher-risk patient groups).[6-17] Unfortunately, the rapid advancement and maturation of CTC ultimately played a role in the conflicting results seen in the set of studies with large study populations (see later) evaluating CTC performance in low-prevalence cohorts as a result of these changing techniques.

CTC TRIALS EVALUATING LOW-PREVALENCE COHORTS

The Initial Four Studies

The promising results from the small series single institution experiences subsequently led to larger single and multiinstitution studies assessing CTC performance in low-prevalence and screening cohorts. Although these studies required larger patient numbers, the CTC performance results seen in these studies could more confidently be extrapolated. The pertinent question concerned the issue of whether the good performance of CTC seen in high polyp–prevalence cohorts be maintained in true screening situations of low polyp prevalence. Unfortunately, confusion regarding the disparate results in several trials, and professional politics, led to disagreements regarding the true performance capabilities of CT colonography. Four trials are commonly referenced from this early time period (Table 7-1).[18-21]

Three of the four studies demonstrated fairly poor sensitivities for CTC, even at the 10-mm threshold, suggesting that polyp detection performance was not adequate when applied in the screening setting. Johnson et al.[18] from the Mayo Clinic in Rochester enrolled 703 asymptomatic individuals in a prospective blinded trial where each participant underwent both CT colonography and optical colonoscopy. In this low polyp–prevalence trial (not a true screening cohort), the per-patient sensitivity for 10 mm or larger polyps was 64% at double reading, with a sensitivity range for individual readers of 35% to 72%. The sensitivity for small polyps was 65% at double reading with a range of 41% to 69% between the readers. The specificity was in a narrow range for large polyps between 97% and 98% for the readers and a somewhat wider range of 88% to 95% for small polyps. The second large series was a multiinstitution study conducted by Cotton et al.[19] Nine institutions enrolled 615 patients over an 18-month period comparing CTC with colonoscopy. The sensitivities at CTC were poor at 55% for 10-mm or greater lesions and 39% at the 6-mm threshold. The third study by Rockey et al.[20] involved a comparison between double contrast barium enema, CT colonography, and optical colonoscopy. Individuals (614) from several institutions underwent all

Table 7-1 ▫ Initial CTC Performance in Low Polyp–Prevalence Cohorts

Study	(n)	Interpretive approach	Tagging agents?	Sensitivity (%)*		Specificity (%)*	
				≥6 mm	≥10 mm	≥6 mm	≥10 mm
Johnson	703	2D	No	65†	64	86	95
Cotton	615	2D	No	39	55	91	96
Rockey	614	2D	No	55	59	89	96
Pickhardt	1233	3D > 2D	Yes	89‡	94‡	80	96

*Per patient calculation.
†Measure reflects a double read for polyps 5 to 9 mm in size rather than a 6-mm threshold.
‡Measure reflects adenomatous polyps.

three examinations. In this study, the sensitivity of CTC was 59% at the 10-mm threshold and 55% at the 6-mm threshold.

In contrast to these three studies, the Department of Defense (DoD) trial led by Pickhardt and colleagues demonstrated excellent performance results for CTC within a screening population.[21] This multiinstitutional study involved three sites (Bethesda Naval Hospital, Walter Reed Hospital, and San Diego Naval Hospital) and enrolled 1233 adults who received both CTC and same-day optical colonoscopy. The CTC protocol included a cathartic regimen that incorporated both stool and fluid tagging with low-density barium and iodine-based agents. Multidetector CT scanners were used with 1.25- to 2.5-mm collimation. A primary 3D interpretation algorithm was used. The sensitivity on a per-patient basis at the 10-mm threshold was 94% for adenomatous polyps, 94% at the 8-mm threshold, and 89% at the 6-mm threshold. In comparison, optical colonoscopy had a sensitivity of 88% at the 10-mm threshold, 92% at the 8-mm level, and 92% at the 6-mm level. CTC detected both cancers, whereas colonoscopy missed one. The authors concluded that CTC with a 3D polyp detection approach was an accurate screening method for average-risk adults and compared favorably with colonoscopy for the detection of clinically relevant lesions.

Some of these studies used an important design element not seen in previous trials. Segmental unblinding of the CTC results at colonoscopy was undertaken. Previously, colonoscopy had been used as the reference standard against which CTC was evaluated. Consequently, any polyp detected at CTC not seen at optical colonoscopy was scored as a CTC false-positive result. With segmental unblinding, once a segment was evaluated at colonoscopy, the results for that segment at CTC were revealed to the colonoscopist. If a polyp was reported at CTC but not seen at colonoscopy, the segment was reexamined for this potential polyp. Segmental unblinding recognized that colonoscopy is an imperfect standard where significant miss rates exist even for large polyps. Tandem colonoscopy studies have reported a 6% miss rate for large adenomas and up to 13% for smaller (6-9 mm) adenomas.[22] It is important to realize that such

rates are an underestimation in which the reference standard is the same method as the examining modality. Thus, the systematic factors that render a lesion difficult to perceive and are missed on one colonoscopic examination would be present for the second. In the DoD trial, when CTC was used as the reference standard, the colonoscopy miss rate for large adenomas doubled from 6% to 12% (Fig. 7-2).[23] More recently, studies with the third-eye retroscope in which endoscopic viewing of the backside of folds is possible during colonic extubation have produced results that support these higher miss rates. In a small series, Triadafilopoulos and Li[24] demonstrated a 12% increase in diagnostic yield from polyps detected only on the retrograde image. In short, the use of segmental unblinding within a study helps to correct, at least partially, for potential false-negative colonoscopy findings that would be interpreted incorrectly as CT colonography false-positive results.

The disparate results among the four trials led to disagreement regarding the true capabilities of CT colonography. Furthermore, the time course of publishing of the studies further confounded results. The promising results from the DoD trial were published at the end of 2003 following Johnson's study. This trial pointed to the potential efficacy for CTC in colorectal cancer screening. However, subsequent published studies from Cotton in 2004 and Rockey in 2005 seemed to suggest that the "more recent" studies of CTC did not confirm satisfactory performance. However, it is important to consider the dates of patient accrual for these studies, which in part explain the poor results of the subsequent studies. Although the Cotton and Rockey studies were published after the 2003 Pickhardt DoD trial, these two studies actually represented older studies in which patient accrual began 2 years prior to the DoD study. Because of slow patient recruitment, the patient accrual time periods extended beyond the DoD trial and led to a publishing date long after the Pickhardt study published in *The New England Journal of Medicine*. Herein lies a significant factor in the poor results. The older Cotton and Rockey studies used older techniques and CTC protocols. For example, the Cotton study used thicker collimation for a number of examinations and did not use contrast tag-

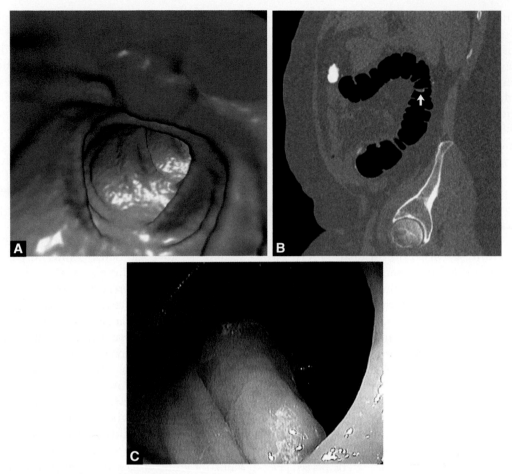

Figure 7-2 **OC false-negative result.** A 14-mm flat polyp in the ascending colon that was not confirmed at subsequent OC was called at CTC during screening of a 59-year-old female at average risk. 3D endoluminal CTC image **(A)** from the vantage point of the cecum looking toward the hepatic flexure demonstrates a large flat lesion in the right colon. Note that it resides on the backside of a colonic fold. 2D sagittal CTC image **(B)** better delineates this relationship of the polyp *(arrow)* to the fold. Given the CTC appearance, the patient was contacted for repeat CTC, which ultimately was done 13 months later. The polyp was again seen at CTC and sent for repeat colonoscopy, which found and removed the large lesion **(C)**. Large misses at optical colonoscopy tend to be right sided.

ging. Similarly, the Rockey study used cathartic-only bowel preparation protocols without contrast tagging. It stands to reason that the Pickhardt study, using newer techniques that included thin slice collimation and contrast tagging agents, would obtain better results.

The differences in CTC performance among the studies, however, involved much more than simply the use of older techniques. A significant part was related to the method of interpretation. The Johnson, Cotton, and Rockey studies were primary 2D trials in which polyp detection occurred through lumen tracking within 2D series, whereas the Pickhardt trial was a primary 3D study in which polyp detection largely occurred through an endoluminal fly-through, with secondary 2D detection. A 3D approach to polyp detection leads to a more sensitive strategy that is less prone to perceptual errors and less fatiguing to use (see Chapter 17). In 2007 Pickhardt and colleagues reexamined the Navy subset (n = 730) of the DoD study trial with a primary 2D approach.[25] Readers undertook polyp detection by using the 2D displays only.

Three-dimensional views were restricted to problem solving to confirm a suspected polypoid morphology. Despite more experienced and well-trained readers compared with the original prospective DoD, the sensitivity dropped to 81% for 10-mm or larger adenomas, in comparison to the original 94% sensitivity achieved by the 3D approach, leading to the conclusion that a primary 2D approach leads to less sensitive detection compared with primary 3D CTC in low-prevalence screening cohorts.

A final reason cited as a contributing factor to poor performance in some trials was related to reader experience and training. In both the Cotton and Rockey trial, the large number of institutions relative to the number of patients in the study population led to decreased numbers of target polyps seen per institution. Typically, large polyps are seen in approximately 5% of patients in a true screening situation.[26,27] For the Cotton trial with nine institutions, there was an average of 68 patients per institution, which would predict a limited experience with patients with large polyps (perhaps 3-4 such patients per institution). In fact, the true number was much lower than this for the majority of the institutions involved because one institution accrued a relatively large fraction of the entire cohort (n = 184). Similarly, in the Rockey trial the median number of patients enrolled per site was 22, with a high of 165 for one institution and a low of 2.[20] Consequently, an institution's experience with large polyps would be limited as a result of the low-prevalence setting. In contrast, in the Pickhardt trial each site enrolled more than 400 participants on average, markedly increasing exposure to large polyps and allowing for a more realistic assessment of performance. A second related issue concerned reader training. In the Cotton study, no formal training was given to the readers prior to the trial. Five studies were required for review for each site to participate to assess technical quality only. No formal assessment of CTC interpretation was made, and participating sites only had to report that 10 CTC examinations were previously preformed at that site prior to the study. In both the Cotton and Rockey trials, no feedback during the trial was given to the readers. It is evident that training was suboptimal for these studies. Studies such as Spinzi et al. have demonstrated the need for training and experience at CTC in which readers in their series demonstrated a sensitivity of 32% in the first 25 cases as compared with 92% for the last 20.[28]

In 2005, two meta-analyses regarding the cumulative published CTC performance data in both high-risk and screening populations were completed.[29,30] The pooled per-patient CTC sensitivity and specificity for large (≥10 mm) polyps was 85% to 93% and 97%, respectively. Pooled sensitivity and specificity for small (6-9 mm) polyps was 70% to 86% and 86% to 93%, respectively. For carcinoma, the sensitivity was 96%, comparable with the reported sensitivity for colonoscopy.[31,32]

Despite the meta-analyses, the discrepant results between the four initial studies led to much confusion and argument regarding the true abilities of CTC. Today, the shortcomings of the three 2D trials are recognized, and the performance characteristics seen in the DoD trial have been validated by subsequent studies. During the early and mid 2000s, however, the capabilities of CTC remained in question as a result of these three primary 2D studies. Unfortunately, there was also an element of professional politics that fueled this debate, in which the negative performance of CTC was emphasized because it was viewed by some as an encroachment on the use of optical colonoscopy in the screening setting.

Subsequent Validation Studies

The announcement of several study results in the fall of 2007 led to validation of the positive CTC performance documented in the DoD trial. The results of the National CT colonography Trial (American College of Radiology Imaging Network [ACRIN] protocol 6664) were announced at the American College of Radiology Imaging Network 2007 fall meeting and published in *The New England Journal of Medicine* in 2008.[33] The aim of this study, which was sponsored and funded in part by the National Cancer Institute, was to assess the performance of CTC for large adenomas and cancer in a large screening cohort by a multiinstitution effort. More than 2500 patients were enrolled by 15 institutions over a 23-month period. Current techniques were used, including cathartic protocols with additional oral tagging agents, colonic distention with automated CO_2 delivery, thin collimation on multidetector scanner, and the use of 2D and 3D techniques in interpretation strategies. Intravenous glucagon was administered as well. Readers were required to demonstrate a level of competency in CTC interpretation by passing an assessment test prior to the study. Several readers required additional testing to pass this entrance examination.

The ACRIN trial reported an overall solid sensitivity for large adenomas (≥10 mm) of 90%. The sensitivity remained very good at the 8-mm threshold at 87% and adequate at the 6-mm threshold at 78%. Specificities were 86%, 87%, and 88%, respectively. The positive predictive value was low at 23% for large adenomas (≥10 mm). Part of this lower than expected number was related to the screening setting with low prevalence of advanced neoplasia, the lack of segmental unblinding in the study design, and the consideration of nonadenomatous polyps as false positives. The negative predictive value for lesion ≥10 mm was excellent at 99%, confirming that a negative CTC examination result effectively excludes a significant large polyp or mass.

In addition to the ACRIN results, similar positive results were announced in two European trials at the 8th International Virtual Colonoscopy Symposium held in Boston. The IMPACT (Italian Multicenter Polyp Accuracy CTC) trial reported a sensitivity of 90% at the 10-mm threshold, whereas the Munich Colorectal Cancer Prevention trial reported a 92% sensitivity at that level.[34,35] The Munich trial has been published,[35] whereas the IMPACT trial is currently in press.

In addition to these validation studies on performance, our group at the University of Wisconsin compared the clinical efficacy of CTC with a selective polypectomy strategy against optical colonoscopy with a universal polypectomy strategy within parallel screening populations.[36] The diagnostic yield of advanced neoplasia of each program was the primary measure of the study. Advanced neoplasia was defined as either an advanced adenoma or cancer. In this study, CTC demonstrated the ability to select out this target from the larger population of colorectal polyps using size as a surrogate measure. From 3120 consecutive patients screened by CTC, 123 advanced neoplastic lesions were obtained (resulting in a prevalence of 3.2%), in comparison with 121 advanced neoplastic lesions in 3163 patients in the colonoscopy group (prevalence of 3.4%). Similar yields of advanced lesions were seen between the screening groups despite a

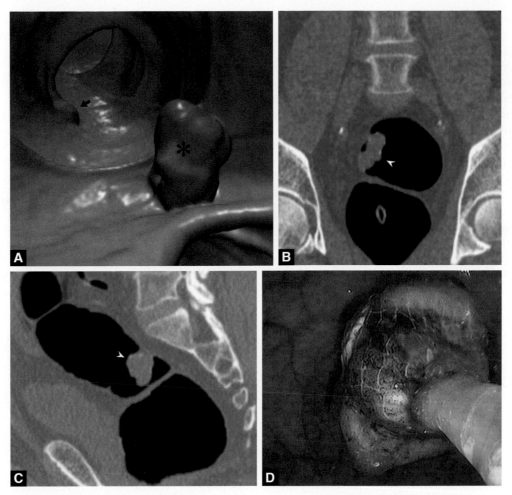

Figure 7-3   CTC screening of average-risk adult male. 3D endoluminal image **(A)** shows a large lobulated rectal polyp *(asterisk)* and a smaller sessile sigmoid polyp in the background *(arrow)*. 2D coronal **(B)** and sagittal **(C)** images of the larger polyp *(arrowheads)* confirm a soft tissue nature. Correlative OC image **(D)** shows the polyp in a retrieval basket. Pathologic evaluation was consistent with a tubulovillous adenoma with high-grade dysplasia. The smaller sessile polyp also demonstrated tubulovillous architecture without high-grade dysplasia. (From Kim DH, Pickhardt PJ, Taylor AJ, et al. CT colonography versus colonoscopy for the detection of advanced neoplasia. *N Engl J Med.* 2007;357(14):1403-1412.)

marked difference in number of polypectomies. Within the CTC cohort, only 561 polypectomies were undertaken because of the selective approach, whereas 2434 polypectomies were needed in the colonoscopy population in which all detected polyps were removed. Not unexpectedly, such differences led to a significant difference in the number of complications in which none were seen in the CTC program and seven perforations were seen in the colonoscopy program. Such results led us to conclude that the use of CTC was supported as a primary screening test before therapeutic OC (Fig. 7-3).

Several studies have also pointed to potential advantages of CTC over colonoscopy in the detection of colon cancers. Both the DoD trial and the Wisconsin advanced neoplasia comparison study demonstrated increased numbers of cancers detected over colonoscopy. In the DoD trial, CTC detected both cancers in the study population, whereas OC missed one.[21] In the Wisconsin study, 14 cancers were seen on the CTC population, whereas only 4 were seen in the colonoscopy population

(p = 0.02) despite populations matched in the important demographic variables.[36] In addition, a large Mayo Clinic study, which was primarily undertaken to compare 2D to 3D detection approaches at CTC, demonstrated that colonoscopy (the colonoscopists were blinded initially to the CTC results) missed 4 of 5 cancers in the series. CTC detected all 5 cancers.[37]

CTC AS A RECOGNIZED SCREENING OPTION

These studies laid the framework for CTC acceptance as a viable screening modality. As a result of these and other studies, CTC was formally included in the latest (2008) revision of the American Cancer Society (ACS) guidelines for colorectal cancer screening.[38] The conclusions stated that based on the accumulation of data since the last revision, the data are sufficient to "include CTC as an acceptable option for CRC screening." It was the opinion of the expert panel that CTC was comparable with colonoscopy for the detection of cancers and polyps of significant size when state-of-the-art techniques were applied (see Chapter 5).

There was another important modification of the 2008 ACS guidelines from previous versions, in which two discrete categories of screening options now exist. One concerns tests of *cancer prevention*, in which the examination detects adenomatous polyps and cancers, and a second concerns *cancer detection*, in which only cancers would be detected. The preferred goal is cancer prevention, but it was recognized that some patients would be unwilling to undergo endoscopy or CTC and tests of cancer detection were preferable to the situation of no screening. CTC was added to the first list of tests of cancer prevention alongside flexible sigmoidoscopy, colonoscopy, and double contrast barium enema. The interval for a negative examination was set at 5 years, and key points for informed decisions included that (1) a complete bowel preparation was required; (2) colonoscopy was recommended for any polyp ≥6mm detected; (3) the risks for CTC were low but rare cases of perforation had been reported; and (4) extracolonic abnormalities could be detected on CTC, requiring further evaluation.

SUMMARY

CTC has moved from the research realm to clinical acceptance in the span of 14 years. It demonstrates effective and generalizable performance in low polyp–prevalence settings as the technology has matured and is now poised for implementation on a national scale. Because of the increasing body of CTC research with excellent performance results and inclusion within the most recent ACS guidelines, both public and scientific sentiment is changing from views held only several years ago. CTC is now considered an effective modality equivalent to colonoscopy, representing a viable screening option for colorectal cancer. Key issues concern maintenance of quality as this screening modality becomes more widely applied.

REFERENCES

1. Hara AK, Johnson CD, Reed JE, et al. Detection of colorectal polyps with CT colography: Initial assessment of sensitivity and specificity. *Radiology.* 1997;205(1):59-65.
2. Dachman AH, Kuniyoshi JK, Boyle CM, et al. CT colonography with three-dimensional problem solving for detection of colonic polyps. *Am J Roentgenol.* 1998;171(4):989-995.
3. Fenlon HM, Nunes DP, Schroy PC, Barish MA, Clarke PD, Ferrucci JT. A comparison of virtual and conventional colonoscopy for the detection of colorectal polyps. *N Engl J Med.* 1999;341 (20):1496-1503.
4. Yee J, Akerkar GA, Hung RK, Steinauer-Gebauer AM, Wall SD, McQuaid KR. Colorectal neoplasia: Performance characteristics of CT colonography for detection in 300 patients. *Radiology.* 2001;219(3):685-692.
5. Royster AP, Fenlon HM, Clarke PD, Nunes DP, Ferrucci JT. CT colonoscopy of colorectal neoplasms: Two-dimensional and three-dimensional virtual-reality techniques with colonoscopic correlation. *Am J Roentgenol.* 1997;169(5):1237-1242.
6. Hara AK, Johnson CD, MacCarty RL, Welch TJ, McCollough CH, Harmen WS. CT colonography: Single-versus multi-detector row imaging. *Radiology.* 2001;219(2):461-465.
7. Fletcher JG, Johnson CD, Welch TJ, et al. Optimization of CT colonography technique: Prospective trial in 180 patients. *Radiology.* 2000;216(3):704-711.
8. Morrin MM, Farrell RJ, Kruskal JB, Reynolds K, McGee JB, Raptopoulos V. Utility of intravenously administered contrast material at CT colonography. *Radiology.* 2000;217(3):765-771.
9. McFarland EG, Pilgram TK, Brink JA, et al. CT colonography: Multiobserver diagnostic performance. *Radiology.* 2002;225(2):380-390.
10. Lefere PA, Gryspeerdt SS, Dewyspelaere J, Baekelandt M, Van Holsbeeck BG. Dietary fecal tagging as a cleansing method before CT colonography: Initial results-polyp detection and patient acceptance. *Radiology.* 2002;224(2):393-403.
11. Pedersen BG, Christiansen TEM, Bjerregaard NC, Ljungmann K, Laurberg S. Colonoscopy and multidetector-array computed-tomographic colonography: Detection rates and feasibility. *Endoscopy.* 2003;35(9):736-742.
12. Taylor SA, Halligan S, Saunders BP, et al. Of multidetector-row CT colonography for detection of colorectal neoplasia in patients referred via the department of health "2-week-wait" initiative. *Clin Radiol.* 2003;58(11):855-861.
13. Pineau BC, Paskett ED, Chen GJ, et al. Virtual colonoscopy using oral contrast compared with colonoscopy for the detection of patients with colorectal polyps. *Gastroenterology.* 2003;125(2):304-310.
14. Hoppe H, Netzer P, Spreng A, Quattropani C, Mattich J, Dinkel HP. Prospective comparison of contrast enhanced CT colonography and conventional colonoscopy for detection of colorectal neoplasms in a single institutional study using second-look colonoscopy with discrepant results. *Am J Gastroenterol.* 2004;99(10):1924-1935.
15. Van Gelder RE, Nio CY, Florie J, et al. Computed tomographic colonography compared with colonoscopy in patients at increased risk for colorectal cancer. *Gastroenterology.* 2004;127(1):41-48.
16. Macari M, Bini EJ, Xue XN, et al. Colorectal neoplasms: Prospective comparison of thin-section low-dose multi-detector row CT colonography and conventional colonoscopy for detection. *Radiology.* 2002;224(2):383-392.
17. Laghi A, Iannaccone R, Carbone I, et al. Detection of colorectal lesions with virtual computed tomographic colonography. *Am J Surg.* 2002;183(2):124-131.
18. Johnson CD, Toledano AY, Herman BA, et al. Computerized tomographic colonography: Performance evaluation in a retrospective multicenter setting. *Gastroenterology.* 2003;125(3):688-695.
19. Cotton PB, Durkalski VL, Benoit PC, et al. Computed tomographic colonography (virtual colonoscopy)—A multicenter comparison with standard colonoscopy for detection of colorectal neoplasia. *JAMA.* 2004;291(14):1713-1719.
20. Rockey DC, Paulson E, Niedzwiecki D, et al. Analysis of air contrast barium enema, computed tomographic colonography, and colonoscopy: prospective comparison. *Lancet.* 2005;365(9456):305-311.
21. Pickhardt PJ, Choi JR, Hwang I, et al. Computed tomographic virtual colonoscopy to screen for colorectal neoplasia in asymptomatic adults. *N Engl J Med.* 2003;349(23):2191-2200.
22. Rex DK, Cutler CS, Lemmel GT, et al. Colonoscopic miss rates of adenomas determined by back-to-back colonoscopies. *Gastroenterology.* 1997;112(1):24-28.

23. Pickhardt PJ, Nugent PA, Mysliwiec PA, Choi JR, Schindler WR. Location of adenomas missed by optical colonoscopy. *Ann Intern Med.* 2004;141(5):352-359.

24. Triadafilopoulos G, Li J. A pilot study to assess the safety and efficacy of the Third Eye Retrograde auxiliary imaging system during colonoscopy. *Endoscopy.* 2008;40(6):478-482.

25. Pickhardt PJ, Lee AD, Taylor AJ, et al. Primary 2D versus primary 3D polyp detection at screening CT Colonography. *Am J Roentgenol.* 2007;189(6):1451-1456.

26. Pickhardt PJ, Taylor AJ, Kim DH, Reichelderfer M, Gopal DV, Pfau PR. Screening for colorectal neoplasia with CT colonography: Initial experience from the 1st year of coverage by third-party payers. *Radiology.* 2006;241(2):417-425.

27. Kim DH, Pickhardt PJ, Taylor AJ. Characteristics of advanced adenomas detected at CT colonographic screening: Implications for appropriate polyp size thresholds for polypectomy versus surveillance. *Am J Roentgenol.* 2007;188(4):940-944.

28. Spinzi G, Belloni G, Martegani A, Sangiovanni A, Del Favero C, Minoli G. Computed tomographic colonography and conventional colonoscopy for colon diseases: A prospective, blinded study. *Am J Gastroenterol.* 2001;96(2):394-400.

29. Mulhall BP, Veerappan GR, Jackson JL. Meta-analysis: Computed tomographic colonography. *Ann Intern Med.* 2005;142(8):635-650.

30. Halligan S, Altman DG, Taylor SA, et al. CT colonography in the detection of colorectal polyps and cancer: Systematic review meta-analysis and proposed minimum data set for study level reporting. *Radiology.* 2005;238(3):893-904.

31. Rex DK, Rahmani EY, Haseman JH, Lemmel GT, Kaster S, Buckley JS. Relative sensitivity of colonoscopy and barium enema for detection of colorectal cancer in clinical practice. *Gastroenterology.* 1997;112(1):17-23.

32. Bressler B, Paszat LF, Vinden C, Li C, He JS, Rabeneck L. Colonoscopic miss rates for right-sided colon cancer: A population-based analysis. *Gastroenterology.* 2004;127(2):452-456.

33. Johnson CD, Chen MH, Toledano AY, et al. Accuracy of CT colonography for detection of large adenomas and cancers. *N Engl J Med.* 2008;359(12):1207-1217.

34. Regge D. Accuracy of CT colonography in subjects at increased risk of colorectal carcinoma: A multicenter study on 1,066 patients (IMPACT). Boston: 8th International Symposium on Virtual Colonoscopy; 2007:108-109.

35. Graser A, Stieber P, Nagel D, et al. Comparison of CT colonography, colonoscopy, sigmoidoscopy, and fecal occult blood tests for the detection of advanced adenoma in an average risk population. *Gut.* 2009;58(2):241-248.

36. Kim DH, Pickhardt PJ, Taylor AJ, et al. CT colonography versus colonoscopy for the detection of advanced neoplasia. *N Engl J Med.* 2007;357(14):1403-1412.

37. Johnson CD, Fletcher JG, MacCarty RL, et al. Effect of slice thickness and primary 2D versus 3D virtual dissection on colorectal lesion detection at CT colonography in 452 asymptomatic adults. *Am J Roentgenol.* 2007;189(3):672-680.

38. Levin B, Lieberman DA, McFarland B, et al. Screening and surveillance for the early detection of colorectal cancer and adenomatous polyps, 2008: A joint guideline from the American Cancer Society, the US Multi-Society Task Force on Colorectal Cancer, and the American College of Radiology. *CA Cancer J Clin.* 2008;58(3):130-160.

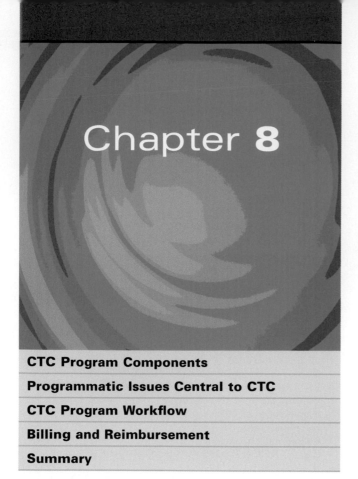

Chapter 8

Building a Clinical CT Colonography Program

DAVID H. KIM, MD
PERRY J. PICKHARDT, MD

INTRODUCTION

Effective population screening by CT colonography (CTC) requires a programmatic approach. Competently performed CTC examinations and interpretations undertaken in a vacuum without coordination lead to less than optimal coverage from a public health standpoint. By comparison, such examinations under the umbrella of a programmatic approach lead to more effective, systematic evaluation of the population at risk. In addition to an optimized examination conducted by a team of professionals, screened individuals would not be "lost to followup" and appropriate surveillance would be coordinated. This chapter explores the components that comprise a clinical CT colonography program and the specific issues central to a well-run program.

CTC PROGRAM COMPONENTS

The physical components that comprise a CTC program include both infrastructure requirements and personnel. In terms of infrastructure, defined space for both the program coordinator and for the physicians interpreting the examination is paramount to an optimally functioning program. An office with a dedicated phone number is essential for the necessary administrative duties. Scheduled screening patients will need a contact number for the program coordinator. Many questions arise between the time the patient is scheduled and the

time examination is performed. Patient education particularly regarding bowel preparation responsibilities is of central importance in obtaining high-quality screening examinations. Although time consuming, these conversations directing how best to proceed with the bowel preparation for a given patient are key elements in maintaining high sensitivity and specificity of the examination. Despite the best streamlined bowel preparation protocol, questions will arise and the subsequent conversations between the program coordinator and scheduled patient will often prevent a misunderstanding that could have a fairly significant impact on the interpretation of the examination (Fig. 8-1). In our experience, nondiagnostic examinations related to poor bowel preparation are much less than 1% of cases because of these preexamination interactions. In addition, answers to these and other questions build rapport with the patient, hopefully improving compliance and the likelihood that the individual would proceed with the examination. Obviously, the program coordinator is a key individual and, along with the CT technologists, becomes the "face" of the program. The office also acts as the central information repository for the program including the patient intake historical forms, the clinical database, and the various scheduling lists, including those regarding patients who are due for follow-up examinations.

Similarly, it is important to have a dedicated area set aside for the interpretation of the examinations. A defined space devoid of the usual traffic of a busy CT reading room is helpful in maintaining reader concentration. Similar to a mammography program, a secluded environment to decrease outside distractions helps to maintain productivity when interpreting a large volume of screening examinations (Fig. 8-2). This area should have ap-

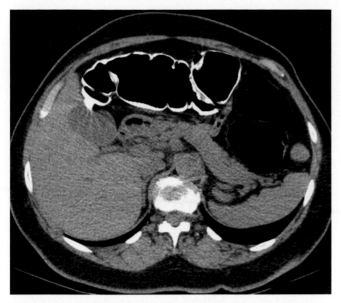

Figure 8-1 Patient confusion with the bowel preparation. This individual switched the order of the tagging agents, taking the diatrizoate prior to the dilute barium. It is hoped that interaction with the patient prior to the examination would prevent these incidents. 2D transverse image demonstrates a cast of barium coating outlining the colon. Because the diatrizoate was given before the barium, this hypertonic agent could not "scrub" off the barium from the normal colonic mucosa as typically occurs (see Chapter 12).

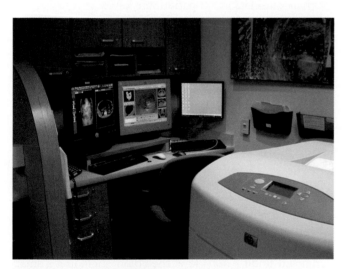

Figure 8-2 CTC work area. Photograph shows the CTC workstation platform *(center)* with adjacent PACS system on the left and voice-recognition dictation system on the right. It is important to have a dedicated space for interpretation away from the normal work flow of CT.

propriate networking capabilities because many different clinical examination sites would likely funnel completed CTC examinations into this area for interpretation by the physician.

Other infrastructure needs include appropriate hardware including a multidetector CT (MDCT) scanner, an automated CO_2 delivery device, and an integrated PACS three-dimensional (3D) workstation. The proximity of the MDCT scanner in relation to the 3D workstation and interpreting physician is not important. Because of the nature of the CTC examination, physician presence during image acquisition is not required for the vast majority of cases (see Chapter 14). This is advantageous for several reasons. These elective screening examinations can be scheduled at times when the MDCT scanner is underused (e.g., very early in the morning when prepped patients are eager to arrive), thus maximizing output of the scanner. In addition, the examinations can be conducted at several sites distant from the central reading area and networked in to allow a small core of physicians to remotely cover a broad region. This would allow examinations to be performed at various outpatient centers—a setting typically more appealing for the group of healthy individuals being screened.

Basic personnel for a CTC program include the program coordinator, the CTC technologist, and the CTC interpreting physician. Each individual holds defined roles and responsibilities that are vital to the success of the program. As noted earlier, the CTC program coordinator is largely the "face" of the clinical CTC program. This person may interact with the patient on multiple occasions from initial scheduling through the postexamination period, answering numerous questions along the way. After the completion of the CTC examination, this person helps to coordinate subsequent evaluation options (e.g., imaging surveillance versus colonoscopy versus routine screening). An effective program coordinator is invaluable at maintaining high patient satisfaction with the screening process, which, it is hoped, translates to future compliance with screening. This person can provide the longitudinal care and attention to ensure that patients are not lost in the system. It is our opinion that this position is best filled by a registered nurse. Many of the conversations with the patient require specific medical knowledge such as the use of one cathartic agent over another and how best to administer the agent. The nurse coordinator can also help educate the individual regarding the significance of the examination results and the potential options available. A nurse coordinator is invaluable at helping the individual undertake an informed decision. In addition to becoming the patient liaison, the coordinator holds several other responsibilities vital to a successful program. This person maintains active lists to reschedule patients who have missed appointments and to send reminders to patients regarding the need to schedule follow-up examinations. Direct conversations with patients who are noncompliant and have missed appointments often can bring these people in off the sidelines and into screening. The coordinator is also a bridge to the referring physician's office, providing education regarding ordering issues. The program coordinator may also help in maintenance of the program's clinical database. Without a coordinator, many of these duties would fall to the physician. Obviously, these responsibilities could not be performed at the same level because of physician time constraints in comparison to a dedicated program coordinator.

CTC technologists are the second key personnel component in a CTC program. It is worthwhile to create a small group of CT technologists trained specifically for CTC. Once properly trained, these individuals hold primary responsibility in acquiring the images and evaluating the technical adequacy of the examination. Physician oversight is minimal, and the physician becomes involved only for unusual circumstances. This separation between image acquisition and interpretation allows the physician to maximize efficiency. Because the physician can concentrate on the interpretation of the examination and is not tied to the performance of each one, the number of CTC examinations that can be completed in a given period markedly increases. Because of the close patient contact, the CTC technologist represents another important "face" of the program from the patient perspective. It is important that the CTC technologist feels comfortable in conducting the examination. Indecision or nervousness on the part of the technologist is readily detected by the patient and can result in significant negative perception of the program as a whole. The CTC technologist holds primary responsibility for the assessment of cathartic effectiveness by direct patient questioning and evaluation of the scout and cross-sectional images. The technologist also is responsible for colonic distention from placing the rectal catheter, to initiating CO_2 instillation, to assessing adequacy of distention. If distention is deemed inadequate by the technologist, this individual determines which potential solution would best lead to a technically optimized examination, including decubitus positioning or room air instillation (see Chapter 13). In our experience, well-trained, competent technologists produce consistently diagnostic examinations. A weak link at this level will considerably hamper overall program effectiveness as a result of missed lesions from suboptimal examinations, the need for patient recall, or for significant physician oversight for examination adequacy.

The final core member of the program is the physician, who holds overall responsibility for the CTC program. Although ultimately responsible for the entire program, the primary function of the CTC physician is in the interpretation of the examination. If this person is able to remain separate from image acquisition, the physician can be very productive and cover several sites that network examinations into the central reading area. The physician holds the ultimate responsibility for relaying significant findings along with specific recommendations to both the patient and referring physician. If the program coordinator is a registered nurse, some of these duties can be passed on to this individual after appropriate training. In our opinion, the CTC physician also is primarily responsible for the integrity of the program database, regardless of who enters the data. A database that records all relevant results is a necessary component and is the foundation of several important program functions including quality control through monitoring of various quality metrics, resolving discordant cases, and maintaining clinical follow-up lists. It is helpful to create a pool of physician readers for the program, which allows for flexibility in scheduling.

PROGRAMMATIC ISSUES CENTRAL TO CTC

Patient Education

Patient education is a key function of the CTC program. Typically, the CTC office fields many calls from both interested unscheduled patients regarding general colorectal cancer (CRC) screening questions and from scheduled patients regarding specific issues of the bowel preparation. A CTC program can be a focal point to increase public awareness of the importance of CRC screening through one-on-one conversations and through various health fairs. The program coordinator plays a central role in this area. For the scheduled patient, education regarding specific issues for the upcoming CTC examination is crucial in optimizing patient preparation for the examination.

Scheduling and the Clinical Database

One of the requirements for scheduling a patient for screening CTC is a physician order for the examination. In contrast to the situation in mammography, patients should not enter a CTC screening program without a referring physician because of the unavoidable incidental examination of extracolonic structures at CTC. This requirement for physician referral to the program ensures that unsuspected significant findings can be relayed to a specific responsible health care provider and can be acted on appropriately. In our experience, approximately 2% to 3% of the screening population will have an unsuspected significant finding outside of the colon, including a small number of asymptomatic cancers and significant vascular aneurysms.[1] The order requirement also allows the referring physician who is familiar with the overall health status of the patient to select the appropriate bowel preparation. Once the order has been generated, scheduling for screening CTC examinations can be undertaken, generally by trained administrative personnel. It is helpful, however, to reserve the program coordinator for scheduling those patients who have missed prior examinations or those who need follow-up examinations. Patient education is key for these individuals and can often lead to increased compliance with screening.

With the initial scheduling, basic historical information is gathered from the patient (Fig. 8-3) in addition to health insurance and other billing issues. This allows assessment of risk and defines the patient population demographics. This information can be then compared to the polyp output of the program to assess whether the results are in the expected range for a given population. For example, for a higher-risk population of older males, a higher prevalence of advanced adenomas would be expected. The scheduling patient intake forms are reviewed by the program coordinator for confirmation of appropriate choice of bowel preparation, appropriate insurance coverage, and potential issues that may arise from the prep from the patient's underlying health status. In our experience, it is helpful to contact the patient to discuss specific strategies during the bowel preparation for patients taking insulin or oral hypoglycemics for diabetes. If an inappropriate bowel preparation was selected

---

Virtual Colonoscopy Intake

Screening

CALLS:

Name: _____ MR#: _____ Sex: Female

Patient Address: _____

Patient Phone #: _____ DOB: _____ Age: _____

Ordering MD: _____ Clinic: _____

Clinic Address: _____ Phone #: _____

Current Diagnosis: Eval for Colorectal Cancer: _____

Reason for Exam: Eval for Colorectal Cancer: _____

Known Medical History: _____

_____

_____

*Insurance: _____ Other: _____

Scheduler's Comments:

(if listed please add to comments)   Date to Scheduling: _____

(To be completed by Scheduler)

Appt. Date: _____ Appt. Time: _____ Arrival Time: _____

Scheduled at: (please select) [ ]   Reschedules:

Questions to ask patient: (select appropriate answers)

Ht. _____ Wt. _____ (kg/lbs)

*Ever diagnosed with bowel disease?   Yes ◯   No ◯

   If "yes", please list: _____

*Parents or siblings diagnosed with colon cancer? Yes ◯   No ◯

   If "yes", specify relation: _____ and age at time of diagnosis: _____

*Patient diagnosed with <u>any</u> cancers?   Yes ◯   No ◯

   If "yes", specify diagnosis: _____ year: _____ Treatment: _____

*Any abdominal surgeries?   Yes ◯   No ◯

   If "yes", please specify: _____

Pharmacy Choice: (please select) [ ]

SCHEDULER: SCROLL DOWN (Long form-2pgs)

Scheduler Comments for VC Office:

Scheduler's Name: _____ Date to RN: _____

Date Rx faxed to Pharmacy: _____ Date to LV: _____ Date to pre-Auth: _____

INSURANCE COVERAGE: Yes ◯ No ◯   *PRIVATE PAYER:* Yes ◯ No ◯

A

Figure 8-3 CTC scheduling intake and results forms. The intake forms (**A** and **B**) establish patient demographics, pertinent medical history, and risk factors.   *Illustration continued on following page*

(To be completed by Scheduler)

—Ever been diagnosed with any kidney or heart condition/problem?   Yes ◯   No ◯

   If yes, list: _____

—Do you have Diabetes?   Yes ◯   No ◯   If yes, insulin dependent?   Yes ◯   No ◯

—Medications [   ]   List ALL: _____

—Are you taking blood thinners?   Yes ◯   No ◯

   (If yes, please choose type(s) & list how often) [   ]

CT QA Data

Prep completed? (select one) [   ]   Staff Verification (Initials): [   ]

Are there incompletely evaluated segments after BOTH 2D/3D supine and prone?   Yes ◯   No ◯

If yes, select segment(s): [   ]   MD PLEASE "cc": [   ]

Classification & Follow-Up: C0 ☐   C1 ☐   C2 ☐   C3 ☐   C4 ☐

Note: See posting for C0–C4 descriptions

Current follow-up for negagive study is 5 years, for 6–7 mm polyp is 2 years, and for 8–9 mm polyp is 1 year.

C0 = Inadequate study (poor prep and/or insufflation) If C0, give reason: [   ]

POLYP FINDINGS:

#	Distance from rectum (cm-Sup/Pr)	Size (mm)	Colonic Segment	Morphology*	Diagnostic Confidence* (1–3)
1					
2					
3					
4					
5					
6					
7					

Note: – Segments: rectum, sigmoid, descending, splenic flexure, trnasverse, hepatic flexure, ascending, cecum
– Size should be longest axis on 3D view
– Morphology: penduculated (stalk present), sessile, or flat (broad-based, plaque-like, height < ½ of width)
– This sheet should also include invasive colon cancers (e.g., "morphology" might be "annular mass")
– Diagnostic conficence: (1) – least certain; (3) – most certain; (2) – intermediate

*OTHER NOTABLE COLONIC Findings: Recommended Colon Follow-Up: [   ]
(e.g., Lipoma, sig. Diverticular dz)

[   ]

EXTRACOLONIC Classification: E0 ☐   E1 ☐   E2 ☐   E3 ☐   E4 ☐

Note: See posting for E0-E4 descriptions

List notable findings (i.e., what will be mentioned in the report):

[   ]

If further work-up is necessary, list: [   ]

2

C

Figure 8-3 (Continued)   **CTC scheduling intake and results forms.** The intake forms (**A** and **B**) establish patient demographics, pertinent medical history, and risk factors. Results from the CTC examination (**C**) are added by the physician to complete the form. All information is subsequently entered into a robust clinical database. This is an electronic (paperless) form at our center.

by the ordering physician, the program coordinator can notify the office to rectify the situation.

A CTC program should create an active clinical database that records all enrolled patients and examination results (Fig. 8-4). The data input should include demographic information, patient historical information, technical and quality parameters of the examination, polyp findings, and subsequent evaluation plan with dates. The information is imperative for several programmatic functions, including maintaining patient follow-up lists, preparing a discordant case list, and monitoring various quality metrics. Many of these analytic functions can be automated, allowing for easy and rapid generation of these reports (Fig. 8-4). Much of the patient demographic data can be entered by the program coordinator or other personnel. However, the primary responsibility for the input of polyp results and reconciliation with OC and pathology findings should rest on the physician.

Polyp Surveillance of Patients at Low Risk

CTC screening is fundamentally different from screening by traditional optical colonoscopy. Screening by CTC is more in the mode of a traditional screening examination, which is one step removed from the therapeutic option. Thus, it makes sense to filter out the patients at low risk and send only those with likely significant polyps for polypectomy, particularly when the majority of high-risk polyps can be identified (here by a surrogate measure of large size) and represent a very small fraction of all colorectal polyps. The few high-risk small polyps left in place within the CTC surveillance group can then be identified by demonstrating interval growth over time.[2] Such a strategy is permissible because of the favorable time course of cancer transformation from a benign target, consisting of many years. The benefits of this approach include conserving limited colonoscopic resources and decreasing the number of adverse events related to polypectomy. With the creation of a polyp surveillance group at CTC, there are inherent duties and responsibilities required of a CTC program. It is important to keep accurate lists of these patients and the scheduled date of the future examination. In our opinion, it is the program's responsibility (and not the referring physician's) to notify individuals regarding followup and to have reminder systems in place if patients do not show up for the examination. A clinical database is helpful in this regard to maintain an accurate active status of these lists. One of the key responsibilities of the University of Wisconsin (UW) CTC program coordinator revolves

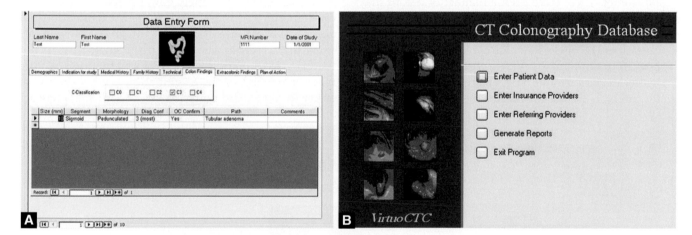

Figure 8-4 CTC clinical database. A Microsoft Access database **(A)** houses information from the scheduling intake forms and the pertinent CTC, colonoscopic, and pathologic data for detected polyps. Dates for needed followup examinations are also entered. Automated reports can be generated **(B),** including lists of patients with scheduled followup **(C).** Note: These patient names are fictitious.

around this important issue of surveillance scheduling and maintenance of compliance.

Discordant Case Resolution and Quality Metrics Monitoring

Discordant case resolution and quality metrics monitoring are important functions for a CTC program to undertake. Discordant cases represent CTC examinations in which a focal abnormality is identified but no structural correlate is seen at subsequent colonoscopy (see Chapter 26). The presumption by some endoscopists may be that the case represents a CTC false-positive result, but an OC false-negative result must also be considered. These cases should be periodically reviewed by the physicians who interpret CTC. A discordant case conference scheduled at regular intervals is an optimal approach. A quorum of interpreting physicians should reach a consensus as to whether the case indeed most likely represents a CTC false positive or if there is a reasonable chance of a colonoscopy false negative. If there is consensus that the polyp reported at CTC may be real, the patient should be scheduled for a repeat CTC examination to assess if the finding persists. If so, the patient should then be resent for another colonoscopy (possibly by a more skilled endoscopist). In our experience, there have been a number of lesions that initially were called CTC false positives in the endoscopy report but were eventually proven to represent OC false negatives after the discordant case conference process (see Chapter 26).

Quality metrics should be generated and reviewed at regular intervals to assess whether the program is main-

taining adequate quality. The discordant case conference is one measure that helps in this regard. Other measures include the C0 or nondiagnostic rate, the colonoscopy correlation rate (CTC positive predictive value), the colonoscopy referral rate, the advanced adenoma prevalence, and the significant complication rate (please see Chapter 28 for details). All of these measures can be calculated from the data entered into the clinical database. Appropriately configured databases can perform these reports on an automatic basis. Regular monitoring of the various metric measures is a key program function to maintain quality.

Integrated CTC–OC Screening Paradigm

A CTC program will have to decide on the philosophy regarding colonoscopic referral. An integrated program in which positive CTC cases are sent for colonoscopic polypectomy on the same day is the optimal option in our opinion. In addition, it has been endorsed by the American Gastroenterological Association as the preferred model in their letter to the Centers for Medicare and Medicaid Services during the national coverage analysis comment period for CTC screening. Such a paradigm allows for a single bowel preparation, even for the minority of instances when both examinations are necessary. More importantly, an integrated program answers the screening question with a single visit. Either the CTC examination is negative and routine screening is recommended, or the examination is positive, leading either to immediate polypectomy later in the afternoon

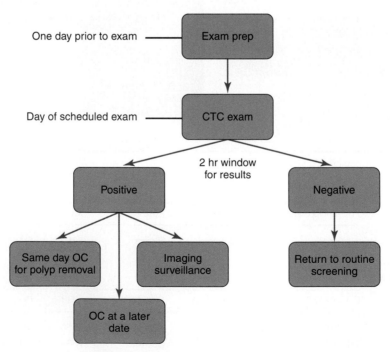

Figure 8-5 Program workflow. Flowchart demonstrates the straightforward workflow of a CTC examination. A team approach involving the program coordinator, CTC technologist, and CTC physician is helpful to maximizing efficiency and throughput.

or a follow-up CTC in 1 to 3 years (Fig. 8-5). In a program that is not integrated, the dissociation from therapeutic OC does make scheduling issues simpler for the endoscopy service. However, patients with positive CTC examination results must endure a second bowel preparation and a second visit to the hospital. An intermediate solution is to leave the patient on a clear-liquid diet and set up the polypectomy on the next day. For the typical screening patient who is a relatively young functioning individual in society, the ability to complete the evaluation with a single visit as opposed to potentially two visits is highly desirable. In our experience, the integrated model is feasible even for busy colonoscopic services. Approximately 8% of screening CTC patients require colonoscopy,[3] translating into an average of less than one add-on patient to the gastrointestinal (GI) schedule per day for every 10 patients screened. The program coordinator is a key individual in coordinating between CTC and OC services when the patient is sent for polypectomy. Various issues such as remaining in a fasting state and securing transportation following colonoscopy (the patient will not be able to drive because of sedation) can be settled. From a physician standpoint, an integrated program does require a relatively rapid turnaround of CTC results, as opposed to the dissociated CTC–OC model in which there essentially is no time limit for interpretation. At UW, we quote a 2-hour window for reporting examination results to allow for a possible same-day OC later in the afternoon if needed (Fig. 8-5).

Relationship with GI and Others

A CTC screening program should function smoothly in parallel with a preexisting OC screening program. With the estimated 40 million individuals eligible for screening in the United States who are currently noncompliant,[4] both programs will be needed to effectively cover this population. Although some models have predicted a siphoning of OC screening volumes by CTC,[5] this has not come to pass in reality for our program. In the UW experience, the number of screening OC examinations has actually increased after the CTC screening program was introduced.[6] With the recognition of this phenomenon leading to the view that CTC is not a competing modality, along with the recognition of the complementary strengths of these modalities, the relationship between radiologists and gastroenterologists has been favorable. It is advantageous to maintain a strong working relationship because good communication between the services ultimately leads to improved patient care. In addition to parallel programs leading to increased capacity for CRC screening, each modality can be used to complement or complete the evaluation initiated by the other modality. For example, CTC can confirm and potentially narrow the differential for suspected submucosal lesions seen at OC. In addition, CTC is often called on to complete an examination that began with colonoscopy in which the entire colon could not be visualized.

It is important to remember that although a favorable relationship with GI is optimal, the gatekeeper of the screening population is the primary care provider. Seamless entry into the CTC program through close communication regarding ordering issues with the primary care office is important to remove barriers to screening for individuals. Education of referring health care providers regarding the various aspects of the CTC examinations will ultimately have a positive impact on program functionality.

PROGRAM WORKFLOW

A smooth workflow reflects an optimized program (Fig. 8-5), which requires seamless interaction of the various program components. For those that adopt a same-day OC arm, good communication with the GI department is paramount in maintaining uninterrupted workflow. In the days prior to the scheduled examination, the program coordinator is the point person handling patients' questions to optimize the bowel preparation and address related medical issues. On the day of the examination, the patient is handed over to the CTC technologist, who holds primary responsibility for performing the examination. The technologist confirms adequacy of the bowel prep, distends the patient's colon with carbon dioxide, and assesses adequacy of the images, performing additional series if necessary. For straightforward cases, this process typically takes 10 to 15 minutes of CT room time for the patient. The examination time, however, may extend to 30 minutes for difficult cases. Once the images are acquired and deemed adequate, the patient is allowed to leave. The patient does not need to remain physically in the imaging department; he or she can provide a contact number. The patient, however, remains fasting until contacted by the program coordinator to proceed to colonoscopy, if needed. In our experience, many patients simply return to work awaiting results. The interpreting CTC physician has a 2-hour turnaround window for examination interpretation and reporting of results. The 3D model build time is now negligible given the marked improvements in computing power, typically requiring only 2 to 3 minutes. Interpretation times range from 5 to 10 minutes for straightforward cases, extending to 20 minutes for difficult ones. All results are recorded in the database or in appropriate forms to be placed in the database at a future time. Once interpreted, the examination results and recommendations are given to the program coordinator to be communicated to the patient. If negative, the patient may eat and resume typical daily activities. At this point, the CTC screening examination has officially concluded. If positive, the recommendations are relayed. If a colonoscopy is required, the program coordinator acts as liaison between GI and the patient to handle the various issues surrounding the scheduling of the examination later in the afternoon (e.g., driver following colonoscopy examination). In our experience, it has been useful to email or send a text message of pertinent images and comments to the colonoscopist. For example, notifying the endoscopist of a tortuous elongated colon or of a potentially difficult polyp location (e.g., behind a fold) is helpful. Ultimately, good communication in both directions aids in optimizing program results.

The program workflow is somewhat different when the CTC program is disassociated from same-day OC. If a dissociated model is used, there is no time pressure to turn around the CTC results because these are elective examinations. The patients may immediately return to normal daily activities following image acquisition. Positive CTC examination results that require colonoscopy can be scheduled for therapeutic removal some time in the future. Although this paradigm is amenable from a scheduling perspective, the major disadvantage to this workflow is the need for two separate bowel preparations and two visits to the hospital to address the screening question—which is a major imposition for otherwise-healthy "patients" who typically are productive members of society.

BILLING AND REIMBURSEMENT

Reimbursement for CTC is currently in a state of evolution and is rapidly changing (see Chapter 10). Currently, some diagnostic indications are broadly covered, although this varies somewhat from state to state. CTC for the purpose of screening is not yet widely covered, but this should change in the near future. The elective nature of CTC examinations allows for great flexibility in scheduling and time to settle billing issues or questions prior to the performance of the examination. All examinations are thus typically preapproved. It is helpful to have an individual skilled in this area to address the pertinent issues regarding reimbursement.

SUMMARY

CTC is best performed by a programmatic approach that leads to more systematic evaluation of the at-risk population. It requires a team approach composed of a program coordinator, CTC technologist, and physician. Each individual has specific responsibilities and all must function at a high level to maintain quality CTC examinations. Programmatic responsibilities include patient and referring physician education, appropriate patient followup, resolution of discordant cases, and quality metrics monitoring. An integrated model with colonoscopy represents an optimal paradigm for CTC screening.

REFERENCES

1. Pickhardt PJ, Hanson ME, Vanness DJ, et al. Unsuspected extracolonic findings at screening CT colonography: Clinical and economic impact. *Radiology*. 2008;249(1):151-159.
2. Pickhardt PJ, Kim DH, Cash BD, Lee AD. The natural history of small polyps at CT colonography. Rancho Mirage, CA: Annual Meeting for the Society of Gastrointestinal Radiologists; 2008.
3. Kim DH, Pickhardt PJ, Taylor AJ, et al. CT colonography versus colonoscopy for the detection of advanced neoplasia. *N Engl J Med*. 2007;357(14):1403-1412.
4. Seeff LC, Tangka FKL. Can we predict the outcomes of national colorectal cancer screening and can predictions help us plan? *Gastroenterology*. 2005;129(4):1339-1342.
5. Hur C, Gazelle GS, Zalis ME, Podolsky DK. An analysis of the potential impact of computed tomographic colonography (virtual colonoscopy) on colonoscopy demand. *Gastroenterology*. 2004; 127(5):1312-1321.
6. Schwartz DC, Dasher KJ, Said A, et al. Impact of a CT colonography screening program on endoscopic colonoscopy in clinical practice. *Am J Gastroenterol*. 2008;103(2):346-351.

Indications for Performing CT Colonography

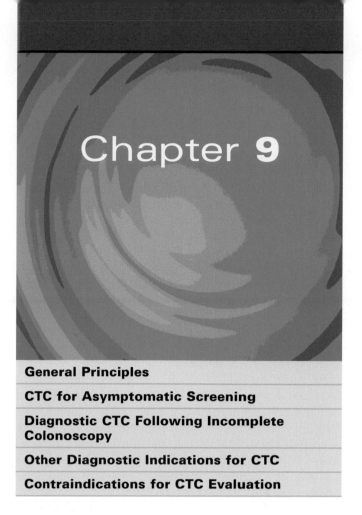

Chapter **9**

PERRY J. PICKHARDT, MD
DAVID H. KIM, MD

General Principles

CTC for Asymptomatic Screening

Diagnostic CTC Following Incomplete Colonoscopy

Other Diagnostic Indications for CTC

Contraindications for CTC Evaluation

GENERAL PRINCIPLES

The appropriate clinical indications for performing CT colonography (CTC) continue to evolve as this diagnostic tool matures (Table 9-1). Many of the indications draw parallels from both barium enema and optical colonoscopy (OC) examinations. In general terms, CTC can be divided into two main clinical entities: screening CTC and diagnostic CTC examinations. Screening CTC refers to the routine evaluation for colorectal polyps in generally asymptomatic adults, whereas diagnostic CTC refers to evaluation for a heterogeneous variety of indications other than routine screening. Completion CTC following incomplete OC currently represents the most common diagnostic indication, but a number of additional diagnostic indications are discussed in this chapter. In particular, CTC for the initial workup following a positive fecal occult blood test

result is being considered by a number of health care systems. The relative and absolute contraindications for performing CTC will also be considered at the end of this chapter.

CTC FOR ASYMPTOMATIC SCREENING

Diagnostic indications aside, screening of asymptomatic adults clearly represents the clinical indication of greatest potential for virtual colonoscopy (Table 9-1). Although colorectal carcinoma (CRC) is largely preventable through effective screening, it remains the second-leading cause of cancer-related death in the United States, largely because so many adults are not being screened at all.[1] In fact, it is estimated that more than 40 million adults in the United States have not been screened,[2] and many more have only been tested for fecal occult blood, which is not an effective means for cancer prevention and even fails to detect many cancers. CTC has recently been shown to represent a highly effective screening tool when properly performed.[3,4] Given this recent evidence, the American Cancer Society (ACS) in 2008 recommended CTC for CRC screening in its guidelines for the first time.[5] Furthermore, the ACS strongly encouraged the use of structural examinations, such as CTC and OC, which can detect precancerous polyps, over the use of fecal-

Table 9-1 ▫ Clinical Indications for Performing CTC

SCREENING INDICATIONS
Asymptomatic adults at average risk
Asymptomatic patients with positive family history*†
Asymptomatic patients at increased risk for colonoscopy†

DIAGNOSTIC INDICATIONS
Following incomplete optical colonoscopy
Evaluation of suspected submucosal lesions
Surveillance of unresected 6-9-mm polyps detected at previous CTC
Unexplained GI bleeding, iron deficiency anemia, or other GI symptoms
Symptomatic patients at increased risk for colonoscopy
Surveillance following resection of polyps or cancer†

*Excluding hereditary polyposis or nonpolyposis cancer syndromes.
†See text for details.

based tests, which largely just detect cancer and are not effective in preventing it.

For the time being, CTC should not be viewed as a replacement for OC screening, but rather as an additional effective option that has the potential to significantly increase overall compliance rates for screening. The introduction of a parallel CTC screening program at our institution has not had a negative impact on referrals for OC screening,[6] which implies that we are bringing in new individuals off the screening "sidelines" rather than simply exchanging one viable test for another. By providing additional screening options to patients, particularly tests such as CTC that are less invasive but still highly effective, it is hoped that the magnitude of the unscreened population will be reduced. We have found that sufficient multidetector CT (MDCT) capacity likely already exists for implementing a robust CTC screening program for the U.S. population.[7] Widespread reimbursement from third-party payers for CTC screening should not only lead to increased demand for this procedure, but may also fuel demand for additional MDCT scanners, which would further increase capacity for population screening. From a purely economic standpoint, the introduction of widespread CTC screening could have profound implications for radiology practices, particularly given the enormous number of adults in need of screening

CTC is ideally suited for the evaluation of average-risk adults, in which the *a priori* risk of having a large polyp necessitating OC is relatively low. In our experience with prospective CTC screening of asymptomatic adults, the prevalence of polyps at the 6- and 10-mm thresholds has remained steady at about 12% to 13% and 4% to 5%, respectively.[3,8] With regard to patient compliance and participation, the ability to provide same-day OC for polypectomy is critical because it avoids the need for a second bowel preparation. The American Gastroenterological Association has endorsed this single-prep, same-day approach as the preferred practice strategy. However, if same-day OC service is not feasible, the possibility of next-day therapy can represent a reasonable alternative whereby patients remain on clear liquids and avoid the need for additional cleansing.

CTC is also a reasonable screening option for asymptomatic patients at somewhat higher-than-average risk for CRC. Patients at slightly increased risk would primarily include those with a positive family history of CRC or a personal history of benign polyps. In our experience, the positivity rate for CTC screening in adults with a family history of CRC in a first-degree relative or with nonspecific gastrointestinal (GI) symptoms is not significantly greater than an average-risk asymptomatic cohort. This does not include patients with a personal history of a hereditary polyposis or a nonpolyposis cancer syndrome. This group is generally at much higher risk for CRC, and direct visualization with OC is generally indicated for possible therapy, particularly given the atypical appearance of lesions associated with some syndromes (e.g., hereditary nonpolyposis colon cancer syndrome).

CTC represents an ideal screening test in asymptomatic patients for whom primary OC screening is unnecessarily risky. A number of preexisting conditions render colonoscopy undesirable or unsuitable as a primary screening test. Prime examples include patients receiving anticoagulation therapy or with an underlying bleeding diathesis, patients at increased risk for sedation (e.g., those with severe chronic obstructive pulmonary disease), patients who are debilitated and/or elderly, and patients with a prior history of a difficult or complicated OC examination. This last group would include future screening for patients following completion CTC for incomplete OC.

DIAGNOSTIC CTC FOLLOWING INCOMPLETE COLONOSCOPY

Chief among the diagnostic indications for performing CTC is the completion of colorectal evaluation following an incomplete OC examination. Using CTC to evaluate the proximal colon following incomplete OC is well established and has been the predominant indication for CTC during the early prescreening era.[9-11] It should be made clear that, although most practices have been largely limited to performing CTC for this indication, this actually represents the most challenging group of patients by far. Reasons for this include the inherent underlying difficulty that lead to incomplete OC in the first place and the lack of effective oral contrast tagging if CTC is performed on the same day. This patient group can be discouraging to radiology practices just getting started with CTC, and this may dampen enthusiasm for large-scale screening. However, it is important to keep in mind that primary CTC screening produces examinations that are much easier to obtain and interpret.

Many factors can contribute to failure to intubate the cecum at OC. In addition to the commonly recognized patient associations of older age, female gender, and prior abdominal surgery,[12] along with endoscopist factors,[13] there are also common associations related to colonic anatomy. In fact, CTC itself also allows for detailed assessment of anatomy in this setting, which has shed some light on certain features associated with incomplete OC. By comparing colonic anatomy at CTC in patients who underwent incomplete versus complete OC, we found significant differences in the average total colonic length (167 cm versus 211 cm), the number of acute-angle bends or flexures (9.6 versus 11.9), and the prevalence of advanced sigmoid diverticular disease (22% versus 34%) (Fig. 9-1).[14] These findings may have relevance for training of endoscopists and for development of new endoscopic technology. Additional reasons for incomplete OC include occlusive cancers, benign strictures, colon-containing hernias, intestinal malrotation, and poor bowel

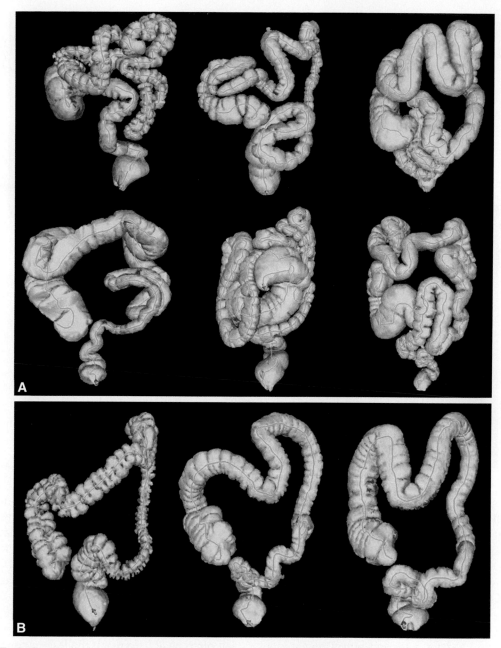

Figure 9-1   Typical colorectal anatomy at CTC in patients with incomplete versus complete OC. Collage of three-dimensional (3D) colon maps **(A)** from six different patients undergoing diagnostic CTC for incomplete OC shows the typical redundancy and tortuosity seen in this clinical setting. By comparison, note the more "classic" colorectal anatomy from three individuals **(B)** who had a complete OC examination as part of the DoD screening trial. (From Hanson ME, Pickhardt PJ, Kim DH, Pfau PR. Anatomic factors predictive of incomplete colonoscopy based on findings at CT colonography. *Am J Roentgenol.* 2007;189:774-779.)

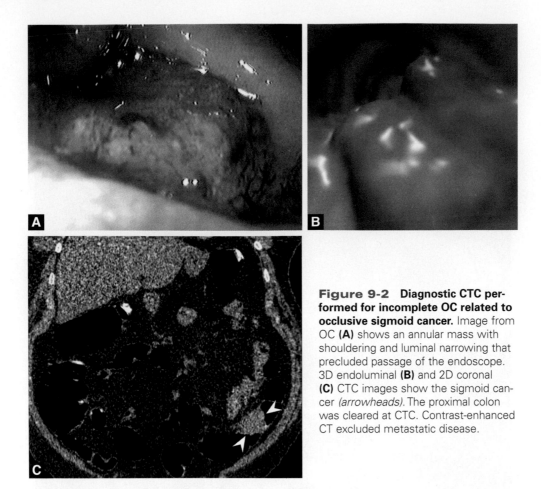

Figure 9-2 Diagnostic CTC performed for incomplete OC related to occlusive sigmoid cancer. Image from OC **(A)** shows an annular mass with shouldering and luminal narrowing that precluded passage of the endoscope. 3D endoluminal **(B)** and 2D coronal **(C)** CTC images show the sigmoid cancer *(arrowheads)*. The proximal colon was cleared at CTC. Contrast-enhanced CT excluded metastatic disease.

preparation (Figs. 9-2 through 9-8). Combinations of these factors will further increase the likelihood of incomplete OC (Fig. 9-7). In patients with persistently inadequate bowel preparation for colonoscopy despite all reasonable efforts, CTC can still generally exclude large polyps and masses as long as oral contrast tagging is used.

Performing CTC after failed colonoscopy presents a number of protocol challenges. From the patient's perspective, same-day CTC is clearly the most convenient because it avoids the need for a second bowel preparation and can often be performed as soon as the patient has recovered from sedation. The main disadvantage to this same-day approach, however, is that attempts at oral contrast tagging are often suboptimal, which can significantly affect the study quality and likely reduce the accuracy of CTC interpretation. Without oral contrast, however, residual untagged stool can lead to false-positive interpretations that are almost never seen when oral contrast tagging is used (Fig. 9-9). Unfortunately, same-day salvage efforts for providing oral contrast tagging have proved to be only moderately successful in our experience. We generally have patients drink a small volume (e.g., 30 mL) of diatrizoate when adequately recovered from OC and wait a couple of hours before scanning (Fig. 9-10). In some cases, excess luminal fluid or streak artifact from dense residual contrast in the stomach significantly degrades the

quality of the study without effectively tagging residual fecal material. Furthermore, the risk for aspiration of hyperosmolar iodinated contrast material may be of concern if attempted too soon after the sedation for OC. Despite these technical challenges related to CTC following incomplete OC, detection of significant pathology beyond the reach of the endoscope is not rare (Figs. 9-10 and 9-11). Once an important proximal finding is detected at CTC after incomplete OC, an experienced colonoscopist will often be able to reach the lesion, armed with the specific knowledge of the anatomic challenges and the increased motivation to reach the CTC-detected lesion (Figs. 9-10 and 9-11).

Possible alternative options to same-day oral contrast tagging include the use of intravenous contrast, rectal enema contrast, or overnight oral contrast dosing, leaving the patient on clear liquids in the interim. Another consideration for the future is the routine use of oral contrast administration as part of the standard bowel preparation for OC. The tagging agents are not a hindrance at colonoscopy and yet are invaluable in the event that completion CTC becomes necessary. From a purely clinical standpoint, having the patient return on another day following a dedicated CTC bowel preparation is currently the best option because it will yield the most accurate examination (Figs. 9-2, 9-6, 9-7, and

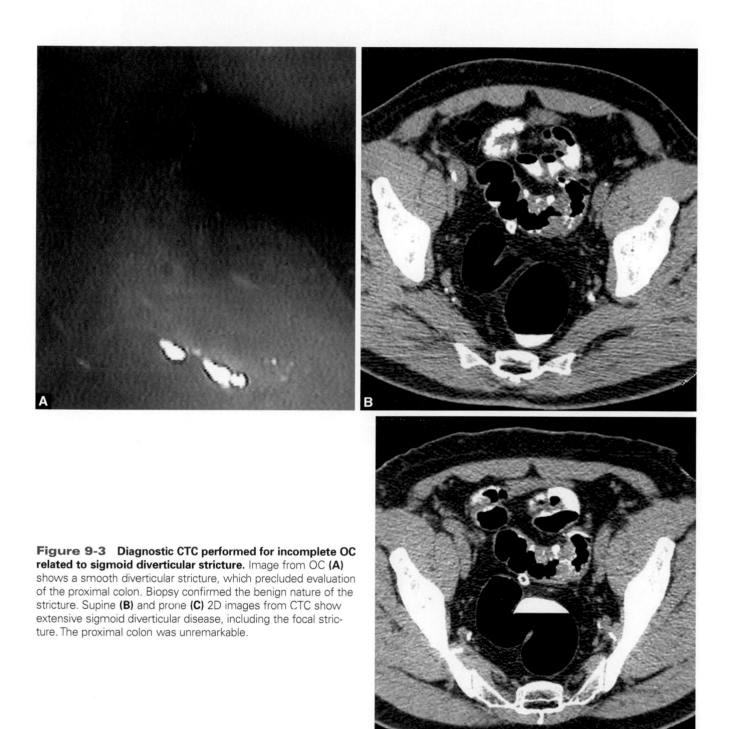

Figure 9-3   Diagnostic CTC performed for incomplete OC related to sigmoid diverticular stricture. Image from OC **(A)** shows a smooth diverticular stricture, which precluded evaluation of the proximal colon. Biopsy confirmed the benign nature of the stricture. Supine **(B)** and prone **(C)** 2D images from CTC show extensive sigmoid diverticular disease, including the focal stricture. The proximal colon was unremarkable.

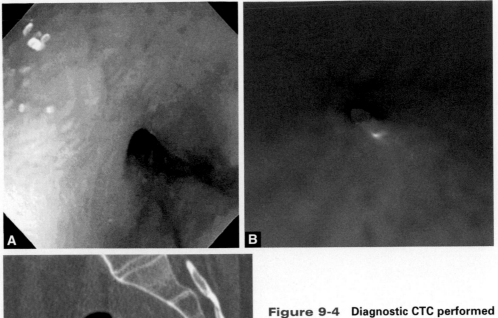

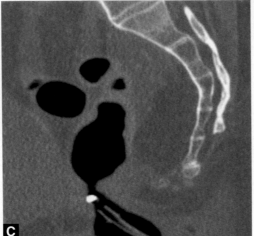

Figure 9-4 Diagnostic CTC performed for incomplete OC related benign high-grade rectal stricture from prior treatment for rectal lymphoma. Image from OC **(A)** shows the stricture within the distal rectum. 3D endoluminal **(B)** and 2D sagittal **(C)** CTC images show the high-grade stricture, which focally narrowed the lumen to 6 mm in diameter. The proximal rectum and colon were cleared by CTC.

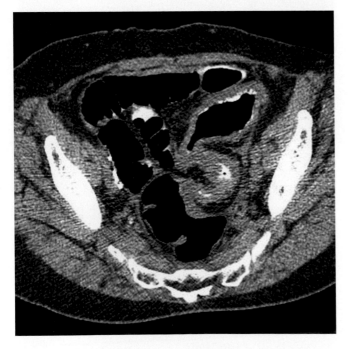

Figure 9-5 Diagnostic CTC performed for multiple prior incomplete OC examinations related to a complex radiation stricture involving the sigmoid colon. 2D transverse CTC image shows long-segment wall thickening and luminal narrowing of the sigmoid colon, associated with a fixed, kinked appearance. No significant lesions were seen in the proximal colon.

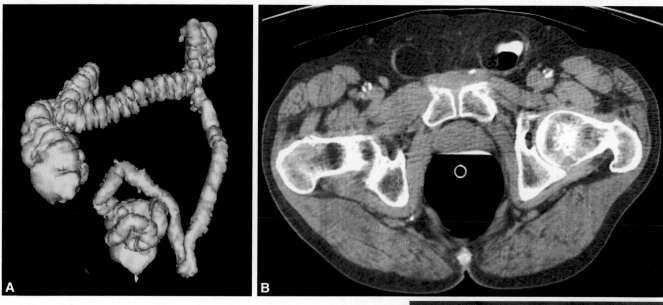

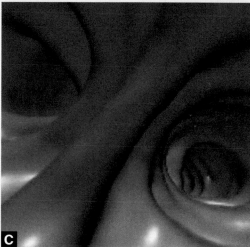

Figure 9-6   Diagnostic CTC performed for incomplete OC related to inguinal herniation of the sigmoid colon. 3D colon map **(A)** shows an abnormally low position of the sigmoid colon, which dips to the level of the anorectal junction. 2D transverse CTC image **(B)** shows the sigmoid colon within the inguinal canal. 3D endoluminal image **(C)** from the vantage of the hernia sac shows good distention of the proximal colon.

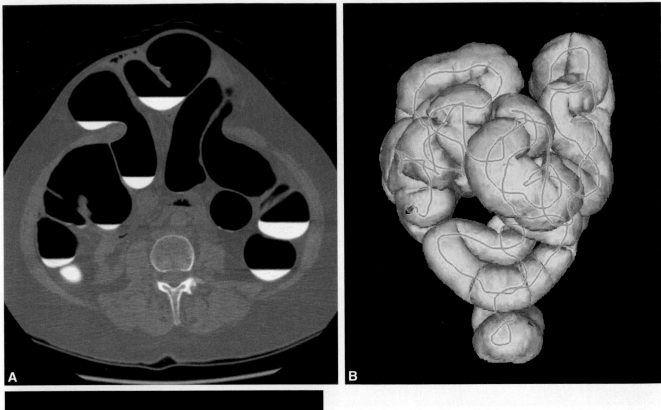

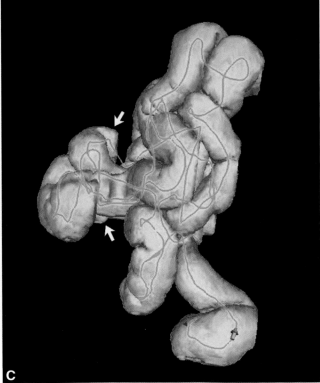

Figure 9-7 **Diagnostic CTC performed for incomplete OC related to both colonic redundancy and ventral herniation of a portion of the colon.** 2D transverse CTC image **(A)** shows several loops of colon extending through a wide-mouth ventral hernia. Note the excellent colonic preparation and distention. Frontal 3D colon map **(B)** shows the marked redundancy of the colon, with a total length of 325 cm. Lateral 3D colon map **(C)** shows the herniated loops of colon *(arrows)*.

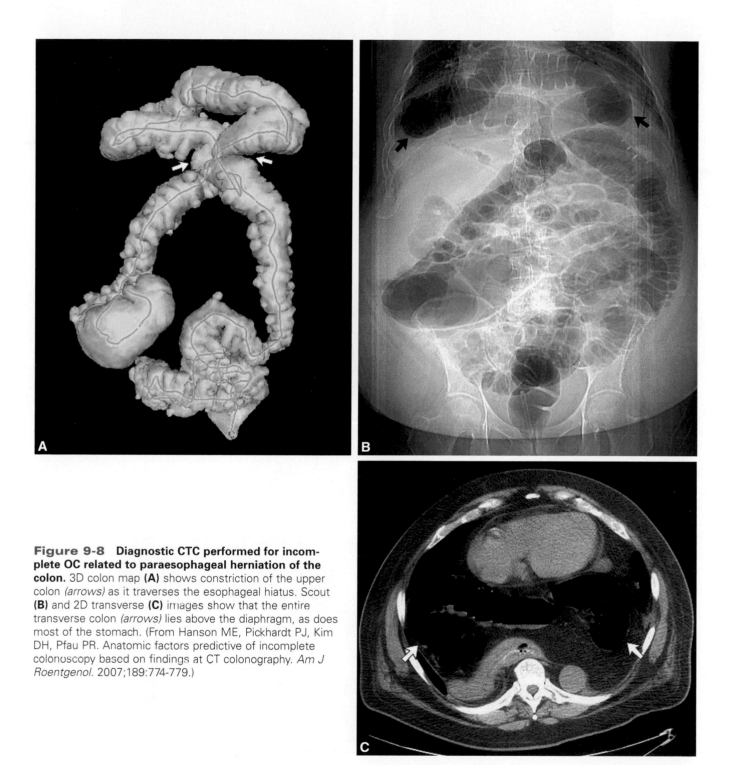

Figure 9-8 Diagnostic CTC performed for incomplete OC related to paraesophageal herniation of the colon. 3D colon map **(A)** shows constriction of the upper colon *(arrows)* as it traverses the esophageal hiatus. Scout **(B)** and 2D transverse **(C)** images show that the entire transverse colon *(arrows)* lies above the diaphragm, as does most of the stomach. (From Hanson ME, Pickhardt PJ, Kim DH, Pfau PR. Anatomic factors predictive of incomplete colonoscopy based on findings at CT colonography. *Am J Roentgenol.* 2007;189:774-779.)

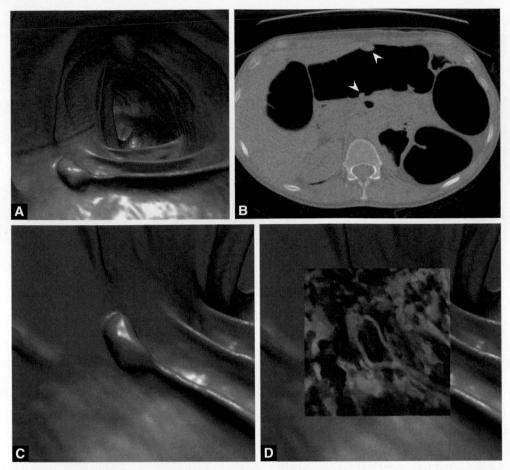

Figure 9-9 **Residual untagged stool on diagnostic CTC performed the same-day after incomplete OC.** 3D endoluminal CTC image **(A)** shows two polypoid lesions within the transverse colon, which have a fairly homogeneous appearance on 2D correlation (**B,** *arrowheads*). 3D endoluminal images without **(C)** and with **(D)** translucency rendering show a nearly homogeneous red core to one of the "lesions." This appearance of adherent untagged stool mimicking true soft tissue polyps can be avoided with oral contrast tagging. (*See associated video clip in DVD.)

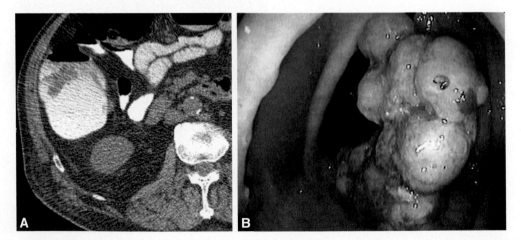

Figure 9-10 **Large right-sided mass (4-cm tubular adenoma) identified in opacified luminal fluid at diagnostic CTC.** The patient had undergone OC preparation with PEG but was deemed medically unfit for invasive endoscopy and was referred for same-day CTC. 2D transverse CTC image **(A)** shows a large amount of residual luminal fluid. However, opacification of the fluid with diatrizoate allowed for the detection of a large lobulated soft tissue match extending along a fold in the ascending colon. Because cancer could not be excluded, the patient underwent subsequent OC **(B)** and ultimately surgical resection.

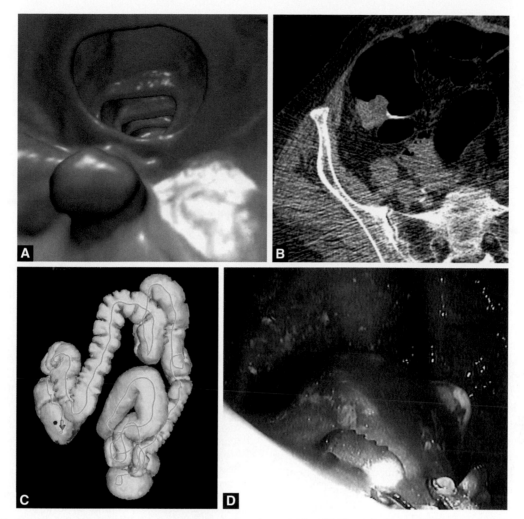

Figure 9-11   **Large cecal mass (3-cm non-Hodgkin's lymphoma) identified at diagnostic CTC performed for incomplete OC.** 3D endoluminal **(A)** and 2D transverse **(B)** CTC images show a large lobulated cecal mass adjacent to the ileocecal valve. 3D colon map **(C)** shows that the left colon is moderately redundant. Repeat OC **(D)** confirmed a large submucosal mass, which proved to be lymphoma. (*See associated video clip in DVD.)

9-11). Despite this, most completion CTC studies are still performed on the same day as the incomplete colonoscopy, with or without contrast, for the sake of patient convenience.

OTHER DIAGNOSTIC INDICATIONS FOR CTC

Beyond incomplete OC, there are a number of other established indications for performing diagnostic CTC (Table 9-1). CTC evaluation for suspected submucosal lesions detected at OC can be valuable in distinguishing a true intramural process from extrinsic impression by an extracolonic structure.[15,16] Such distinction can be surprisingly difficult at strictly luminal examinations such as OC, and attempts at endoscopic biopsy are generally nondiagnostic and possibly even dangerous. CTC evaluation of submucosal lesions is discussed in detail in

Chapter 22. Surveillance of unresected small (6-9 mm) polyps initially detected at a previous CTC examination is an evolving indication that has been recognized in consensus statements and screening guidelines.[5,17] One or two small polyps correspond to C-RADS category C2,[17] for which 3-year CTC surveillance appears to be a reasonable option, especially given the low rate of advanced histology in these lesions and the high costs associated with OC polypectomy.[18] Furthermore, only a small minority of 6- to 9-mm polyps will demonstrate interval growth at short-term surveillance.[3,19,20] Long-term management of subcentimeter polyps that fail to grow at CTC followup can probably return to routine screening intervals. Specifics on the natural history of small colorectal polyps can be found in Chapter 2.

CTC represents a reasonable test for the initial evaluation of unexplained GI bleeding, iron-deficiency anemia, or certain other nonspecific GI complaints in some

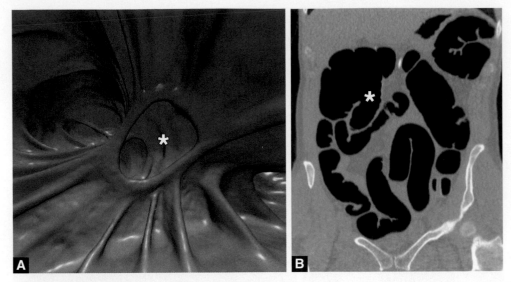

Figure 9-12   CTC evaluation in patient with prior ileocecal resection. 3D endoluminal **(A)** and 2D coronal **(B)** images show the ileocolic anastomosis *(asterisk),* which is widely patent. Colonic distention was excellent despite the absence of the ileocecal valve.

patients. This includes patients of screening age with a positive fecal occult blood test (FOBT) result. Although OC has been traditionally used in this clinical setting, the relatively low specificity of a positive FOBT or other GI symptoms in relation to colorectal polyps and cancer, along with the expense, invasiveness, and limited capacity of OC, makes CTC an attractive option for excluding significant pathology. In fact, some centralized health systems are considering widespread use of CTC for patients with a positive FOBT result. As with asymptomatic screening noted earlier, CTC in the presence of a preexisting condition that makes primary OC unsuitable would also apply to most diagnostic indications. The role of CTC for postpolypectomy surveillance or following CRC treatment has not been well established. In general, OC surveillance strategies are currently recommended for these patient groups.[5] In addition, there is some evidence that missed polyps or regrowth of polyps found in patients after a clearing OC examination may be more difficult to detect at surveillance CTC.[21] However, IV (intravenous) contrast-enhanced CTC has been shown to be an effective surveillance tool by some following curative-intent surgery for CRC.[22] In general, we have had good success in achieving diagnostic distention in patients with a history of partial colectomy, including ileocecal resection and right hemicolectomy, in which the ileocecal valve is absent (Fig. 9-12).

CONTRAINDICATIONS FOR CTC EVALUATION

Most contraindications for performing CTC are relative and not absolute (Table 9-2). The absolute contraindications are analogous to those for barium enema exami-

Table 9-2 ▫ Relative and Absolute Contraindications for Performing CTC

Fulminant colitis
Any symptomatic acute colitis
Acute diarrhea
Acute diverticulitis
Pregnancy
Recent colorectal surgery
Colon-containing inguinal hernia
Recent deep endoscopic biopsy or polypectomy
Known or suspected colonic perforation
Symptomatic or high-grade bowel obstruction
Routine followup of inflammatory bowel disease
Hereditary polyposis or nonpolyposis cancer syndromes*

*Unless part of a carefully orchestrated surveillance strategy alternating with OC.

nation and generally include any condition for which there is a high likelihood for colonic perforation. Prime examples include any severe acute fulminant or toxic colitis, regardless of the cause; recent colonic surgery; and recent known or suspected colonic perforation from any cause. Acute colonic diverticulitis represents another contraindication for CTC. Four to 6 weeks is probably an appropriate minimum time interval for waiting to perform routine CTC following conservative treatment for uncomplicated diverticulitis. In general, a conservative time delay between any acute colonic event or disease and CTC evaluation is prudent because this examination is almost never urgently needed. Inguinal herniation of the sigmoid colon is a relatively rare finding but can result in a closed-loop obstruction and even perforation if manual room air distention is used. In fact, four of the seven colonic perforations reported in an Israeli CTC experience were related to inguinal herniation of the sigmoid colon.[23] The risk of sigmoid perforation with low-pressure automated CO_2 delivery is probably extremely low, but recognition of the inguinal hernia is critical because inappropriate conversion to manual room air might be otherwise considered (Fig. 9-13). Most other colon-containing hernias are wide-mouthed and unlikely to cause significant problems at CTC, but they may result in incomplete evaluation at OC (Figs. 9-7 and 9-8).

The risk of performing CTC immediately after an incomplete OC largely hinges on the complexity and difficulty of the preceding endoscopic examination. If a deeply penetrating biopsy was performed at OC, we prefer to wait 4 to 6 weeks before proceeding with CTC. However, we will often perform same-day completion

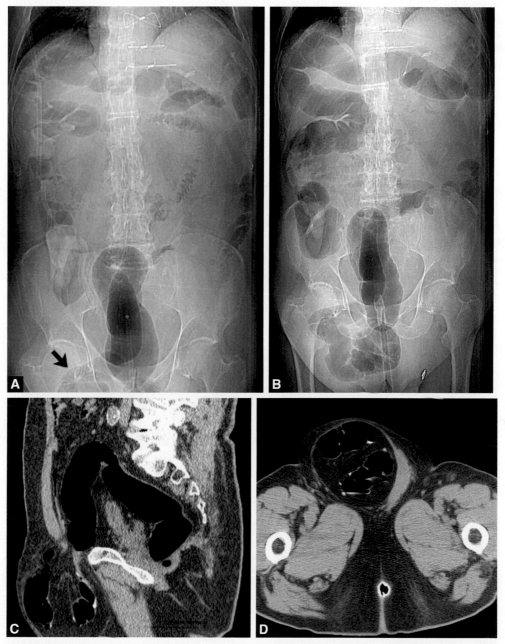

Figure 9-13 **Inguinal herniation of sigmoid colon at primary CTC evaluation.** Initial scout view **(A)** shows good rectal distention but very little gas within the proximal colon. The air-filled sigmoid loop projecting over the right groin *(arrow)* was not appreciated by the technologist. Repeat scout view **(B)** after a larger-caliber rectal balloon catheter was placed more clearly shows the herniated loop of sigmoid. Some proximal distention is now present. 2D sagittal **(C)** and transverse **(D)** CTC images show the inguinal herniation. Except for focally collapsed areas extending through the inguinal canal, the examination was diagnostic.

CTC when only superficial biopsies are taken. Given the wide array of endoscopic biopsy techniques for polypectomy, we primarily rely on the colonoscopist to determine whether a "superficial" or "deep" biopsy was performed. If an incomplete OC was felt to be particularly difficult or traumatic, but there is a strong desire to perform same-day CTC, we may still proceed but use appropriate caution. For example, we may take a preliminary scout and selected cross-sectional CT images prior to CO_2 distention to exclude a preexisting perforation. Of note, unsuspected perforation following incomplete OC may be detected at CTC with preliminary imaging in about 1% of cases.[24] If preliminary imaging is not performed prior to CTC following a difficult incomplete OC examination, the presence of extraluminal gas may be (incorrectly) blamed on CTC (Fig. 9-14). In our experience, most cases of perforation from OC will manifest with extraperitoneal gas that may not be obvious on conventional radiography.[25]

The role of CTC in patients with inflammatory bowel disease (ulcerative colitis and Crohn's disease) is controversial. For any patient with a suspected acute flareup of inflammatory bowel disease, CTC is probably contraindicated. Routine CT (or MR) without colonography technique is excellent in this setting, whether using enterography technique or not. CTC is generally not indicated for patients with hereditary colon cancer syndromes, whether polyposis or nonpolyposis in nature, as noted earlier. However, it is conceivable that CTC may eventually prove useful as an alternating surveillance strategy with OC in patients with either inflammatory bowel disease or a hereditary cancer syndrome because of the complementary nature of these two diagnostic tools (Fig. 9-15).

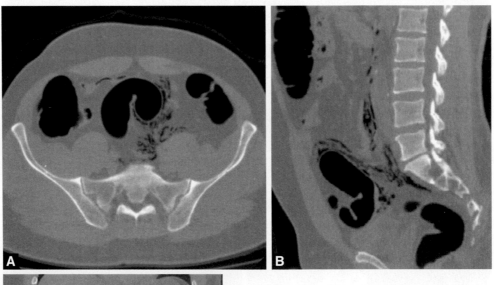

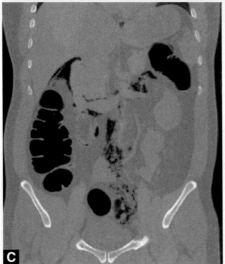

Figure 9-14 **Unsuspected colonic perforation at incomplete OC diagnosed at same-day diagnostic CTC.** Transverse **(A)**, sagittal **(B)**, and coronal **(C)** 2D CTC images show extraluminal gas extending along the sigmoid mesentery and superiorly along retroperitoneal fascial planes. Incomplete OC earlier the same day was difficult and included sigmoid polypectomy. (Case courtesy of Joel Bortz, MD.)

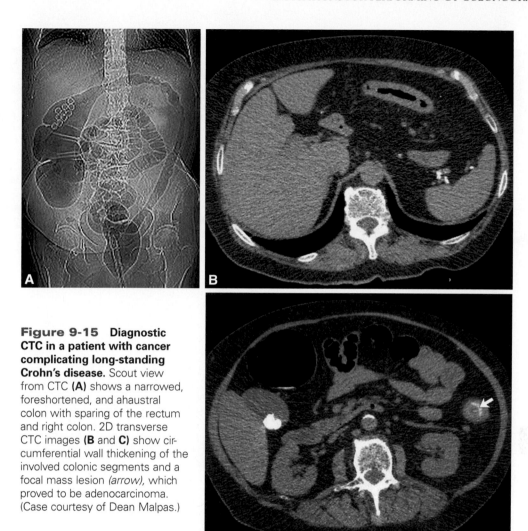

Figure 9-15 Diagnostic CTC in a patient with cancer complicating long-standing Crohn's disease. Scout view from CTC **(A)** shows a narrowed, foreshortened, and ahaustral colon with sparing of the rectum and right colon. 2D transverse CTC images **(B** and **C)** show circumferential wall thickening of the involved colonic segments and a focal mass lesion *(arrow),* which proved to be adenocarcinoma. (Case courtesy of Dean Malpas.)

REFERENCES

1. Jemal A, Siegel R, Ward E, Murray T, Xu JQ, Thun MJ. Cancer statistics, 2007. *CA Cancer J Clin.* 2007;57(1):43-66.
2. Seeff LC, Manninen DL, Dong FB, et al. Is there endoscopic capacity to provide colorectal cancer screening to the unscreened population in the United States? *Gastroenterology.* 2004;127(6): 1661-1669.
3. Kim DH, Pickhardt PJ, Taylor AJ, et al. CT colonography versus colonoscopy for the detection of advanced neoplasia. *N Engl J Med.* 2007;357(14):1403-1412.
4. Pickhardt PJ, Choi JR, Hwang I, et al. Computed tomographic virtual colonoscopy to screen for colorectal neoplasia in asymptomatic adults. *N Engl J Med.* 2003;349(23):2191-2200.
5. Levin B, Lieberman DA, McFarland B, et al. Screening and surveillance for the early detection of colorectal cancer and adenomatous polyps, 2008: A joint guideline from the American Cancer Society, the US Multi-Society Task Force on Colorectal Cancer, and the American College of Radiology. *CA Cancer J Clin.* 2008;58(3):130-160.
6. Schwartz DC, Dasher KJ, Said A, et al. Impact of a CT colonography screening program on endoscopic colonoscopy in clinical practice. *Am J Gastroenterol.* 2008;103(2):346-351.
7. Pickhardt PJ, Hassan C, Laghi A, et al. Is there sufficient MDCT capacity to provide colorectal cancer screening with CT colonography for the US population? *Am J Roentgenol.* 2008;190(4):1044-1049.
8. Pickhardt PJ, Taylor AJ, Kim DH, Reichelderfer M, Gopal DV, Pfau PR. Screening for colorectal neoplasia with CT colonography: Initial experience from the 1st year of coverage by third-party payers. *Radiology.* 2006;241(2):417-425.
9. Macari M, Berman P, Dicker M, Milano A, Megibow AJ. Usefulness of CT colonography in patients with incomplete colonoscopy. *Am J Roentgenol.* 1999;173(3):561-564.
10. Morrin MM, Kruskal JB, Farrell RJ, Goldberg SN, McGee JB, Raptopoulos V. Endoluminal CT colonography after an incomplete endoscopic colonoscopy. *Am J Roentgenol.* 1999;172(4):913-918.
11. Copel L, Sosna J, Kruskal JB, Raptopoulos V, Farrell RJ, Morrin MM. CT colonography in 546 patients with incomplete colonoscopy. *Radiology.* 2007;244(2):471-478.
12. Dafnis G, Granath F, Pahlman L, Ekbom A, Blomqvist P. Patient factors influencing the completion rate in colonoscopy. *Digest Liver Dis.* 2005;37(2):113-118.
13. Harewood GC. Relationship of colonoscopy completion rates and endoscopist features. *Dig Dis Sci.* 2005;50(1):47-51.
14. Hanson ME, Pickhardt PJ, Kim DH, Pfau PR. Anatomic factors predictive of incomplete colonoscopy based on findings at CT colonography. *Am J Roentgenol.* 2007;189(4):774-779.

15. Pickhardt PJ, Kim DH, Menias CO, Gopal DV, Arluk GM, Heise CP. Evaluation of submucosal lesions of the large intestine: Part 1. Neoplasms. *Radiographics*. 2007;27(6):1681-1692.

16. Pickhardt PJ, Kim DH, Menias CO, Gopal DV, Arluk GM, Heise CP. Evaluation of submucosal lesions of the large intestine: Part 2. Nonneoplastic causes. *Radiographics*. 2007;27(6):1693-1703.

17. Zalis ME, Barish MA, Choi JR, et al. CT colonography reporting and data system: A consensus proposal. *Radiology*. 2005;236(1):3-9.

18. Pickhardt PJ, Hassan C, Laghi A, et al. Small and diminutive polyps detected at screening CT colonography: A decision analysis for referral to colonoscopy. *Am J Roentgenol*. 2008;190(1):136-144.

19. Pickhardt PJ. The natural history of colorectal polyps and masses: Rediscovered truths from the barium enema era. *Am J Roentgenol*. 2007;188(3):619-621.

20. Pickhardt PJ, Kim DH, Cash BD, Lee AD. The natural history of small polyps at CT colonography. Annual Meeting. Society of Gastrointestinal Radiologists: Rancho Mirage, CA; 2008.

21. MacCarty RL, Johnson CD, Fletcher JG, Wilson LA. Occult colorectal polyps on CT colonography: Implications for surveillance. *Am J Roentgenol*. 2006;186(5):1380-1383.

22. Choi YJ, Park SH, Lee SS, et al. CT Colonography for follow-up after surgery for colorectal cancer. *Am J Roentgenol*. 2007;189(2):283-289.

23. Sosna J, Blachar A, Amitai M, et al. Colonic perforation at CT colonography: Assessment of risk in a multicenter large cohort. *Radiology*. 2006;239(2):457-463.

24. Hough DM, Kuntz MA, Fidler JL, et al. Detection of occult colonic perforation before CT colonography after incomplete colonoscopy: perforation rate and use of a low-dose diagnostic scan before CO_2 insufflation. *Am J Roentgenol*. 2008;191(4):1077-1081.

25. Kim DH, Pickhardt PJ, Taylor AJ, Menias CO. Imaging evaluation of complications at optical colonoscopy. *Curr Probl Diagn Radiol*. 2008;37(4):165-177.

Economic Aspects of CT Colonography

PERRY J. PICKHARDT, MD
DAVID H. KIM, MD

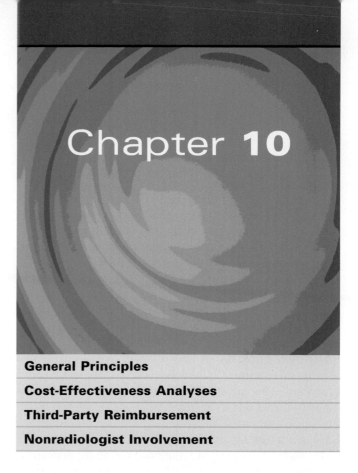

Chapter 10

- General Principles
- Cost-Effectiveness Analyses
- Third-Party Reimbursement
- Nonradiologist Involvement

GENERAL PRINCIPLES

The economic aspects of CT colonography (CTC) unavoidably affect all levels of consideration, from the individual clinical radiologist or group trying to decide whether including CTC in their practice makes good fiscal sense to the health care policymakers trying to determine whether screening with CTC is cost effective from a population standpoint. A cost-effectiveness analysis (CEA) can be an important tool for assessing and comparing different colorectal cancer (CRC) screening tests. However, one must carefully consider the various input assumptions driving each model, the type of modeling that is used, and even the potential for bias among the investigators (i.e., is there an *a priori* agenda?). In the United States, third-party reimbursement dominates the economic landscape for practicing radiologists. Without such insurance coverage in place, a large-volume screening CTC practice simply cannot exist. Although we had hoped for a grassroots movement pushing local third-party payers to cover screening CTC, similar to what we accomplished at the University of Wisconsin (UW) back in April 2004, it now appears more likely that a typical top-down approach starting with Medicare coverage and/or other national payers will transpire. Still other issues worthy of consideration are the impact of potential nonradiologist involvement, including both interpretation and outright ownership of CTC. Because of the rapid evolution of CTC itself and its role in clinical practice, this chapter will probably be rendered obsolete before it is even in print. Furthermore, we do not feign to be either proper medical economists or business experts, so this chapter will be more of our layman's view of cost-effectiveness and business analysis regarding CTC.

COST-EFFECTIVENESS ANALYSES

CEA studies and other economic analyses generally strive to quantify the cost for achieving a specific health outcome. For analyses involving CRC screening, this is typically the cost per life year gained from specific screening interventions. Some studies report in terms of cost per "quality-adjusted life year" (QALY) gained. Regardless, this outcome is generally more valuable than reporting the cost per individual screened, cost per CRC detected, or other such measure. The threshold for what constitutes a "cost-effective" CRC screening test is arbitrary. Although values of $100,000 or $50,000 per life year gained compared with no screening are often generically used in CEA studies, these turn out to be soft targets for CRC screening, in which much lower values are typically seen. In general, one must always keep in mind that CEA models are artificial attempts to capture complex real-life events, and the results can be exquisitely sensitive to the input variables, many of which represent "best guesses." Other economic analyses beyond cost-effectiveness considerations, such as cost-utility, cost-benefit, and cost-minimization studies, will not be addressed in this brief review.

When assessing a CEA study, some key elements to consider include the model type, analytic perspective (e.g., societal or payer), time horizon, specific study population, interventions being compared, data source for input assumptions, and specific costs that are—or are not—included.[1] CEA studies may use a Markov model, microsimulation model, or decision tree analysis in evaluating CRC screening tests, making comparison of different CEA studies more challenging. "Markov" seems to be a powerful buzzword for some when considering CEA studies. However, just because such an analysis was performed is absolutely no guarantee of either study quality or accurate reflection of reality. A well-done decision tree analysis is much more useful than a poorly executed Markov analysis. With analyses related to CRC screening, a given intervention will often be compared with no screening (in terms of cost per life year gained). As noted earlier, given the favorable aspects of CRC in terms of screening and prevention, nearly all tests will generally be cost effective relative to doing nothing. When one screening test is compared with another, the incremental cost-effectiveness ratio (ICER) represents the additional cost per life year gained, assuming the more costly option is also more clinically effective. When one screening test is both more clinically effective (i.e., a relative gain of life years) and more cost effective compared with another test, it is said to be *dominant*—or the inferior test is said to be *dominated*. The primary results reported from a CEA study reflect the baseline input assumptions that were made. A "sensitivity analysis" is usually performed in addition, which evaluates the effect of varying certain key input variables over a plausible range.

For better or worse, nearly all CTC-related CEA studies prior to 2008 were largely conducted by gastroenterology groups with little or no radiology input.[2-6] Most of these Markov studies showed that CTC was cost effective compared with no intervention, which is important assuming that CTC would increase overall compliance and not simply replace optical colonoscopy (OC). However, the main focus of these studies was often on the direct comparison between CTC and OC, for which the latter generally came out ahead. Without going into fine detail for each model or study, a number of factors contributed to these predictable findings, including pessimistic assumptions for CTC performance, optimistic values for OC performance, inaccurate cost estimates, skewed natural history assumptions, and so on. In the sensitivity analyses of many of these works, which can be important but often get buried deep in the text, there are many plausible or even preferable input assumptions for which CTC appeared very favorable. In particular, the CTC/OC cost ratio was an important variable, with very favorable results when a ratio of 0.6 or less was used. Compliance is another critical variable in some studies. One critical flaw common to many or all of these initial studies was the lack of any provision for a polyp size threshold that would trigger referral from CTC screening to OC polypectomy, which would reflect actual clinical practice.

In 2006, an opportune communication with Cesare Hassan, an Italian gastroenterologist and expert in mathematical modeling and cost-effectiveness analyses, ultimately led to a fruitful and enduring collaboration, resulting in a number of publications relevant to CRC screening.[7-13] The impetus behind contacting Dr. Hassan in the first place was related to the need for improving the cost-effectiveness modeling of CTC screening, which included, among other things, proper handling of diminutive lesions. This led to our first CEA collaboration that was published in *Cancer* in 2007.[12] To match published consensus guidelines and our own clinical practice,[14,15] we assumed nonreporting of isolated diminutive lesions at CTC screening. In addition, we were able to update many other input assumptions to better reflect reality. By comparing CTC, OC, and flexible sigmoidoscopy (FS) in a hypothetical screening cohort of 100,000 individuals, our Markov analysis showed that CTC with a 6-mm reporting threshold was the safest and most cost-effective screening option, costing only $4361 per life year gained compared with no screening intervention (Table 10-1). Reporting of diminutive lesions at CTC raised the CRC prevention rate only about 1% (from 36.5% to 37.8%), with an ICER of more than $100,000 per life year gained. CTC screening resulted in a 78% reduction in invasive endoscopic procedures compared with primary OC screening (39,374 versus 175,911) and more than 1000 fewer OC-related complications from perforation or bleeding. We concluded that removal of diminutive lesions carries an unjustified burden of costs and complications relative to the minimal gains in CRC prevention.

We have built on this initial CEA collaboration with a number of subsequent publications,[7-11,13,16] some of which we will briefly review here. To evaluate the impact of sending small and diminutive CTC-detected polyps to OC, we constructed a decision analysis model incorporating the expected polyp distribution, advanced adenoma prevalence, CRC risk, CTC performance, and costs related to CRC screening and treatment.[10] It is important to note that the model conservatively assumed that CRC risk was independent of advanced adenoma size, which clearly overestimates the risk of subcentimeter polyps. Here, a *3-mm* tubulovillous adenoma would carry the same cancer risk as a *3-cm* villous adenoma with high-grade dysplasia. Nonetheless, we found that the number of diminutive, small, and large polyps that needed to be removed to avoid leaving behind one advanced adenoma was 562, 71, and 2.5, respectively; similarly, 2352, 297, and 10.7 polypectomies would be needed, respectively, to prevent one CRC over 10 years (Table 10-2). The estimated 10-year CRC risk for unresected diminutive, small, and large polyps was found to be 0.08%, 0.7%, and 15.8%, respectively. The incremental cost-effectiveness ratio of removing all diminutive and small CTC-detected polyps was $464,407 and $59,015 per life year gained, respectively. Polypectomy for large CTC-detected polyps was cost saving at $151 per person screened. We concluded that the very low likelihood of advanced neoplasia and the high costs

Table 10-1 ◻ Modeled Outcomes at Baseline Assumptions for a Variety of CRC Screening Tests[12]

Variable	CTC 6-mm Reporting Threshold	CTC No Reporting Threshold	FS	OC
Cases of CRC prevented	1073	1110	924	1187
CRC prevention	36.5%	37.8%	31.4%	40.4%
Life years gained	4266	4372	3609	4641
Procedures				
CTC	141,176	140,052		
FS			141,246	
OC	39,374	61,849	50,838	175,9511
OC-related complications	351	691	610	1463
Bleeding event	253	525	455	1036
Perforation	98	166	154	427
Without advanced lesion	301	642	566	1415
Total cost	$116,581,633	$129,183,146	124,705,103	$140,582,839
Cost per life year gained*	$4361	$7138	$7407	$9180

CRC, colorectal cancer; CTC, CT colonography; FS, flexible sigmoidoscopy; OC, optical colonoscopy.
*Compared with no screening. The cost of no screening was $97,976,886.
(From Pickhardt PJ, Hassan C, Laghi A, Zullo A, Kim DH, Morini S. Cost-effectiveness of colorectal cancer screening with computed tomography colonography—The impact of not reporting diminutive lesions. *Cancer.* 2007;109:2213-2221.)

Table 10-2 ◻ Number of CTC-Detected Polyps Needed to be Removed at Colonoscopy and the Associated Cost Implications[10]

Polyp Size Category	Number of Polypectomies		Estimated 10-Year CRC Risk of Unresected Polyp (%)	Incremental Cost-Effectiveness Ratio (cost per life year gained)
	Per Advanced Adenoma Removed	Per CRC Prevented over 10 Years		
Diminutive (≤5 mm)	562	2352	0.08	$464,407
Small (6-9 mm)	71	297	0.7	$59,015
Large (≥10 mm)	2.5	10.7	15.7	−$151 per person (cost savings)

(From Pickhardt PJ, Hassan C, Laghi A, et al. Small and diminutive polyps detected at screening CT colonography: A decision analysis for referral to colonoscopy. *Am J Roentgenol.* 2008;190:136-144.)

associated with polypectomy argue against colonoscopic referral for diminutive polyps, whereas removal of large CTC-detected polyps was highly effective. The yield of colonoscopic referral for small polyps was relatively low, suggesting that CTC surveillance may represent a reasonable management option.

We modified our Markov CEA model to include the additional clinical and economic impact of extracolonic evaluation at CTC for detecting unsuspected extracolonic cancers and abdominal aortic aneurysms (AAA).[8] We also compared the findings against a competing screening intervention of OC with or without abdominal ultrasound for AAA detection (OC-ultrasound [US] strategy). We found that CTC was the dominant screening strategy, (i.e., more clinically effec-

tive and more cost effective) over both the OC and OC-US strategies (Table 10-3). The additional gain in life years for CTC in this study was largely the result of a decrease in AAA-related deaths, whereas the modeled benefit from extracolonic cancer downstaging was a relatively minor factor. At sensitivity analysis, OC-US became more cost effective only when the CTC sensitivity for large polyps dropped to 61% or when broad variations of costs were simulated (Fig. 10-1). Even with pessimistic and probably unrealistic assumptions about the health effects of radiation, the estimated mortality from CT-induced cancer was still less than estimated colonoscopy-related mortality (8 versus 22 deaths), both of which were minor when compared with the positive benefit from screening.

Table 10-3 ◨ Incremental Cost-Effectiveness Ratios (ICERs) for CRC Screening with CTC, OC, and OC Combined with US[8]

Screening Strategy	No Screening	OC	OC-US
CTC	$12,025	−$266, OC–dominated*	−$449, OC-US–dominated*
OC-US	$16,350	$18,338	NA
OC	$16,165	NA	NA

CTC, computed tomographic colonography; NA, not applicable; OC, colonoscopy; US, abdominal ultrasonography for abdominal aortic aneurysm detection.
*Dominance implies that CTC is less expensive and more effective, resulting in the listed earnings (cost savings) per person.
(From Hassan C, Pickhardt P, Laghi A, et al. Computed tomographic colonography to screen for colorectal cancer, extracolonic cancer, and aortic aneurysm. *Arch Intern Med.* 2008;168:696-705.)

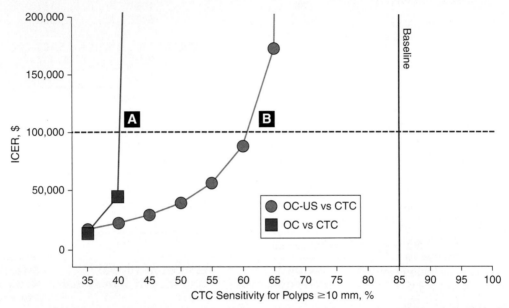

Figure 10-1 **Incremental cost-effectiveness ratio (ICER) of CTC as compared with OC and combined OC-US strategies according to CTC sensitivity for large polyps.** Data beyond 70% (OC-US) and 44% (OC) sensitivity, including the baseline value of 85%, are not shown because OC-US and OC were dominated at these levels. At less than 70% and 44% CTC sensitivity, OC-US and OC become more clinically effective, but only at lower values (*points* **A** and **B**) does the ICER drop below a $100,000 threshold. (From Hassan C, Pickhardt P, Laghi A, et al. Computed tomographic colonography to screen for colorectal cancer, extracolonic cancer, and aortic aneurysm. *Arch Intern Med.* 2008;168:696-705.)

To address the controversial issue of CTC surveillance of small (6-9 mm) polyps, we constructed a decision analysis model to compare the clinical and economic impact of immediate polypectomy versus 3-year CTC.[11] The hypothetical cohort in this study was a concentrated group of 100,000 individuals, all with 6- to 9-mm polyps, evaluated over a 5-year time horizon. We used our initial clinical results with actual CTC surveillance to model the short-term natural history of small polyps. For the CTC surveillance strategy, only cases with measurable growth (≥1 mm) at follow-up CTC were referred for polypectomy. We found that without any intervention, the estimated 5-year CRC death rate from a 6- to 9-mm polyp was 0.08%, which already represents a sevenfold decrease over the 0.56% CRC risk for the general unselected screening population. The death rate was further reduced to 0.03% with the CTC surveillance strategy and 0.02% with im-

mediate colonoscopy referral. However, for each additional cancer-related death prevented with immediate polypectomy versus CTC follow-up, 9977 colonoscopy referrals would be needed, resulting in 10 additional perforations and an incremental cost-effectiveness ratio of $372,853 (Table 10-4). We concluded that for individuals with only 6- to 9-mm polyps detected at CTC screening, the exclusion of large polyps (≥10 mm) already confers a very low CRC risk. Furthermore, the high costs, additional complications, and relatively low incremental yield associated with immediate polypectomy of 6- to 9-mm polyps support the practice of 3-year CTC surveillance, which allows for selective noninvasive identification of small polyps at risk.

We evaluated the potential impact of the use of computer-aided detection (CAD) on CTC screening.[13] At the baseline assumptions, the addition of CAD re-

Table 10-4 ◘ Model Outputs Comparing Strategies of CTC Surveillance, Immediate OC, and No Intervention for Small (6-9 mm) Polyps Detected at CTC Screening[11]

Output	No Intervention	3-year CTC Surveillance	Immediate Colonoscopy
CRC cases	115	87	50
CRC deaths	78	28	18*
Life years lost	1880	685	445
Cost	$8,049,486	$68,290,291	$157,984,989
ICER[†]			
Compared with no intervention	–	$50,418	$104,456
Compared with 3-year CTC	–	–	$372,853

Note: Data are numbers unless otherwise indicated. Dash (–) indicates not applicable.
CRC, colorectal cancer; CTC, CT colonography; ICER, incremental cost-effectiveness ratio.
*Six deaths were related to colonoscopy-related complications.
[†]In cost per life year gained.
(From Pickhardt PJ, Hassan C, Laghi A, et al. Clinical management of small [6- to 9-mm] polyps detected at screening CT colonography: A cost-effectiveness analysis. *Am J Roentgenol.* 2008;191:1509-1516.)

sulted in small incremental increases in the CRC prevention rate compared with CTC without CAD, which was more pronounced for inexperienced versus experienced readers (9% and 2%, respectively). Assuming a CAD cost of $50 per CTC, the overall program costs increased by only 3% to 5%, largely because of the substantial reduction in CRC-related costs. The incremental cost effectiveness of CTC with CAD compared with CTC without CAD was $8661 and $61,354 per life year gained for inexperienced and experienced readers, respectively. OC was not a cost-effective alternative to CTC with CAD by experienced readers, with an incremental cost effectiveness of $498,668 per life year gained. CTC with CAD for inexperienced readers was more effective and cost effective than FS. At sensitivity analysis, CAD-CTC sensitivity for ≥6 mm polyps was the most meaningful variable. We concluded that the addition of CAD to CTC screening improves the CRC prevention rate, resulting in advantageous cost effectiveness for screening.

We have also evaluated the potential impact of adding a chest evaluation to CTC, resulting in whole-body CT screening,[16] which has been a controversial topic of unproven scientific merit. At base-case analysis, our Markov model estimated a 22% increase in life years gained for whole-body CTC screening versus CTC alone, primarily as a result of cardiovascular prevention and early detection of lung cancer. However, the total cost of the whole-body CT screening program was about 50% higher compared with CTC alone, mainly because of false-positive evaluations, resulting in an ICER of more than $164,000. We concluded that the addition of chest CT to CTC screening may increase the overall clinical efficacy, but its unfavorable cost-effectiveness profile and other uncertainties preclude its recommended use in current clinical practice.

Although not an actual cost-effectiveness analysis, we have also modeled the multidetector CT (MDCT) capacity for providing mass CTC screening in both the United States and Europe.[7,9] Because this issue has clear economic implications, we will briefly discuss our findings for the United States. Mathematical and Markov models were used to assess the mean number of CTC procedures per MDCT scanner per day (CTC/MDCT unit/day) necessary for both a startup and steady-state phase of a nationwide screening effort. Plausible ranges were applied to a number of variables in the sensitivity analysis. The number of existing CT scanners in the United States was based on the 2006 CT Benchmark Report from the IMV Medical Information Division. At the baseline analysis, assuming gradual increases in compliance, CTC penetrance, and MDCT capacity, we calculated that a total of 37,227,541 U.S. adults would need to undergo CTC screening over a 10-year startup period, corresponding to 1.2 to 1.6 CTC/MDCT unit/day. Assuming a 5-year routine screening interval between the ages of 50 and 80 years, the number of CTC studies needed to be performed in the steady-state period was 1.2 CTC/MDCT unit/day. These estimates were sensitive to variations in compliance, MDCT capacity, population size, interval for startup phase, and routine CTC screening interval. Our conclusion was that MDCT capacity in the United States appears to be adequate for handling the potential demand related to mass population screening with CTC, even without assuming a specific CTC-driven increase in MDCT supply.

In addition to the works discussed here, cost-effectiveness analyses or reviews for CTC screening from other groups have been performed.[17-19] In 2008 the Institute for Clinical and Economic Review released its study, which reported a cost per life year gained (versus no screening) of only $1500—a remarkably low figure.[19] For CTC to be cost effective relative to OC screening, however, the cost of CTC would need to be about 40% of the OC cost, a condition that is easily met in our practice but perhaps not by Medicare.

THIRD-PARTY REIMBURSEMENT

In the United States, third-party payers such as Medicare determine what medical procedures will be reimbursed, which largely determines the viability of most procedures and practices. In other countries such as Canada and throughout Europe, national health services generally determine what services are allowable. In either case, it is clear that CTC screening cannot seriously compete with other screening modalities if individuals are forced to pay directly out of pocket for the test. Despite what is known about the benefit of CRC prevention through polyp detection, a number of countries are currently pushing for the use of fecal occult blood testing for screening, which is no longer a preferred option according to the American Cancer Society guidelines.[20]

The current status and potential future role for CTC will vary by country, but we will now focus on third-party payer coverage in the United States. As with most CTC-related topics, a clear distinction must be made between diagnostic indications and asymptomatic screening. The main diagnostic indication—prior incomplete OC—generally enjoys broad coverage from third-party payers, including positive local coverage determinations (LCD) from Medicare in nearly every state. In our local four-state region (Wisconsin, Michigan, Minnesota, and Illinois), we successfully lobbied for even broader coverage for diagnostic CTC indications by meeting with representatives from Medicare Parts A and B at our hospital. Examples of acceptable diagnostic indications beyond incomplete OC include diverticular disease, colonic tortuosity, suspected submucosal abnormality, anticoagulation therapy, and prior difficult or complicated OC (even if complete).

Unlike the nationwide success story related to third-party coverage for diagnostic CTC following incomplete OC, the story for asymptomatic screening has been much different. In terms of Medicare, coverage of a new colorectal screening test requires either a national coverage determination (NCD) by the Centers for Medicare and Medicaid Services (CMS) or legislative action from Congress. In 2004, the prospects for any sort of widespread or national coverage for CTC screening by third-party payers were slim. Therefore, we decided to act locally at UW, with the hope that success could ultimately lead to coverage at other "centers of excellence" through a grassroots approach. Because of our proven results for CTC screening, we convinced several local medical care organizations to initiate coverage for CTC screening at UW, marking the beginning of the implementation era.[14,21] Although coverage was specifically limited to our medical center, in 2006 we added another statewide payer that allowed for coverage at other CTC "centers of excellence" in Wisconsin. Unfortunately, few centers have achieved this designation, which was not well defined. Furthermore, a full 4 years after initiation of screening at UW, no other program in the United States

had yet achieved this important goal. Therefore, because the grassroots approach was stagnating, a more "top-down" approach at the national level was pursued.

We worked closely with Representative Barbara Cubin, Congresswoman from Wyoming, on a bill that would mandate Medicare coverage of CTC screening, which was introduced to the U.S. House of Representatives in December 2007. Shortly thereafter, the revised screening guidelines from the American Cancer Society, in conjunction with the major gastrointestinal (GI) and radiology societies, included CTC as a newly recommended screening test.[20] The momentum for national coverage continued in June 2008, when CMS announced the commencement of a national coverage analysis (NCA), potentially leading to an NCD before 2010. Either one of these parallel tracks (i.e., the congressional bill or the NCA/NCD process) could result in the ultimate goal of Medicare coverage. Unfortunately, the proposed decision memo from CMS indicated non-coverage for CTC screening, with the final decision still pending at the time of this writing. Of course, once Medicare initiates coverage for CTC screening, the expectation would be that the other major national payers would follow suit. Even without Medicare coverage, a number of national-level payers have initiated coverage in 2008 and 2009. However, before we assume that the floodgates will immediately swing open, another important consideration will be the actual reimbursement rate that is determined, which will have a direct impact on a practice decision of whether to incorporate CTC. This includes the relative breakdown between technical and professional components of reimbursement. At UW, our radiology group successfully negotiated with the hospital for a larger percentage of the professional component because CTC requires more time to interpret and all "3D reconstruction" is handled by the physician.

A topic that is not directly linked to reimbursement, yet is nonetheless related to compensation, is the Current Procedural Terminology (CPT) coding process, which is governed by the American Medical Association (AMA). For the first decade of CTC, no specific CPT code existed, which was actually beneficial because the generic codes for abdominal and pelvic CT without contrast (74150 and 72192, respectively), in conjunction with the code for 3D reconstruction (76375), could generally be applied.[22] These are Category I CPT codes, which are familiar to most radiologists, and signify that the procedure has been assigned a value by the Relative Value Update Committee (RUC) of the AMA. This value is critical because it is generally used to establish the reimbursement rate from third-party payers. However, in July 2004 the CPT Editorial Panel created Category III "tracking codes" for both screening (0066T) and diagnostic (0067T) CTC, the use of which was mandatory. In the short term, this was a mixed blessing for clinical practice. On one hand, this signified that CTC was maturing and "on the radar" for an eventual Category I code, contributing to ultimate reimbursement. However, because Category III codes do not graduate to the RUC, there is no associated value and therefore generally no compensation. CTC is currently under consideration for Category I CPT code designation, which may be in place before 2010. Controversy between radiology and GI organizations surrounding the issue of split codes for colorectal and extracolonic interpretation has impeded progress somewhat. In our opinion, split codes would unnecessarily complicate an already-complex process and there is simply no precedent for such an action. Any radiologist who interprets body CT understands that many organ systems interact and cannot be artificially extricated from the global interpretation.

Other issues related to reimbursement deserve some consideration. Unlike OC, considerable attention has been given to building in quality metrics for CTC screening at the front end (see Chapter 28). In fact, quality assurance may ultimately be tied to reimbursement by some payers. It is uncertain at this time if quality assurance for CTC will take the form of individual "self-policing," defined centers of excellence, or outright accreditation. Regarding third-party payment, one intriguing model that should be considered is an integrated CRC screening program that involves both radiologists and gastroenterologists working closely together. With this arrangement, a single bundled payment could be made for "colon care" of the patient, whether that includes primary CTC or primary OC evaluation. This payment structure encourages efficient use of the combined resources. By working together and getting paid together, the "turf" issues between radiologists and gastroenterologists would disappear and the choice of examination will be based more on effective, noninvasive, and cost-effective detection. Finally, it is unclear if CAD will ultimately be reimbursed separately (as is the case with mammography), as part of the global CTC charge, or perhaps not reimbursed at all.

One could be easily frustrated by the seemingly slow pace for obtaining reimbursement for CTC screening in the United States. However, it is useful to briefly review the history of reimbursement for OC screening to appreciate how far we have come in a relatively short time. Although it did not have to go through the rigorous CMS NCA/NCD process, it may come as a surprise to some that Medicare has only reimbursed for screening OC since 2001. OC was not included in the screening guidelines from the U.S. Preventive Services Task Force (USPSTF) until 2002. Since that time, there has been rapid growth of OC screening in ambulatory surgery centers, which not only delivers such an outpatient service more efficiently, it has until recently also enjoyed higher reimbursement rates, further encouraging entrepreneurial efforts by gastroenterologists. At the same time, low reimbursement rates have significantly undercut the use of flexible sigmoidoscopy in the United States, although

it is still used for screening by some groups. Considering that OC has been around for decades yet has only enjoyed widespread reimbursement for screening since 2001, this perhaps puts the time course for CTC screening coverage in a more positive light.

NONRADIOLOGIST INVOLVEMENT

The precise role that a given gastroenterologist assumes within a clinical CTC program could range from simply receiving the referrals from positive CTC (and sending incomplete OC cases to CTC), to controlling part or all of the CTC practice or even interpreting the CTC examination. Our sense is that no single approach will be universal, although in our experience the gastroenterologists at both UW and National Naval Medical Center (Bethesda, MD) have proved to be active members of a collaborative CRC screening team but have little or no interest in actual CTC interpretation. This healthy collaboration has facilitated same-day polypectomy for positive CTC cases and streamlined referral to CTC following incomplete OC.[14,23] This is not to imply that some gastroenterologists would not pursue ownership of the entire CTC process. It is also possible that some gastroenterologists will be capable of adequate colorectal interpretation at CTC, although it would require acquiring a cross-sectional skill set to provide quality interpretations. However, we believe that a relatively small minority of gastroenterologists will have the time and motivation necessary to truly become proficient enough with advanced cross-sectional image interpretation, which typically requires radiology residency training. Besides, gastroenterologists are trained to remove polyps via therapeutic OC, which will hopefully be in ever-increasing demand. A broad range of intermediate strategies and partnerships may be possible between radiologists and gastroenterologists in an integrated CRC screening program. GI ownership of the MDCT scanner would provide them with the technical revenue stream, but obtaining such an expensive piece of equipment may prove risky compared with a radiology practice, where a wide array of diagnostic uses is possible.

One must not underestimate the current financial importance of CRC screening to many gastroenterology practices because screening OC represents a substantial revenue stream. Therefore, some of the interest or concern that gastroenterologists have demonstrated for the impending widespread implementation of CTC may be driven in part by the (irrational) fear that primary OC screening volume will immediately fall off. There have even been theoretical models put forward by GI researchers to help raise this fear.[24] However, for a number of reasons, these concerns do not appear to be justified. For one, primary OC screening at UW continues unabated by the parallel CTC screening program, with progressive increases in screening referrals and number of studies performed.[25] Because parallel OC and CTC screening allows for an individual choice between examinations, it appears a significant percentage will continue to opt for OC for primary screening. Furthermore, referral from CTC for therapeutic polypectomy represents a high-yield and well-compensated OC examination, which is essentially served up on a platter for the gastroenterologist. Finally, it is important to remember that a substantial majority of the general screening population have not had (and likely will not ever acquiesce to have) a primary OC for CRC screening. Most of our primary CTC referrals come from this majority and are not siphoned away from primary OC screening. CTC therefore acts to bring additional individuals off the "screening sidelines," thereby increasing overall compliance.

Beyond gastroenterologists, radiographers and CT technologists represent another clinical component of CTC beyond the radiologist. At our institution, the CTC technologist (i.e., a CT technologist trained and experienced in CTC) obtains the entire examination and performs the key online quality assessment. Although it is important for them to differentiate between invasive cancer and segmental collapse for obtaining a diagnostic examination, they have no formal role in CTC interpretation. In the United States, this is typically the limit of involvement for technologists, unless they happen to also serve as the CTC program coordinator. The situation is different in the United Kingdom, where radiographers often perform and interpret barium enema studies, usually in conjunction with an over-read or double-read by a consultant radiologist. A similar approach to CTC has also been applied, with radiographers providing an initial "wet read" that can facilitate same-day OC if an obvious cancer is found.[26] In the United States, the medicolegal implications of CTC interpretation by technologists may restrict this practice, although nurse practitioners have been performing flexible sigmoidoscopy for years.[27]

On a final note, CAD has often been heralded as the magic bullet that will allow for successful nonradiologist interpretation of CTC, whether by gastroenterologists, radiographers, or other medical personnel. Although it is true that CAD will be more beneficial in improving sensitivity for less experienced or less skilled readers, this is only part of the picture. Achieving an adequate specificity is now the real challenge with CTC interpretation when state-of-the-art primary 3D evaluation is applied because polyp detection is relatively easy. It is important to understand that the specificity of current CAD systems is essentially 0% because false-positive "hits" are present in virtually every case, including the majority of cases in which no true polyps are present. Therefore, successful CTC interpretation requires the appropriate skills to recognize the many pitfalls leading to false-positive diagnosis.[28] Without substantial experience in general CT interpretation, this skill set will be lacking and CAD will not be an adequate substitute.

REFERENCES

1. Pignone M, Saha S, Hoerger T, Lohr KN, Teutsch S, Mandelblatt J. Challenges in systematic reviews of economic analyses. *Ann Intern Med.* 2005;142(12):1073-1079.
2. Heitman SJ, Manns BJ, Hilsden RJ, Fong A, Dean S, Romagnuolo J. Cost-effectiveness of computerized tomographic colonography versus colonoscopy for colorectal cancer screening. *Can Med Assoc J.* 2005;173(8):877-881.
3. Sonnenberg A, Delco F, Bauerfeind P. Ts virtual colonoscopy a cost-effective option to screen for colorectal cancer? *Am J Gastroenterol.* 1999;94(8):2268-2274.
4. Ladabaum U, Song K, Fendrick AM. Colorectal neoplasia screening with virtual colonoscopy: when, at what cost, and with what national impact? *Clin Gastroenterol Hepatol.* 2004; 2(7):554-563.
5. Vijan S, Hwang I, Inadomi J, et al. The cost-effectiveness of CT colonography in screening for colorectal neoplasia. *Am J Gastroenterol.* 2007;102(2):380-390.
6. Hassan C, Zullo A, Laghi A, et al. Colon cancer prevention in Italy: Cost-effectiveness analysis with CT colonography and endoscopy. *Digest Liver Dis.* 2007;39(3):242-250.
7. Hassan C, Laghi A, Pickhardt PJ, et al. Projected impact of colorectal cancer screening with computerized tomographic colonography on current radiological capacity in Europe. *Aliment Pharmacol Ther.* 2008;27(4):366-374.
8. Hassan C, Pickhardt P, Laghi A, et al. Computed tomographic colonography to screen for colorectal cancer, extracolonic cancer, and aortic aneurysm. *Arch Intern Med.* 2008;168(7):696-705.
9. Pickhardt PJ, Hassan C, Laghi A, et al. Is there sufficient MDCT capacity to provide colorectal cancer screening with CT colonography for the US population? *Am J Roentgenol.* 2008;190(4):1044-1049.
10. Pickhardt PJ, Hassan C, Laghi A, et al. Small and diminutive polyps detected at screening CT colonography: A decision analysis for referral to colonoscopy. *Am J Roentgenol.* 2008;190(1):136-144.
11. Pickhardt PJ, Hassan C, Laghi A, et al. Clinical management of small (6- to 9-mm) polyps detected at screening CT colonography: A cost-effectiveness analysis. *Am J Roentgenol.* 2008; 191(5):1509-1516.
12. Pickhardt PJ, Hassan C, Laghi A, Zullo A, Kim DH, Morini S. Cost-effectiveness of colorectal cancer screening with computed tomography colonography—The impact of not reporting diminutive lesions. *Cancer.* 2007;109(11):2213-2221.
13. Regge D, Hassan C, Pickhardt PJ, et al. Impact of computer-aided detection on the cost-effectiveness of CT colonography. *Radiology.* 2009;250(2):488-497.
14. Pickhardt PJ, Taylor AJ, Kim DH, Reichelderfer M, Gopal DV, Pfau PR. Screening for colorectal neoplasia with CT colonography: Initial experience from the 1st year of coverage by third-party payers. *Radiology.* 2006;241(2):417-425.
15. Zalis ME, Barish MA, Choi JR, et al. CT colonography reporting and data system: A consensus proposal. *Radiology.* 2005;236(1):3-9.
16. Hassan C, Pickhardt PJ, Laghi A, et al. Impact of whole-body CT screening on the cost-effectiveness of CT colonography. *Radiology.* 2009;251:156-165.

17. Mavranezouli I, East JE, Taylor SA. CT colonography and cost-effectiveness. *Eur Radiol.* 2008;18(11):2485-2497.

18. Arnesen RB, Ginnerup-Pedersen B, Poulsen PB, et al. Cost-effectiveness of computed tomographic colonography: A prospective comparison with colonoscopy. *Acta Radiol.* 2007;48(3):259-266.

19. Scherer R, Knudson A, Pearson SD. CT colonography for colorectal cancer screening—Final appraisal document. Boston: Institute for Clinical and Economic Review; 2008.

20. Levin B, Lieberman DA, McFarland B, et al. Screening and surveillance for the early detection of colorectal cancer and adenomatous polyps, 2008: A joint guideline from the American Cancer Society, the US Multi-Society Task Force on Colorectal Cancer, and the American College of Radiology. *CA Cancer J Clin.* 2008;58(3):130-160.

21. Pickhardt PJ, Taylor AJ, Johnson GL, et al. Building a CT colonography program: Necessary ingredients for reimbursement and clinical success. *Radiology.* 2005;235(1):17-20.

22. Duszak R Jr. CT colonography and virtual reimbursement. *J Am Coll Radiol.* 2004;1(7):457-458.

23. Pickhardt PJ. Screening CT colonography: How I do it. *Am J Roentgenol.* 2007;189(2):290-298.

24. Hur C, Gazelle GS, Zalis ME, Podolsky DK. An analysis of the potential impact of computed tomographic colonography (virtual colonoscopy) on colonoscopy demand. *Gastroenterology.* 2004; 127(5):1312-1321.

25. Schwartz DC, Dasher KJ, Said A, et al. Impact of a CT colonography screening program on endoscopic colonoscopy in clinical practice. *Am J Gastroenterol.* 2008;103:346-351.

26. Burling D, Moore A, Marshall M, et al. Virtual colonoscopy: Effect of computer-assisted detection (CAD) on radiographer performance. *Clin Radiol.* 2008;63(5):549-556.

27. Maule WF. Screening for colorectal cancer by nurse endoscopists. *N Engl J Med.* 1994;330(3):183-187.

28. Pickhardt PJ. Differential diagnosis of polypoid lesions seen at CT colonography (virtual colonoscopy). *Radiographics.* 2004;24(6): 1535-1556.

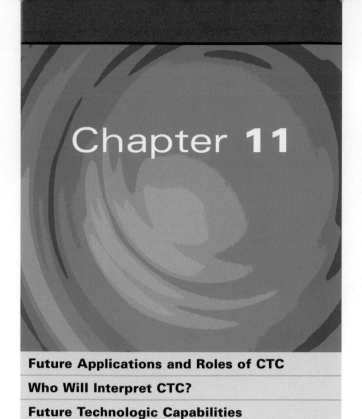

Chapter 11

Future Directions for Virtual Colonoscopy

DAVID H. KIM, MD

PERRY J. PICKHARDT, MD

Future Applications and Roles of CTC

Who Will Interpret CTC?

Future Technologic Capabilities

Concluding Statements

INTRODUCTION

CT colonography (CTC) has matured and considerably advanced since its initial introduction back in 1994. The path of development has included many unexpected twists and turns. Advances in software visualization algorithms, CT scanner technology, and underlying computer hardware have propelled this technology. Whereas it was difficult to visualize this technique as an effective population screening tool in the mid-1990s, it has subsequently demonstrated polyp sensitivities equivalent to optical colonoscopy (OC) in low polyp–prevalence cohorts only a mere decade later. This is a time of significant change for CTC, in which it is currently poised for implementation on a national scale and fulfillment of the role of a population screening tool. What are the future directions for CTC? Such predictions are fraught with difficulty, but certainly some trends seem likely. This chapter discusses these potential areas of future change, including how this modality may be used within the screening algorithm in the coming years, which groups will interpret the examination, and possible areas of future technologic advances.

FUTURE APPLICATIONS AND ROLES OF CTC

For Screening

With the inclusion of CTC within the most recent American Cancer Society (ACS) guidelines as a preferred modality for colorectal cancer (CRC) prevention alongside colonoscopy,[1] it is anticipated to be one of the major options chosen by a person for screening in the near future. It is clear that additional effective screening modalities are needed. It is estimated that there are more than 40 million individuals older than age 50 years eligible for screening that are currently noncompliant.[2] The current colonoscopic capacity is estimated to fall far short of this number. On the CTC side, Markov and mathematic modeling suggest that multidetector CT (MDCT) capacity is able to absorb these numbers.[3] Training to increase sufficient number of CTC readers will be a key issue as screening rolls out.

What will be the role of CTC in screening? Initially, it will likely hold a parallel role with colonoscopy as a front-line examination. Both modalities will likely be needed to effectively screen the large numbers of currently unscreened patients in a reasonably short time period. In addition, both modalities would likely be necessary because the patient population is a heterogeneous group with differing preferences—some would prefer CTC, whereas others would favor OC. The University of Wisconsin program experience suggests that noncompliant patients are indeed being pulled off the sidelines because the total screening volume has increased with the institution of the CTC program alongside the preexisting colonoscopy-based program (Fig. 11-1).[4] A similar experience has been seen with the Colon Health Initiative at the National Naval Medical Center (NNMC) in Bethesda, MD. Here, the addition of CTC as a screening option has increased overall CRC screening rates by 33% over a 3-year period. In addition, the OC volume has increased by 25% despite decreasing gastroenterology staffing.[5] In the future, CTC may ultimately move to more of a front-line screening role, reserving OC for selected high-risk cases and for therapy. CTC represents a much less invasive modality with a nearly nonexistent

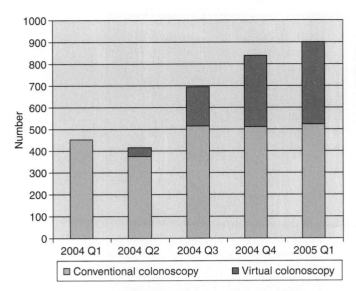

Figure 11-1 **CRC screening volumes at the University of Wisconsin.** Bar graph demonstrates the number of people screened by OC *(blue)* and CTC *(red)* by quarter. Note that the total number screened progressively increased, with a doubling from the first quarter of 2004 to the first quarter of 2005, with CTC constituting about 40% of that volume. The OC volume remained overall stable to slightly increased over this time interval, suggesting that additional people were being pulled into screening.

perforation risk.[6] It uses fewer resources because of the lack of need for sedation and recovery. Thus, it stands to reason that a screening strategy based on CTC holds marked advantages. Our program results have demonstrated that CTC can effectively serve as a filter to determine those who need therapeutic colonoscopy.[7] Advanced adenoma yields can be maintained while significantly decreasing colonoscopic resources, complications, and costs.

As another possibility, perhaps a strategy of alternating screening by both CTC and OC will evolve, in which an individual is evaluated by one modality, followed by the other at the next routine follow-up interval. The rationale would be to decrease the miss rate for significant lesions. Both CTC and colonoscopy are not perfect examinations. Although long considered the gold standard with a "100%" sensitivity, a miss rate exists for colonoscopy that is not insignificant even for large lesions—up to 12% when CTC is used as the reference standard.[8] Similarly, CTC is not perfect, with sensitivities ranging from 90% to 92% for large polyps.[9-11] An alternating strategy takes advantage of the fact that these two modalities are largely complementary in that the areas of difficulty ("the blind spots") for one modality are typically not an area of difficulty for the other. For example, the back side of colonic haustra has areas for potential missed lesions at colonoscopy, which are not a problem area at CTC because of the lack of directional constraints. However, the optical cues of color difference between the lesion and normal colonic mucosa aid OC

in detection of lesions that may be difficult to see on morphologic criteria alone—a potential weakness at CTC. Another area of weakness for OC is the right colon,[12] which tends to be well evaluated at CTC and may in part explain observed differences in cancer detection rates.[7] Consequently, a lesion missed in a difficult area on one test would more likely be picked up by the other modality on the subsequent examination. Such an alternating strategy would presumably lead to a synergistic effect, and the miss rate for the combined approach would be much less than for the single modality alone.

Over the coming years, it is likely that CTC will continue to drive research regarding the natural history of small adenomas and serrated polyps (Fig. 11-2). This technology is well suited for this task. It allows for precise size measurements with little interobserver variation, which allows for accurate determination of interval change. In addition, CTC allows for precise localization of a given polyp because of the ability to visualize the polyp within the colon in the context of both the colonic and extracolonic environment. Consequently, a polyp can be confidently determined as the same polyp between examinations. Both of these tasks can be difficult at OC. Because of surveillance, CTC will provide a unique opportunity to study the accumulation of genetic changes of polyps of differing histologies over time—knowledge that is currently unavailable because of the universal polypectomy strategy of screening OC. For example, what are the genetic changes that arise in an adenoma that has been growing as opposed to one that has remained stable or regressed during surveillance? This knowledge, along with the observational surveillance data, will be of critical importance to effectively craft appropriate selective polypectomy strategies and determine optimal surveillance intervals at screening CTC for the various polyp subgroups. A judicious approach to polypectomy will be needed to minimize use of critical limited medical resources and to minimize unnecessary complications in this group.

In Preoperative Planning and Staging

CTC may play a larger role in preoperative planning for identified colorectal cancers in the coming years. Issues such as tumor localization, evaluation for synchronous cancers, local staging, and the search for metastatic disease are currently addressed through both imaging and surgical methods. CTC alone can address many of these issues. CTC holds superior ability over colonoscopy in localizing colonic tumors.[13] Whereas determining the location of a cancer may be difficult at colonoscopy, particularly as the colon lengthens and becomes more tortuous, such is not the case with CT colonography. As mentioned in the previous paragraph, this is a result of the ability of CTC to visualize the colonic lesion within

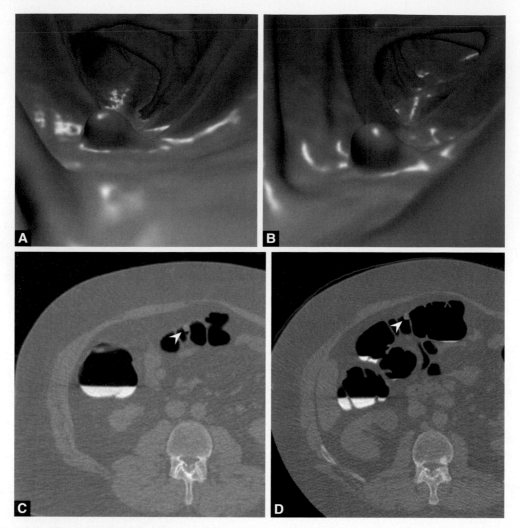

Figure 11-2 Polyp (8 mm) in CTC surveillance. Subcentimeter polyp seen in the transverse colon on CTC, where the patient elected imaging follow-up. 3D endoluminal CTC image from the index examination **(A)** shows an 8-mm sessile polyp, which did not demonstrate interval growth at 2 years **(B).** This was confirmed at 2D, in which the polyp did not change from the original **(C)** to the followup **(D)** examination *(arrowheads).* Additional followup was subsequently extended for an additional 3 years. Note how CTC is well suited to determine that the polyp in followup correlates to the original polyp and that accurate determination of interval change (or the lack thereof) can be made.

the colon in relation to the colonic anatomy and extracolonic environment (Fig. 11-3). In addition, CTC is useful for the evaluation of synchronous cancers and significant polyps. The rate for synchronous cancers is not insignificant and has been estimated to be approximately 3% from large multiinstitutional databases.[14] At colonoscopy, this evaluation may not be possible where the constricting cancer does not allow advancement of the endoscope to the cecum. Even in these situations, however, CTC examination is often possible. The carbon dioxide can easily pass through the area of stricture to allow adequate evaluation of the more proximal colon. CTC is also excellent at evaluating for distant metastases. Increasing the technique to standard doses and using intravenous (IV) contrast allow CTC to evaluate for distant metastases as it essentially becomes a standard diagnostic CT scan.

What are the current areas of weakness with this modality and areas of potential development? They revolve around local staging of the cancer including (1) the assessment of the depth of tumor invasion, specifically distinguishing a cancer contained by the muscularis propria layer (T2) from a tumor that extends past this layer (T3), and (2) the detection of a tumor in regional lymph nodes when the lymph nodes are not enlarged. Similar to other imaging modalities, including endoscopic ultrasound, CTC has difficulty in both areas. It is difficult to distinguish between a T2 and T3 cancer on imaging—overstaging can occur as a result of inflammatory fibrosis or understaging through microscopic extension. Also, malignant involvement of regional lymph nodes can occur with micrometastases in normal-sized nodes. The thin section technique, colonic distention, and use of IV contrast at CTC do help in some regard

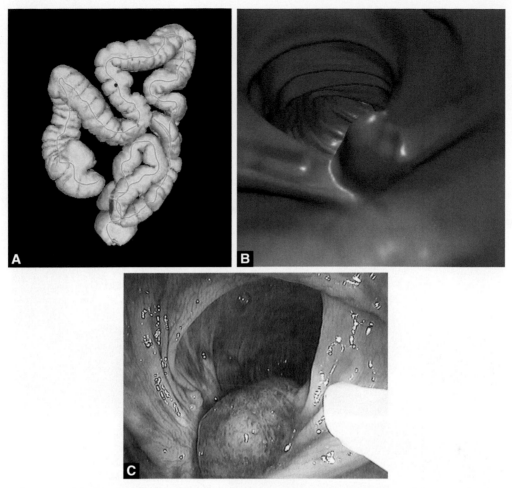

Figure 11-3 **Value of CTC in polyp localization.** A 62-year-old male for screening CTC with a long and tortuous colon seen on the 3D colon map **(A).** One of the benefits of CTC is exquisite localization of polyps. Whereas localization may be difficult at OC and lead to an erroneous reported location, this is not the case at CTC, where this transverse polyp is easily localized because the colon can be viewed in the context of the colonic and extracolonic environment. 3D endoluminal CTC image **(B)** shows a 17-mm polyp, which was subsequently confirmed at OC **(C).** A villous tumor with invasive carcinoma was seen at polypectomy with positive margins, ultimately requiring an extended right hemicolectomy. (From Kim DH, Pickhardt PJ. CT colonography: Pertinent issues for the colorectal surgeon. *Semin Colon Rectal Surg.* 2007;18:88-95.)

(Fig. 11-4). Ultimately, new technology will be needed to help in both areas. Perhaps future markers demonstrating some physiologic aspect of the tumor or determining the molecular makeup of the cancer in combination with the anatomic information of CTC will help in this evaluation. Radioiodinated phospholipid ether analogs hold intriguing promise demonstrating selective uptake in various cancer lines in animal models.[15]

Along the same lines, CTC may play a future role in assessing local response to neoadjuvant chemoradiation for rectal cancer prior to surgery, possibly through assessment of interval change in tumor volume or perfusion. T2 versus T3 determination will remain a difficult issue, particularly following radiation in which postprocedure scarring may mimic a tumor. Again, the combination of CTC with physiologic markers may hold the key here.

In Other Diagnostic Indications

CTC presumably will play a larger role in niche situations replacing colonoscopy and barium enema for specific diagnostic indications. For example, an excellent use of CTC is for screening patients receiving anticoagulation therapy or with other bleeding diatheses. Whereas the anticoagulation requires reversal for colonoscopy, this is not necessary for CTC. The patient does not have to endure the risk of coming off of anticoagulation. Only the small minority with a positive CTC examination result will need reversal for removal of a significant polyp at colonoscopy. Other situations in which CTC is preferred would include patients at a relatively high risk for complication at OC (including sedation-related complications) or a history of previously difficult or incomplete OC. In the coming years, the indications for use of CTC in diagnostic settings should continue to expand. At a

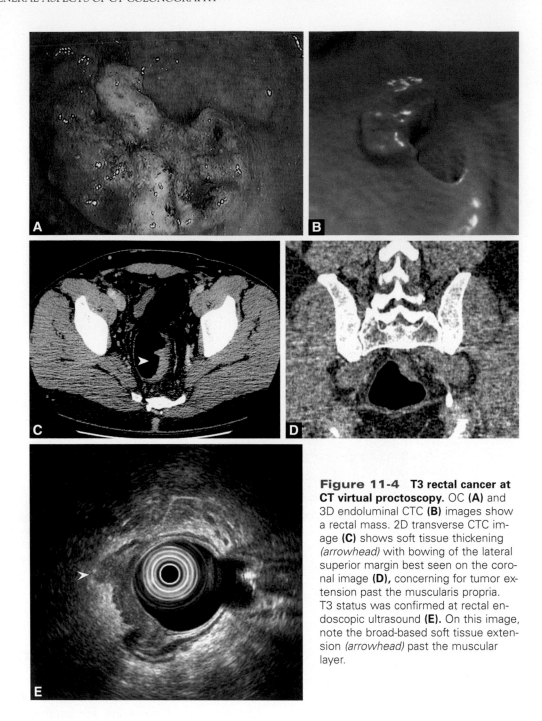

Figure 11-4   T3 rectal cancer at CT virtual proctoscopy. OC **(A)** and 3D endoluminal CTC **(B)** images show a rectal mass. 2D transverse CTC image **(C)** shows soft tissue thickening *(arrowhead)* with bowing of the lateral superior margin best seen on the coronal image **(D),** concerning for tumor extension past the muscularis propria. T3 status was confirmed at rectal endoscopic ultrasound **(E).** On this image, note the broad-based soft tissue extension *(arrowhead)* past the muscular layer.

minimum, CTC should replace all indications for which the double contrast barium enema is performed because of its markedly improved performance characteristics.

WHO WILL INTERPRET CTC?

Control over CTC interpretation is an area that is vigorously contested between the disciplines of *Radiology* and *Gastroenterology.* The ultimate outcome remains uncertain. In our opinion, whether these individuals are from a radiology or gastroenterology background (or both) is not important. The crucial issue is whether these individuals are capable of providing quality interpreta-

tions. Quality interpretations include the ability to manipulate the three-dimensional (3D) sequences to maximize polyp detection and to correctly evaluate the source 2D images for polyp confirmation (see Chapter 16). Simply detecting focal "bumps" on the endoluminal 3D flythrough does not equate with complete CTC interpretation. It is simply a specific task to generate a list of potential polyps—one that requires little skill or training to undertake. However, the application of cross-sectional skills required to allow confirmation of the few true polyps extracted from this list of potential polyps is critical. If this skill set is not present, both the colonic portion and extracolonic portion of the CTC interpretation suffer. On the colonic side, there will be an unacceptably high number of false-positive results, and on the extracolonic side, significant findings will be missed. In our estimation, when readers report that they are uncomfortable reading extracolonic findings, they are indicating that they do not have the requisite skill set to read the colonic side as well. Although this cross-sectional skill set can be acquired by nonradiologists, this represents a significant undertaking, and, beyond formal radiology training, it is unclear what the minimal level of training would be to ensure quality interpretations.

So who will read CTC examination in the coming years? It is hoped that it will be some combination of interested, properly trained individuals from both specialties. Perhaps the field will transform to one in which a CRC screening specialist (initially from either *Radiology* or *Gastroenterology*) performs both CTC and OC. The synergies in knowledge about the two modalities may substantially increase the expertise of the physician for both modalities.

The United Kingdom provides a glimpse of a potential alternative future. There is research into radiology technologists aided by CAD (computer-aided detection) to perform these interpretations. This has been driven by the limited physician capacity to provide CTC in the United Kingdom and the large numbers of people that need to be evaluated. Currently, the radiology technologists help fill the colon cancer screening role in England by performing and interpreting many of the barium enemas. Perhaps the future will follow a third option, in which the interpretation will be undertaken completely by computer algorithms without any human interaction to interpret and report out these examinations (see Chapter 24).

FUTURE TECHNOLOGIC CAPABILITIES

Predicting future technologic developments for CTC is difficult. It is a rapidly evolving modality with surprises on the horizon. Some likely incremental changes include (1) movement to volume measurements for polyp size, (2) advancements in dose reduction, and (3) use of noncathartic regimens.

Current polyp management uses size as the guiding feature. By convention, this has been undertaken by using the longest linear measurement of a polyp (excluding the stalk on a pedunculated lesion). This convention has served fairly well, but the improvement in computer abilities for quality automated volume measurements suggests that such measurements may supplant linear distance. Volume measurements are more sensitive to change, which is important in the assessment of interval growth or stability in surveillance protocols.[16] In addition, lesion volume may correlate better with clinical significance than linear size does. For example, in our experience, flat adenomas tend to demonstrate less aggressive histology compared with polypoid lesions of the same linear size, but such histology may correlate better in terms of tumor volume. Improvements that allow easy, automated volume calculations that are accurate and reproducible will likely propel this change (Fig. 11-5).

Exposure to ionizing radiation from medical imaging has garnered increasing attention in recent years.[17] In the case of CTC, the already low-dose nature makes quantification of future theoretic risk difficult. Indeed, many argue that at these levels, CTC likely holds no relevant risk.[18] However, further decreases without sacrificing imaging quality would always be welcomed. Dual-energy protocols and novel iterative reconstruction algorithms may allow for such dose reductions. Both allow for "denoising" of the data to maintain image quality at lower doses. Currently, iterative reconstruction algorithms are not clinically feasible, requiring up to 8 hours to process the data. This reconstruction time will progressively decrease as processing capabilities increase.

One of the biggest hurdles to patient compliance with colorectal cancer screening involves the cathartic bowel preparation.[19-21] There is active interest in using noncathartic or "prepless" regimens. These protocols, which are not truly prepless, have yet to be validated in low-prevalence cohorts but have demonstrated initial promising results in high polyp–prevalence populations.[22] A noncathartic approach to CTC would likely increase compliance further but is unlikely to represent a singular solution because same-day polypectomy is not possible.[23] In addition to refining the noncathartic protocol in terms of the specific agents, timing, and amounts, continued advancement in electronic subtraction and digital cleansing to decrease associated artifacts and perhaps improve polyp detection may be helpful (Fig. 11-6). Potentially, applications such as CAD will play a more important role with noncathartic examinations.

CAD represents another area of future development. CAD shows promise in helping particularly inexperienced readers in polyp detection (Fig. 11-7). Unfortunately, it appears to increase sensitivity at the expense of decreased specificity.[24] What will be the ultimate role of CAD in CTC? Will it remain an adjunct to interpretation with a niche role aiding inexperienced readers in improving performance, or will it develop capabilities that ultimately supplant the final assessment by the human reader in which the output of the CAD device is the final interpretation? Certainly, incremental steps such as minimizing decreases in specificity will be important in the further development of CAD.

Other less certain predictions include the addition of physiologic information to this anatomically based examination, as mentioned earlier. Assessment of perfusion may be ultimately proved clinically useful by quantifying tumor enhancement. Parameters such as blood volume, blood flow, and permeability–surface

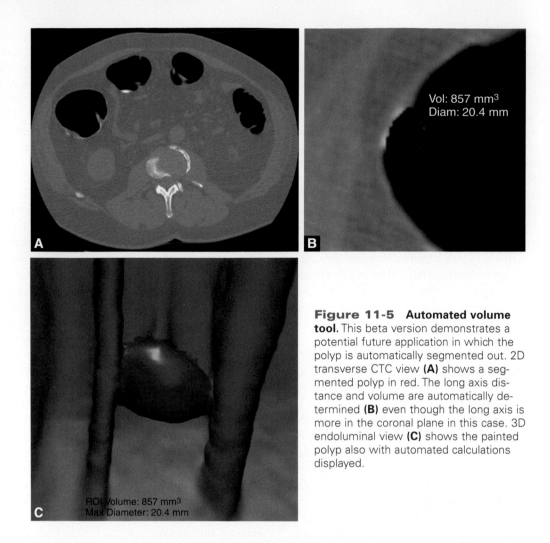

Vol: 857 mm³
Diam: 20.4 mm

ROI Volume: 857 mm³
Max Diameter: 20.4 mm

Figure 11-5 Automated volume tool. This beta version demonstrates a potential future application in which the polyp is automatically segmented out. 2D transverse CTC view **(A)** shows a segmented polyp in red. The long axis distance and volume are automatically determined **(B)** even though the long axis is more in the coronal plane in this case. 3D endoluminal view **(C)** shows the painted polyp also with automated calculations displayed.

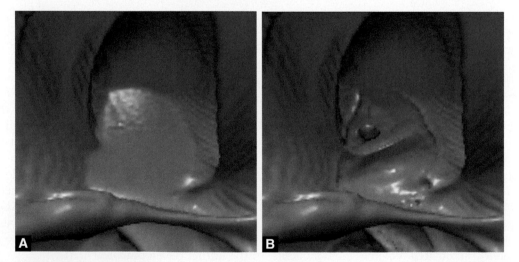

Figure 11-6 Electronic cleansing. Future versions of electronic cleansing may allow for a time-efficient 3D approach free of artifact. Currently, this is not possible with postprocessing introducing a layer of artifact that hampers such evaluation. It remains an area of active research because it would help in the interpretation of noncathartic protocols. 3D endoluminal CTC image **(A)** shows a residual fluid pool that is subtracted out electronically **(B).** The ileocecal valve is present in the foreground. In this case, the artifact is not too distracting, with just a "bathtub ring" seen at the edges. Note that the electronically cleansed image uncovers a polyp hidden in the pool.

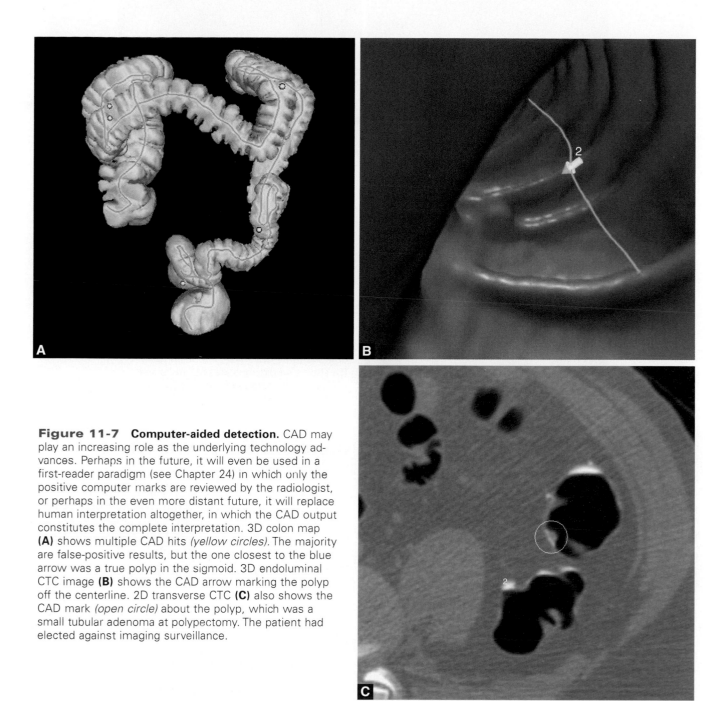

Figure 11-7 Computer-aided detection. CAD may play an increasing role as the underlying technology advances. Perhaps in the future, it will even be used in a first-reader paradigm (see Chapter 24) in which only the positive computer marks are reviewed by the radiologist, or perhaps in the even more distant future, it will replace human interpretation altogether, in which the CAD output constitutes the complete interpretation. 3D colon map **(A)** shows multiple CAD hits *(yellow circles)*. The majority are false-positive results, but the one closest to the blue arrow was a true polyp in the sigmoid. 3D endoluminal CTC image **(B)** shows the CAD arrow marking the polyp off the centerline. 2D transverse CTC **(C)** also shows the CAD mark *(open circle)* about the polyp, which was a small tubular adenoma at polypectomy. The patient had elected against imaging surveillance.

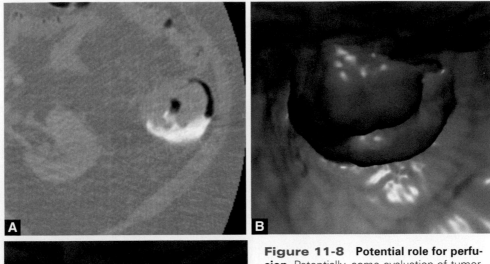

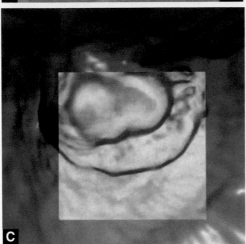

Figure 11-8 Potential role for perfusion. Potentially, some evaluation of tumor perfusion may play a role in CRC evaluation at CTC. Currently, there are rudimentary tools that can grossly assess increased vascularity. Diagnostic CTC performed in a 69-year-old woman with near-obstructing colonic mass. Transverse 2D CTC images **(A)** demonstrate the known mass in the proximal descending colon. Note that intravenous contrast was given for the supine series on this diagnostic examination *(left kidney enhancing on image)*. 3D endoluminal CTC image **(B)** again demonstrates this mass. Perfusion tool **(C)** shows serpiginous areas of red signal suggestive of increased "vascularity" or enhancement of the mass.

area products are some measures that can be currently crudely calculated. Perhaps a role in tumor response to various therapies may evolve for future perfusion tools. Some workstations have a translucency-like function that demonstrates areas of increased enhancement (Fig. 11-8). Alternatively, perhaps a combination with molecular markers or other entities such as radio-iodinated phospholipid ether analogs that tag malignancy may be in the future for CTC.

CONCLUDING STATEMENTS

CTC is poised to join colonoscopy in the effort of colorectal cancer prevention. Rapid advancements in only 14 years have propelled this modality into an effective screening modality equivalent to its optical counterpart. The future holds great promise in its potential impact on this preventable disease. The ultimate role of this imaging modality and ultimate capabilities remain to be seen.

REFERENCES

1. Levin B, Lieberman DA, McFarland B, et al. Screening and surveillance for the early detection of colorectal cancer and adenomatous polyps, 2008: A joint guideline from the American Cancer Society, the US Multi-Society Task Force on Colorectal Cancer, and the American College of Radiology. CA Cancer J Clin. 2008;58(3):130-160.
2. Seeff LC, Manninen DL, Dong FB, et al. Is there endoscopic capacity to provide colorectal cancer screening to the unscreened population in the United States? Gastroenterology. 2004;127(6):1661-1669.
3. Pickhardt PJ, Hassan C, Laghi A, et al. Is there sufficient MDCT capacity to provide colorectal cancer screening with CT colonography for the US population? Am J Roentgenol. 2008;190(4):1044-1049.
4. Pickhardt PJ, Taylor AJ, Kim DH, Reichelderfer M, Gopal DV, Pfau PR. Screening for colorectal neoplasia with CT colonography: Initial experience from the 1st year of coverage by third-party payers. Radiology. 2006;241(2):417-425.
5. Cash BD, Barlow DS. Computed tomographic colonography: A model for gastroenterology and radiology collaboration. AGA Perspectives. August/September 2008.
6. Pickhardt PJ. Incidence of colonic perforation at CT colonography: Review of existing data and implications for screening of asymptomatic adults. Radiology. 2006;239(2):313-316.
7. Kim DH, Pickhardt PJ, Taylor AJ, et al. CT colonography versus colonoscopy for the detection of advanced neoplasia. N Engl J Med. 2007;357(14):1403-1412.
8. Pickhardt PJ, Nugent PA, Mysliwiec PA, Choi JR, Schindler WR. Location of adenomas missed by optical colonoscopy. Ann Intern Med. 2004;141(5):352-359.

9. Pickhardt PJ, Choi JR, Hwang I, et al. Computed tomographic virtual colonoscopy to screen for colorectal neoplasia in asymptomatic adults. *N Engl J Med.* 2003;349(23):2191-2200.

10. Johnson CD, Chen MH, Toledano AY, et al. Accuracy of CT colonography for detection of large adenomas and cancers. *N Engl J Med.* 2008;359(12):1207-1217.

11. Regge D. Accuracy of CT colonography in subjects at increased risk of colorectal carcinoma: A multicenter study on 1,066 patients (IMPACT). Boston: 8th International Symposium on Virtual Colonoscopy; 2007:108-109.

12. Baxter NN, Goldwasser MA, Paszat LF, Saskin R, Urbach DR, Rabeneck L. Association of colonoscopy and death from colorectal cancer: A population-based, case-control study. *Ann Intern Med.* 2009;150(1):1-8.

13. Kim JH, Kim WH, Kim TI, et al. Incomplete colonoscopy in patients with occlusive colorectal cancer: Usefulness of CT colonography according to tumor location. *Yonsei Med J.* 2007;48:934-941.

14. Passman MA, Pommier RF, Vetto JT. Synchronous colon primaries have the same prognosis as solitary colon cancers. *Dis Colon Rectum.* 1996;39(3):329-334.

15. Pinchuk AN, Rampy MA, Longino MA, et al. Synthesis and structure-activity relationship effects on the tumor avidity of radioiodinated phospholipid ether analogues. *J Med Chem.* 2006;49(7):2155-2165.

16. Pickhardt PJ, Lehman VT, Winter TC, Taylor AJ. Polyp volume versus linear size measurements at CT colonography: Implications for noninvasive surveillance of unresected colorectal lesions. *Am J Roentgenol.* 2006;186(6):1605-1610.

17. Brenner DJ, Hall EJ. Current concepts—Computed tomography—An increasing source of radiation exposure. *N Engl J Med.* 2007;357(22):2277-2284.

18. Radiation risk in perspective. Position statement of the Health Physics Society. Adopted January 1996, revised August 2004. McLean, VA: Health Physics Society; 2004.

19. Edwards JT, Mendelson RM, Fritschi L, et al. Colorectal neoplasia screening with CT colonography in average-risk asymptomatic subjects: Community-based study. *Radiology.* 2004;230(2):459-464.

20. Gluecker TM, Johnson CD, Harmsen WS, et al. Colorectal cancer screening with CT colonography, colonoscopy, and double-contrast barium enema examination: Prospective assessment of patient perceptions and preferences. *Radiology.* 2003;227(2):378-384.

21. Harewood GC, Wiersema MJ, Melton LJ. A prospective, controlled assessment of factors influencing acceptance of screening colonoscopy. *Am J Gastroenterol.* 2002;97(12):3186-3194.

22. Iannaccone R, Laghi A, Catalano C, et al. Computed tomographic colonography without cathartic preparation for the detection of colorectal polyps. *Gastroenterology.* 2004;127(5):1300-1311.

23. Pickhardt PJ. Colonic preparation for computed tomographic colonography: Understanding the relative advantages and disadvantages of a noncathartic approach. *Mayo Clin Proc.* 2007;82(6):659-661.

24. Petrick N, Haider M, Summers RM, et al. CT colonography with computer-aided detection as a second reader: Observer performance study. *Radiology.* 2008;246(1):148-156.

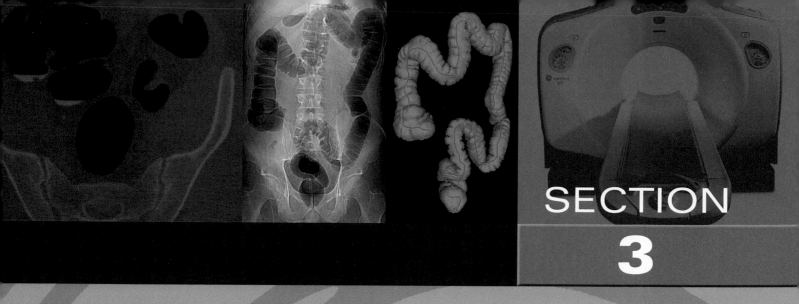

CT Colonography Technique

Bowel Preparation for CT Colonography

DAVID H. KIM, MD
PERRY J. PICKHARDT, MD

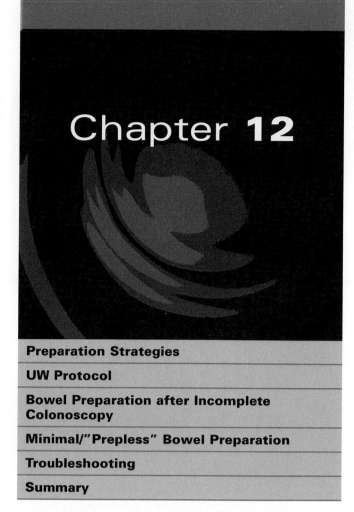

Chapter 12

INTRODUCTION

One of the key components of effective polyp detection at CT colonography (CTC) involves the bowel preparation for the study. Without adequate preparation, CTC is destined to perform poorly despite optimization of all other aspects of the examination. Unfortunately, despite its central importance for the examination, there is no standardized use of agents or protocols, with wide variation in overall preparation strategy. This chapter will delineate the major bowel preparation strategies including cathartic-only, tagging-only, and complete (cathartic and tagging) approaches. The rationale for the complete bowel preparation, which we believe is the optimal approach, will be highlighted. We will then focus on the specific agents and protocol used in the University of Wisconsin (UW) CTC screening program. This bowel preparation protocol is an integral reason behind our effective polyp detection capabilities and strong program results.

PREPARATION STRATEGIES

The purpose of the bowel preparation for CTC is to minimize or eliminate the negative effect of stool on the interpretation of the examination. Three major approaches have been undertaken: (1) cathartic-only, (2) tagging-only, and (3) complete cathartic/tagging strategies. Whereas the first two approaches have demonstrated adequate polyp sensitivities in high-prevalence cohorts, only the complete cathartic/tagging strategy has demonstrated effective polyp detection rates in the intended cohorts of low-prevalence or screening populations.[1,2]

The *cathartic-only approach* was the major approach used early on in the CTC experience. It involves purging the colon with cathartic agents. No oral contrast tagging agents are given. The major drawback to this approach concerns the fact that no matter how well the colon is cleansed; there will often be some residual stool particles and fluid. Unfortunately, residual solid stool often has a grayish appearance at CTC when a tagging agent is not given, thus mimicking a soft tissue polyp. Stool can only be distinguished from a polyp by demonstrating either internal heterogeneity (e.g., the presence of air) or by movement between the supine and prone series (Fig. 12-1). Thus, any homogenous adherent stool would likely result in a CTC false-positive result. Similarly, any residual luminal fluid would pose problems in which the gray appearance of the fluid would obscure a submerged polyp on that series (Fig. 12-2). For this reason, research had previously concentrated on minimizing residual fluid by using cathartics that promoted a relatively "dry prep."[3] With regimens that add tagging agents (see later), the issues of increased residual fluid are of less concern. The cathartic-only approach can lead to effective detection in a reasonable proportion of cases, but in the cases in which the catharsis is not optimal, the examination quickly becomes tedious to interpret because multiple pseudopolyps related to stool must be interrogated. Sensitivity for polyp detection ultimately decreases as a result.

The *tagging-only approach* is a more recent approach that has developed to address one of the recognized majors factors behind noncompliance with colorectal cancer screening—that is, use of the cathartic agent.[4-6] Often the term "prepless" has been affixed to these non-

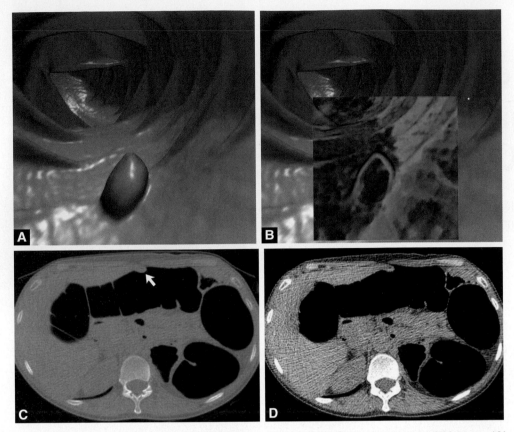

Figure 12-1 **Appearance of untagged stool with cathartic-only approach.** 3D endoluminal CTC image **(A)** shows residual untagged stool. The same 3D image with translucency rendering applied **(B)** shows that the untagged stool matches the red color signature of a true soft tissue polyp. 2D transverse images with polyp **(C)** and soft tissue **(D)** windowing also show that distinguishing the stool *(arrow)* from a polyp is difficult without contrast tagging. Untagged stool can only be confirmed in this case by movement to a dependent location between the supine and prone series. *Illustration continued on following page*

cathartic regimens, although this is a misnomer because this approach represents a true bowel preparation. "Tagging-only" or "noncathartic" descriptors represent more correct designations. In this strategy, there is alteration of the individual's diet to low-residue foods and ingestion of tagging agents at various intervals. No cathartic agents are administered. The aim is to tag all fecal material (Fig. 12-3). The examination is interpreted by either a 2D approach or a 3D approach, with or without postprocessing with electronic subtraction algorithms (see subsequent section on minimal preparation).

The final approach is the *complete bowel preparation strategy*, which uses both catharsis and tagging. The aim is to clean out the colon as completely as possible and then tag any residual stool or fluid. This strategy is the one that has demonstrated consistently high accuracies for polyp detection in low-prevalence cohorts and is the basis of the UW protocol. Similar to the cathartic-only approach, a clean colon allows for facile and effective interpretation because there are few pseudopolyps related to stool that need to be evaluated. The key difference involves the application of tagging agents. Whereas the residual stool and fluid following catharsis cause a problem in the approach without tagging, this is not the case for the complete bowel preparation. The ad-

ministered tagging agents interact with any remaining colonic residue to significantly raise the attenuation values and allow for easy differentiation from the soft tissue attenuation of true polyps and potential detection of submerged polyps (Fig. 12-4). In addition to promoting an effective nontaxing search pattern for polyp detection, the complete bowel preparation also allows for the ability to refer patients to same-day optical colonoscopy (OC) for removal of significant lesions. Thus, this bowel protocol allows for an integrated CTC–OC model, which in turn allows the clinical question to be answered and addressed in a single medical encounter with a single bowel preparation.

UW PROTOCOL

The UW prep is based on the complete bowel preparation approach, which uses the benefits of both catharsis and tagging (Fig. 12-5). Since the inception of this approach with the Department of Defense screening trial, the protocol has gradually evolved to its current optimized state. The amount of the cathartic and tagging agents has been minimized and the timing of administration has been greatly simplified. In addition, there has been a recent shift to magnesium citrate from sodium

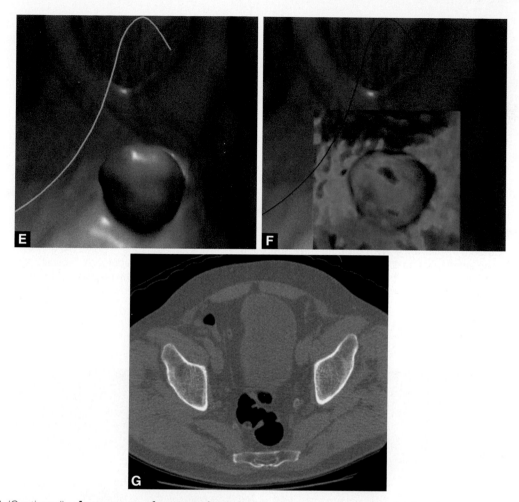

Figure 12-1 (Continued)   **Appearance of untagged stool with cathartic-only approach.** In other cases, untagged stool can also be diagnosed by demonstrating internal heterogeneity **(E-G).** 3D endoluminal CTC image **(E)** shows an apparent large rectal polyp that fails to demonstrate a soft tissue red core at translucency **(F)** and shows internal heterogeneity on the 2D transverse image **(G).** Internal heterogeneity reflects internal low-density foci and thus confirms stool. Unfortunately, this appearance is not frequently seen with small subcentimeter stool particles. *(*See associated video clip in DVD.)*

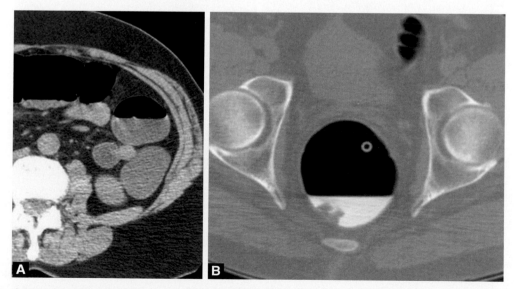

Figure 12-2   Appearance of untagged versus tagged colonic fluid. 2D transverse image **(A)** shows the gray appearance of untagged fluid as would be seen in a cathartic-only approach. Note that any submerged polyp would be concealed on this view, whereas with fluid tagging **(B),** such polyps would be visible. This tagged case demonstrates a large submerged tubulovillous adenoma.

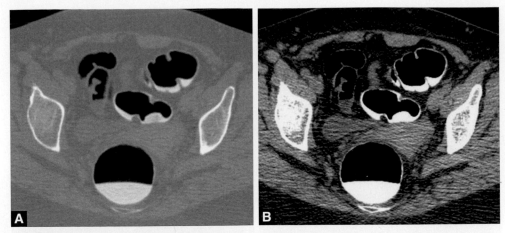

Figure 12-3 Colonic appearance with tagging-only approach. 2D transverse images in polyp **(A)** and soft tissue **(B)** windows demonstrate the appearance of the colon with a typical noncathartic, barium-tagging approach. Typically, low-residue diets are followed to decrease fecal bulk, with various regimens used to tag stool and fluid to allow primary 2D search algorithms or electronic subtraction (for 3D approaches).

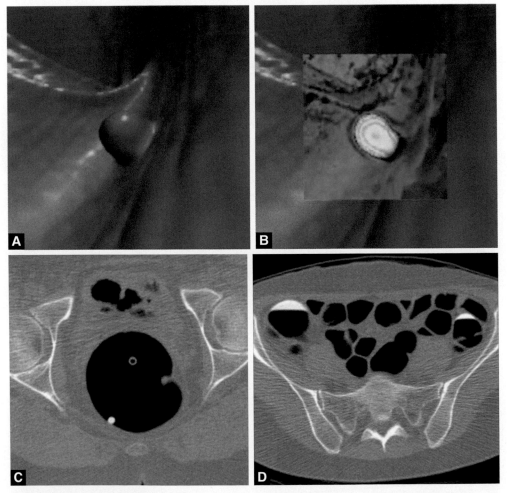

Figure 12-4 Value of the complete prep. 3D endoluminal view **(A)** shows a potential polyp that is easily discounted as adherent tagged stool with translucency **(B)** and 2D transverse imaging **(C)**. Because residual fluid is tagged as well **(D)**, the importance of a "dry prep" is minimized because submerged polyps can still be seen.

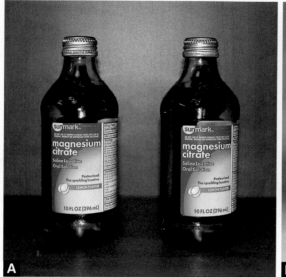
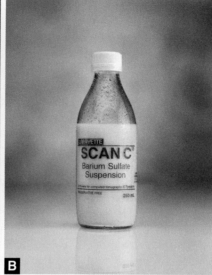
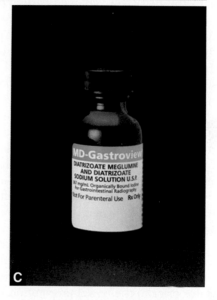

Figure 12-5   Components of standard UW bowel preparation for CTC. Magnesium citrate **(A)**, 2% barium **(B)**, and diatrizoate **(C)** are taken sequentially the evening before CTC examination (see text for details).

phosphate as the default cathartic agent. Use of this specific regimen has led to consistently robust bowel preparations for CTC interpretation. The following sections will examine the specific cathartic and tagging agents in use with this protocol followed by the timing of administration of these agents.

Cathartic Agents

Three different cathartic agents have been used for CTC at UW. These include magnesium citrate, sodium phosphate, and polyethylene glycol (PEG). Each specific cathartic agent carries certain advantages and disadvantages. Small-volume osmotic cathartics (magnesium citrate and sodium phosphate) are easier to ingest but create relatively large fluid shifts in the individual, whereas large-volume osmotically balanced preparations (PEG) are much more difficult for the patient to complete but are generally safer for debilitated patients with tenuous fluid balances.

Magnesium citrate is a low-volume, osmotic cathartic agent. It has been in use as a bowel preparation agent for barium enema examinations since the 1960s. It is typically given in liquid form and has a fairly palatable taste. A standard dose is 300 mL (10 oz), which contains approximately 3 g of magnesium (Sunmark, San Francisco, CA). As opposed to the barium enema, in which a single dose is administered, a split, double-dose protocol is used at CTC (see later). Its cathartic action works primarily through the high osmolarity of the solution, which draws large amounts of fluid into the colonic lumen, creating a large effluent for catharsis. In addition, there is probable stimulation of fluid excretion by cholecystokinin release and activation of smooth muscle peristalsis to secondarily aid in clearing colonic material.[7] The time of onset can be as early as 30 minutes, with a mean onset time of

2 hours from the administered dose. The duration of action may last up to 4 hours.[8] When multiple doses are administered, the cleansing ability has been shown equivalent to other preparations at endoscopic evaluation.[9,10] One of the recognized keys for efficacious cleansing is related to the individual's hydration status. As is true of all cathartics that act through an osmotic nature to pull fluid into the colonic lumen, a well-hydrated state promotes cleansing activity, whereas a dehydrated status retards cathartic action, presumably as a result of a decreased effluent volume.[7]

One interesting observation from the barium enema era regarding magnesium citrate cathartic preparations may have an impact on CTC. It has been observed that magnesium interacts with barium suspensions in which there is increased barium coating of the colon. It is felt that residual magnesium cations within colonic mucus can associate with the negatively charged barium particles.[11] For barium enema, this has resulted in alterations in protocol to decrease the propensity for excessive coating. For CTC, it emphasizes the importance of the use of diatrizoate within the preparation protocol (see later). Without the secondary cathartic effects of diatrizoate, right-sided adherent barium would presumably be increased with magnesium citrate–based preparations.

The advantages of magnesium citrate include a relatively small required volume administration and palatable taste, which both lead to improved patient compliance. The disadvantages are related to its osmotic nature, in which pulling fluid into the colon creates fluids shifts, ultimately from the intravascular space. Thus, this preparation should be avoided in patients with intolerance to changes in fluid balance related to significantly diminished renal or cardiac function. It should also be used with caution in patients eating a low-sodium diet. In general, a well-hydrated status prior to the bowel preparation is recommended to decrease risks of orthostasis. In addition, it is important to remember that the induced colonic catharsis will further affect the patient's fluid status, thus requiring adequate oral fluid intake during this period to maintain a well-hydrated status. Holte and colleagues demonstrated a median weight loss of slightly more than 1 kg with use of an osmotic-based cathartic regimen despite a median fluid intake of close to 4 L over this time.[12]

Overall, magnesium citrate is felt to be a safe cathartic option that is well tolerated. Indeed, it has had a long track record of use at barium enema for several decades. In addition, the use of a double dose at CTC is likely very safe in the general population. Picosalax (sodium picosulphate with magnesium citrate) has been widely used in Europe as a cathartic agent since the early 1980s. This regimen administers the equivalent of a double dose of magnesium citrate (3.5 g of magnesium in each sachet; two sachets are given in total). Contraindications to magnesium citrate administration include patients with abdominal pain or hemorrhage, intestinal obstruction, and renal failure.[13] Because the major route of excretion is through the urinary

system, use of this agent should be avoided in patients with significant renal dysfunction because it could potentially lead to severe hypermagnesemia. Severe, even fatal, consequences have been reported with magnesium citrate use with patients with frank renal failure.[14]

In the UW program, magnesium citrate was initially used as the secondary cathartic option within the bowel preparation protocol, constituting approximately 10% of the patients. Magnesium citrate was reserved for patients with relative contraindications for administering sodium phosphate. Sodium phosphate had been favored over magnesium citrate because of its excellent cleansing properties with only a single 45-mL dose. Recently, we changed over to magnesium citrate as the primary cathartic option following the outcome of a direct comparison of efficacy between the two regimens in which equivalency was seen[15] and because of the emerging concerns for acute phosphate nephropathy associated with sodium phosphate use (see later).

Sodium phosphate is a buffered saline osmotic cathartic containing both monobasic and dibasic forms. It is typically given in liquid form, although it is also available in tablets. Its cathartic action works through the high osmolarity of the solution, which draws large amounts of fluid into the colonic lumen with resultant large effluent and catharsis. The average time to onset of bowel activity is within 2 hours, although the response often occurs much sooner.[16] It is highly effective in colonic cleansing and considered equivalent or superior to other cathartics such as PEG.[17-19] As with other osmotic cathartics, the mechanism of action creates large fluid shifts within the individual, which may become problematic in people with limited cardiac or renal functioning. Traditionally, sodium phosphate for optical colonoscopy preparation has been administered in two 45-mL doses separated by 5 to 12 hours.[20] We initially used a double-dose protocol for CTC[1]; however, a prospective comparison between single- and double-dose sodium phosphate demonstrated that the dose could be reduced to a single 45-mL administration at CTC with equivalent cleansing results.[21] Such a reduction was possible as a result of the additional cathartic effects of the diatrizoate tagging agent given during CTC bowel preparation (see later).

The major advantage of sodium phosphate is related to its low-volume 45-mL administration. It is substantially lower than even the low-volume magnesium citrate–based regimen (two doses of 300 mL). Several studies have demonstrated increased compliance in completing the cathartic regimen compared to the 4-L large-volume PEG regimens.[17] Disadvantages are primarily related to the lower safety margin. Sodium phosphate creates large fluid shifts in individuals and has demonstrated electrolyte changes including transient hyperphosphatemia and potential hypocalcemia. However, in the past, studies have shown an overall favorable safety profile in the typical healthy screening individual.[17-20,22,23] Most adverse events were felt to be related to inappropriately administered, higher-than-recommended doses or given to inappropriate patient groups.[20] Sodium phosphate use is contraindicated in patients with significant renal insufficiency and other conditions in which rapid fluid and electrolyte shifts are risky, such as congestive heart failure and cirrhosis.

In recent years, a rare but significant complication has been identified with sodium phosphate use.[24,25] Small numbers of individuals with previously normal renal function subsequently developed renal failure following sodium phosphate use that was largely irreversible. This rare event (termed acute phosphate nephropathy) is currently poorly understood, but patients who have developed this condition following sodium phosphate administration have demonstrated worsening renal failure with histologic findings of acute/chronic tubular injury and abundant calcium phosphate deposition. Persons at risk include older individuals with a history of hypertension taking angiotensin-converting enzyme inhibitors, angiotensin receptor blockers, or diuretic medications. Dehydration is felt to be a potential contributing factor.[26]

In our program, sodium phosphate had long stood as the main cathartic of choice, accounting for nearly 90% of our patients. It was very effective in colonic cleansing with a high compliance rate among patients because of the need for only a small volume for ingestion. In healthy, middle-aged adults of whom a typical screening population represents, it was felt to be a safe agent to administer; the safety margin was further increased by use of a single dose (as opposed to the standard split double-dose regimen for colonoscopy). Nonetheless, we shifted over to a magnesium citrate–based protocol to simplify the cathartic options from a programmatic standpoint and to address the emerging concerns regarding sodium phosphate use. Several months later, safety warnings were issued by the Food and Drug Administration, leading to the voluntary recall of all over-the-counter sodium phosphate products for bowel cleansing.

PEG is a third option for colonic cleansing. It is an osmotically balanced solution containing various electrolytes and a high molecular weight nonabsorbable polymer. This cathartic is nonabsorbable with negligible fluid and electrolyte shifts across the colonic mucosa. Because of the osmotic pressure created by the polymer, the electrolyte solution remains intraluminal and can then act as a colonic cleanser via lavage.[27] Time to onset is typically 30 minutes to 1 hour. It is effective for cleansing the colon and has been in use for colonoscopy for many years but requires a large-volume administration of 4 L. The main advantage is the lack of appreciable fluid or electrolyte shifts as a result of its nonabsorbed nature. It does, however, lead to a large amount of residual colonic fluid ("a wet prep"), which is not ideal but not a major problem for CTC interpretation when tagging agents are administered to opacify the fluid. The major disadvantage revolves around patient compliance because complete ingestion of the solution is difficult because of its poor palatability and

large volume. The 4-L administration translates into sixteen 8-ounce cups taken every 10 minutes. More recently, PEG preps consisting of 2-L administration have been introduced, which should improve patient compliance but may degrade the prep quality.

In our program, PEG is used infrequently, in less than 1% of patients. It is reserved for patients who are significantly debilitated and/or cannot tolerate any fluid shifts. Most patients enrolled in our screening program are typically fairly healthy outpatients, and low-volume osmotic cathartic preparations are more suitable for them.

Tagging Agents

Two tagging agents are administered *after* the cathartic agent to complete the UW CTC bowel preparation. These include a 2% w/v barium sulfate suspension and an iodine-based solution of diatrizoate meglumine and diatrizoate sodium. These agents mix with any stool and colonic fluid left behind after catharsis to markedly increase the attenuation of the residual material. Consequently, the residual stool particles and colonic fluid have a white appearance at CT, which allows for both easy differentiation from the soft tissue attenuation of a polyp and detection of polyps submerged within colonic pools.

The 2.1% w/v barium sulfate suspension is a dilute mixture of barium that is typically used at routine CT. It is inert with no appreciable absorption by the body.[28] It is given as a single 250-mL dose several hours after the cathartic. It is likely the main agent that tags the particulate stool, mixing with residual material to increase the attenuation (Fig. 12-4). It plays a smaller role in opacifying residual luminal fluid, typically leading to a suboptimal gradient of dense material in more dependent positions from sedimentation effects. One interesting effect noticed at image interpretation has been the thin surface coating of polyps by contrast (Fig. 12-6).[29] This is a common appearance in which a soft tissue polyp has a thin uniform layer of overlying contrast, similar to a polyp that is "etched-in-white" at a barium enema. This fortuitous phenomenon has been helpful for increasing the conspicuity of polyps at CTC. With our prep, the tagging agent is generally not seen lining the normal colonic wall, which is likely a result of the mini-cathartic effect of the diatrizoate. It is important to note that the dilute nature of the 2% barium suspension has not posed a problem at potential same-day colonoscopy, whereas higher density 40% barium preparations have reportedly obscured polyps at endoscopy and have affected the equipment by clogging various channels of the scope at same-day evaluation.

The iodine-based water-soluble tagging agent of diatrizoate is a hypertonic solution of approximately 1400 mOsm/kg and contains 370 mg of organically bound iodine per milliliter.[28] It is given as a single 60-mL administration after both the cathartic and barium tagging agents. Diatrizoate is felt to be the primary component for

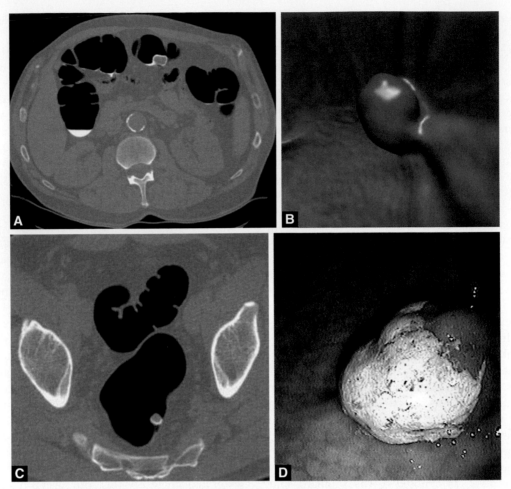

Figure 12-6 Surface coating of a polyp by the tagging agent. 2D transverse view **(A)** shows a thin rim of contrast outlining a tubulovillous adenoma. This characteristic phenomenon aids in both characterization and detection of soft tissue polyps. Note how the tagging agent washes away from the adjacent normal colonic mucosa. 3D endoluminal CTC image **(B)** in another patient shows a rectal polyp. 2D transverse view **(C)** shows contrast clinging to the polyp surface, which is seen at colonoscopy **(D)** as a yellowish film. (Figs B, D from Pickhardt PJ. Screening CT colonography: How I do it. *Am J Roentgenol.* 2007;189:290-298.)

tagging residual colonic fluid. With the administration of diatrizoate, the opacification of the colonic fluid pools is much more homogenous than with barium alone (Fig. 12-4). Diatrizoate likely plays a lesser role in tagging of residual solid stool and the surface coating of true polyps. Diatrizoate serves a second vital function in the overall bowel preparation protocol. The hypertonic nature of the solution draws fluid into the colonic lumen along similar principles of the osmotic cathartics. In addition, it also stimulates intestinal peristalsis. Together, there is a second mini-catharsis, which helps to scrub away any adherent residual tagged stool from the colonic wall (Fig. 12-7). The stool can then be either expelled prior to imaging or remain mobile in the colonic fluid pool.

Protocol Timing

The bowel preparation protocol begins 1 day prior to the scheduled CTC examination as a simple, straightforward regimen (Fig. 12-8). The protocol is optimized to create as minimal a disruption to the individual's routine as possible. The beginning of the preparation allows the person to engage in normal daily activities including regular work hours until the true cathartic portion begins in the late afternoon/early evening. Cathartics are administered before the tagging agents to remove the bulk of the stool. Consequently, only minimal amounts of tagging agents are required, as opposed to a reverse approach in which large doses would be required if the bulk stool was tagged before catharsis.

On the day prior to the CTC examination, the individual restricts his or her diet to clear liquids beginning at midnight. Consequently, breakfast is limited to a clear-liquid diet (which can include black coffee to help minimize the disruption for those accustomed to morning caffeine). Hydration is stressed with recommendations to drink 4 to 6 cups of carbohydrate/electrolyte replenishment drinks during the morning and mid afternoon prior to catharsis for the reasons discussed in the saline-based cathartics section. Red-colored liquids are to be avoided because they may potentially interfere with a colonoscopy if required (such liquids purportedly

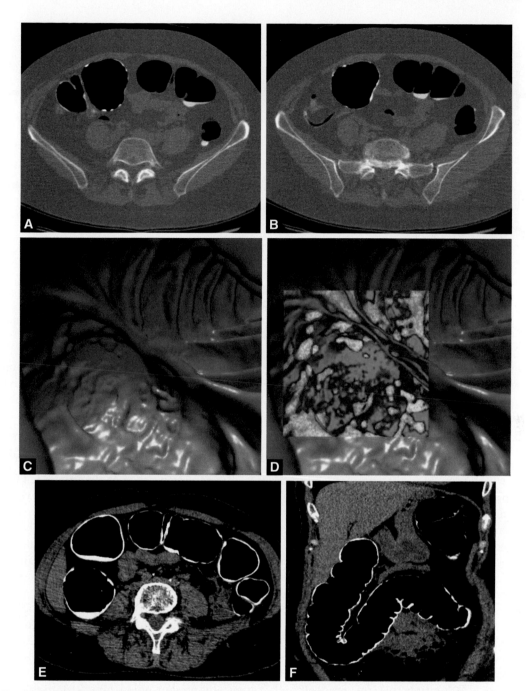

Figure 12-7 Absence of diatrizoate in bowel prep. Note the adherent barium-tagged stool that remains in this individual who did not take the diatrizoate. 2D transverse images (**A** and **B**) demonstrate scattered punctuate foci of tagged residual stool, which appear as polypoid structures on the 3D endoluminal view (**C**). Translucency rendering at 3D CTC (**D**) confirms tagged stool. 2D transverse and coronal images (**E** and **F**) in another patient without diatrizoate show a cast of barium-tagged stool covering the mucosal surface. Cases such as these underscore the importance of the cathartic nature of the diatrizoate agent in addition to its fluid tagging properties. (*See associated video clip in DVD.)*

can stain the mucosa). In the late morning, the patient ingests two tablets of bisacodyl for the magnesium citrate or sodium phosphate–based protocols (not given for the PEG-based regimen). This stimulant laxative does not typically produce immediate diarrhea, generally requiring 6 to 8 hours before inducing a bowel movement. Consequently, the individual may continue usual daily activities during this period. It is postulated that this

medication may "prepare" the colon and improve the overall effect of the subsequent cathartic medications.

Beginning in the late afternoon or early evening, the true cathartic portion of the examination begins in which the patient may need to restrict normal activities and have access to a restroom. One of the cathartic choices is administered (now, typically magnesium citrate). After a 3-hour window, the first tagging agent is

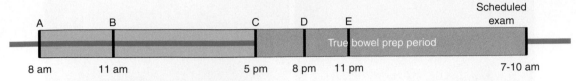

Schedule of prep agents

A: Clear liquid diet beginning with breakfast
B: Two bisacodyl tablets (5 mg each) by mouth
C: Cathartic agent given.* (typically, magnesium citrate)
D: First tagging agent given (250 mL 2% barium). A second dose of
   magnesium citrate is given here with the barium.
E: Second tagging agent given (60 mL diatrizoate). Bowel prep complete.
A-E: Patient should maintain good oral hydration until midnight.

* May begin prep as early as 2 pm. Space each administered agent by 3
  hours. If polyethylene glycol is used as the cathartic, the first dose should
  be given around noon to complete the prep that evening (16 eight-
  ounce cups, one every 10 minutes). For the noncathartic prep, 60 mL
  diatrizoate is substituted here for the cathartic agent.

Figure 12-8 **Standard bowel preparation protocol schedule.** Note the relatively simple, straightforward nature of this low-volume protocol with administration of the three agents each separated by approximately 3 hours.

taken, in which a single dose of 250 mL of 2% barium suspension is administered. A second dose of magnesium citrate is also automatically given at this time for the multidose regimen. After a second 3-hour period, the second tagging agent of diatrizoate is taken as a single 60-mL dose. Throughout the afternoon and night, the individual must maintain hydration with ingestion of 2 to 3 L of fluid, which translates into approximately 8 to 12, 8-ounce cups, to replace fluid loss associated with catharsis. After midnight, the patient remains fasting to include liquids and the examination is then conducted the following morning.

One issue concerning bowel preparation for CTC has concerned the idea of "dry" versus "wet" preparations related to the amount of residual colonic fluid.[3] Low-volume osmotic cathartics such as magnesium citrate and sodium phosphate are considered dry preparations with only minimal remaining colonic fluid, whereas polyethylene glycol is considered to be a wet preparation with large amounts of residual fluid. The dry preparations have been generally favored at CTC, citing that the residual fluid could potentially obscure polyps despite supine and prone positioning. However, such an argument carries less weight when fluid tagging is used because soft tissue polyps are clearly seen within the opacified colonic fluid pool (Fig. 12-2). One disadvantage with dry preparations is the potential for adherent dessicated residual stool. When untagged, such particulate matter may be indistinguishable from true polyps. When tagged, they are easily characterized as stool but still may preclude a 3D search pattern because the multiplicity of "polyps" would require too-frequent 2D correlation. The protocol we advocate typically uses a low-volume osmotic cathartic that would tend toward a dry preparation. However, the use of diatrizoate as one of the tagging agents appears to convert it to somewhat of a wetter preparation with more fluid than is seen in untagged cathartic preparations. One apparent advantage is that the dessicated adherent stool that can be seen with dry preparations is not typically a problem.

BOWEL PREPARATION AFTER INCOMPLETE COLONOSCOPY

We are often asked to undertake CTC following incomplete colonoscopy. For patient convenience, we typically perform the examination on the same day to preclude the need for a separate complete bowel preparation and an additional visit to the hospital. This approach, however, does create some difficulty in interpretation. The bowel preparation at optical colonoscopy is a cathartic-only approach with no tagging agents administered. Consequently, any residual stool may mimic a polyp unless it demonstrates movement between supine and prone positioning or discernible internal heterogeneity. In addition, for those individuals who received a PEG-based preparation, a large amount of colonic fluid is typically present unless aspirated at colonoscopy, which potentially could obscure a polyp because of its untagged state. To improve sensitivity and specificity, we typically administer 30 mL of diatrizoate by mouth once the patient has recovered from anesthesia (it is important that the patient is fully awake because aspiration of this hypertonic solution could lead to pulmonary edema). This is followed by the patient drinking one to two glasses of water; then the patient is placed right side down to promote clearance from the stomach. The patient is then imaged approximately 2 hours (if possible) after administration. There have been variable results in colonic tagging with this salvage approach (Fig. 12-9). Alternatively, another option (although less convenient for the patient) is to keep the patient on clear liquids, administer oral contrast tagging that evening, and proceed with

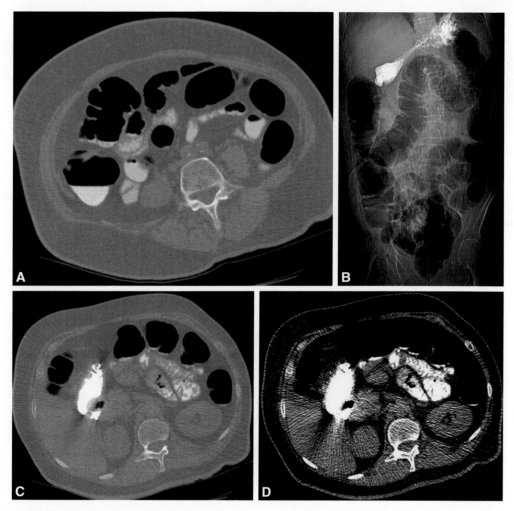

Figure 12-9 CTC after incomplete colonoscopy. 2D transverse image **(A)** shows that the diatrizoate has reached the colon, allowing tagging of residual fluid and stool in this case. CTC scout **(B)**, however, also shows retention of the tagging agent in the stomach, which is relatively undiluted. 2D transverse images in polyp **(C)** and soft tissue **(D)** windows show streak artifact related to the concentrated diatrizoate in the gastric antrum, which is less pronounced on polyp windows.

CTC the following day. This avoids the need for additional cathartics while ensuring the benefits of tagging. Finally, rescheduling the patient at a future date with a complete bowel preparation with cathartic and tagging agents could be done if acceptable to the referring physician and patient.

MINIMAL/"PREPLESS" BOWEL PREPARATION

Alternative bowel preparations for CTC are under investigation. One of the major reasons cited by individuals for decreased colorectal cancer screening compliance concerns the perceived difficulties with the bowel preparation related to the cathartic agents.[6] Consequently, elimination of the cathartic could potentially remove a significant barrier to screening. Although these regimens are sometimes termed "prepless," this is a misnomer because all of these alternative CTC bowel protocols require some form of preparation before

the examination, which can sometimes be more onerous than our routine cathartic preparation. This approach is typically in the form of fecal tagging with oral contrast agents; a more appropriate term for these alternative regimens may be *noncathartic* or *tagging-only* bowel preparations.

The underlying principle for this approach is to tag all intraluminal colonic contents with a contrast agent prior to the CTC examination. This has been accomplished by either using barium suspensions[30-32] or iodine-based solutions[33] given with meals 24 to 72 hours before the examination. Frequently, a low-residue diet is also followed during this time. The intended appearance of the colon at CTC is to have homogenously tagged stool without any untagged areas (Fig. 12-10). A 2D search pattern is then used for polyp detection. Alternatively, additional postprocessing techniques have been investigated including digital electronic subtraction of the tagged stool to allow for primary 3D methods of polyp detection.[34]

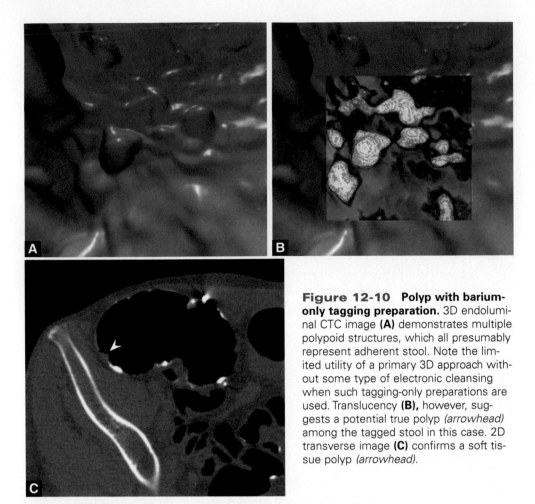

Figure 12-10 Polyp with barium-only tagging preparation. 3D endoluminal CTC image **(A)** demonstrates multiple polypoid structures, which all presumably represent adherent stool. Note the limited utility of a primary 3D approach without some type of electronic cleansing when such tagging-only preparations are used. Translucency **(B),** however, suggests a potential true polyp *(arrowhead)* among the tagged stool in this case. 2D transverse image **(C)** confirms a soft tissue polyp *(arrowhead).*

There is some debate as to which tagging agent is more favorable within these regimens. Barium suspensions have the advantages of improved taste and tolerability over iodine-based solutions. In addition, barium is inert, whereas iodine theoretically could incite an allergic reaction in susceptible individuals because trace amounts can be absorbed across the colonic mucosa. However, barium has difficulty tagging colonic fluid homogenously. Both agents tag stool well, although barium may be better in this regard. Iodine-based agents that are hypertonic also cause a mild catharsis, which is beneficial to the fidelity of the prep but may be detrimental to its "noncathartic" billing. Patient discomfort scores between barium-based agents and nonionic iodine solutions have been shown equivalent.[35]

Although there have been some promising initial results with both noncathartic tagging approaches,[30,33] such protocols remain in the investigatory realm. The performance characteristics in a large-scale, low polyp–prevalence population have not been evaluated. Currently, the presence of large amounts of stool, even when tagged, presents difficulties in polyp detection. Primary 3D search algorithms cannot be easily used (unless with additional postprocessing techniques) because of the multiplicity of potential polyp candidates that must be characterized at 2D. Although electronic subtraction can be performed, the addition of these and other postprocessing techniques introduce an additional layer of potential artifacts that affect both sensitivity and specificity. Consequently, primary 2D remains the default polyp detection method for noncathartic protocols, with its inherent limitations. Even in well-cleansed, well-tagged colons, this method as a primary detection strategy has performed poorly compared to primary 3D protocols.[1,36-38] In the case of an uncleansed colon, such search patterns become even more difficult and presumably would perform at a level less than the optimal cleansed situation.

At UW, we use a variation of the minimal preparation approach. The default protocol used in the majority of patients is the complete bowel preparation. However, for those symptomatic patients who are elderly and/or frail in which the primary indication is generally cancer detection (colorectal or otherwise), as opposed to colorectal polyp detection/cancer prevention, a noncathartic tagging-only approach based on diatrizoate and barium is used (Fig. 12-8). A low-residue diet combined with the tagging agents is undertaken. An extra dose of diatrizoate is substituted for the cathartic agent. In addition, intravenous contrast is generally used with this approach because extracolonic evaluation is often indicated to help explain patient symptoms. Although this preparation is

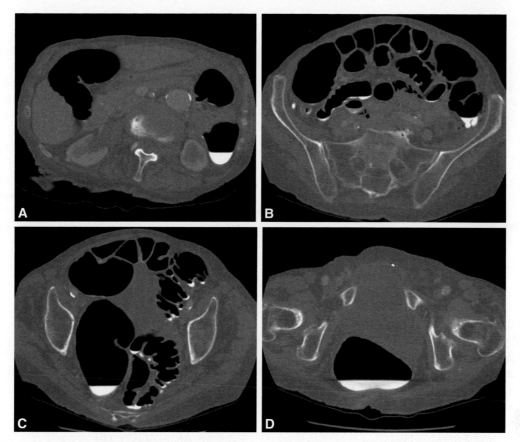

Figure 12-11 UW noncathartic CTC prep. 2D transverse views **(A-D)** show a well-cleansed and tagged colon in this individual, although a true cathartic was not used. Currently, this prep is used when the target of CTC is a large polyp or cancer in a debilitated symptomatic patient. IV contrast is often used in this setting to evaluate for extracolonic pathology.

technically noncathartic, it is important to realize that there are mild cathartic effects from the diatrizoate. In some individuals the colon may be very well cleansed with this protocol (Fig. 12-11).

TROUBLESHOOTING

Questions often arise regarding the bowel preparation. The following is a partial list restricted to the more common questions we have encountered in our program. They are intended to represent a guide for possible solutions and not absolute answers. When at least some combination of cathartic and contrast agents were taken but there is still some uncertainty regarding fidelity of the prep, our typical approach is to lean toward performing the examination if at all possible because the majority prove to be of diagnostic quality.

Questions Relating to:
Diet Restriction

I didn't read the instructions until now and I have already eaten breakfast. Can I still have the examination?

This is a common question. Some patients do not read the bowel preparation instructions until the morning before CTC, not realizing that the clear-liquid diet restric-

tion began earlier (after midnight). The restriction thus includes breakfast on the day before the examination. If the patient has eaten a full breakfast, it is probably best to reschedule the examination. In our experience, there is an increased proportion of suboptimal preparations in this circumstance. Although there is the inconvenience of rescheduling, the patient has yet to begin the cathartic and most difficult portion of the preparation. If the patient has eaten only a small amount (e.g., a single piece of toast), we often will continue with the preparation and examination, with generally good results.

Is coffee a clear liquid?

Yes. However, the patient should not add milk products to the coffee. Additional acceptable options for the clear liquid diet include the following:
- Sport carbohydrate/electrolyte replenishment drinks
- Water, tea, coffee, lemonade
- Bouillon or broth
- Gelatin, popsicles
- Apple, white grape, or white cranberry juice
- Soda
- Clear hard candy

Juice with pulp such as orange or grapefruit juice should be avoided.

I see you can't have red clear liquids, but are orange and purple okay?

Patients are asked to avoid drinking clear liquids with red coloring such as red gelatin (Jell-O) or cranberry juice to help prevent potential difficulties at colonoscopy. For those few patients that may need a same-day colonoscopy in the afternoon, it is purported that the red coloring can stain the mucosa and may make visualization for polyps more difficult. In practice, this probably is not a major problem and we are therefore somewhat lax on this restriction (and for other food coloring). We ask that patients stay away from red-colored liquids but indicate that other colors are permissible. If the patient has accidentally ingested a red-colored food, it would not be a contraindication to continuing with the study.

Medications

Can I take my medicine for high blood pressure?

This is a common question. Patients often call about individual medications and whether to continue. As a rule, we advise patients to continue their typical medications, altering administration times to 1 hour before or after the cathartic dose to maximize absorption.

I was prescribed an antibiotic recently by my doctor. Can I still take these with the prep?

Yes. Please see previous response.

Should I continue taking my Coumadin?

Unless discussed specifically with the patient's physician, we continue warfarin (Coumadin) and clopidogrel (Plavix). It is advantageous that the individual can continue the benefits of the needed anticoagulation and still undergo effective CRC screening. If a significant lesion is seen at CTC, the patient can then be reversed for a future colonoscopy. Fortunately, only a small minority of patients will require subsequent colonoscopy.[2] In addition, the polyp size threshold for colonoscopy referral may be increased in this patient cohort.

Can I take my iron supplements?

We typically hold iron supplements, which can cause tarry black stool residue even after the cathartics. We also restrict multivitamins. Although they would not affect the CTC examination, they potentially may cause difficulty at OC. We also advise patients to discontinue any fiber supplements.

I took ibuprofen yesterday. Can I have the examination?

If only a single dose was taken and the patient is not chronically using this medication, we would likely proceed with the examination with the idea of allowing the patients to undergo referral for same-day polypectomy if needed. It is somewhat dependent on the colonoscopist whether it would preclude same-day OC. We advise that patients do not take aspirin, antiinflammatory medications, or antiarthritic medications for 5 days prior to the examination. If they have been taken, the patient is made aware that same-day polypectomy may not be an option and a second bowel preparation and visit may be required to remove the polyp. Acetaminophen (Tylenol) is an appropriate substitute for pain relief.

I have diabetes. What should I do with my insulin?

We typically refer the patient to his or her physician in charge of diabetes management to develop a specific plan for insulin dosing or oral diabetes medications during the clear-liquid diet. We advise the patient to monitor blood sugar levels more frequently. If serum glucose is less than 70 mg/dL or the patient is symptomatic, the patient is instructed to drink 4 ounces of a clear liquid with sugar (e.g., apple juice) or ingest glucose tablets. If unable to maintain serum glucose levels without solid food, the preparation may need to be terminated and the patient will need to be rescheduled with an altered diabetic management plan.

Timing Issues

I have something to do tonight. Can I start the prep at 9:00 pm?

No. Beginning the cathartics at 9:00 pm would end the preparation too late—at 3:00 am in the best-case scenario. In our experience, this is insufficient time for the diatrizoate tagging to effectively opacify the residual colonic fluid. Arguably, the interval between the three prep agents could be shortened to 2 hours, but this has not been adequately tested.

I am going to an interview this morning and going to take the laxative (bisacodyl). How long does it take to work?

The bisacodyl effect is variable. It is a stimulant laxative that typically does not cause immediate diarrhea, but it does cause a bowel movement in approximately 6 to 8 hours. Consequently, we advise patients that they can continue normal daily routines such as work until the afternoon when the cathartics are taken. We have noticed that a few patients (typically men), however, have experienced more immediate effects.

I took the diatrizoate first by mistake. Does it matter?

Yes. This will require the patient to restart the bowel preparation. If the diatrizoate is taken before the cathartic, the fluid tagging will be lost. If the diatrizoate is taken out of order before the barium but after the cathartics, the mini-cathartic value of diatrizoate to scrub away residual barium tagged stool is lost. This often leads to a barium-tagged stool coating of the right colon (Fig. 12-7).

Cathartic Agents

If I am having bowel movements after taking the first bottle of magnesium citrate, do I have to take the second one?

Yes. The entire cathartic regimen must be taken to optimize the preparation.

I took the all the cathartic medications as written, but I am still not having any bowel movements. What should I do?

Given its excellent safety margin, we typically add polyethylene glycol (4 L), calling in a prescription for the individual. The tagging agents begin 1 hour after this cathartic is completed. In our experience, some women may have a delayed response to the cathartics.

When will the effects from the laxative wear off?

It is not uncommon to have continued loose stools and diarrhea following the CTC examination, but this should taper off over the remainder of the day.

I have had a colonoscopy before and they told me I wasn't cleaned out enough. Is this prep going to be enough? I don't want to do this again.

We typically find out what preparation did not work and whether there were any confounding factors that may account for the poor response. Potential modifiers to increase success include instituting a low-residue diet a few days before the clear-liquid diet, extending the clear-liquid diet for 2 days, and occasionally adding PEG (often given as MiraLAX) to an initial osmotic cathartic regimen.

Tagging Agent

I am allergic to shellfish and iodine and was told I can't have dye. Does any of this prep contain iodine?

The diatrizoate is administered orally and not intravenously. Absorption of the diatrizoate from the gut lumen is theoretically possible but generally negligible. Thus, typical "dye allergies" (which incidentally are not truly related to iodine but rather the associated binding molecule) generally do not apply. Our precautions mirror the same that we take for water-soluble iodine-based enemas. If the patient has a true documented serious allergy (e.g., anaphylaxis) to intravenous contrast, the diatrizoate may be dropped from the preparation with barium tagging alone to alleviate patient anxiety. However, there will likely be adherent barium-tagged colonic residue particularly in the right colon that decreases sensitivity. It would be advantageous in these cases to take steps to maximize the catharsis to minimize any residual stool. Other minor allergies, asthma, or atopic history do not preclude the use of diatrizoate (given the importance to the preparation and the oral route of administration). Short-term steroid preparation may be a consideration in these cases depending on the individual case, but we rarely use this approach.

I took barium before and I was told to take a laxative after so I don't get constipated. Do you recommend I take a laxative after the examination?

No. The barium used is a very dilute preparation (2%) that is typically used for CT and is not constipating.

Miscellaneous

What if I get a cold or am sick before I am supposed to have the examination? Can I still do the prep and have the examination?

The CTC portion can be done if the patient has a cold or fever. However, if the patient has an elevated temperature or has respiratory symptoms, a colonoscopy (if needed) may not be performed because of the sedative medications that are given with this procedure.

A medication in my kit is expired. Can I still take it?

No.

SUMMARY

Optimal bowel preparation is an essential component to maintain effective polyp detection capabilities. Currently, a complete bowel preparation approach including both cathartic and tagging agents is required for high polyp sensitivity in low-prevalence or screening populations. There is wide variability in specific approaches and protocols. The UW prep is a simple, straightforward regimen that has been shown to give consistently good results.

References

1. Pickhardt PJ, Choi JR, Hwang I, et al. Computed tomographic virtual colonoscopy to screen for colorectal neoplasia in asymptomatic adults. *N Engl J Med.* 2003;349(23):2191-2200.
2. Kim DH, Pickhardt PJ, Taylor AJ, et al. CT colonography versus colonoscopy for the detection of advanced neoplasia. *N Engl J Med.* 2007;357(14):1403-1412.
3. Macari M, Lavelle M, Pedrosa I, et al. Effect of different bowel preparations on residual fluid at CT colonography. *Radiology.* 2001;218(1):274-277.
4. Edwards JT, Mendelson RM, Fritschi L, et al. Colorectal neoplasia screening with CT colonography in average-risk asymptomatic subjects: Community-based study. *Radiology.* 2004;230(2):459-464.
5. Gluecker TM, Johnson CD, Harmsen WS, et al. Colorectal cancer screening with CT colonography, colonoscopy, and double-contrast barium enema examination: Prospective assessment of patient perceptions and preferences. *Radiology.* 2003;227(2):378-384.
6. Harewood GC, Wiersema MJ, Melton LJ. A prospective, controlled assessment of factors influencing acceptance of screening colonoscopy. *Am J Gastroenterol.* 2002;97(12):3186-3194.
7. Bartram CI. Bowel preparation—Principles and practice. *Clin Radiol.* 1994;49(6):365-367.
8. Taylor E, Waye J, Palmon R. Magnesium citrate (MagC) preparation for colonoscopy: Onset and duration of bowel activity. *Am J Gastroenterol.* 2008:S1243.
9. Delegge M, Kaplan R. Efficacy of bowel preparation with the use of a prepackaged, low fibre diet with a low sodium, magnesium citrate cathartic vs. a clear liquid diet with a standard sodium phosphate cathartic. *Aliment Pharmacol Ther.* 2005;21(12):1491-1495.
10. Berkelhammer C, Ekambaram A, Silva RG. Low-volume oral colonoscopy bowel preparation: Sodium phosphate and magnesium citrate. *Gastrointest Endosc.* 2002;56(1):89-94.
11. Conry BG, Jones S, Bartram CI. The Effect of Oral Magnesium-Containing Bowel Preparation Agents on Mucosal Coating by Barium-Sulfate Suspensions. *Br J Radiology.* 1987;60(720):1215-1219.
12. Holte K, Nielsen KG, Madsen JL, Kehlet H. Physiologic effects of bowel preparation. *Dis Colon Rectum.* 2004;47:1397-1402.
13. Barkun A, Chiba N, Enns R, et al. Commonly used preparations for colonoscopy: Efficacy, tolerability and safety—A Canadian

Association of Gastroenterology position paper. *Can J Gastroenterol*. 2006;20(11):699-710.

14. Schelling JR. Fatal hypermagnesemia. *Clin Nephrol*. 2000;53(1):61-65.

15. Agriantonios D, Kim D, Pickhardt P, Hinshaw J. Bowel preparation for computed tomographic colonography (CTC): A comparison of single dose sodium phosphate and magnesium citrate (abstr). *Radiol Soc North Am*. 2008.

16. Curran MP, Plosker GL. Oral sodium phosphate solution - A review of its use as a colorectal cleanser. *Drugs*. 2004;64(15):1697-1714.

17. Cohen SM, Wexner SD, Binderow SR, et al. Prospective, Randomized, Endoscopic-Blinded Trial Comparing Precolonoscopy Bowel Cleansing Methods. *Dis Colon Rectum*. 1994;37(7):689-696.

18. Kolts BE, Lyles WE, Achem SR, Burton L, Geller AJ, Macmath T. A Comparison of the Effectiveness and Patient Tolerance of Oral Sodium-Phosphate, Castor-Oil, and Standard Electrolyte Lavage for Colonoscopy or Sigmoidoscopy Preparation. *Am J Gastroenterol*. 1993;88(8):1218-1223.

19. Vanner SJ, Macdonald PH, Paterson WG, Prentice RSA, Dacosta LR, Beck IT. A Randomized Prospective Trial Comparing Oral Sodium-Phosphate with Standard Polyethylene Glycol-Based Lavage Solution (Golytely) in the Preparation of Patients for Colonoscopy. *Am J Gastroenterol*. 1990;85(4):422-427.

20. Hookey LC, Depew WT, Vanner S. The safety profile of oral sodium phosphate for colonic cleansing before colonoscopy in adults. *Gastrointest Endosc*. 2002;56(6):895-902.

21. Kim DH, Pickhardt PJ, Hinshaw JL, Taylor AJ, Mukherjee R, Pfau PR. Prospective blinded trial comparing 45-mL and 90-mL doses of oral sodium phosphate for bowel preparation before computed tomographic colonography. *J Comp Assist Tomog*. 2007;31(1):53-58.

22. Hsu CW, Imperiale TF. Meta-analysis and cost comparison of polyethylene glycol lavage versus sodium phosphate for colonoscopy preparation. *Gastrointest Endosc*. 1998;48(3):276-282.

23. Hunyh T, Vanner S, Paterson W. Safety profile of 5-h oral sodium phosphate regimen for colonoscopy cleansing: lack of clinically significant hypocalcemia or hypovolemia. *Am J Gastroenterol*. 1995;90(1):104-107.

24. Markowitz GS, Nasr SH, Klein P, et al. Renal failure due to acute nephrocalcinosis following oral sodium phosphate bowel cleansing. *Hum Pathol*. 2004;35(6):675-684.

25. Markowitz GS, Stokes MB, Radhakrishnan J, D'Agati VD. Acute phosphate nephropathy following oral sodium phosphate bowel purgative: An underrecognized cause of chronic renal failure. *J Am Soc Nephrol*. 2005;16(11):3389-3396.

26. Lichtenstein GR, Cohen LB, Uribarri J. Review article: bowel preparation for colonoscopy—The importance of adequate hydration. *Aliment Pharmacol Ther*. 2007;26(5):633-641.

27. Belsey J, Epstein O, Heresbach D. Systematic review: Oral bowel preparation for colonoscopy. *Aliment Pharmacol Ther*. 2007;25(4):373-384.

28. Gore R, MS L, eds. *Textbook of gastrointestinal radiology*. 2nd ed: Philadelphia: WB Saunders; 2000.

29. O'Connor SD, Summers RM, Choi JR, Pickhardt PJ. Oral contrast adherence to polyps on CT colonography. *J Comp Assist Tomog*. 2006;30(1):51-57.

30. Callstrom MR, Johnson CD, Fletcher JG, et al. CT colonography without cathartic preparation: Feasibility study. *Radiology*. 2001;219(3):693-698.

31. Lefere P, Gryspeerdt S, Baekelandt M, Van Holsbeeck B. Laxative-free CT colonography. *Am J Roentgenol*. 2004;183(4):945-948.

32. Lefere PA, Gryspeerdt SS, Dewyspelaere J, Baekelandt M, Van Holsbeeck BG. Dietary fecal tagging as a cleansing method before CT colonography: Initial results-polyp detection and patient acceptance. *Radiology*. 2002;224(2):393-403.

33. Iannaccone R, Laghi A, Catalano C, et al. Computed tomographic colonography without cathartic preparation for the detection of colorectal polyps. *Gastroenterology*. 2004;127(5):1300-1311.

34. Zalis ME, Perumpillichira J, Del Frate C, Hahn PF. CT colonography: Digital subtraction bowel cleansing with mucosal reconstruction—Initial observations. *Radiology*. 2003;226(3):911-917.

35. Zalis ME, Perumpillichira JJ, Magee C, Kohlberg G, Hahn PF. Tagging-based, electronically cleansed CT colonography: Evaluation of patient comfort and image readability. *Radiology*. 2006;239(1):149-159.

36. Cotton PB, Durkalski VL, Benoit PC, et al. Computed tomographic colonography (virtual colonoscopy)—A multicenter comparison with standard colonoscopy for detection of colorectal neoplasia. *JAMA*. 2004;291(14):1713-1719.

37. Johnson CD, Toledano AY, Herman BA, et al. Computerized tomographic colonography: Performance evaluation in a retrospective multicenter setting. *Gastroenterology*. 2003;125(3):688-695.

38. Rockey DC, Paulson E, Niedzwiecki D, et al. Analysis of air contrast barium enema, computed tomographic colonography, and colonoscopy: prospective comparison. *Lancet*. 2005;365(9456):305-311.

Colonic Distention for CT Colonography

DAVID H. KIM, MD
PERRY J. PICKHARDT, MD

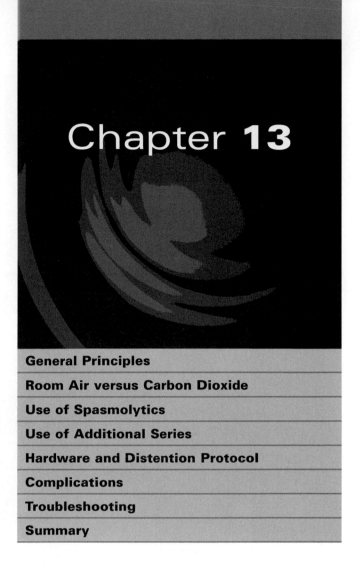

Chapter 13

INTRODUCTION

Another key component to effective polyp detection at CT colonography (CTC) concerns optimized colonic distention. Poor distention generally leads to decreased sensitivity, and no interpretation strategy can compensate for problems in this area of technique (Fig. 13-1). In addition to obscuring large polyps, underdistention can either obscure or mimic the appearance of annular carcinomas, leading to both underdiagnosis and overdiagnosis. Originally, the insufflation of room air by manual methods was favored, but more recently, automated carbon dioxide (CO_2) delivery has become the preferred standard for colonic distention. This chapter will explore the pertinent issues regarding this portion of the technique.

GENERAL PRINCIPLES

Optimized colorectal distention refers to the tenet that the large intestine is distended throughout its length to allow easy, effective detection of colorectal polyps. In the normal colon, the colonic walls are thus well separated, with the cecum representing the most capacious segment. With adequate distention, the walls are thin and nearly imperceptible, allowing polyps to clearly stand out (Fig. 13-2). It is important to note that optimized distention may not correlate with maximal distention in the setting of an abnormal underlying colonic wall. A common example is a diverticular-diseased colonic segment, which may only moderately distend because of the deposition of fibroelastic material in the muscular layer (Fig. 13-3). It is important to recognize that in most cases, the colon can be adequately assessed in these types of situations. In addition, adequate distention does not imply complete distention of all segments in all series. As long as all segments of colon are adequately distended on at least one series, diagnostic evaluation of the colon can be achieved. If a segment remains collapsed on all series, the examination would then be nondiagnostic in that area.

The ideal method of distention would be easy to achieve and easy to reproduce from patient to patient. High-quality results would be operator and patient independent. There would be minimal discomfort to the patient with a very low complication rate. Typically, gases such as room air or carbon dioxide are favored over aqueous media such as water or contrast enemas. Gases are much easier to administer than fluids and allow excellent contrast between the marked low attenuation of a gas-filled lumen from the soft tissue density of a polyp protruding into this space. This high contrast allows for a low-dose technique at CT colonography while maintaining excellent polyp sensitivities. In the case of carbon dioxide, the active resorption of this gas across the colonic mucosa also helps decrease postprocedure discomfort for the individual.

ROOM AIR VERSUS CARBON DIOXIDE

One of the major issues regarding colonic distention is the use of room air or carbon dioxide for the distention media. Early on in CTC, room air was favored because it

131

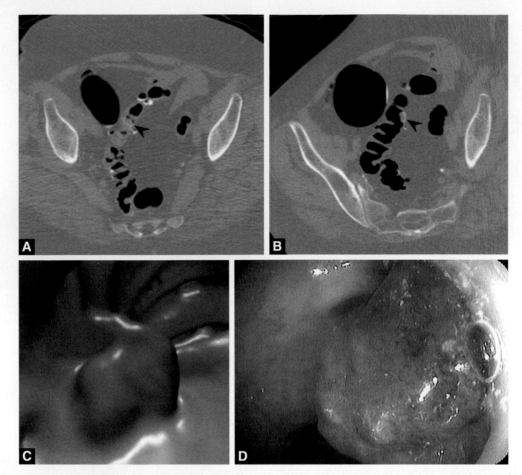

Figure 13-1 Poor luminal distention affects interpretation. 2D transverse CTC image **(A)** shows a poorly distended sigmoid obscuring a large 15-mm advanced adenoma *(arrowhead)*. If all series are collapsed, this lesion would be missed regardless of the interpretation algorithm. Decubitus 2D transverse **(B)** and 3D endoluminal **(C)** views with good distention identify this polyp *(arrowhead)*, which was later removed at OC **(D)**. *(*See associated video clip on DVD.)*

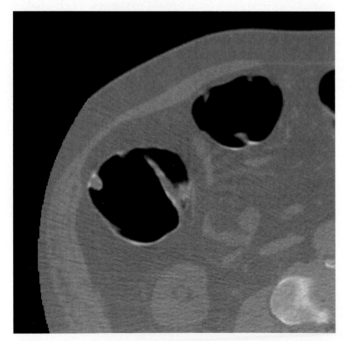

Figure 13-2 Optimal luminal distention. 2D transverse CTC image shows a well-distended ascending colon in which the wall is imperceptible, allowing the large tubular adenoma to easily stand out. Notice the thin skirt of contrast tag at the base, which is frequently seen.

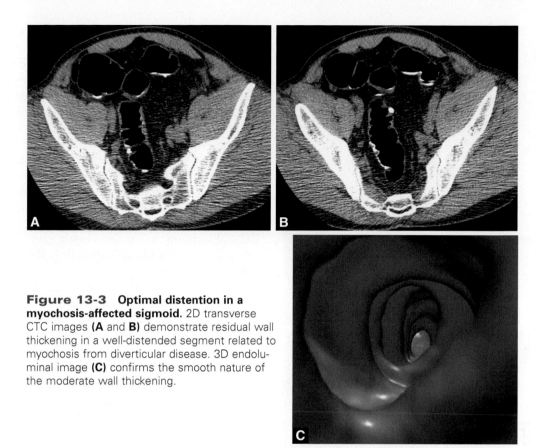

Figure 13-3 Optimal distention in a myochosis-affected sigmoid. 2D transverse CTC images (**A** and **B**) demonstrate residual wall thickening in a well-distended segment related to myochosis from diverticular disease. 3D endoluminal image (**C**) confirms the smooth nature of the moderate wall thickening.

is cheap, ever present, and perceived as relatively easy to administer. Previous longstanding experience with air insufflation at barium enema and conventional endoscopy perhaps increased its initial acceptance at CTC. For such administration, a rectal enema tip is inserted and a bulb apparatus is used to manually insufflate air into the colon by the radiologist, technologist, or patient (self-inflated).[1,2] Excellent distention could be achieved, but there was considerable variation from examination to examination, depending on certain patient and technical factors. Unlike barium enemas, in which the amount of distention could be assessed real-time under fluoroscopy, air administration at CTC was done in a blind fashion. Typically, insufflation was to patient tolerance. Adequacy was then determined by the scout view just prior to series acquisition. It is not surprising that there was wide variability in results dependent on the operator and the specific patient. In addition, this was a labor-intensive approach in which each patient required coaching and education to provide appropriate feedback for the assessment of adequate administration. Because nitrogen (the main component of air) is an inert gas not absorbed by the colonic mucosa, it often led to postprocedure discomfort and bloating for the patient until expelled several hours later, unlike carbon dioxide (Fig. 13-4).

The advent of automated carbon dioxide delivery has significantly changed colonic distention. Once experience was gained with this medium, the advantages were quickly realized and the majority of institutions now use this method. Although CO_2 is more expensive than room air and requires additional equipment, it allows for consistently better distention with less effort. As opposed to nitrogen, CO_2 is actively reabsorbed across the colonic mucosa. This property allows rapid decompression of the colon following the procedure with resultant decreased discomfort and abdominal distention immediately following the procedure (Fig. 13-4).[3-5] It also illustrates the need for continual automated delivery and why manual bulb insufflation would be insufficient because the colon rapidly decompresses once the flow of CO_2 stops. Consequently, manual CO_2 administration (in which there is not continuous inflow) often leads to poor colonic distention, as demonstrated in a prior study using CO_2 from the barium enema era.[6] Automated delivery allows for a constant low-pressure infusion of CO_2 to maintain distention.[7] Ultimately, an equilibrium results between CO_2 *infusion* and CO_2 *loss*, which comprises active resorption, potential loss around the rectal catheter, and potential reflux into the small bowel (in cases with an incompetent ileocecal valve). As long as this equilibrium is maintained, the colon will remain distended. Thus, even in the situation of an incompetent (or surgically absent) ileocecal valve with substantial reflux into the small bowel, good colonic distention can generally be obtained (Fig. 13-5).

From a technical standpoint, CO_2 administration is much less labor intensive. After a small-caliber flexible

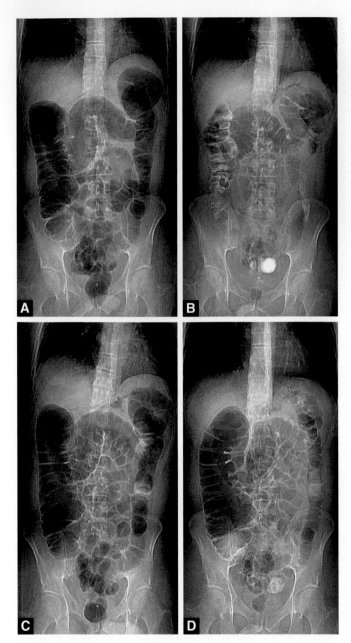

Figure 13-4 Carbon dioxide versus room air. Screening CTC individual who volunteered to space out supine and prone series to permit distention with both CO_2 and room air with scout films repeated 15 minutes after scanning each series. CTC scout **(A)** shows excellent colonic distention with carbon dioxide on the supine series that largely resolves at 15 minutes **(B)**. CTC scout **(C)** with room air distention for the prone series also demonstrates good distention. However, significant residual colonic air persists on the repeat scout 15 minutes later **(D),** which may lead to substantial postprocedure discomfort until expelled by the patient. The rapid resorption of CO_2 allows patients to avoid the postprocedure cramping associated with room air. (From Shinners TJ, Pickhardt PJ, Taylor AJ, Jones DA, Olsen CH. Patient-controlled room air insufflation versus automated carbon dioxide delivery for CT colonography. *Am J Roentbenol.* 2006;186:1491-1496.)

rectal tube is inserted, the flow of CO_2 is begun. Whereas manual room air requires instruction and coaching of the patient for optimal distention, automated CO_2 delivery does not. Instead, it simply consists of monitoring the intracolonic pressure measurements obtained by the insufflator. Once certain levels are reached, the scout is initiated. The patients are simply cautioned that they may experience some cramping when the colon distends but that it will quickly resolve after the machine is turned off. High-quality examinations are easier to obtain and more reproducible because the procedure is largely operator- and patient-independent.

In the past, there has been some concern regarding CO_2 absorption in patients with chronic obstructive pulmonary disease. Carbon dioxide is absorbed across the colonic mucosa into the colonic venous circulation and ultimately expelled from the lungs. However, to our knowledge, no published studies have documented an increased risk. In addition, the NORCCAP (NORwegian Colorectal CAncer Prevention) study demonstrated no increase in end-tidal CO_2 measurements with the use of carbon dioxide insufflation at colonoscopy.[8] We have not experienced complications related to CO_2 absorption in our screening program at the University of Wisconsin (UW) in more than 5000 patients to date.

USE OF SPASMOLYTICS

Spasmolytics such as glucagon or buscopan (hyoscine N-butylbromide) remain an area of relative controversy. In the United States spasmolytics are typically not recommended for routine use in CT colonography, particularly with the available agent of glucagon. Glucagon is a polypeptide hormone produced in the pancreas with smooth muscle relaxant effects. The theoretic advantages include bowel hypotonia to increase distention and to decrease colonic spasm for decreased patient discomfort. In practice, no significant difference in colonic distention has been seen with glucagon administration.[9] In addition, the relaxant effects on the ileocecal valve may paraxodically decrease distention because of reflux into the small bowel (although this is a less important factor when automated CO_2 is used, in which distention can be maintained even in the face of an incompetent ileocecal valve; Fig. 13-6). Buscopan is an anticholinergic agent that acts on the postganglionic parasympathetic smooth muscle receptors to cause relaxation. Studies have demonstrated increased colonic distention, although without significant improvement in polyp detection.[10,11] Many investigators in Europe and Canada feel that this medication is helpful in improving the examination overall and recommend its use in routine CTC. Even if buscopan has beneficial effects, it is not available in the United States because it does not have FDA approval. In our experience, the use of spasmolytics is not warranted.

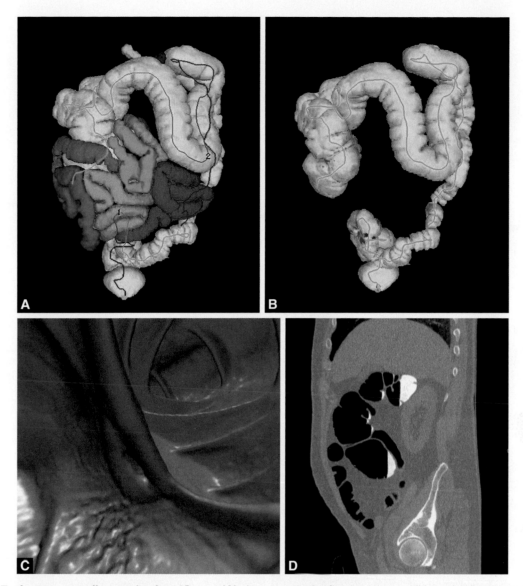

Figure 13-5 **Incompetent ileocecal valve.** 3D map **(A)** shows marked reflux into the small bowel. With the small bowel segmented out **(B),** the colon is seen to be well distended despite an incompetent valve. 3D endoluminal CTC image **(C)** demonstrates a patulous ileocecal valve. 2D sagittal CTC image **(D)** demonstrates the well-distended right colon and refluxed gas within the terminal ileum.

Current automated CO_2 delivery leads to very few collapsed segments without the adjunctive use of spasmolytics. In addition, small bowel reflux resulting from ileocecal valve relaxation could theoretically hamper examinations. In our estimation, the use of such medications does not lead to significantly improved polyp detection to compensate for the increase in patient anxiety (use of a needle), time, and expense.

USE OF ADDITIONAL SERIES

Standard series acquisitions include supine and prone positioning (see Chapter 14 for additional details). Series are obtained in end expiration to decrease the effects of air-filled lungs on the transverse colon. Both series are needed at a minimum for effective polyp detection.[12,13] If an abnormality is obscured by unopacified fluid (if untagged or poorly tagged) or by collapse on one view, it is often apparent on the other as a result of the shifting of fluid and gas in response to gravity (Fig. 13-7). In addition, the identification of a possible polyp at the same location within the colon on both views significantly increases the reader confidence of a true finding. However, movement by a potential nonpedunculated polyp between the series is consistent with stool mimicking a true polyp.

Additional series and maneuvers may be needed when the standard series do not allow complete evaluation of the colon. Infrequently, a segment of bowel (typically the sigmoid colon) will remain collapsed on both the supine

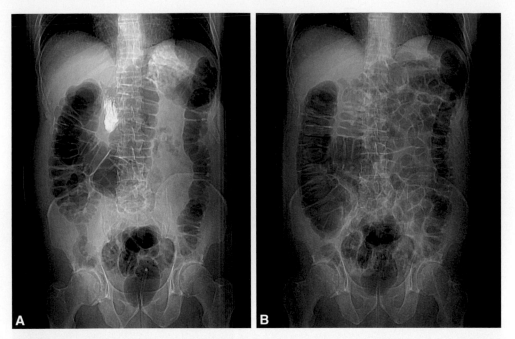

Figure 13-6 Small bowel reflux with glucagon. Scout from initial CTC study **(A)** shows a fairly well-distended colon with minimal reflux into small bowel. This study was performed without spasmolytics per routine for incomplete OC earlier the same day. Follow-up CTC **(B)** was performed with glucagon. Note that colonic distention was not significantly improved, but there is now marked reflux into the small bowel.

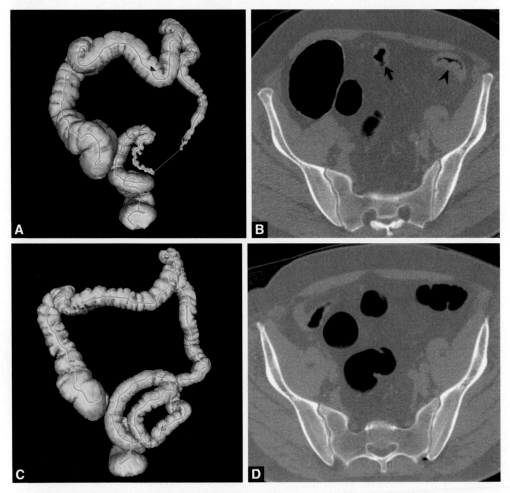

Figure 13-7 Complementary nature of supine and prone series. 3D map **(A)** shows sigmoid collapse on supine series. Supine 2D transverse CTC **(B)** image confirms collapse in proximal sigmoid *(arrowhead)* and relative underdistention in distal sigmoid *(arrow)*. With prone positioning, the sigmoid colon distends out nicely **(C)**, which is also demonstrated on 2D imaging **(D)**.

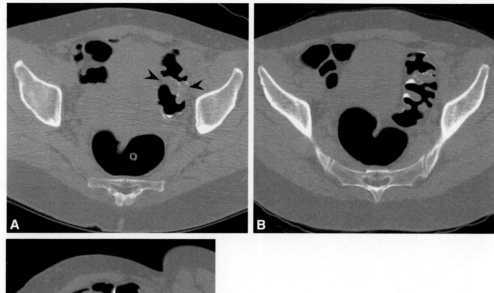

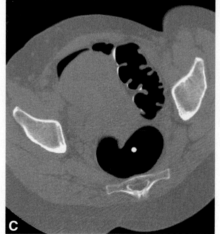

Figure 13-8   Value of the decubitus series.
2D transverse CTC images with standard positioning demonstrates focal sigmoid collapse *(arrowheads)* on both the supine **(A)** and prone **(B)** series. Right lateral decubitus series **(C)**, however, allows for confident evaluation of the sigmoid. (From Pickhardt PJ. Screening CT colonography: How I do it. *Am J Roentgenol.* 2007;189:290-298.)

and prone views. In this situation, an additional series can be done with the patient in the right lateral decubitus position (right side down) (Fig. 13-8). In our experience, this often opens the area of collapse. The need for additional series occurs in about 1 of every 10 to 15 examinations, and typically this is a result of focal collapse of the sigmoid colon on both standard series. The left lateral decubitus view rarely may be helpful if a right lateral decubitus is unsuccessful.

Each series is typically undertaken with automated CO_2. In certain situations, however, it may be advantageous to substitute room air to optimize distention. Manual room air insufflation can generate higher pressures to allow relatively collapsed segments to distend. The clinical situation in which this is most effective is in patients who are morbidly obese. The abdominal and intraperitoneal fat can restrict full distention of the colon. The low-pressure instillation of CO_2 often cannot overcome this restriction. After the decision has been made to convert to room air, the flexible tubing connecting the rectal catheter to the insufflator can be cut and a bulb apparatus can be inserted to insufflate the colon with room air. Insufflation should be performed with care to patient tolerance (Fig. 13-9).

HARDWARE AND DISTENTION PROTOCOL

Central to the distention protocol is the CO_2 automated delivery device. Currently, there is a single machine for use in CT colonography (PROTOCO$_2$L, Bracco Diagnostics; Fig. 13-10). The description herein applies to this machine, but the principles should carry over to other machines as they become available. The device allows for continuous infusion of CO_2 regulated by pressure measurements. Safety measures include an electronic pressure-controlled cutoff at 50 mm Hg and a mechanical valve release at 75 mm Hg. A variable instillation rate is used in which there is a ramp up in flow rate over time to minimize patient discomfort: 1 L/min for the first 0.5 L, 2 L/min for the next 0.5 L, and a maximum rate of 3 L/min after a volume of 1 L is instilled. A maximal instillation pressure is set (typically at 20 mm Hg to start) at the beginning of the examination; if the increasing flow rates exceed this pressure, the flow ceases until the pressure drops below this level. This instillation pressure can be altered as required to minimize patient discomfort. For now, total volume cutoffs are in place at 4 L and every 2 L thereafter, requiring

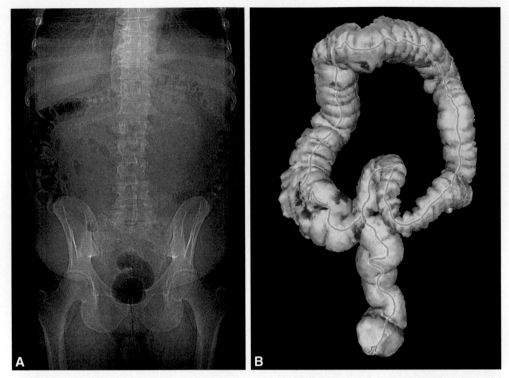

Figure 13-9 **Value of combined decubitus positioning and room air.** Screening CTC in an individual who is obese. Prone CTC scout **(A)** shows poor distention. Conversion to room air allowed for increased distention pressures. 3D colon map **(B)** in the decubitus position after room air administration shows good luminal distention.

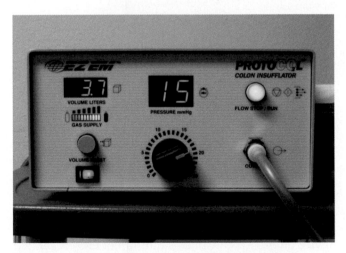

Figure 13-10 **Automated CO₂ colonic insufflator.** Closeup image of the insufflator. The instillation pressure maximum can be set by the middle dial (set at 19 mm Hg in this case). The pressure measurement window in the middle documents the rectal intraluminal pressures from the end of the rectal catheter. Typically, this value is in the mid-teens when the colon is filling. Note the total volume readout in the upper lefthand corner.

the operator to manually restart the flow. This safety measure unfortunately may lead to decreased distention at imaging (discussed later).

The preferred rectal catheter is a disposable flexible latex-free 20-Fr catheter with a 30-mL low-pressure retention cuff included with the delivery system. A stan-

dard rectal enema tip with the large balloon is not typically used but can be substituted in patients with poor sphincter tone or who have difficulty retaining the carbon dioxide that results in leakage about the standard small-caliber catheter.

The following distention protocol is used:[14-16]

- The patient is first asked to use the restroom to evacuate any excess retained material. The procedure is described to the patient. It is important to inform the patient that CO₂ may cause crampy discomfort but that it will quickly resolve after the conclusion of the examination.
- The patient is placed in the left lateral decubitus position on the scanner table. The rectal catheter is placed and the retention cuff is insufflated. The retention cuff does not need to be maximally inflated because it is not intended to help prevent leakage of CO₂ but simply to keep the catheter from migrating out of the rectum. Gently pull back on the catheter to confirm that the catheter will not easily displace.
- The instillation pressure is set at 20 mm Hg for most patients. It is adjusted downward to 17 mm Hg for smaller patients.
- The colon is filled to a volume of approximate 1.5 L. The patient is then placed in the right lateral decubitus position for another 1.5 L to 2 L.
- The patient is then rolled supine and a CT scout is taken once equilibrium pressures are reached. The CT scout can assess overall distention adequacy (the sig-

moid and distal descending colon may be relative blind spots; see following bullets).

- During the examination, the flow of CO_2 is restarted when a volume cutoff level is reached to maintain a constant low-level infusion throughout the examination. For example, the 4-L mark triggering the volume cutoff safety measure is typically reached after the supine scout acquisition, which requires restarting the flow prior to acquiring the supine images series.
- If distention is deemed adequate, the scan is initiated in end expiration. End expiration is preferred to decrease the mass effect of lungs on the transverse colon. Review of the transverse two-dimensional (2D) images is mandatory to assess adequacy of distention for the descending and sigmoid colon.[16a] Assessment of the scout is often insufficient in this area. Because of

tortuosity, overlapping loops of sigmoid may create the appearance of good distention when in fact it is focally collapsed (Fig. 13-11). Only in some cases can the scout alone assess the distention of the sigmoid colon (typically a short, nontortuous sigmoid).

- The patient is rolled prone and the imaging sequence (scout to scan) is repeated.
- If required, an additional right lateral decubitus series is obtained.
- After the last series, the CO_2 delivery is stopped, the cuff is deflated, and the rectal catheter is removed.

Several important issues must be considered with this protocol to optimize distention. *Most importantly, CO_2 should be infusing during image acquisition.* If CO_2 instillation ceases for too long, the colon will decompress and distention will be less than optimal with collapsed segments.

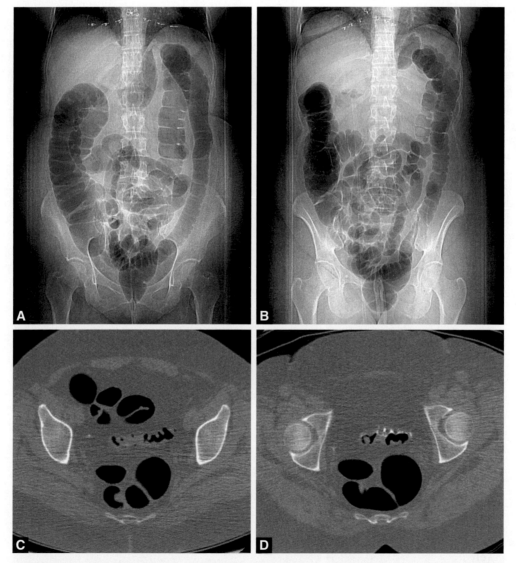

Figure 13-11   Inadequate assessment of sigmoid colon distention on scout view. CTC scout views from supine **(A)** and prone **(B)** series suggest that the sigmoid colon is well distended. However, 2D transverse images in the supine **(C)** and prone **(D)** positions demonstrate that it is actually largely collapsed on both views, and a decubitus is therefore required. An overlying loop gave the false appearance of adequate sigmoid distention on the scout views. We require our CT technologists to assess sigmoid distention on the 2D images at the console.

Consequently, the volume cutoff safety measure may cause poor distention. A common scenario occurs when the safety cutoff at 4 L has been reached, typically after the supine scout image has been obtained. This image then demonstrates excellent distention. However, if the CO_2 is not restarted and the series acquisition is delayed (for even 30 to 60 seconds), the distention suffers considerably (Fig. 13-12). It is important to restart the flow at the various cutoff values (4 L, 6 L, 8 L, 10 L, etc) and image during active CO_2 inflow.

For the prone series, the transverse colon can be compressed by the patient's body habitus in this position. Particularly in individuals with a protuberant abdomen, it is helpful to place towel rolls under the shoulder and hips to create some space and decrease pressure on the transverse colon (Fig. 13-13). In some cases, however, a right lateral decubitus may be needed, particularly in very large individuals (Fig. 13-14). In this situation, a series with room air may be necessary because higher pressures can be generated.

The intrarectal pressure measurements are an important indirect guide during CO_2 instillation. In the filling phase, the measurements range from 12 to 18 mm Hg. During spasm, the numbers may increase to 35 mm Hg to 40 mm Hg. It is often helpful to coach the patient with deep breathing to help relieve the spasm. When the patient has reached equilibrium between CO_2 inflow and outflow, the numbers range from 22 mm Hg to 28 mm Hg. This typically correlates with optimal distention. In a typical straightforward case, this occurs somewhere around the 4-L mark for instilled volume. The scout should then be taken for initial assessment of adequacy.

The total volume of gas delivered is not as important. Ultimately, the patient reaches an equilibrium phase between inflow and outflow. In most patients, the total volume instilled ranges from 4 L to 6 L at the conclusion of the examination. However, it is not uncommon for total volumes to exceed 10 L if the patient has an incompetent ileocecal valve or is losing CO_2 about the rectal catheter.

The distention protocol, image acquisition, and assessment of adequacy are typically undertaken by an experienced CT technologist. There is little involvement on the part of the interpreting physician unless an unusual situation or question arises. Attention to the previously mentioned details will result in optimal distention on a regular basis. In our experience, nondiagnostic distention is seen in much less than 1% of cases.

COMPLICATIONS

Pneumatic distention of the large intestine at CTC is safe, particularly with carbon dioxide. As opposed to manual room air administration, in which fairly high intraluminal pressures can be generated, automated CO_2 delivery is a low-pressure delivery process. Measured intrarectal pressures at CO_2 instillation (used as a surrogate for overall intracolonic pressures) rarely exceed 40 mm Hg for more than a few seconds. Human cadaveric colon models suggest that much higher pressures are generally needed for perforation.[17] The documented symptomatic perforation rate for CTC is extremely low at 0.005%, as reported in a survey of the Working Group on Virtual Colonoscopy encompassing 21,923 examinations.[18] In fact, when only examinations using carbon dioxide were considered, no perforations were seen in 8857 individuals. For a measure of comparison, typical perforation rates at optical colonoscopy range from 0.1% to 0.2%.[19-21] It is important to real-

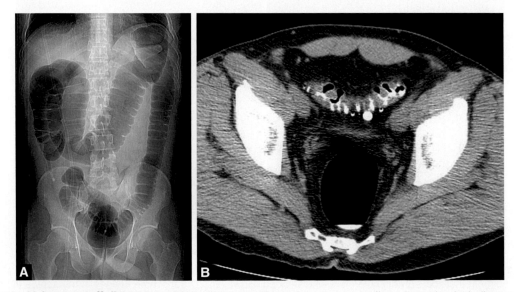

Figure 13-12 **Volume cutoff distention pitfall.** CTC scout **(A)** demonstrates excellent distention including a nontortuous sigmoid. An extended time interval occurred between the scout and series acquisition during which the CO_2 inflow was stopped because a total volume cutoff was reached. The sigmoid colon is now completely decompressed on the 2D image **(B)**, causing a discrepancy between scout and scan.

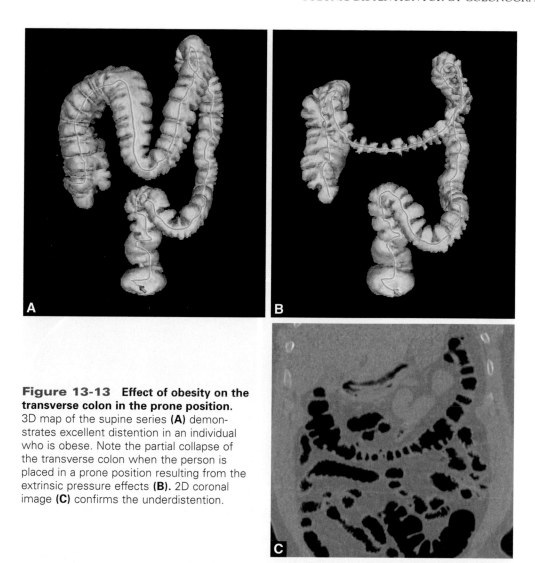

Figure 13-13 Effect of obesity on the transverse colon in the prone position. 3D map of the supine series **(A)** demonstrates excellent distention in an individual who is obese. Note the partial collapse of the transverse colon when the person is placed in a prone position resulting from the extrinsic pressure effects **(B)**. 2D coronal image **(C)** confirms the underdistention.

ize, however, that certain clinical situations significantly increase the risk for perforation at CTC. Colonic distention in the face of an inguinal hernia containing a loop of sigmoid significantly increases the possibility for a serious complication. The Israeli experience (with manual room air insufflation) emphasizes this point because four of the seven perforations occurred in patients with a colon-containing left inguinal hernia.[22] We have trained our technologists to scrutinize the CT scout for abnormal collections of air in this region, particularly if the patient reports focal pain (Fig. 13-15). A CTC examination with CO_2 can potentially still be completed if monitored carefully, but room air in which higher pressures are usually generated should be avoided. All of the Israeli perforations in the setting of inguinal hernia involved manual room air insufflation. Other situations that increase risk include recent prior "deep" biopsy/polypectomy or recent bout of acute diverticulitis. These patients are typically rescheduled because of the increased risk of complication. For a deep biopsy in the setting of same-day referral from incomplete colonoscopy, we generally wait 4 to 6 weeks, unless the gastroenterologist performing the procedure asserts

that only a superficial biopsy was taken. For diverticulitis, we wait a similar time period after complete treatment and resolution of the acute episode.

A newly described phenomenon at CTC concerns incidental colonic pneumatosis. It is important to recognize because this finding is a self-limited benign process. This infrequent occurrence has been noted in asymptomatic individuals following CTC with a prevalence of 0.11%. When first identified, it can be disconcerting. The pneumatosis typically involves the right colon. The intramural gas is characterized as lucent foci dissecting in a fairly linear fashion along the colonic wall (Fig. 13-16). No free air or significant foci of air distant to the colonic wall in the surrounding mesentery or pericolonic fat are present. Most important, the patient is completely asymptomatic and is doing well other than the CT imaging finding. Obviously, the initial fear is that the patient has suffered a perforation. However, this finding appears to be separate from a true perforation, which typically results in symptoms and often the need for surgical repair. In our series, all patients with incidental colonic pneumatosis remained asymptomatic

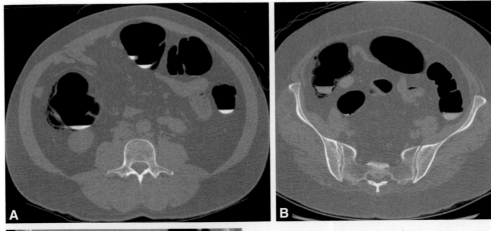

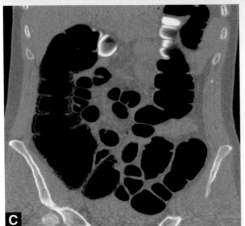

Figure 13-16 **Incidental colonic pneumatosis.** 2D CTC images **(A-C)** from three different patients all demonstrate right-sided pneumatosis with coalescing foci of air seen within the colonic wall in a relatively linear configuration. All patients were asymptomatic and developed no complications at long-term followup. (Pickhardt PJ, Kim DH, Taylor AJ. Asymptomatic pneumatosis at CT colonography: A benign self-limited imaging finding distinct from perforation. *Am J Roentgenol.* 2008;190(2):W112-W117.)

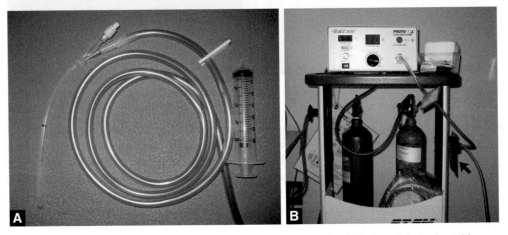

Figure 13-17 **Fluid block in tubing.** Excessive residual fluid may cause a fluid block to CO_2 in the tubing connecting the rectal catheter **(A)** to the insufflator **(B).** This fluid should be milked back to the collection bag *(arrow)* to clear the tubing.

severe underdistention. A common scenario occurs because of the volume cutoff safety measure on the CO_2 machine. When a predetermined volume limit is reached (at 4 L, 6 L, 8 L, etc.), the flow is automatically stopped and must be manually restarted. If the volume cutoff is reached and not recognized, scanning can occur during this time of decompression. For example, often the 4-L limit is reached just after the CT scout for the supine series has been taken. The scout demonstrates excellent distention. If it takes a few minutes for the supine series to be set up and scanned, the flow has ceased and the colon decompresses in that interval, leading to poor results.

Persistently Collapsed Sigmoid Colon

The most common problem segment for luminal collapse is (by far) the sigmoid colon. Automated CO_2 delivery has significantly decreased the number of collapsed sigmoid segments. Often the prone series is the best series for sigmoid distention. If a segment is collapsed at the same point on both views, a decubitus series (typically right lateral decubitus) should be performed. Consideration of substitution with room air can be given for individuals who are obese. We rarely go on to a fourth series (the other decubitus position), but this may be considered in special cases. We do not use spasmolytics. In our opinion, the yield for these additional final maneuvers is low and simply adds time, radiation, anxiety, and frustration. Often, there is a pathologic reason why a persistently "collapsed" segment will not open, such as a diverticular stricture or involvement with endometriosis. A flexible sigmoidoscopy may be needed to evaluate the sigmoid in these cases, which can be done as a same-day procedure without sedation. It is important to note that a segment needs only to be distended on one series to confidently clear it.

Groin Pain

Focal groin pain and swelling should alert the technologist to stop CO_2 inflow and alert the physician. The possibility of an inguinal hernia–containing sigmoid colon should be considered. Albeit rare, this scenario significantly raises the possibility of perforation, as demonstrated by the aforementioned Israeli experience.

History of Recent Polypectomy, Biopsy, Active Diverticulitis, or Colitis

If the patient has had a recent "deep" biopsy (typically occurs in the setting of an incomplete colonoscopy sent to CTC for completion of the colonic evaluation), CTC should not be performed in the immediate setting. It is important to inquire about this possibility because it may significantly increase the possibility of perforation. We typically wait 4 to 6 weeks to ensure healing of the polypectomy site. One potential exception is where the endoscopist ensures that it was a small superficial biopsy/polypectomy.

CTC, which is a non-emergent examination, should also not be performed in patients with an active inflammatory condition of the large intestine because of the increased risk of complications. We typically wait 4 to 6 weeks after the resolution and treatment of the active process.

Vaginal Intubation

Similar to barium enema, unrecognized inadvertent vaginal intubation may lead to confusion as to why the colon will not distend (Fig. 13-18). On the CTC scout, it is helpful to recognize that the presumed CO_2-filled rectum is more anterior than usual. The situation should be immediately obvious on the 2D images.

SUMMARY

Colonic distention is a key component of effective polyp detection at CTC. Without optimized technique, sensitivity suffers regardless of the interpretation strategy used. CO_2 holds many advantages over room air including improved reproducible colonic distention that is less dependent on operator and patient factors and decreased patient discomfort following the examination. It is vitally important that there is not a large time delay between CO_2 infusion and image acquisition to optimize distention. Overall, it is a low-pressure delivery system with a very low risk of perforation. Incidental asymptomatic colonic pneumatosis is a newly recognized entity infrequently seen at CTC that is distinct from a true perforation and without significant negative sequela.

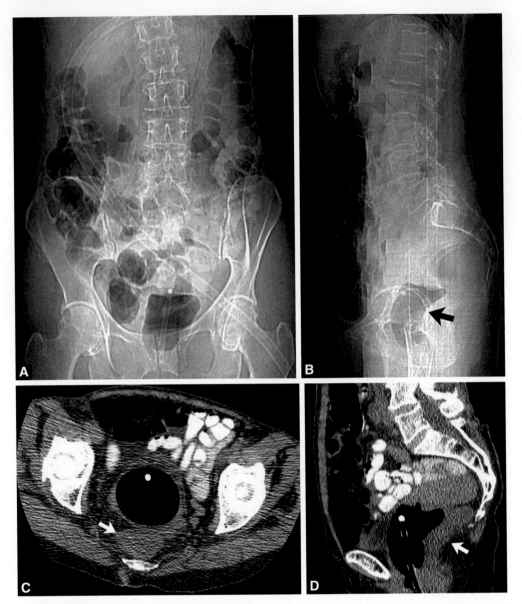

Figure 13-18 **Vaginal intubation.** Diagnostic CTC performed "after hours" following incomplete OC by a CT technologist with relatively little CTC experience. Frontal **(A)** and lateral **(B)** CTC scout views show poor distention of colon. Notice the gas-filled "rectum," which is more anterior than usual *(arrow)*. 2D transverse **(C)** and sagittal **(D)** CTC images confirm vaginal intubation with a collapsed rectum seen posteriorly *(arrows)*.

REFERENCES

1. Ristvedt SL, McFarland EG, Weinstock LB, Thyssen EP. Patient preferences for CT colonography conventional colonoscopy, and bowel preparation. *Am J Gastroenterol.* 2003;98(3):578-585.
2. Shinners TJ, Pickhardt PJ, Taylor AJ, Jones DA, Olsen CH. Patient-controlled room air insufflation versus automated carbon dioxide delivery for CT colonography. *Am J Roentgenol.* 2006;186(6):1491-1496.
3. Sumanac K, Zealley I, Fox BM, et al. Minimizing postcolonoscopy abdominal pain by using CO_2 insufflation: A prospective, randomized, double blind, controlled trial evaluating a new commercially available CO_2 delivery system. *Gastrointest Endosc.* 2002;56(2):190-194.
4. Church J, Delaney C. Randomized, controlled trial of carbon dioxide insufflation during colonoscopy. *Dis Colon Rectum.* 2003;46(3):322-326.
5. Robson NK, Lloyd M, Regan F. The use of carbon-dioxide as an insufflation agent in barium enema—Does it have a role. *Br J Radiol.* 1993;66(783):197-198.
6. Scullion DA, Wetton CWN, Davies C, Whitaker L, Shorvon PJ. The use of air or CO_2 as insufflation agents for double contrast barium enema (DCBE): Is there a qualitative difference? *Clin Radiol.* 1995;50(8):558-561.
7. Burling D, Taylor SA, Halligan S, et al. Automated insufflation of carbon dioxide for MDCT colonography: Distension and patient experience compared with manual insufflation. *Am J Roentgenol.* 2006;186(1):96-103.

8. Bretthauer M, Thiis-Evensen E, Huppertz-Hauss G, et al. NORC-CAP (Norwegian colorectal cancer prevention): A randomised trial to assess the safety and efficacy of carbon dioxide versus air insufflation in colonoscopy. *Gut.* 2002;50(5):604-607.

9. Yee J, Hung RK, Akerkar GA, Wall SD. The usefulness of glucagon hydrochloride for colonic distention in CT colonography. *Am J Roentgenol.* 1999;173(1):169-172.

10. Rogalla P, Lembcke A, Ruckert JC, et al. Spasmolysis at CT colonography: Butyl scopolamine versus glucagon. *Radiology.* 2005;236(1):184-188.

11. Taylor SA, Halligan S, Goh V, et al. Optimizing colonic distention for multi-detector row CT colonography: Effect of hyoscine butylbromide and rectal balloon catheter. *Radiology.* 2003;229(1):99-108.

12. Yee J, Kumar NN, Hung RK, Akerkar GA, Kumar PRG, Wall SD. Comparison of supine and prone scanning separately and in combination at CT colonography. *Radiology.* 2003;226(3):653-661.

13. Fletcher JG, Johnson CD, Welch TJ, et al. Optimization of CT colonography technique: Prospective trial in 180 patients. *Radiology.* 2000;216(3):704-711.

14. Pickhardt PJ, Kim DH. CT colonography (virtual colonoscopy): A practical approach for population screening. *Radiol Clin North Am.* 2007;45(2):361-375.

15. Kim DH, Pickhardt PJ, Hoff G, Kay CL. Computed tomographic colonography for colorectal screening. *Endoscopy.* 2007;39(6):545-549.

16. Pickhardt PJ. Screening CT colonography: How I do it. *Am J Roentgenol.* 2007;189(2):290-298.

16a. Choi M, Taylor AJ, VonBerge JL, Bartels CM, Pickhardt PJ. Can the CT scout reliably assess for adequate colonic distention at CT colonography? *Am J Roentgenol.* 2005;184:21-22.

17. Kozarek RA ED, Silverstein ME, Smith RG. Air-pressure-induced colon injury during diagnostic colonoscopy. *Gastroenterology.* 1980;78:7-14.

18. Pickhardt PJ. Incidence of colonic perforation at CT colonography: Review of existing data and implications for screening of asymptomatic adults. *Radiology.* 2006;239(2):313-316.

19. Levin TR, Zhao W, Conell C, et al. Complications of colonoscopy in an integrated health care delivery system. *Ann Intern Med.* 2006;145(12):880-886.

20. Anderson ML, Pasha TM, Leighton JA. Endoscopic perforation of the colon: Lessons from a 10-year study. *Am J Gastroenterol.* 2000;95(12):3418-3422.

21. Kim DH, Pickhardt PJ, Taylor AJ, et al. CT colonography versus colonoscopy for the detection of advanced neoplasia. *N Engl J Med.* 2007;357(14):1403-1412.

22. Sosna J, Blachar A, Amitai M, et al. Colonic perforation at CT colonography: Assessment of risk in a multicenter large cohort. *Radiology.* 2006;239(2):457-463.

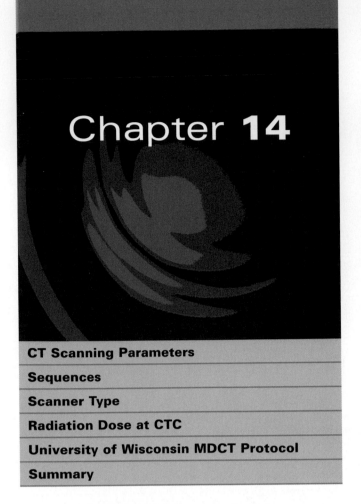

Chapter 14

MDCT Protocol for CT Colonography

DAVID H. KIM, MD
PERRY J. PICKHARDT, MD

INTRODUCTION

The technologic advances involving the computed tomography (CT) scanner in the 1990s and early 2000s were underlying factors that allowed CT colonography (CTC) to develop as a viable modality. CTC was not realistically feasible without the volumetric acquisition of data. Even with the favorable imaging characteristics of colorectal screening (i.e., marked contrast of a soft tissue polyp against the adjacent luminal air within a stationary environment), conventional nonspiral incremental scanners with multiple breath holds did not lead to effective protocols. The advent of spiral scanning with volumetric data was a major step toward modern-day CTC. However, issues of coverage existed with a single-detector spiral scanner because fairly long breath holds necessitated a thicker-slice collimation to allow the entire colon to be imaged. The emergence of multidetector CT (MDCT) scanner technology allowed coverage of the entire colorectum with thin collimation and breath holds of very short duration. Thus, because of these advances, the CT scanner is no longer the limiting factor in the CTC evaluation sequence. This chapter will examine the effect of various scanning parameters on the CTC examination used on current scanners. We will also outline an optimized MDCT protocol for CTC with the aim of maximizing polyp detection sensitivity while minimizing radiation dose to the patient.

CT SCANNING PARAMETERS

Collimation

For MDCT, collimation refers to the collimated slice thickness, which is equal to the width of a single section/row (of either a single detector or combination of detectors) used by the scanner. The final effective slice thickness is related to the collimated slice thickness but can be a larger value because of the spiral interpolation reconstruction process and pitch. Collimation helps to determine longitudinal (z-axis) resolution of the image, which in turn determines the detectability of a lesion of a given size (in-plane resolution in the x-y direction is not a limiting factor for lesion detectability). Thin collimation is required for effective CT colonography. What constitutes thin collimation has changed with advancing scanner technology. As a result of prior scanner constraints, collimation up to 5 mm was used for CTC in the past. This slice thickness is not optimal and does not constitute thin collimation in today's terms. Multislice scanners from 4 to 16 rows of detectors have allowed collimation to narrow to the 1.25 mm to 2.5 mm range. Scanner technology with 64-detector row CT scanners now allows for coverage of the abdomen with submillimeter collimation with reasonable breath holds. However, a tradeoff exists where noise is increased at the same dose profile, which may offset the improved z-axis resolution. To offset the increased noise at thinner collimations, dose must be increased, which is not desirable for CTC screening.

What is the optimal collimation for CTC? It is highly dependent on the size of the target lesion of CTC. The true target of CTC screening concerns large polyps ($\geq$10 mm), but the detection of smaller (6-9 mm) lesions is currently considered relevant because there is a small proportion with advanced neoplasia in this group. The issue of surveillance versus immediate polypectomy for polyps of this size category remains controversial (see Chapter 2). There is consensus in the CTC research community that diminutive lesions (≤5 mm) should not be an aim of detection given their clinical insignificance.[1,2] Hence, the thinnest collimation should be directed at maximizing the sensitivity for detection of polyps 6 mm or greater where the z-axis resolution obtained from the inherent thinness of a slice is balanced against the noise (which incrementally increases as the collimation decreases). Intuitively, the collimation should be less than that of the intended target for detection. A collimation larger than the target would automatically introduce volume averaging artifact with adjacent structures and thus decrease resolution (Fig. 14-1). How

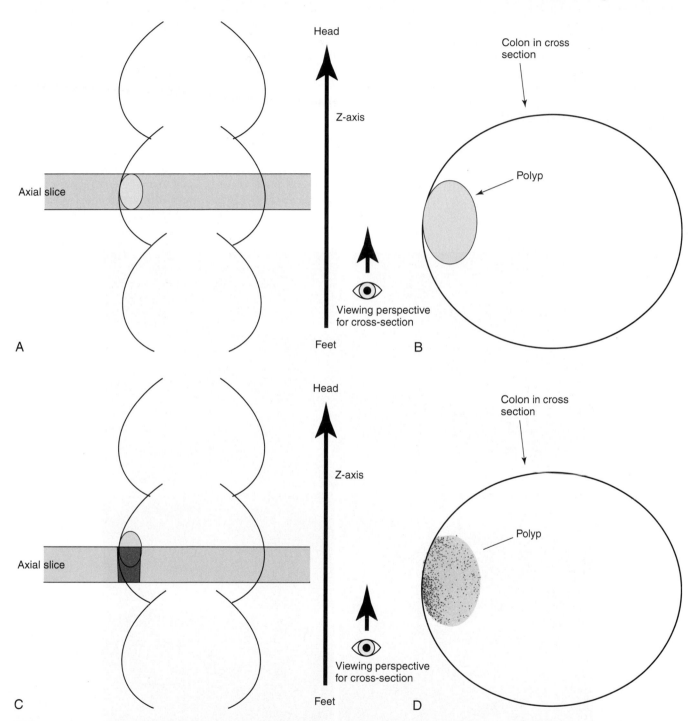

Figure 14-1 Collimation and volume averaging artifact. Schematic drawings show how thick collimation along the z-axis can result in substantial volume averaging artifact. For example, when the collimation equals the polyp size and is centered on the polyp in the z-axis **(A)**, there is minimal volume averaging and the polyp is well seen, as demonstrated in a transverse schematic **(B)**. However, when a collimation of similar thickness is off-center relative to the polyp along the z-axis **(C)**, the adjacent gas is volume averaged along with the polyp to generate the image *(dark purple region)* and the polyp would be less apparent on the transverse view **(D)**. As collimation become thinner in relation to the polyp, this artifact decreases.

much narrower than 6 mm should the collimation be? As collimation narrows relative to the target size, the potential effect of volume averaging on visualization decreases. The meta-analysis by Mulhall et al. suggested that as collimation increased by 1 mm, the sensitivity for polyp detection decreased by 5%.[3] Similarly, Taylor and colleagues demonstrated a 7% difference in nondiminutive polyp detection rates between 1.25 mm and 2.5 mm collimation within an ex vivo colectomy specimen.[4] From a practical standpoint, several studies have shown excellent polyp detection rates using thin collimation between 1.25 and 2.5 mm (Fig. 14-2).[5,6] It is our opinion that the optimal collimation is 1.25 mm, offering the best compromise between z-axis resolution and noise. Use of submillimeter collimation (although possible on current 64-slice/scanners) does not appear to significantly increase detection for the target lesion size of 6 mm and would lead to unnecessary dose increases to maintain a certain noise level.

Pitch

Pitch is an MDCT scanning parameter that relates table movement to gantry rotation and slice collimation (Fig. 14-3). In other words, how far does the table move in the longitudinal (z-axis) during a single gantry rotation? This parameter was first developed for single-detector CT scanners. In this setting, a pitch of 1 correlates to a situation where the distance of the table increments equals the slice collimation with a single complete rotation of the gantry. With a pitch less than 1, there is imaging overlap where the table moves less than the slice collimation with a gantry rotation. With a pitch greater than 1, the table moves a larger distance than the slice collimation and a gap in imaging of the object is present. Unfortunately, early in the MDCT setting, the definition was initially altered where the slice collimation could refer to a single detector or refer to the entire width of the multidetector scanner array

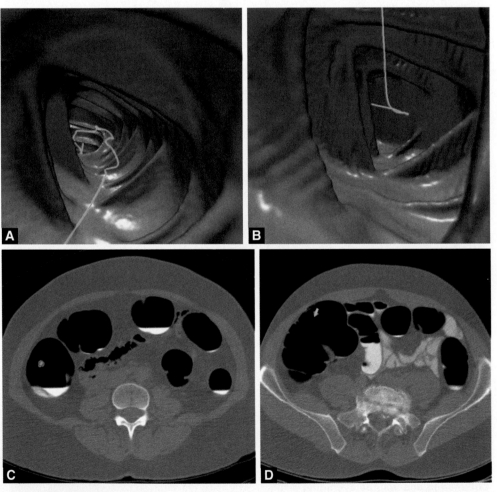

Figure 14-2 **1.25-mm versus 2.5-mm slice collimation.** The difference in collimation between these two levels is illustrated. 3D endoluminal CTC image **(A)** with 1.25-mm collimation depicts the typical appearance of the colonic lumen. Note the rippled or ridged appearance of the endoluminal image **(B)** with 2.5-mm collimation. Similarly, note the difference on the 2D transverse CTC images where the 1.25-mm collimation **(C)** is in sharper focus than the 2.5-mm collimated image **(D),** which is slightly blurred or ghosted. The 2.5-mm collimation images are diagnostic, but this artifact can become fairly pronounced in some areas of the colon.

$$p = TF/W$$

- p: pitch
- TF: table feed per rotation
- W: total width of the collimated beam

Figure 14-3 **Equation for pitch.** Pitch relates the distance of table movement to gantry rotation and total width of the collimated beam. This definition applies to both single-detector and multidetector CT. For pitches greater than 1, there is a gap in the helical data acquisition; for pitches less than 1, there is overlap in the z-axis.

4-Slice MDCT

1.25	1.25	1.25	1.25	1.25	1.25	1.25	1.25	1.25	1.25	1.25	1.25	1.25	1.25	1.25	1.25

By single detector width and a table feed of 7.5 mm:

- p = table feed/detector width
- p = 7.5/1.25 = 6

By activated array width and a table feed of 7.5 mm:

- p = table feed/act. array width
- p = 7.5/5 = 1.5

Figure 14-4 **The differing definitions for pitch.** Unfortunately, multiple definitions of pitch arose with the introduction of multidetector scanners. The schematic demonstrates a four-detector row MDCT array with uniform detector width where the four central channels of 1.25-mm collimation are activated. With a table feed of 7.5 mm during a complete revolution of the scanner, one definition (given in terms of a single activated detector width) would report the pitch to be 6, whereas the other definition (in terms of the width of the entire activated array) would give a pitch of 1.5. The second definition is preferred because it correlates with the traditional definition of pitch. The former should be relegated to a historic footnote.

(Fig. 14-4). It is preferable to define pitch in terms of the entire width of the scanner array used.[7] This definition is directly comparable to the traditional definition of pitch for single-slice scanners and maintains the relationships among pitch, dose, and image quality as documented for the single-slice scanners. For example, a 16-detector row scanner with 1.25-mm sections would have a total scanner array width of 20 mm. Consequently, if the table moved 40 mm during a single rotation, the pitch would be 2.

Traditionally, increasing the pitch broadened the slice sensitivity profile, resulting in decreased z-axis resolution. This was true for single-slice and early multislice scanners, which used linear interpolation reconstruction algorithms. In addition, stair-stepping and rippling artifacts increase, which contribute to decreased lesion conspicuity.[8] This relationship of slice broadening and increasing pitch remains true for some current MDCT 16-slice scanners that provide discrete optimized pitch values (e.g., 0.5625, 0.9375, 1.375, 1.75) as they continue to use linear interpolation reconstruction approaches. However, for other MDCT scanners that use Z-filter approaches and other reconstruction algorithms that account for cone-beam geometry, this relationship is no longer valid where longitudinal (z-axis) resolution is independent of pitch. In these scanners, the same effective section width is seen at all pitch values up to 2.[9] In addition, for all MDCT scanners, the dose to the patient does not change with increasing pitch.[10,11] It is true that dose should decrease when pitch increases with a constant tube current. However, in contrast to single-slice scanners, current MDCT scanners alter dose with pitch to maintain a constant noise level. Thus, optimized pitch holds less importance for CTC with MDCT than in the era of single-slice scanners and early MDCT. Traditionally, a pitch of 1.5 to 2.0 was felt to result in diagnostic images. Taylor et al.[4] explored pitch in MDCT and CT colonography. Using a colon phantom created from a colectomy specimen from a patient with familial polyposis coli, they found that detection of polyps greater than 5 mm was unaffected by changes of pitch up to 1.5 when collimation was kept constant at 1.25 mm.[4] Most protocols keep pitch at or under 1.5.

Reconstruction Interval

Overlapping reconstructions have been shown to increase lesion detection in a number of settings such as in detection of pulmonary nodules.[12] Interpolated slices allow decrease in volume averaging artifact and also help in smoothing multiplanar and 3D projections. Previously, 60% overlap was recommended at CT colonography.[13] Such overlapping intervals were much more important in the single-slice era where the z-axis resolution was much poorer than in-plane resolution. With MDCT, this is much less of a concern given the thin collimation that is possible. However, reconstruction intervals with modest overlap remain helpful, with protocols varying between 0% and 25% overlap.

Tube Current/Potential

Minimizing tube current is a goal of CT colonography protocols with MDCT so as to decrease radiation dose to the patient. This examination is used in an otherwise-healthy population; thus, any potential risks related of radiation should be kept at the lowest possible level (see Chapter 15). Optimizing this parameter minimizes administered dose but at the expense of increased image mottle or noise. Initially, this was accomplished by using the minimal mAs level possible while producing diagnostic images, typically between 35 and 75 mAs per series.[5,14] With the advent of tube current modulation, protocols can concentrate on setting an appropriate noise level to minimize dose. Here, the mA is altered dynamically during image acquisition to maintain a preset acceptable level of noise. The tube current is then automatically decreased when progressing through areas of less density and increased in areas more dense, such as the pelvis, to maintain this noise level. With some systems, such as Smart-mA by GE Medical Systems, dose is modulated in both along the z-axis and within the x-y plane. This results in efficient dose delivery with an overall decrease in the total dose administered. What is the maximal noise level that is acceptable? In our experience, it is dependent more on the effects seen at the three-dimensional (3D) reconstruction than on the 2D images. As the noise increases because of decreased technique, the colonic walls on the 3D fly-through become more heterogenous and mottled, which decreases sensitivity for lesions before a similar decrease in image quality is seen at 2D (Fig. 14-5). We set the noise index level at 50 (for comparison, standard abdominal CT protocols have noise index levels offset at 10-12). In addition, a minimum and maximum tube current value is set. The minimum mA is set at 30 to maintain the image quality at 3D. A ceiling of 300 mA is set as the maximum value. On average, this results in a dose of 2.5 mSv per series. At these levels, the walls at 3D are relatively smooth, with a few areas that may become somewhat mottled but remain diagnostic. There is less impact on 2D images, but it is important to realize that beam hardening and quantum mottle on this low-dose scan may cause heterogeneity in true soft tissue lesions that can mimic stool or even a lipoma (see Chapter 20).

Tube potential is set at 120 kV_p (the default value for standard abdominal CT). Tube potential affects both contrast and noise. Decreasing kVp increases contrast and noise while decreasing dose. To date, there has been

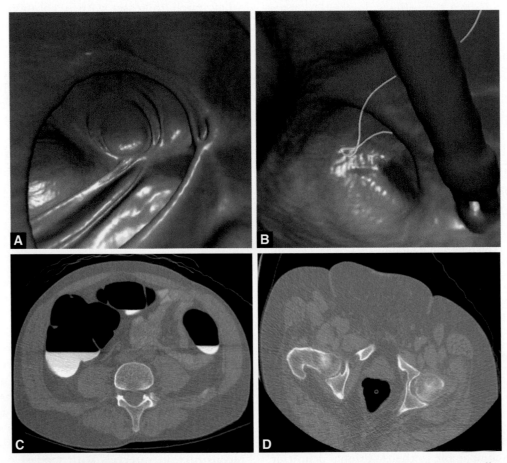

Figure 14-5   The effect of decreased mA. Decreasing mA results in increased noise, which objectively affects the 3D image to a greater degree than the 2D image. 3D endoluminal CTC image **(A)** shows very smooth, "shiny" colonic walls with older higher technique protocols. Note the change in the smoothness of the colonic walls with increased texturing with the current lower dose technique **(B)**. This decreased mA has little effect on the 2D image with higher **(C)** and lower **(D)** mA.

little research at CTC investigating altered kV_p values to assess benefits from the standard value. However, one low-dose CTC protocol currently under research at UW consists of using 140 kV_p to potentially decrease overall dose. Here, the increased dose from the higher kV_p is offset by decreases in dose from an increased noise index to 70 and decreased mA ceiling to 150.

Gantry Rotation

Speed of gantry rotation is not a key factor for CTC. It is a major determinant of temporal resolution—the ability to freeze motion. As opposed to coronary CT angiography in which temporal resolution is important to adequately image a coronary artery on a beating, moving heart, such is not the case with CTC in which the large intestine is a relatively static organ. Rotation speeds, such as 0.4 to 0.5 second per rotation, are not necessary for imaging. Much slower rotations can be used if needed, up to 0.8 to 1.0 second per revolution.

SEQUENCES

At a minimum, both supine and prone acquisitions are required for a complete CTC examination. There is complementary luminal distention and shifting of gas and fluid between the two series that are necessary for optimal polyp detection (Fig. 14-6). The supine series tends to distend the transverse colon better, whereas the sigmoid colon is more consistently distended on the prone series. Several studies including one from the Mayo Clinic in Rochester have demonstrated increased polyp detection with the use of both series as opposed to a single one only. Fletcher et al.[15] showed that sensitivity increased from 70% to 85% for large polyps ($\geq$10 mm) and from 75% to 88% for polyps 5 mm or greater when the prone series was added to the interpretation. Each series is obtained in end-expiration. This is preferred over end-inspiration to minimize compressive effects of inflated lungs on the transverse colon. In addition to the standard supine and prone series, a decubitus series may

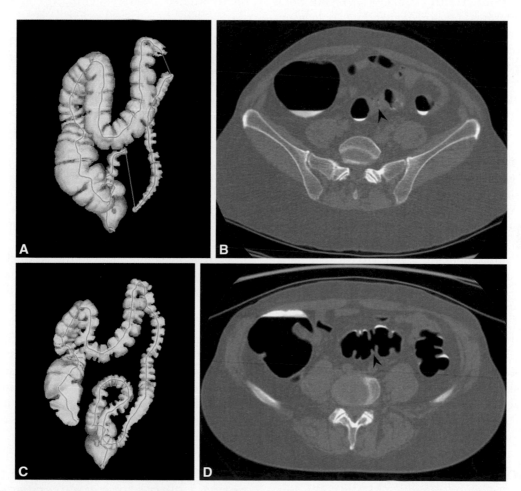

Figure 14-6 Supine and prone acquisitions. At a minimum, both supine and prone series are required as a result of the complementary shifting of gas and fluid. 3D colon image **(A)** shows excellent distention of the right and transverse colon on the supine view with collapse and marked underdistention of the left colon and sigmoid. Supine 2D transverse CTC image **(B)** nicely confirms this situation where there is collapse *(arrowhead)* of the portion of the sigmoid colon. With prone positioning, there is suboptimal but adequate distention with a complete air column in the left colon, allowing for diagnostic evaluation **(C)**. Prone 2D transverse CTC image **(D)** shows that the previous area *(arrowhead)* of sigmoid collapse is now adequately distended.

be added if a segment of colon remains collapsed on both standard views. Typically, it is performed in the right lateral decubitus position (or right side down). In our experience, this will occur in approximately 1 out of every 10 to 15 examinations.

SCANNER TYPE

An MDCT scanner is required for adequate CT colonography. Single-slice scanners cannot support a narrow-enough collimation while maintaining coverage of the entire colorectum. At a minimum, a 4-slice scanner can be used to perform this examination with acceptable polyp-detection capabilities. A 2.5-mm collimation used in a 4-slice scanner allows for diagnostic images. An 8-slice scanner allows for the preferred thinner collimation of 1.25 mm. Breath holds, however, remain on the longer side at 35 to 40 seconds with these parameters. The optimal scanner is a 16-slice scanner where 1.25-mm collimation can be used with short breath holds of 15 to 20 seconds. A 64-slice scanner can be substituted with even shorter breath holds but may be better used by more demanding applications such as coronary artery depiction. Although submillimeter collimation is possible on these scanners (and on the 16-slice scanners), the increase in longitudinal resolution is not worth the increased noise (or increased mA to maintain equivalent noise levels) of the thinner collimation in our opinion.

In addition, there is improved geometric efficiency and thus decreased dose with 8- or 16-slice scanners in comparison to a 4-slice scanner. Geometric efficiency refers to the percentage of wasted radiation. For MDCT, there is radiation that passes adjacent to the active detectors that is not used in image generation (the penumbra). The width of the penumbra is fairly constant at between 1 and 3 mm.[16] Consequently, the percentage of "wasted" radiation is higher in relation to the used radiation when thinner collimation is used at a 4-slice scanner as opposed to thicker collimation. The geometric efficiency also improves with decreased wasted radiation as the number of slices increases (e.g., 8 or 16).

For CTC, the optimal scanner is a 16-slice scanner in our opinion. It allows thin collimation (1.25 mm) with reasonable breath holds and improved geometric efficiency. It also is widely available in the United States. A 64-slice scanner can be used but holds capabilities that exceed the requirements of the examination and is a more expensive scanner.

RADIATION DOSE AT CTC

CTC is a low-dose examination. A survey of the CTC protocols of 34 institutions active in CTC demonstrated a median effective dose at 5.7 mSv (2.8 mSv supine; 2.5mSv prone) for screening protocols.[17] There is active research

in ultra-low–dose techniques that remain investigational. The protocol used at the University of Wisconsin (UW) delivers about 2.5 mSv per series or 5.0 mSv for a typical examination with supine and prone series. The actual risk for future cancer induction, if present, remains controversial.[18,19] However, even proponents of the linear-no-threshold model of risk agree that the benefits of colorectal cancer screening greatly outweigh these small theoretic risks.[18] Chapter 15 discusses such issues in greater detail.

UNIVERSITY OF WISCONSIN MDCT PROTOCOL

Several MDCT CTC protocols are in use for a 16-slice scanner at UW, including both fixed mA and tube current modulation protocols. In addition, differing protocols are in place for screening (by far, the majority of examinations) and diagnostic indications *versus* evaluation of a known or highly suspected cancer, where intravenous contrast is given. The low-dose protocol currently under investigation that uses 140 kV_p and noise index of 70 is not shown here. Visit www.virtuoctc.com for updates.

CTC Protocol: Screening and Most Diagnostic Indications (no IV contrast)

Pre-scan: Make sure the patient has been prepped properly. Encourage use of restroom.

Patient Setup: Place the patient on the CT table on his or her left side to insufflate the colon with CO_2 (left decubitus for approx 1.5 L, right decubitus to 3.0 to 3.5 L total volume, then supine until equilibrium reached).

Scan Description: Scan is performed supine and prone.

Series 1: Anteroposterior (AP) and lateral *supine* scouts diaphragm through pubic symphysis (check colon distention).

Series 2: Supine: Start above the highest flexure of the colon and scan through the rectum. Review 2D images to check for proper colonic distention, and pay special attention to sigmoid distention.

Series 3: Posteroanterior (PA) and lateral *prone* scouts diaphragm through pubic symphysis (check colon distention).

Series 4: Prone: Start above the highest flexure of the colon and scan through the rectum. Review 2D images to check for proper colonic distention.

Consider right decubitus **Series 5** if areas of collapse are present on both views at 2D review.

Scan Factors (for supine and prone series using static mA protocol)

Series 2: Supine (acquire in end-expiration)
- Scan type: Helical
- Gantry rotation: 0.5 sec

- Collimation: 1.25 mm
- Table speed: 27.5 mm
- Pitch: 1.375:1
- Reconstruction interval: 1 mm
- Scan FOV: Large
- kV_p: 120
- Static mA: 100 (BMI <25); 300 (BMI >40); 100-300 (BMI = 25-40; linear scale)
- DFOV: Large
- Recon type: Standard; 1.25 mm thick/1-mm interval
- Recon2 (supine only): 5-mm thick/3-mm interval (for extracolonic evaluation)

Series 4 (Prone): Same scan factors as above. Acquire in end-expiration.

Series 5 (Rt. decubitus, if needed): Same scan factors as above. Acquire in end-expiration.

————OR————

Scan Factors (for supine and prone series using modulated dose protocols: Smart mA)

Series 2: Supine (acquire in end-expiration)
- Scan type: Helical
- Gantry rotation: 0.5 sec
- Collimation: 1.25 mm
- Table speed: 27.5 mm
- Pitch: 1.375:1
- Reconstruction interval: 1 mm
- Scan FOV: Large
- kV_p: 120
- Noise index: 50
- Smart mA range: 30-300
- DFOV: Large
- Recon type: Standard; 1.25-mm thick/1-mm interval
- Recon2 (supine only): 5-mm thick/3-mm interval (for extracolonic evaluation)

Series 4 (Prone): Same scan factors as above. Acquire in end-expiration.

Series 5 (Rt. decubitus, if needed): Same scan factors as above. Acquire in end-expiration.

CTC Protocol: Evaluation of Known Colorectal Cancer (with IV contrast)

Indications: Occlusive CRC and/or cancer staging.

Prescan: Make sure the patient has been prepped properly. Encourage use of restroom.

Patient setup: Place the patient on the CT table on his or her left side to insufflate the colon with CO_2 (left decubitus for approx 1.5 L, right decubitus to 3.0 to 3.5 L total volume, then supine until equilibrium reached). *Place patient prone for the initial noncontrast series.*

IV contrast/rate: 100 mL with a 50-mL saline chase, 3 mL per second (supine series).

Scan Description: Scan is performed prone without IV contrast, then supine with IV contrast

Series 1: PA and lateral *prone* scouts diaphragm through pubic symphysis (check colon distention).

Series 2: Prone without IV contrast. Start above the highest flexure of the colon and scan through the rectum. Review 2D images to check for proper colonic distention, and pay special attention to sigmoid distention.

Series 3: AP and later *supine* scouts diaphragm through pubic symphysis (check colon distention).

Series 4: Smart prep: Center over the liver. Put three regions of interest (ROIs) in the liver. Threshold 50 HU. No longer than 80-second delay.

Series 5: Supine with IV contrast. Start at the diaphragm and scan through pubic symphysis. Review images to check for proper colonic distention.

Scan Factors

Series 2: Prone without IV contrast (acquire in end-expiration)
- Scan type: Helical
- Gantry rotation: 0.5 sec
- Slice thickness: 1.25 mm
- Table speed: 27.5 mm
- Pitch: 1.375:1
- Reconstruction interval: 1 mm
- Scan FOV: Large
- kV_p: 120
- *If* static mA: 100 (BMI <25); 300 (BMI >40); 100-300 (BMI = 25-40; linear scale)
- *If* smart mA: Noise index = 50 (mA range: 30-300)
- DFOV: Large
- Recon type: Standard; 1.25-mm thick/1-mm interval

Series 5: Supine with IV contrast (acquire in end-expiration). Portal venous phase acquisition.
- Scan type: Helical
- Gantry rotation: 0.5 sec
- Slice thickness: 1.25 mm
- Table speed: 27.5 mm
- Pitch: 1.375:1
- Reconstruction interval: 1 mm
- Scan FOV: Large
- kV_p: 120
- Smart mA range: 80-440 (80-660 on 64-detector row)
- Noise index = 12
- DFOV: Large
- Recon type: Standard; 1.25-mm thick/1-mm interval
- Recon2 (supine only): 5-mm thick/3-mm interval

SUMMARY

Modern-day MDCT has allowed for the development of CT colonography. The volumetric acquisition of data with thin collimation and a reasonably short breath hold have been keys to effective examinations. Current capabilities of MDCT scanners exceed the requirements of the examination. A desirable CTC protocol maximizes polyp-detection capabilities by the optimization of scanning parameters (including collimation, pitch, reconstruction, mA, kV_p) while minimizing dose to the patient. This requires a tradeoff in various parameters. In our opinion, such an optimized protocol can be readily accomplished with 16-slice MDCT scanners.

REFERENCES

1. Barish MA, Soto JA, Ferrucci JT. Consensus on current clinical practice of virtual colonoscopy. *Am J Roentgenol.* 2005;184(3):786-792.
2. Zalis ME, Barish MA, Choi JR, et al. CT colonography reporting and data system: A consensus proposal. *Radiology.* 2005;236(1):3-9.
3. Mulhall BP, Veerappan GR, Jackson JL. Meta-analysis: Computed tomographic colonography. *Annals Intern Med.* 2005;142(8):635-650.
4. Taylor SA, Halligan S, Bartram CI, et al. Multi-detector row CT colonography: Effect of collimation, pitch, and orientation on polyp detection in a human colectomy specimen. *Radiology.* 2003;229(1):109-118.
5. Pickhardt PJ, Choi JR, Hwang I, et al. Computed tomographic virtual colonoscopy to screen for colorectal neoplasia in asymptomatic adults. *N Engl J Med.* 2003;349(23):2191-2200.
6. Kim DH, Pickhardt PJ, Taylor AJ, et al. CT colonography versus colonoscopy for the detection of advanced neoplasia. *N Engl J Med.* 2007;357(14):1403-1412.
7. Silverman PM, Kalender WA, Hazle JD. Common terminology for single and multislice helical CT. *Am J Roentgenol.* 2001;176(5):1135-1136.
8. Whiting BR, McFarland EG, Brink JA. Influence of image acquisition parameters on CT artifacts and polyp depiction in spiral CT colonography: In vitro evaluation. *Radiology.* 2000;217(1):165-172.
9. Flohr TG, Schaller S, Stierstorfer K, Bruder H, Ohnesorge BM, Schoepf UJ. Multi-detector row CT systems and image-reconstruction techniques. *Radiology.* 2005;235(3):756-773.
10. Mahesh M, Scatarige JC, Cooper J, Fishman EK. Original report—Dose and pitch relationship for a particular multislice CT scanner. *Am J Roentgenol.* 2001;177(6):1273-1275.
11. Rydberg J, Liang Y, Teague SD. Fundamentals of multichannel CT. *Radiol Clin North Am.* 2003;41(3):465-474.
12. Diederich S, Lentschig MG, Winter F, Roos N, Bongartz G. Detection of pulmonary nodules with overlapping vs non-overlapping image reconstruction at spiral CT. *Eur Radiol.* 1999;9(2):281-286.
13. McFarland EG, Brink JA, Loh J, et al. Visualization of colorectal polyps with spiral CT colography: Evaluation of processing parameters with perspective volume rendering. *Radiology.* 1997;205(3):701-707.
14. Pickhardt PJ, Kim DH. CT colonography (virtual colonoscopy): A practical approach for population screening. *Radiol Clin North Am.* 2007;45(2):361-375.
15. Fletcher JG, Johnson CD, Welch TJ, et al. Optimization of CT colonography technique: Prospective trial in 180 patients. *Radiology.* 2000;216(3):704-711.
16. Cody DD, Mahesh M. AAPM/RSNA physics tutorial for residents—Technologic advances in multidetector CT with a focus on cardiac imaging. *Radiographics.* 2007;27(6):1829-1837.
17. Liedenbaum MH, Venema HW, Stoker J. Radiation dose in CT colonography—Trends in time and differences between daily practice and screening protocols. *Eur Radiol.* 2008;18(10):2222-2230.
18. Brenner DJ, Georgsson MA. Mass screening with CT colonography: Should the radiation exposure be of concern? *Gastroenterology.* 2005;129(1):328-337.
19. Radiation risk in perspective. Position statement of the Health Physics Society. Adopted January 1996, revised August 2004. McLean, VA: Health Physics Society; 2004.

Potential Complications of CT Colonography

DAVID H. KIM, MD
PERRY J. PICKHARDT, MD

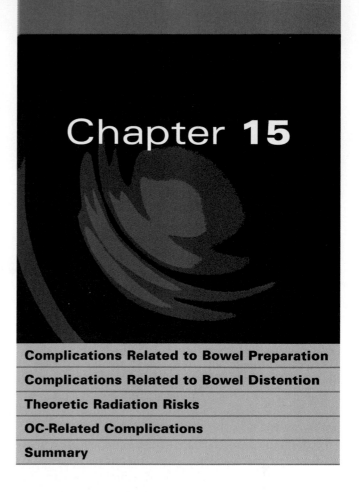

INTRODUCTION

Complications are inherent in medical tests and interventions. All modalities carry a certain level of risk for complications that vary in significance and severity. In the screening situation, morbidity and mortality related to the diagnostic modality should ideally be nonexistent. Screening is applied to healthy individuals without a defined medical problem and is performed to identify people at risk for a presymptomatic or future pathologic condition. Even a very low rate of complications can be detrimental for a screening modality because it may be applied to large segments of the population. Fortunately, CT colonography (CTC) is a safe, minimally invasive procedure in which the complications are rare and mild in significance. From this perspective, CTC is much better suited for screening than optical colonoscopy (OC), which holds a higher risk of severe complications because of its invasive nature and need for sedation. Potential complications at CTC can be divided into several categories, including those related to bowel preparation, those related to colonic distention, and those related to image acquisition. From a programmatic standpoint, it is important to consider the complications related to therapeutic OC for CTC-detected polyps. This chapter will explore the various complications that may infrequently arise with CTC.

COMPLICATIONS RELATED TO BOWEL PREPARATION

Current state-of-the-art CTC requires the administration of both cathartic agents and oral tagging agents within the bowel preparation protocol. Although rare, potential complications can be related to both groups of agents. In a large survey of several U.S. and international institutions active in CTC, the complication rate from the bowel preparation was near nonexistent at 0.009% (2/21,923), representing half of all significant complications seen at CTC.[1]

Among the cathartic agents, complications are more likely related to the osmotic formulations rather than the isoosmolar preparations. Saline osmotic cathartics such as magnesium citrate or sodium phosphate hold certain advantages over their isoosmolar counterparts as a result of their low volume administration; these advantages result in improved compliance by patients (see Chapter 12). Osmotic cathartics, however, create varying degrees of fluid shifts as the hypertonic solutions draw fluid into the colonic lumen. Individuals unable to tolerate such shifts may be at risk for complications related to relative intravascular hypovolemia. Consequently, these agents are generally reserved for individuals without significant renal or cardiac insufficiency.

Sodium phosphate is acknowledged to hold a lower safety profile than magnesium citrate and the isoosmolar cathartics (e.g., polyethylene glycol). The administration of sodium phosphate causes a transient hyperphosphatemia. In a small proportion of individuals, a resultant hypocalcemia related to the hyperphosphatemia has been documented. A meta-analysis of eight randomized controlled trials (n = 1286 combined patients) comparing sodium phosphate and polyethylene glycol reported a lack of clinically significant adverse effects with sodium phosphate use.[2] Two trials within the meta-analysis did report transient hypocalcemia without associated cardiac events. Recently, a condition termed acute phosphate nephropathy has been described with sodium phosphate use.[3,4] This rare circumstance is characterized by medullary nephrocalcinosis and tubular injury. At least some individuals afflicted with this condition have experienced progressive loss of renal function. The exact mechanism is unknown but may be related to calcium phosphate precipitation and deposition. The recognition of this entity has led to recent safety warnings from the Food and Drug Administration with the subsequent voluntary recall of over-the-counter sodium phophate-based cathartics.

When used correctly in healthy individuals, osmotic cathartics are very safe agents with few complications. Magnesium citrate, in particular, has an extensive history of safe use at barium enema. One recognized protective measure to further decrease risk involves adequate hydration both prior to and during bowel preparation. In addition to a well-hydrated state prior to the bowel preparation, it is important that fluid intake during the regimen account for the cathartic-induced fluid loss. For example, it is estimated that each 45-mL dose of sodium phosphate results in 1.0 to 1.8 L of fluid loss to the individual.[5] Similar fluid losses occur with magnesium citrate administration. In the specific case of sodium phosphate, another protective measure involved reducing the cathartic dose. One postulated mechanism of acute phosphate nephropathy concerned a dose dependent phenomenon; it was hoped that decreasing the amount of sodium phosphate administered would decrease the risk of this rare but serious complication. Reduction to a single 45-mL dose from the split double dose regimen traditionally used in optical colonoscopy has been shown to be feasible in the setting of CTC.[6] Adequate colonic cleansing at CTC was possible despite this reduction as a result of the secondary cathartic effects related to the tagging agent diatrizoate used in the CTC bowel preparation. However, with the recent voluntary recall, sodium phosphate cleansing products are no longer a realistic option.

Albeit a very low possibility, complications may also potentially arise from the tagging agents (dilute barium and diatrizoate) within the preparation. Barium is an inert substance and not systemically absorbed. Theoretically, there should be no risk for allergy or adverse reaction. However, patients can and have anecdotally reacted presumably to the additives within the barium preparation.[7] The dilute concentration (2% w/v) has not led to any substantial problems of constipation following the procedure in our experience. The denser barium preparations (40% w/v) have reportedly caused problems at same-day OC in terms of clogging endoscopic ports. Diatrizoate holds a very small possibility for an allergic reaction. It is an iodine-based agent that potentially may be minimally absorbed across the colonic mucosa. It is estimated that 1% to 2% may be absorbed. Consequently, it carries a theoretic risk for allergic reaction for those with documented severe allergies to iodinated intravenous (IV) contrast agents. In our experience with more than 7000 patients (University of Wisconsin and Department of Defense), this particular complication has not occurred.

The bowel preparation regimen may also precipitate complications in patients with comorbidities. One such common disease process is diabetes. Because patients are limited to a liquid diet during the bowel preparation, there are alterations in caloric intake during this time. It is important to adjust insulin and oral hypoglycemic regimens accordingly to prevent adverse events. Another common issue involves medications for various conditions (e.g., antibiotics for an infection). It is important to space out these medications either 1 hour prior to or 1 hour following the administration of the cathartic agent to maximize absorption of the medication.

COMPLICATIONS RELATED TO BOWEL DISTENTION

CTC requires distention of the large bowel with a gaseous medium after placement of a rectal catheter. Consequently, potential complications include mechanical injury of the anus and rectum from the catheter placement and perforation secondary to barotrauma related to luminal distention. Both are very rare events. For the former, the risk of injury is minimized because only a small-caliber flexible catheter is required. A retention balloon is insufflated with placement, but it is a small-volume balloon used only to prevent the catheter from slipping out. When a more rigid barium enema tip is substituted for distention, typically as a result of loss of gas around the catheter in patients with poor tone, the possibility for injury increases. The risk, however, remains very low and decreases with appropriate training and experience.

Colonic perforation at CTC is a very rare event. The prevalence remains much less than that for OC. OC is an invasive procedure requiring sedation to allow manipulation of an endoscope throughout the length of the colon to the cecum, whereas CTC requires only the placement of a small-caliber catheter a few centimeters into the rectum for instillation of a gaseous medium. The perforation rate at OC typically ranges from 0.1% to 0.2%.[8,9] As for CTC, two large surveys and one multicenter series have reported the prevalence at this modality.[1,10,11] A large U.S. and international survey of institutions active in CTC reported a total perforation rate of 0.009% (2/21,923).[1] The symptomatic perforation rate, which is the clinically relevant figure to be compared with OC, was 0.005% (1 case). Both perforations occurred in CTC undertaken for diagnostic indications and not in screening individuals. In addition, both perforations occurred with staff-controlled room air insufflation; none occurred in the automated carbon dioxide administered group. These observations suggest that in a screening population with use of low-pressure CO_2 delivery, the true incidence of perforation is likely even lower—

approaching zero. Two studies encapsulating the United Kingdom and Israeli experiences reported higher perforation rates, ranging from 0.06% to 0.08%.[10,11] However, these populations reflected an older population at high risk for colorectal cancer using methods and techniques likely to increase risk compared to currently automated carbon dioxide delivery. These numbers are likely confounded by the probable inclusion of asymptomatic colonic pneumatosis (see later).

The United Kingdom and Israeli experiences provide important lessons to further improve the already wide safety profile of CTC. Four of seven of the Israeli perforations occurred in patients with a left-sided inguinal hernia containing the sigmoid colon.[11] It is important to be cognizant of this rare occurrence, particularly if there is apparent difficulty during instillation and/or the patient reports groin pain and swelling. Confirmation then can be undertaken on the cross-sectional images. The Israeli perforations all occurred with staff-controlled room air insufflation, which is known to generate much higher intracolonic pressures than the low-pressure automated delivery of CO_2. Thus, the use of CO_2 would likely help to decrease the risk of perforation even if the colon is distended in the presence of a colon-containing inguinal hernia (Fig. 15-1). These studies also point to the need to exercise care when a rigid large-caliber catheter typically used in barium enema is used at CTC. This tip can rarely perforate the rectum as seen in these series and cause significant injury from the balloon insufflation given its blind technique at CTC without real-time fluoroscopy. The specifically designed catheters for CTC should be used in the majority of cases given their small caliber and flexible nature. The rigid barium enema tips with large retention cuffs should be reserved for special situations where the patient cannot hold onto the gas with large amounts of leakage about the catheter.

It is important to recognize one clinical situation where a perforation may be inappropriately attributed to CTC—for examination following an incomplete OC (Fig. 15-2). Ideally, patients are sent on the same day to CTC following recovery from sedation to preclude the need for a second bowel preparation. In these cases, it is important to realize that a perforation at OC may be clinically silent or unrecognized. Hough et al. described their experience at the Mayo Clinic in Rochester where they examined 262 consecutive patients who underwent completion CTC following incomplete OC.[12] As part of the clinical protocol, all patients underwent a low-dose CT scan prior to colonic distention for CTC. In their series, 2 of 262 patients demonstrated an unsuspected OC perforation that was clinically unrecognized (0.8%). This rate presumably increases if polypectomy is attempted or the OC examination was difficult. Thus, it is important to recognize the likely cause of perforation in these situations and not incorrectly assign it to CTC. Furthermore, in the case of incomplete colonoscopy *where deep biopsy, electrocautery, or snare polypectomy* was performed, it is prudent to reschedule these patients (in 4-6 weeks) to decrease the risk of perforation at CTC.

The imaging appearance of colonic perforation related to CTC (Fig. 15-3) is similar to those seen at OC, which will be described in greater detail in the subsequent section. However, incidental colonic pneumatosis rarely can be seen at CTC, which may be misinterpreted as a perforation but likely represents a separate entity with no clinical significance.[13] *CTC-related asymptomatic colonic pneumatosis* is therefore an important imaging finding to be aware of so as not to mistake it as a true perforation and to reassure the patient of its benign clinical course (see Chapter 13). When first encountered, this finding can be alarming and the obvious concern is for a true perforation. However, the patient will generally be completely asymptomatic and will require no intervention. Early in our experience, we more closely monitored these cases, but all patients with this incidental imaging finding have remained asymptomatic and required no support or intervention. Benign colonic pneumatosis may occur in approximately 1 per 1000 patients at CTC.[13] In our experience, all have been right sided and with CO_2 distention, and none have been with room air. The etiology is unknown, but we postulate mild barotrauma with subtle mucosal or serosal injury without a frank tear or perforation. Theoretically, it makes sense that this would occur in the cecum given the higher forces seen at colonic distention related to the increased diameter of this structure relative to other colonic segments, as predicted by Laplace's Law. The increased permeability of CO_2 across the mucosa then results in pneumatosis. The imaging appearance is characterized by

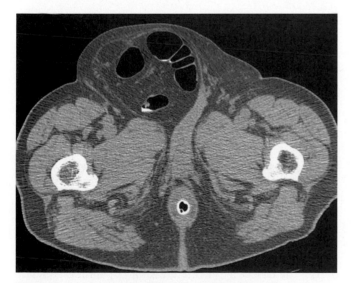

Figure 15-1   Inguinal hernia containing colon. Two-dimensional (2D) transverse CTC image shows an unsuspected large right inguinal hernia containing sigmoid in an 80-year-old patient referred for CTC evaluation. Such a situation increases risk for perforation, especially with room air administration. In this case, CTC was able to be completed with CO_2 and careful monitoring.

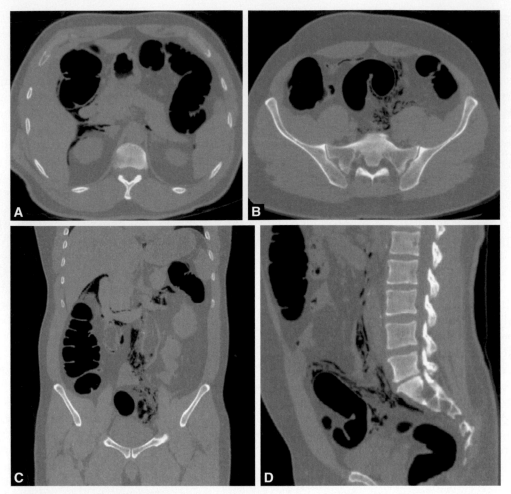

Figure 15-2 **Perforation at incomplete OC.** 2D transverse (**A** and **B**), coronal (**C**), and sagittal (**D**) CTC images show an unrecognized colonic perforation from incomplete colonoscopy that was sent for same-day CTC. Extraperitoneal air is seen dissecting along the sigmoid mesentery along retroperitoneal fascial planes. It is important to recognize this as an OC complication and not to falsely attribute this perforation to CTC. (Case courtesy of Dr. Joel Bortz.)

thin linear gas collections within the wall of the right colon (Fig. 15-4). There may be variable degrees of involvement extending to become circumferential. No frank free intraperitoneal or retroperitoneal air is present. This entity likely occurs with OC but is underrecognized because asymptomatic patients would not be imaged with CT after complete OC examination.

Other minor potential complications include vasovagal reactions related to rapid colonic distention. Patients may become nauseous with emesis, diaphoresis, and bradycardia. This is an infrequent minor complication that is self-limited. It rarely requires intervention past supportive measures including stopping the insufflation. A vasovagal event may, however, require additional imaging series if the reaction occurs during image acquisition. In the U.K. survey, this occurred in 3 of 17,067 patients (0.02%).[10] The use of automated CO_2 may further decrease this risk where rapid distention of the colon is less likely to occur as a result of the low pressure and slow infusion of this technique. It is also important to note that, although CO_2 is actively reabsorbed across the colonic mucosa and ulti-

mately expelled through respiratory system, no untoward events have been reported related to its use in patients with chronic obstructive pulmonary disease. In colonoscopy trials, no elevation in rise of the pCO_2 in end-tidal measurements were seen in large series of patients.[14] In our experience, we have also not seen a significant adverse reaction in this regard.

THEORETIC RADIATION RISKS

Radiation exposure associated with CTC is comparable or less than the levels received during a typical barium enema examination. To put these exposure levels in perspective, the dose is less than twice the background dose from cosmic radiation received over a 1-year period. In addition, the dose is applied to an adult population typically older than 50 years of age (and not an adolescent group in which risk of a future induced cancer is more of a concern) and the majority of the chest is not imaged (which increases the theoretic risk of bronchogenic cancers). At the University of Wisconsin, tube current modulation is used

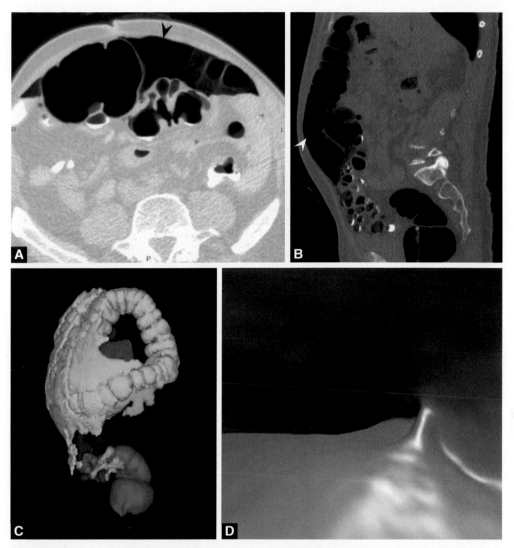

Figure 15-3   Rare perforation at CTC (asymptomatic). 2D thick slab transverse **(A)** and sagittal **(B)** CTC images show intraperitoneal air *(arrowheads)* related to a colonic perforation. 3D colon map **(C)** depicts the amorphous anterior intraperitoneal air surrounding colonic loops and 3D view **(D)** from an intraperitoneal vantage point shows the smooth outline of the falciform ligament. This patient remained asymptomatic and recovered with supportive antibiotic coverage only. He was discharged home after an uneventful hospital stay. Perforation at CTC is a rare event and to date has not occurred in our experience at the University of Wisconsin. To our knowledge, there have been no cases of symptomatic perforation related to CTC screening with automated CO_2 distention. (Case courtesy of Dr. Duncan Barlow.)

to further decrease dose. Each series typically delivers a dose of 2.5 mSv to the patient with a total dose of 5.0 mSv for the standard examination. With optimized low-dose techniques including tube current modulation, other institutions have reported similar numbers ranging from 4.3 to 5.8 mSv.[15] The Health Physics Society position statement reports that at such low doses, any potential risk is too small to be reliably quantified and may be nonexistent.[16] Even noted proponents of the linear, no-threshold model of radiation risk conclude that the benefit–risk ratio of CTC screening is large.[17] Consequently, there is general consensus that the documented real benefits from screening for colorectal cancer greatly outweigh the very small theoretic risk of a future induced cancer.

OC-RELATED COMPLICATIONS

For those patients with positive CTC examinations that are sent on to therapeutic OC for polypectomy, additional adverse events are possible, including perforation, hemorrhage, injury to adjacent organs, and issues related to sedation. When approached from the standpoint of a potential therapeutic option, such risks are justified, particularly when patients at low risk are filtered out and only those with a clinically relevant lesion are sent for polypectomy. When OC is used as a stand-alone screening modality, however, the inherent invasive nature of this modality narrows the benefit–risk ratio in this circumstance.

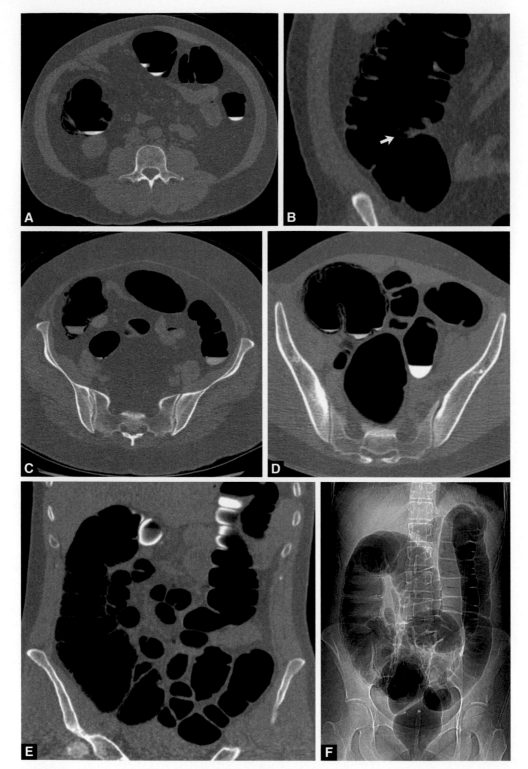

Figure 15-4   CTC-related asymptomatic colonic pneumatosis. 2D transverse **(A)** and coronal **(B)** CTC images demonstrate linear coalescing foci of intramural gas in the ascending colon and ileocecal valve *(arrow)* in an otherwise-well 54-year-old man following screening CTC. 2D transverse CTC image **(C)** in a 64-year-old woman demonstrates similar findings following diagnostic CTC for incomplete optical colonoscopy several months earlier. 2D transverse **(D)** and coronal **(E)** CTC images in a 30-year-old woman demonstrate extensive pneumatosis (the most extensive case in our experience), which could be seen on the CT scout **(F).** All three individuals remained asymptomatic following the CTC examination and did not require any medical intervention. (From Pickhardt PJ, Kim DH, Taylor AJ. Asymptomatic pneumatosis at CT colonography: A benign self-limited imaging finding distinct from perforation. *Am J Roentgenol.* 2008;190(2):W112-W117.)

Of all potential complications, perforation is the most feared. When this occurs, the consequences can be devastating to the individual (see later). Reported rates at colonoscopy typically range from 0.1% to 0.2%.[8,9] There are three major mechanisms for perforation. Colonoscopy requires the mechanical intubation of the cecum, followed by subsequent withdrawal of the instrument, at which time the primary search for polyps begin. Consequently, one route for perforation involves mechanical injury as a result of direct trauma from the end of the endoscope or as a result of the abrasive effects of the side of the scope as the scope is advanced or withdrawn. In addition, traction on areas of colonic attachment can occur with these movements. Maneuvers such as the slide-by technique (where the lumen is not directly visualized as the scope is advanced) and straightening the sigmoid colon increase risk for injury. Perforations from this mechanism typically involve the sigmoid and left colon[18,19] and are more frequent causes than injuries related to barotrauma. Barotrauma related to colonic distention is a second route for perforation. Colonoscopy may generate wall pressures up to 140 mm Hg, which has been demonstrated to create colonic tears in animal and ca-

daveric studies.[20] The serosal layer of the colonic wall is typically involved with injury along the longitudinal axis of the colon. This allows herniation and thinning of the mucosa through these tears, ultimately leading to a perforation. Injuries from this mechanism are typically right sided and most often involve the cecum. Perforations from this route can lead to massive amounts of free air.[21] Polypectomy represents the third mechanism for perforation. This therapeutic maneuver increases the risk for perforation from the baseline risk associated with a diagnostic examination and accounts for the higher end of perforation rates reported in colonoscopic series of approximately 0.4%.[8] Perforations result from through-and-through injury related to the act of polyp removal. Perforations at OC typically hold serious clinical consequences. Although a small percentage may be treated conservatively, the majority will require surgical exploration and repair. A large series from the Mayo Clinic in Rochester looked at more than 250,000 colonoscopies where 180 perforations occurred (0.1%). Of the 180 perforations, 165 (92%) required operative repair. There were significant adverse sequela with substantial morbidity in 36% (Fig. 15-5) and an overall mortality of 7%.[22]

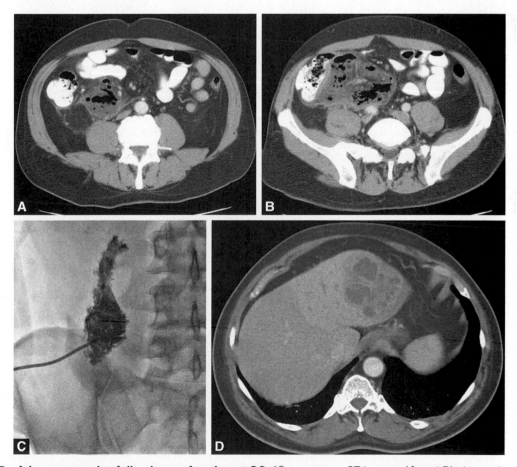

Figure 15-5 **Adverse sequelae following perforation at OC.** 2D transverse CT images **(A** and **B)** show a large pericolonic abscess in a patient who presented with shaking fevers and chills several days after a screening OC. Contrast injection **(C)** of a subsequently placed drain depicts the abscess cavity. 2D transverse CT image **(D)** in another patient shows a multiloculated hepatic abscess following a prior screening OC with hepatic flexure polypectomy several days earlier. (From Kim DH, Pickhardt PJ, Taylor AJ, Menias CO. Imaging evaluation of complications at optical colonoscopy. *Curr Probl Diagn Radiol.* 2008;37(4):165-177.)

The imaging appearance of perforation manifests with two main patterns of extraluminal air: intraperitoneal versus extraperitoneal. Perforation leading to free intraperitoneal air can easily be identified on both CT and upright (or decubitus) abdominal radiographs. On CT, there may be small foci of air and minimal fluid seen about a particular area of colon. which may point to the possible site of perforation (Fig. 15-6).[23] With larger perforations, fluid and extravasated oral contrast may collect in dependent areas such as the hepatorenal fossa, paracolic gutters, and rectovesical space. On upright or decubitus abdominal radiographs, pneumoperitoneum presents as lucency under the diaphragm (Fig. 15-7). When large amounts are present, free air can be identified on supine conventional radiographs as generalized lucency and outline various structures such as the bowel wall (i.e., Rigler's sign) and the falciform ligament.[24] Typically, perforations with this imaging appearance occur at the level of intraperitonealized colonic segments such as the cecum, transverse colon, and sigmoid colon.

A much more common yet under-recognized presentation of perforation involves the extraperitoneal dissection of gas, which may or may not have associated intraperitoneal free air (Fig. 15-8). This presentation may be subtle to detect on conventional radiographs. CT is much more sensitive in this regard, where even tiny amounts of gas related to a small perforation can be readily detected (Fig. 15-9). A perforation involving extraperitoneal segments such as the ascending colon, descending colon, and rectum are more likely to result in this appearance. It is im-

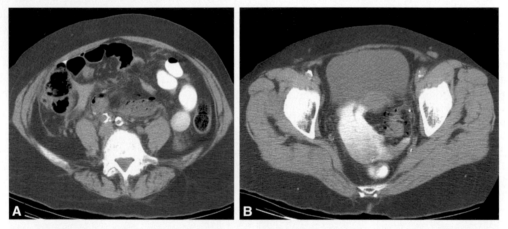

Figure 15-6 Cecal perforation at OC. 2D transverse CT image **(A)** demonstrates minimal fluid and stranding adjacent to the right colon, which may point to the site of perforation. Free extravasated contrast is seen layering dependently in the pelvis on a lower transverse CT image **(B)**. (From Kim DH, Pickhardt PJ, Taylor AJ, Menias CO. Imaging evaluation of complications at optical colonoscopy. *Curr Probl Diagn Radiol.* 2008;37(4):165-177.)

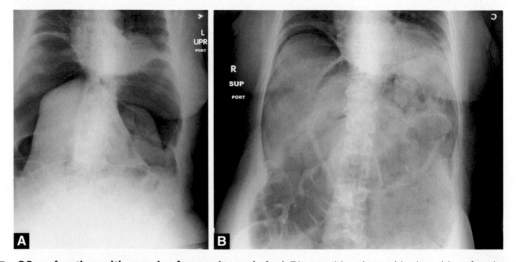

Figure 15-7 OC perforation with massive free peritoneal air. A 74-year-old patient with sigmoid perforation at incomplete colonoscopy. Upright radiograph **(A)** shows lucency beneath the diaphragm consistent with massive pneumoperitoneum. Given the extensive amount of free air, it is visible even with the patient supine **(B).** The patient underwent subsequent sigmoid colectomy. (B from Kim DH, Pickhardt PJ, Taylor AJ, Menias CO. Imaging evaluation of complications at optical colonoscopy. *Curr Probl Diagn Radiol.* 2008;37(4):165-177.)

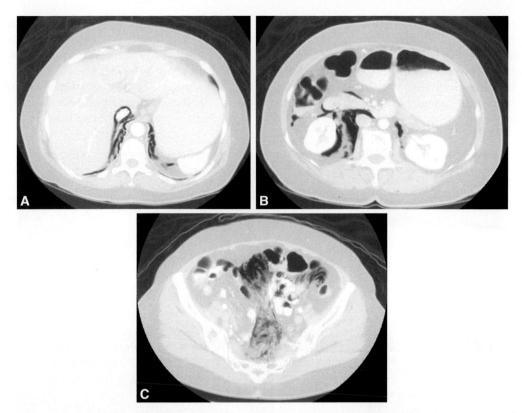

Figure 15-8   OC perforation with extraperitoneal air. Three 2D transverse CT images **(A-C)** demonstrate an extraperitoneal pathway of dissecting gas following perforation at screening OC. Air is present within the sigmoid mesentery and retroperitoneum. This is a very common yet under-recognized pattern of extraluminal gas from OC perforation. (From Kim DH, Pickhardt PJ, Taylor AJ, Menias CO. Imaging evaluation of complications at optical colonoscopy. *Curr Probl Diagn Radiol.* 2008;37(4):165-177.)

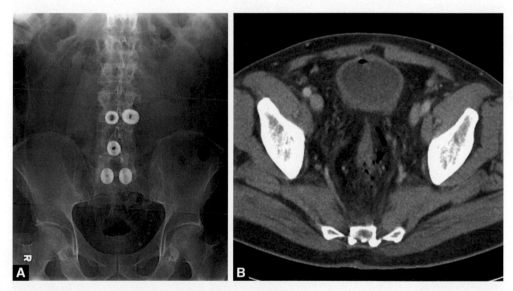

Figure 15-9   Perforation following rectal polypectomy. Note the value of CT for assessment of small extraperitoneal gas collections. Abdominal radiograph **(A)** is grossly negative but 2D transverse CT image **(B)** clearly depicts the extraluminal foci of air, consistent with a rectal perforation. (From Kim DH, Pickhardt PJ, Taylor AJ, Menias CO. Imaging evaluation of complications at optical colonoscopy. *Curr Probl Diagn Radiol.* 2008;37(4):165-177.)

portant to note, however, that this pattern can also occur with intraperitoneal colonic segments where the perforation leads to air dissecting back along the mesentery, as opposed to diffusing freely in the intraperitoneal cavity. On CT, such perforations result in gas dissecting in the subperitoneal spaces contained by peritoneal ligaments and spaces. The gas may track in extraperitoneal and ret-

roperitoneal spaces and into the mediastinum of the chest and in the subcutaneous tissues of the neck and chest. There may also be extension into the intraperitoneal cavity and thus "free air" (Fig. 15-10).

Hemorrhage is a complication that occurs predominantly in the setting of polypectomy. Bleeding rates at therapeutic colonoscopy range from 1% to 2%.[25-27] Most

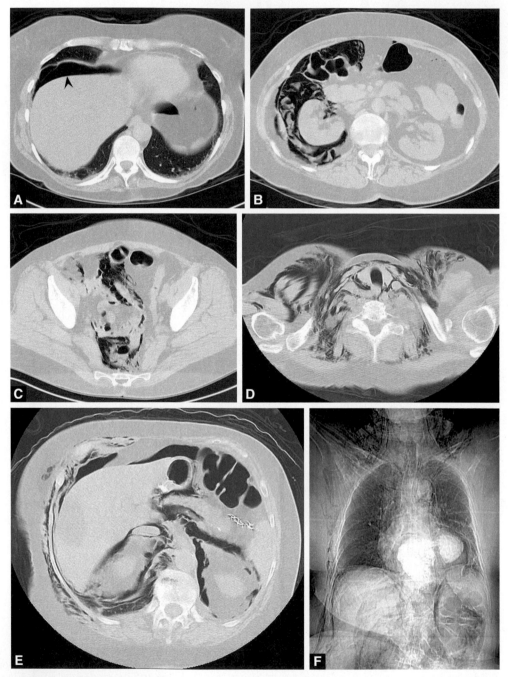

Figure 15-10 **Extensive retroperitoneal extension of air following OC perforation.** Two patients each demonstrate large amounts of air dissecting in retroperitoneal and other extraperitoneal planes. Three 2D transverse CT images in one patient **(A-C)** demonstrate air tracking from the from the extraperitoneal tissues about the rectum (the level of perforation) to surround the perinephric space about the right kidney. Note the extension into the peritoneal cavity *(arrowhead)*. In a second patient, there is extension from the retroperitoneum into the subcutaneous tissues of the chest and neck **(D** and **E)**. This gas is obvious even on the CT scout **(F)**. (From Kim DH, Pickhardt PJ, Taylor AJ, Menias CO. Imaging evaluation of complications at optical colonoscopy. *Curr Probl Diagn Radiol.* 2008;37(4):165-177.)

cases of bleeding can be managed with supportive measures only. It can present during the procedure or present as a delayed phenomenon (defined as after the periprocedural period and within 12 days of the colonoscopy) related to either a sloughing of the healed tissue plug or subsequent progression of the initial injury into the deeper tissues. Bleeding may present from a localized hematoma in the wall of the colon (Fig. 15-11), hemorrhage into the colonic lumen (Fig. 15-12), or high-attenuation ascites representing blood in the peritoneal cavity (Fig. 15-13).

Postpolypectomy syndromes represent another major category of complications. They can be subdivided into *postpolypectomy distention syndrome* and *postpolypectomy coagulation syndrome*. These represent diagnoses of exclusion in which the potentially significant sequelae of perforation or large bleed have been excluded. Postpolypectomy distention syndrome is applied to patients with severe abdominal pain with a distended, rigid abdomen related to a dilated air-filled colon where evaluation for perforation and hemorrhage is negative.[28] It is a somewhat subjective diagnosis because all patients will have an element of colonic distention following colonoscopy (Fig. 15-14). Positioning the patient prone or in right lateral decubitus has been reported to help by allowing the trapped air to move distally and be expelled. Postpolypectomy coagulation syndrome is related to electrocautery injury during polypectomy where there is transmural involvement. It is also known as serositis of transmural burn. On CT there may be minimal localized wall thickening and soft tissue stranding of the adjacent pericolonic fat (Fig. 15-15). The injury is self-limited and typically resolves within 48 hours without therapeutic measures.

Injury to adjacent organs is a reported rare circumstance, although it is not too uncommon in our experience. In particular, the spleen may be lacerated either by direct injury from the endoscope or, more likely, by traction on the phrenicocolic ligament (Fig. 15-16).[29] Traction may also lead to other injuries such as mesenteric hematomas (Fig. 15-17).

Sedation is typically given when colonoscopy is performed to minimize the discomfort associated with this invasive procedure. The level of sedation falls into the moderate conscious category using a combination of intravenous benzodiazepine (e.g., midazolam) and intravenous narcotic pain medication (e.g., fentanyl). The patients are monitored during the sedation and require recovery prior to release. Potential complications include oversedation and may result in cardiopulmonary depression. This has been reported to occur in 0.5% of cases (Fig. 15-18).[30] In addition, oversedation or simply deep sedation may increase the possibility of complications of perforation or bleeding as a result of the patient's blunted ability to respond to pain.

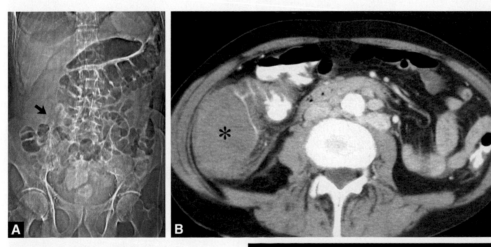

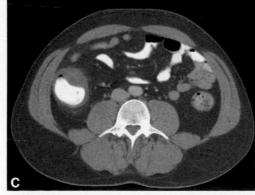

Figure 15-11 Intramural hematoma following biopsy. CT scout **(A)** demonstrates deviation of the colon air column *(arrow)*. 2D transverse image **(B)** confirms a large hematoma *(asterisk)* involving the wall of the ascending colon following polypectomy. Retroperitoneal lymphadenopathy was from metastatic melanoma. CT image in another patient **(C)** shows a smaller intramural hematoma involving the right colon. (From Kim DH, Pickhardt PJ, Taylor AJ, Menias CO. Imaging evaluation of complications at optical colonoscopy. *Curr Probl Diagn Radiol.* 2008;37(4):165-177.)

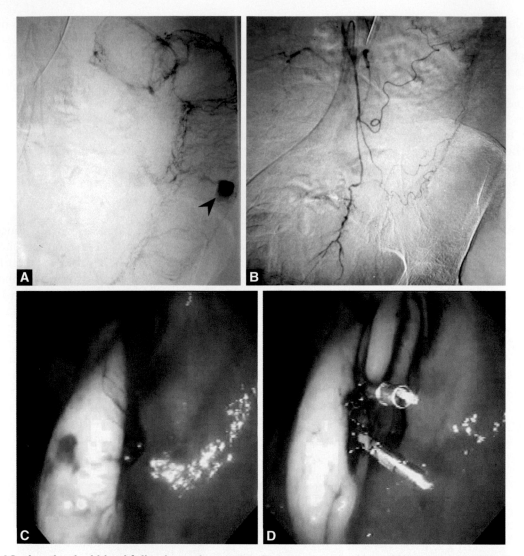

Figure 15-12 Intraluminal bleed following polypectomy. Digital subtraction image **(A)** shows active bleeding into the lumen of the descending colon characterized by a rounded collection of contrast *(arrowhead)*. Postpitressin **(B)** image demonstrates subsequent control of the bleed. Endoscopic image **(C)** in a different patient shows an intraluminal bleed following polypectomy that is treated with placement of hemostatic clips **(D)**. (From Kim DH, Pickhardt PJ, Taylor AJ, Menias CO. Imaging evaluation of complications at optical colonoscopy. *Curr Probl Diagn Radiol.* 2008;37(4):165-177.)

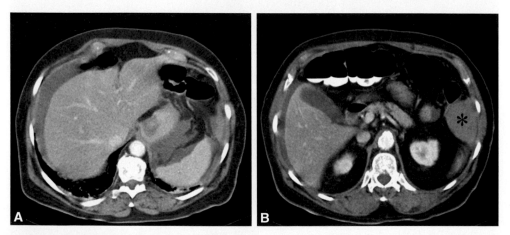

Figure 15-13 Intraperitoneal hematoma following polypectomy. Transverse CT image **(A)** demonstrates mixed attenuation ascites about the liver and spleen consistent with hemorrhage. CT image from a lower section **(B)** shows a focal hematoma *(asterisk)* contiguous with the descending colon and the likely source of the bleed. (From Kim DH, Pickhardt PJ, Taylor AJ, Menias CO. Imaging evaluation of complications at optical colonoscopy. *Curr Probl Diagn Radiol.* 2008;37(4):165-177.)

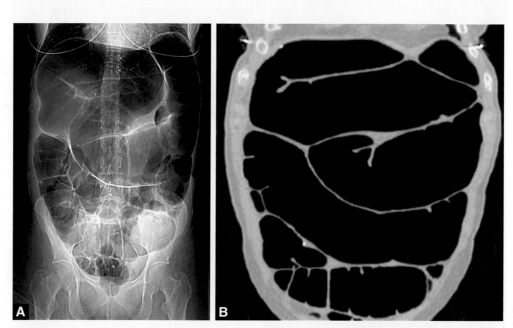

Figure 15-14 **Postpolypectomy distention syndrome mimic.** CT scout radiograph **(A)** and coronal 2D CTC image **(B)** show a markedly dilated colon. If the patient were postcolonoscopy with abdominal pain, a diagnosis of postpolypectomy distention syndrome would likely be given after the exclusion of perforation or bleeding. These images are actually from a CTC examination in an asymptomatic individual who has a large-caliber colon. (From Kim DH, Pickhardt PJ, Taylor AJ, Menias CO. Imaging evaluation of complications at optical colonoscopy. *Curr Probl Diagn Radiol.* 2008;37(4):165-177.)

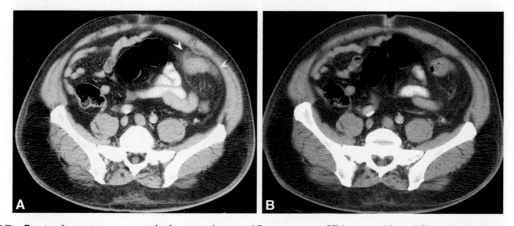

Figure 15-15 **Postpolypectomy coagulation syndrome.** 2D transverse CT images **(A** and **B)** demonstrate mild soft tissue stranding *(arrowheads)* adjacent to the sigmoid colon consistent with "serositis of transmural burn." The patient was managed with supportive measures including antibiotic coverage. (From Kim DH, Pickhardt PJ, Taylor AJ, Menias CO. Imaging evaluation of complications at optical colonoscopy. *Curr Probl Diagn Radiol.* 2008;37(4):165-177.)

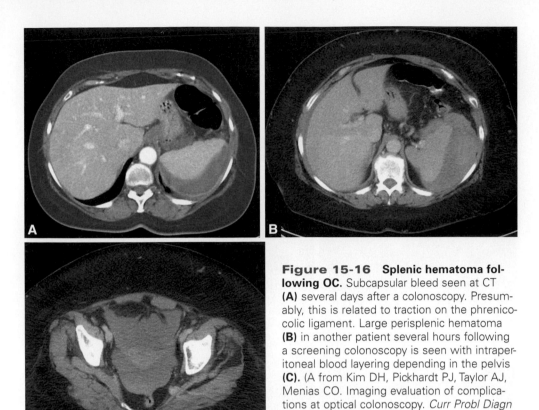

Figure 15-16 Splenic hematoma following OC. Subcapsular bleed seen at CT **(A)** several days after a colonoscopy. Presumably, this is related to traction on the phrenicocolic ligament. Large perisplenic hematoma **(B)** in another patient several hours following a screening colonoscopy is seen with intraperitoneal blood layering depending in the pelvis **(C)**. (A from Kim DH, Pickhardt PJ, Taylor AJ, Menias CO. Imaging evaluation of complications at optical colonoscopy. *Curr Probl Diagn Radiol.* 2008;37(4):165-177.)

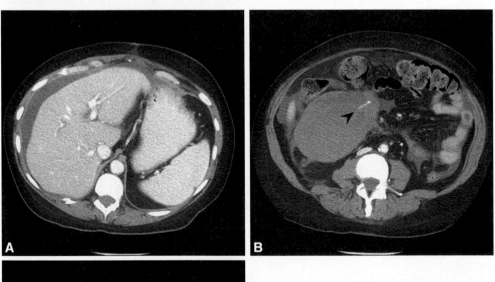

Figure 15-17 Mesenteric hematoma following OC. Three transverse CT images **(A-C)** show a large mesenteric bleed with associated intraperitoneal hemorrhage following OC. Note the active bleeding into the mesenteric hematoma *(arrowhead).* Presumably, this is related to a traction injury with shearing of mesenteric vessels. This patient had prior abdominal surgery with probable adhesions, which likely increased the risk for this traction injury.

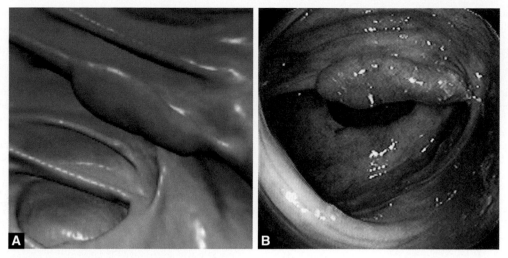

Figure 15-18 A 75-year-old man oversedated at OC. Oversedation led to hypotension resulting in an incomplete OC. Subsequent CTC undertaken at a later date **(A)** showed a large polyp in the ascending colon confirmed and removed at repeat colonoscopy **(B)**. Pathology showed a villous adenoma. (From Kim DH, Pickhardt PJ, Taylor AJ, Menias CO. Imaging evaluation of complications at optical colonoscopy. *Curr Probl Diagn Radiol.* 2008;37(4):165-177.)

SUMMARY

CT colonography is a safe screening modality of minimal invasiveness. Complications are rare and can be further minimized by appropriate training. This is advantageous particularly in the screening setting because the modality is applied to a population of healthy individuals without a defined medical problem for the primary aim of preventing a future serious clinical condition. Complications are inherent in any medical intervention, and it is important to consider them in the overall benefit–risk ratio. This reinforces the selective polypectomy strategies used at CTC-based screening to minimize the risks of therapeutic colonoscopy for those individuals with a positive CTC examination.

REFERENCES

1. Pickhardt PJ. Incidence of colonic perforation at CT colonography: Review of existing data and implications for screening of asymptomatic adults. *Radiology.* 2006;239(2):313-316.
2. Hsu CW, Imperiale TF. Meta-analysis and cost comparison of polyethylene glycol lavage versus sodium phosphate for colonoscopy preparation. *Gastrointest Endosc.* 1998;48(3):276-282.
3. Markowitz GS, Nasr SH, Klein P, et al. Renal failure due to acute nephrocalcinosis following oral sodium phosphate bowel cleansing. *Hum Pathol.* 2004;35(6):675-684.
4. Markowitz GS, Stokes MB, Radhakrishnan J, D'Agati VD. Acute phosphate nephropathy following oral sodium phosphate bowel purgative: An underrecognized cause of chronic renal failure. *J Am Soc Nephrol.* 2005;16(11):3389-3396.
5. Schiller LR. Clinical pharmacology and use of laxatives and lavage solutions. *J Clin Gastroenterol.* 1999;28(1):11-18.
6. Kim DH, Pickhardt PJ, Hinshaw JL, Taylor AJ, Mukherjee R, Pfau PR. Prospective blinded trial comparing 45-mL and 90-mL doses of oral sodium phosphate for bowel preparation before computed tomographic colonography. *J Comp Assist Tomogr.* 2007;31(1):53-58.
7. Thomas AMK, Kubie AM, Britt RP. Acute angioneurotic-edema following a barium meal. *Br J Radiol.* 1986;59(706):1055-1056.
8. Levin TR, Zhao W, Conell C, et al. Complications of colonoscopy in an integrated health care delivery system. *Ann Intern Med.* 2006;145(12):880-886.
9. Gatto NM, Frucht H, Sundararajan V, Jacobson JS, Grann VR, Neugut AI. Risk of perforation after colonoscopy and sigmoidoscopy: A population-based study. *J Nat Cancer Inst.* 2003;95(3):230-236.
10. Burling D, Halligan S, Slater A, Noakes MJ, Taylor SA. Potentially serious adverse events at CT colonography in symptomatic patients: National survey of the United Kingdom. *Radiology.* 2006;239(2):464-471.
11. Sosna J, Blachar A, Amitai M, et al. Colonic perforation at CT colonography: Assessment of risk in a multicenter large cohort. *Radiology.* 2006;239(2):457-463.
12. Hough DM, Kuntz MA, Fidler JL, et al. Detection of occult colonic perforation before ct colonography after incomplete colonoscopy: Perforation rate and use of a low-dose diagnostic scan before CO_2 insufflation. *Am J Roentgenol.* 2008;191(4):1077-1081.
13. Pickhardt PJ, Kim DH, Taylor AJ. Asymptomatic pneumatosis at CT colonography: A benign self-limited imaging finding distinct from perforation. *Am J Roentgenol.* 2008;190(2):W112-W117.
14. Gondal G, Grotmol T, Hofstad B, Bretthauer M, Eide TJ, Hoff G. The Norwegian Colorectal Cancer Prevention (NORCCAP) screening study. *Scand J Gastroenterol.* 2003;38(6):635-642.
15. Liedenbaum MH, Venema HW, Stoker J. Radiation dose in CT colonography—Trends in time and differences between daily practice and screening protocols. *Eur Radiol.* 2008;18(10):2222-2230.
16. Radiation risk in perspective. Position statement of the Health Physics Society. Adopted January 1996, revised August 2004. McLean, VA: Health Physics Society; 2004.
17. Brenner DJ, Georgsson MA. Mass screening with CT colonography: Should the radiation exposure be of concern? *Gastroenterology.* 2005;129(1):328-337.
18. Anderson ML, Pasha TM, Leighton JA. Endoscopic perforation of the colon: Lessons from a 10-year study. *Am J Gastroenterol.* 2000;95(12):3418-3422.

19. Farley DR, Bannon MP, Zietlow SP, Pemberton JH, Ilstrup DM, Larson DR. Management of colonoscopic perforations. *Mayo Clin Proc.* 1997;72(8):729-733.

20. Kozarek RA ED, Silverstein ME, Smith RG. Air-pressure-induced colon injury during diagnostic colonoscopy. *Gastroenterology.* 1980;78:7-14.

21. Han SY, Tishler JM. Perforation of the colon above the peritoneal reflection during the barium-enema examination. *Radiology.* 1982;144(2):253-255.

22. Iqbal CW, Cullinane DC, Schiller HJ, Sawyer MD, Zietlow SP, Farley DR. Surgical management and outcomes of 165 colonoscopic perforations from a single institution. *Arch Surg.* 2008;143(7):701-706.

23. Hainaux B, Agneessens E, Bertinotti R, et al. Accuracy of MDCT in predicting site of gastrointestinal tract perforation. *Am J Roentgenol.* 2006;187(5):1179-1183.

24. Levine MS, Scheiner JD, Rubesin SE, Laufer I, Herlinger H. Diagnosis of pneumoperitoneum on supine abdominal radiographs. *Am J Roentgenol.* 1991;156(4):731-735.

25. Waye JD, Lewis BS, Yessayan S. Colonoscopy—A prospective report of complications. *J Clin Gastroenterol.* 1992;15(4):347-351.

26. Dafnis G, Ekbom A, Pahlman L, Blomqvist P. Complications of diagnostic within a defined population and therapeutic colonoscopy in Sweden. *Gastrointest Endosc.* 2001;54(3):302-309.

27. Silvis SE, Nebel O, Rogers G, Sugawa C, Mandelstam P. Endoscopic complications—Results of 1974 American Society for Gastrointestinal Endoscopy Survey. *JAMA.* 1976;235(9):928-930.

28. Waye JD, Kahn O, Auerbach ME. Complications of colonoscopy and flexible sigmoidoscopy. *Gastrointest Endosc Clin North Am.* 1996;6:343-377.

29. Kavic SM, Basson MD. Complications of endoscopy. *Am J Surg.* 2001;181(4):319-332.

30. Keeffe E, O'Connor K. 1989 A/S/G/E survey of endoscopic sedation and monitoring practices. *Gastrointest Endosc.* 1990;36:S13-18.

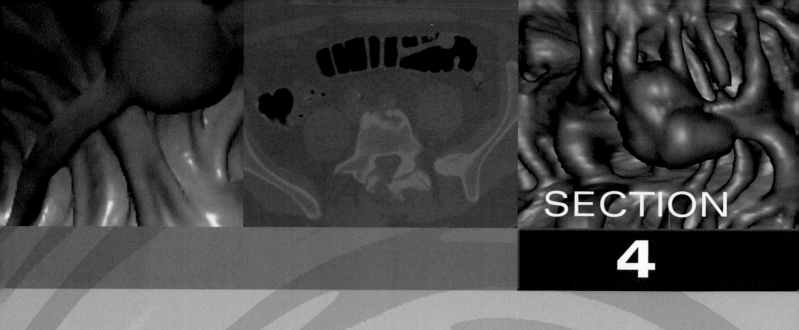

CT Colonography
Interpretation

CTC Interpretation: An Overview

DAVID H. KIM, MD
PERRY J. PICKHARDT, MD

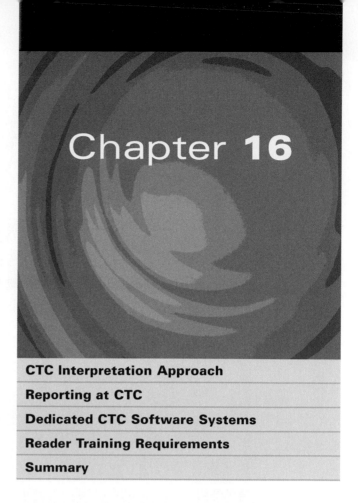

Chapter 16

- CTC Interpretation Approach
- Reporting at CTC
- Dedicated CTC Software Systems
- Reader Training Requirements
- Summary

INTRODUCTION

CT colonography (CTC) interpretation is a key component to the success of the examination. The primary focus involves the detection and confirmation of colorectal polyps. However, it involves more than simply the intraluminal evaluation of colorectum; it also includes the evaluation of the extracolonic structures. The specific software platforms largely determine which particular interpretation strategies can be effectively used. Although there is a learning curve, accurate interpretation can be readily achieved with appropriate training and experience. This overview will introduce basic concepts and issues related to interpretation strategy, the issues of standardized reporting at CT colonography, and reader training requirements. Each area will be further expanded in greater detail in the subsequent chapters comprising this section of the book.

CTC INTERPRETATION APPROACH

Interpretation at CTC can be divided into two major areas of evaluation. The intraluminal evaluation represents the primary focus of interpretation, whereas the extracolonic evaluation represents an unavoidable secondary but nonetheless important aspect of the examination. Both areas must be addressed in a responsible fashion to benefit the patient. For example, if interpretation leads to an unacceptably high false positive rate for polyps or to an excessive work-up rate for benign extracolonic findings, many unnecessary medical interventions will be undertaken, leading to increased costs and risk of complications to the patient.

Intraluminal Examination: Polyp Detection and Characterization

The main purpose of the CTC examination is to identify relevant colorectal precursor lesions for subsequent removal at therapeutic colonoscopy. The large polyp (≥10 mm) is the accepted surrogate for this precursor target at CTC (see Chapter 1). Smaller polyps (6-9 mm) can be detected but generally do not represent the primary CTC target lesion. There is broad consensus that these small polyps represent low-risk lesions, but the management remains controversial (i.e., surveillance versus immediate removal). The process of identifying a colorectal soft tissue polyp at CTC involves two discrete tasks. The first concerns the detection of potential polyp candidates and the second involves winnowing this list to the true soft tissue polyps, separating out the pseudopolyps related to stool or other false lesions. Interpretation strategies vary, with some emphasizing a primary role for two-dimensional (2D) polyp detection and others emphasizing a primary 3D approach. In truth, the optimal interpretation strategy involves use of both 3D and 2D polyp detection because each holds particular strengths and weaknesses.

In our opinion, a primary 3D approach is the preferred method for the task of initial polyp detection whenever possible. Certainly, there has been much debate between the primary 3D versus primary 2D approaches. However, it is evident through reader performance in the literature, and through our personal experience, that a 3D approach is more effective.[1-5] The search algorithm by a 3D approach is easier to implement and less fatiguing for the reader. As opposed to the careful scrutiny required to detect a polyp at 2D where the polyp may reside on only a few images within a 400- to 500-image dataset, a polyp will remain in view for a much longer period on the 3D

endoluminal fly-through display. At 2D, the reader must be vigilant so as not to mistake a polyp for a haustral fold or to misperceive a fold for a polyp. This is a difficult task because the reader must continually mentally translate the 2D data into a 3D structure. At 3D, this is not a concern because this translation is undertaken automatically by the computer (Fig. 16-1). It is important to note

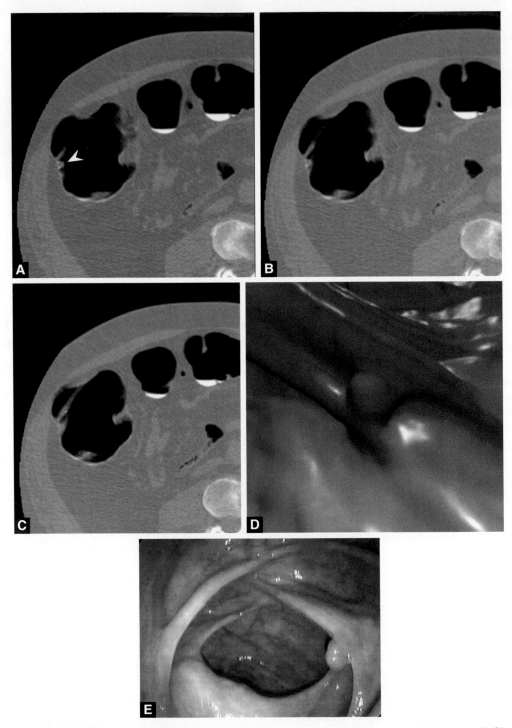

Figure 16-1 Perceptual difficulties in polyp detection at 2D. Contiguous 2D transverse CTC images **(A-C)** show a small polyp *(arrowhead)* that could be mistaken for a colonic fold. 3D endoluminal CTC image **(D)** clearly shows this abnormality as a focal polyp between two haustral folds. Note that the mental translation of the 2D images into a 3D structure is not needed when viewing a 3D volume-rendered image. OC image **(E)** confirms a small polyp, which proved to be a tubular adenoma. *(*See associated video clip in DVD.)*

that a primary 3D approach does not preclude 2D evaluation within the overall detection strategy. In fact, 2D images are always reviewed to supplement the 3D search for polyps and masses, with particular attention to areas where the 3D search may underperform. The 2D images are also scanned quickly for the presence of large annular constricting masses, which may mimic areas of underdistention on the 3D display. This can be rapidly completed much in the same way that a cross-sectional imager would run the bowel on a standard body CT examination. Then, more careful 2D scrutiny is given to areas covered by tagged residual fluid to exclude submerged polyps and also to the capacious cecum and rectum to exclude flat carpet lesions. Thus, the secondary 2D review assesses areas of potential weakness at 3D. In particular, carpet lesions, which often are large and villous in nature, can be fairly subtle at 3D.

This approach to polyp detection at CTC is effective for several reasons. It requires multiple interactions of the dataset from differing viewpoints, including 3D fly-throughs and scrolling through the 2D transverse dataset on both the supine and prone series. This redundancy increases the chance of polyp detection where the lesion needs to be initially identified on only one of the multiple views. Although it may sound time consuming, this approach can be quickly completed in a time-efficient manner. In our experience, the typical straightforward case can be completed in 5 to 10 minutes. This approach combines the strengths of both the 3D and 2D reviews where the relative weaknesses of one view are compensated by the other. In addition, the tedious nature of primary 2D-only polyp detection is avoided. Our approach that emphasizes 3D polyp detection is much less fatiguing for the reader. This is an important concern in the screening realm where a reader may need to interpret a relatively large number of examinations in a short time. A tedious, fatiguing 2D-only search pattern would ultimately have a negative impact on sensitivity.

CTC interpretation is not complete after just the generation of potential polyp candidates. Indeed, this simply represents beginning the intraluminal interpretation process. These potential lesions must be studied to separate the true soft tissue lesions from the pseudopolyps. It is this step of interpretation that requires a specialized skill set of a quality reader. If this second task of interrogation is not performed effectively, the number of CTC false positives will be unacceptably high. The task of polyp characterization occurs by review of the 2D source images. Whereas 3D visualization tools such as translucency rendering (see Chapter 19) may suggest a soft tissue polyp, examination of the suspected polyp on the 2D images is ultimately required for confirmation. On 2D, a true soft tissue polyp must fulfill two basic criteria: (1) it should be of homogenous soft tissue attenuation and (2) its site of attachment to the wall should remain fixed in location between the supine and prone series (Fig. 16-2). Many of the skills used for polyp confirmation are similar to the skills used by cross-sectional imagers in reading a standard body CT examination. Thus, the reader must understand the basic concepts of cross-sectional imaging to interpret the examination. For example, if a polyp candidate demonstrates apparent movement between the two positional views, the reader must determine whether such movement is related to shifting of a pedunculated polyp, rotation of the involved colonic segment, or true dependent movement of residual stool (Fig. 16-3). It is this step of CTC interpretation that will often separate out quality readers from the suboptimal ones.

As is the case with colonoscopy, CTC cannot reliably distinguish between the different histologies for true soft tissue polyps. Indeed, the CTC interpretation strategy is designed to simply separate out the true soft tissue polyps from pseudopolyps related predominantly to stool. Whereas the lack of histologic differentiation has led to a policy of universal polypectomy for colonoscopy-based screening, more refined filtering strategies can be effectively used at CTC by using size thresholds to direct patient management, such as immediate removal for large lesions versus CTC surveillance for smaller lesions (see Chapter 2). The noninvasive nature of CTC and the robust polyp measurement and localization abilities of this modality allow such interpretation algorithms to be effective. The advantages of such a strategy include decreased societal costs, logical use of limited colonoscopy resources for high-yield polypectomies, and decreased numbers of complications.

Extracolonic Evaluation

The evaluation of extracolonic structures is an unavoidable yet important aspect of CTC interpretation. Although the CTC examination has been optimized for the identification of colorectal polyps, the cross-sectional nature of the examination also allows for evaluation of abdominal and pelvic structures in addition to the large intestine despite its low-dose, non-intravenous contrast nature. Although the examination is limited in comparison to a standard diagnostic CT, significant extracolonic pathology can still be detected. Judicious handling of extracolonic "findings" will largely determine whether such evaluation becomes a net benefit or detriment to the patient. On one hand, many "findings" can often be incidentally seen that are generally of little or no consequence to the individual. It has been shown that more than 60% of individuals can demonstrate some sort of extracolonic "finding" on CTC examination.[6] Workup can result in a cascade of additional tests for these largely inconsequential findings, leading to unnecessary costs, potential complications, and undue anxiety for the patient. On the other hand, significant pathology including unsuspected extracolonic cancers and aortic aneurysms can be detected. In our experience, 2% to 3% of asymptomatic adults undergoing screening will harbor an important

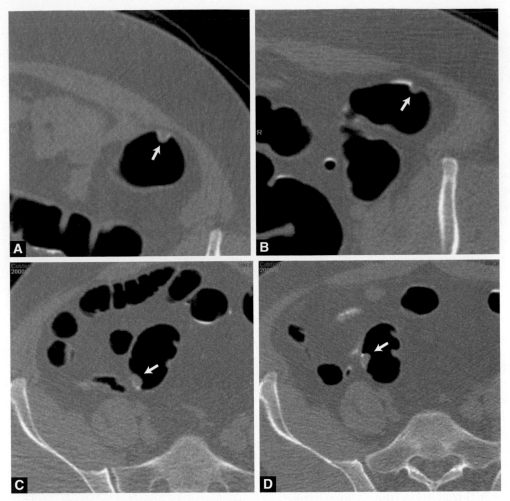

Figure 16-2 **Soft tissue polyp confirmation.** Supine **(A)** and prone **(B)** 2D transverse CTC images show a polyp candidate *(arrows)* that fulfills both confirmation criteria, including homogenous soft tissue attenuation on both series and a fixed location on the anterior wall of the sigmoid colon. Note that the internal attenuation of the polyp can be compared to muscle as an internal control. Supine **(C)** and prone **(D)** 2D transverse CTC images from another individual show a large potential polyp *(arrows)* in the distal sigmoid colon. Note the homogenous appearance similar to the adjacent psoas muscle. The polyp is fixed in the location of attachment but pivots somewhat in response to gravity (likely indicating a short stalk).

unsuspected extracolonic finding.[7] The extracolonic cancer rate for our screening program at the University of Wisconsin has remained steady at about 1 unsuspected case for every 300 individuals screened. The rate of abdominal aneurysms is about the same. A careful balance is needed where the obviously benign lesions are not sent for further work-up, while the potentially significant ones are. A logical decision tree for indeterminate extracolonic findings can be very helpful. Classification schema such as one found in the CT colonography reporting and data system (C-RADS) provides a standardized categorization of extracolonic findings.

REPORTING AT CTC

Standardized reporting at CTC screening is an essential component of quality interpretation given the clinical environment in which this examination oper-

ates. As opposed to the setting where a patient presents with a defined medical problem and individualized nuances in the report may be necessary to optimally summarize the findings and recommendations, CTC in the setting of asymptomatic screening is a very different situation. Here, the examination is applied to a large eligible portion of the population that is otherwise healthy. Standardization is a key factor to allow valid comparisons between different institutions, both clinically and in research. C-RADS will be helpful in this regard (see Chapter 28). C-RADS is a consensus statement from the Working Group on Virtual Colonoscopy that creates a standard lexicon and various categories for polyp findings and extracolonic findings. The lexicon includes a defined set of polyp descriptors that can be applied to each identified lesion. Standardized conventions are set to maintain consistency in the application of the descriptors (e.g., how to measure the size of

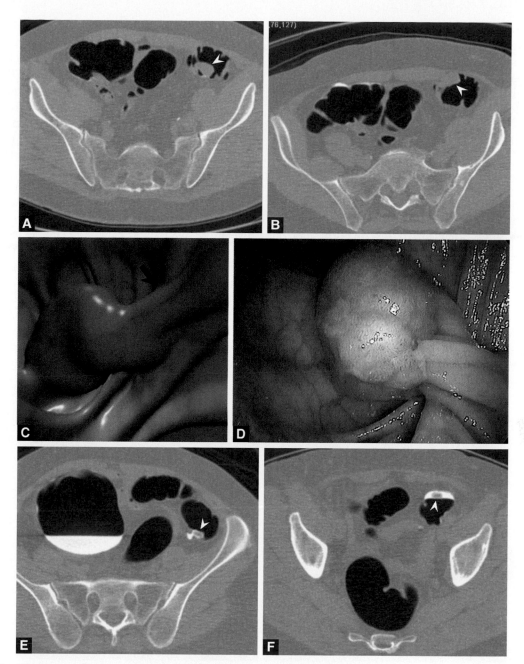

Figure 16-3 Shifting position of a pedunculated polyp versus movement of stool. Supine **(A)** and prone **(B)** 2D transverse CTC images demonstrate dependent movement of a pedunculated polyp *(arrowheads),* which could presumably be mistaken for untagged stool if the stalk is not appreciated. This is typically not a problem on the 3D endoluminal view **(C)** where the stalk is more apparent *(arrow).* OC image **(D)** confirms the pedunculated nature of this advanced adenoma. Supine **(E)** and prone **(F)** 2D transverse CTC images from another individual demonstrate dependent luminal movement of untagged stool. Note that the "lesion" *(arrowhead)* moves from adjacent to a diverticulum along the posterior wall on the supine view to the fluid pool along the opposite wall on the prone view *(arrowhead).* This "polyp" thus represents untagged mobile stool. *(*See associated video clip in DVD.)*

a lesion). Various categories are set for polyp findings and for extracolonic findings to standardize definitions and management. The intended purpose and function is to mirror that of BI-RADS (breast imaging reporting and data system) in mammography. In addition, aspects of C-RADS can be used to formulate program quality metrics.

DEDICATED CTC SOFTWARE SYSTEMS

CTC software platforms affect the manner of CTC interpretation and strategies used. Although the functional capabilities are progressively merging among different software platforms, currently there remain differences whereby some platforms are better suited for a primary 3D approach. Consequently, the use of a specific platform can determine to a certain extent the particular interpretation strategy used. Hopefully, these differences will become negligible in the coming years whereby both 3D and 2D techniques can be used in a primary mode by all systems.

Within the 3D realm, advanced imaging displays include the standard 3D endoluminal fly-through to more exotic options including the static virtual dissection view, the dynamic perspective filet view, the undistorted "clam-shell" dissection view, and the unfolded cube view. In addition, an increased field-of-view angle can be applied to the standard endoluminal view. All of these advanced displays allow for visualization of both sides of folds without the need for bidirectional fly-through (see Chapter 23). Often, there is an important tradeoff with these more exotic displays between increased speed of interpretation (over the standard endoluminal fly-through) and the penalty of increased distortion. For example, viewing static colonic strips from a virtual dissection display is very quick and can potentially result in a significant time savings over the endoluminal fly-through. However, there is spatial distortion introduced within these images that may negatively affect polyp detection. To create a flat strip, the image is unavoidably distorted, particularly at the edges and at the flexures. A reader must learn to recognize these distortion artifacts to maintain effective polyp detection. Likewise, increasing the field-of-view angle at standard endoluminal fly-through increases the amount of colonic mucosa visualized but with the cost of distortion at the periphery of the image (Fig. 16-4).

Despite differences, all usable platforms should be able to perform several basic functions well. The reader should be able to locate points within the colon very easily between the 3D and 2D views and be able to transition between views seamlessly (Fig. 16-5). There should be a bookmarking function to allow recording of important locations (typically of suspected polyps). The software should allow measurement in both the 2D and 3D environment. For the 2D views, the functionality should be similar to that of a PACS system, including functions such as window-level settings, scrolling in cine stack mode, Hounsfield unit measurements, pan/zoom, and so forth.

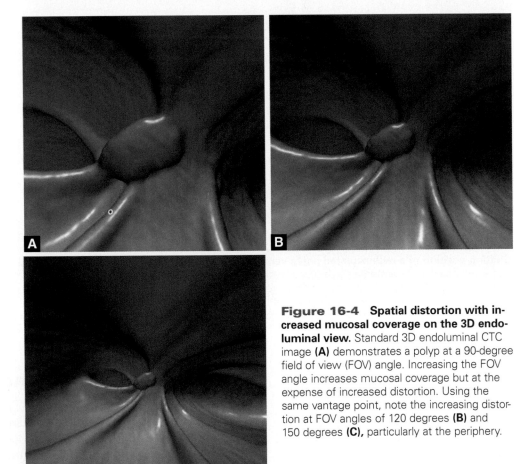

Figure 16-4 Spatial distortion with increased mucosal coverage on the 3D endoluminal view. Standard 3D endoluminal CTC image **(A)** demonstrates a polyp at a 90-degree field of view (FOV) angle. Increasing the FOV angle increases mucosal coverage but at the expense of increased distortion. Using the same vantage point, note the increasing distortion at FOV angles of 120 degrees **(B)** and 150 degrees **(C)**, particularly at the periphery.

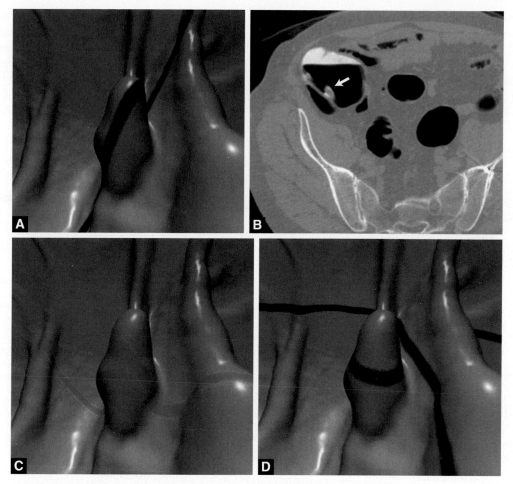

Figure 16-5 **Translation between 3D and 2D environments.** This particular CTC software platform (V3D, Viatronix, Inc.) allows easy localization between 3D and 2D views where a color-coded line on the 3D image corresponds to the 2D MPR orientation and slice. 3D endoluminal view **(A)** demonstrates a red line corresponding to the transverse plane at 2D **(B),** which represents the optimized orthogonal plane for 2D measurement of the depicted polyp *(arrow)*. Similarly, the orientation and slice location in the sagittal **(C)** and coronal **(D)** planes are also color coded on the 3D view.

READER TRAINING REQUIREMENTS

Training and experience are both required for expertise in CTC interpretation. Although the skill set of a cross-sectional imager fits reasonably well with CT colonography, additional specialized skills are required with this examination. For example, such additional skills include the ability to localize a specific point between the 3D and 2D environments and between the supine and prone series. A fairly steep learning curve has been demonstrated, particularly for primary 2D interpretive approaches.[8,9] Primary 3D approaches appear to be easier to learn but still require exposure to endoscopically proven cases.[10] A minimal set of 50 to 75 cases is recommended to gain this experience.[11,12] However, it is becoming evident that interaction with pathologically proven cases alone is not enough to gain true expertise. Burling et al.[13] demonstrated a fairly poor sensitivity of 65% for large polyps in a test series administered to a group of experienced community readers who self-reported a lack of formal training. Similarly, the ACRIN (American College of Radiology Imaging Network) I trial demonstrated significant differences in primary 2D performance independent of reader experience.[3] Specific CTC training appears to be one of the components needed to gain the requisite expertise. Training allows exposure to common and uncommon scenarios and the myriad of diagnostic pitfalls, potentially shortening the learning curve. Evidence suggests, however, that training may not ensure improved performance in all individuals.[14] Thus, some individuals also advocate that some formal testing following training and experience is needed to ensure true competence.

SUMMARY

High-quality interpretation at CTC is a key factor for the overall success of this screening tool. It involves much more than simply the detection of focal protrusions into the colonic lumen that may represent potential polyps. Rather, it is a complex interaction between detection of potential candidates and confirmation of true polyps using a combination of 3D and 2D techniques. Cross-sectional skills are a firm requirement for successful interpretation of this CT-based examination. Software platforms should allow the reader to perform the necessary interpretive

tasks in a time-efficient and easy-to-understand manner. The evaluation and appropriate recommendations for potentially significant extracolonic findings are an important area to judiciously address. Training specific to CTC is a pertinent issue and standardized reporting is necessary to maintain consistency between institutions and to allow valid comparisons clinically and in research.

REFERENCES

1. Pickhardt PJ, Lee AD, Taylor AJ, et al. Primary 2D versus primary 3D polyp detection at screening CT colonography. *Am J Roentgenol.* 2007;189(6):1451-1456.
2. Pickhardt PJ, Choi JR, Hwang I, et al. Computed tomographic virtual colonoscopy to screen for colorectal neoplasia in asymptomatic adults. *N Engl J Med.* 2003;349(23):2191-2200.
3. Johnson CD, Toledano AY, Herman BA, et al. Computerized tomographic colonography: Performance evaluation in a retrospective multicenter setting. *Gastroenterology.* 2003;125(3):688-695.
4. Cotton PB, Durkalski VL, Benoit PC, et al. Computed tomographic colonography (virtual colonoscopy)—A multicenter comparison with standard colonoscopy for detection of colorectal neoplasia. *JAMA.* 2004;291(14):1713-1719.
5. Rockey DC, Paulson E, Niedzwiecki D, et al. Analysis of air contrast barium enema, computed tomographic colonography, and colonoscopy: Prospective comparison. *Lancet.* 2005;365(9456):305-311.
6. Yee J, Kumar NN, Godara S, et al. Extracolonic abnormalities discovered incidentally at CT colonography in a male population. *Radiology.* 2005;236(2):519-526.
7. Pickhardt PJ, Hanson ME, Vanness DJ, et al. Unsuspected extracolonic findings at screening CT colonography: Clinical and economic impact. *Radiology.* 2008;249(1):151-159.
8. Thomeer M, Carbone I, Bosmans H, et al. Stool tagging applied in thin-slice multidetector computed tomography colonography. *J Comp Assist Tomog.* 2003;27(2):132-139.
9. Gluecker TM, Fletcher JG, Welch TJ, et al. Characterization of lesions missed on interpretation of CT colonography using a 2D search method. *Am J Roentgenol.* 2004;182(4):881-889.
10. Pickhardt PJ. Screening CT colonography: How I do it. *Am J Roentgenol.* 2007;189(2):290-298.
11. ACR Practice Guideline for the Performance of Computed Tomography (CT) Colonography in Adults. Reston, VA: American College of Radiology; 2006.
12. Rockey DC, Barish M, Brill JV, et al. Standards for gastroenterologists for performing and interpreting diagnostic computed tomographic Colonography. *Gastroenterology.* 2007;133(3):1005-1024.
13. Burling D, Halligan S, Atchley J, et al. CT colonography: Interpretative performance in a non-academic environment. *Clin Radiol.* 2007;62(5):424-429.
14. Taylor SA, Halligan S, Burling D, et al. CT colonography: Effect of experience and training on reader performance. *Eur Radiol.* 2004;14(6):1025-1033.

Polyp Detection at CTC: 2D versus 3D Evaluation

PERRY J. PICKHARDT, MD
DAVID H. KIM, MD

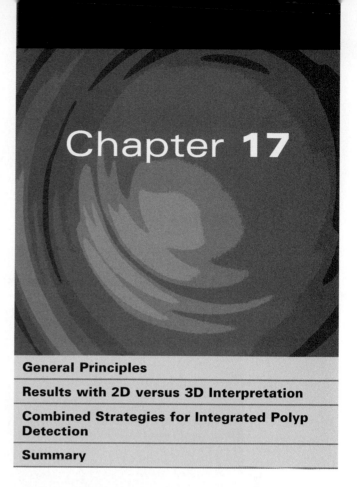

Chapter 17

General Principles

Results with 2D versus 3D Interpretation

Combined Strategies for Integrated Polyp Detection

Summary

INTRODUCTION

From its inception, CT colonography (CTC) has always included a three-dimensional (3D) component in addition to the more standard 2D imaging, hence the alternate moniker of "virtual colonoscopy." As such, the terms "2D CTC" and "3D CTC" are somewhat ambiguous and probably best avoided because they imply that 3D and 2D correlation, respectively, are not used. A very real and important distinction, however, resides with whether one interprets CTC by primarily using a 2D display for *initial polyp detection* (i.e., "primary 2D CTC") or by using a 3D display for initial polyp detection (i.e., "primary 3D CTC"). Considerable confusion has surrounded the debate on whether to use a primary 2D or primary 3D approach to polyp detection at CTC.[1-6] Perhaps this confusion stems in part from the fact that both 2D and 3D visualization modes are generally used to some degree with both reading approaches. For example, after a potential lesion is found on primary 2D CTC analysis, a limited 3D display may be used for "problem solving."[7] Likewise, for potential abnormalities detected on primary 3D CTC, 2D correlation is needed for confirmation of a true soft tissue polyp because there are a host of polypoid-appearing entities that can simulate true polyps on the 3D display (see Chapter 20).[8] Technically, the term "virtual colonoscopy" only applies to primary 3D endoluminal evaluation because the virtual reality fly-through is what simulates conventional endoscopy, whereas primary 2D evaluation with limited 3D problem solving does not. For the reasons discussed in this chapter, we strongly favor a primary 3D approach to CTC interpretation because it allows for effective and facile detection of the vast majority of relevant colorectal polyps. Of course, primary 2D evaluation remains an important adjunct, particularly in the setting of suboptimal colonic preparation or distention.[1]

GENERAL PRINCIPLES

Primary 2D Polyp Detection

Evaluation of the 2D multiplanar reformations (MPR) in the standard orthogonal transverse, coronal, and sagittal planes is a familiar task for virtually any radiologist performing CT interpretation. In the context of CTC, primary 2D evaluation consists of manual cine-mode review of the cross-sectional CT images by carefully tracking back and forth along the tortuous path of the large bowel lumen. Such evaluation generally extends from rectum to cecum or vice versa. The transverse 2D display is most often used for this "lumen tracking" mode, which necessarily includes evaluation of both the supine and prone datasets. Some have advocated the need to continually zoom and pan during the primary 2D polyp search, but we find this approach somewhat cumbersome and generally reserve magnification for interrogating suspected abnormalities. Our preferred "polyp window" for 2D polyp detection consists of a relatively wide width of 2000 HU centered at 0 HU, which provides excellent contrast resolution at the soft tissue–air interface and offers some distinction between soft tissue and fat attenuation. Others have used a window width of 1500 HU centered at −200 HU. Of note, we have found that lower-level settings that resemble a lung window provide too little soft tissue detail and tend to overaccentuate the soft tissue–air interface for polyp detection. Slice thickness should generally not exceed 2.5 mm collimation but need not be submillimeter either. A 1.0- to 1.25-mm reconstruction interval is optimal in our opinion and generally results in about 400 images per series, or less than 1000 images per study (supine and prone).

For suspected lesions detected on the wide polyp window setting, a narrower soft tissue window setting (e.g., width 350 HU, level 40 HU) can be useful to either confirm the soft tissue nature of a true polyp or demonstrate internal attenuation that is inconsistent with a polyp, such as densely tagged adherent stool. For the majority of tagged particulate stool, however, the internal high attenuation will already be apparent on the polyp window setting. One pitfall with the low-dose protocols currently used for CTC is that true polyps often demonstrate a somewhat mottled appearance on the soft tissue window setting, which could potentially be mistaken for untagged stool (Fig. 17-1). This pitfall can generally be avoided with the use of oral contrast tagging, where the presence of adherent untagged stool is rare, and also by noting the homogeneous appearance and smooth border to the lesion on the polyp window setting. 3D "problem solving" consists of focused interrogation limited to a potential 2D abnormality and should not be confused with primary 3D polyp detection. Endoluminal 3D correlation is particularly useful for thickened folds or a confluence of folds, which can appear polypoid or masslike at 2D evaluation (Fig. 17-2), and for polyps located on a fold (Fig. 17-3).

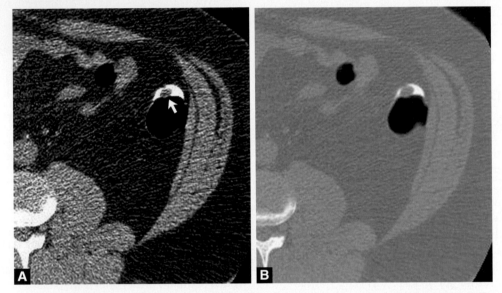

Figure 17-1 **Polyp heterogeneity on 2D soft tissue windowing related to low-dose technique.** Prone 2D transverse image **(A)** from low-dose CTC with soft tissue window settings (width 400 HU, level 50 HU) shows an internal heterogeneous appearance to the 11-mm polyp (tubulovillous adenoma) in the descending colon *(arrow)*. This heterogeneity related to the low-dose technique could be confused for untagged stool, but note the similarity with the abdominal musculature. The homogeneous appearance on the polyp window settings **(B,** width 2000 HU, level 0 HU) and the presence of contrast tagging allow for a confident polyp diagnosis.

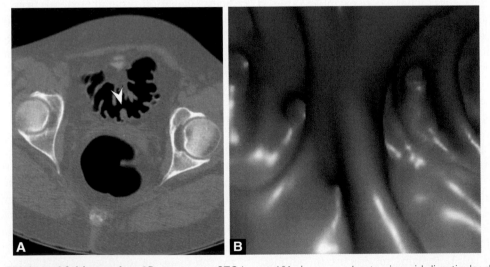

Figure 17-2 **Thickened fold complex.** 2D transverse CTC image **(A)** shows moderate sigmoid diverticular disease, but one bulbous-appearing polyp or fold stands out *(arrowhead)*. The 3D endoluminal view **(B)** clearly shows that the 2D finding correlates with a thickened fold that actually represents a convergence of folds. (From Pickhardt PJ. Differential diagnosis of polypoid lesions seen at CT colonography (virtual colonoscopy). *Radiographics.* 2004;24:1535-1559.)

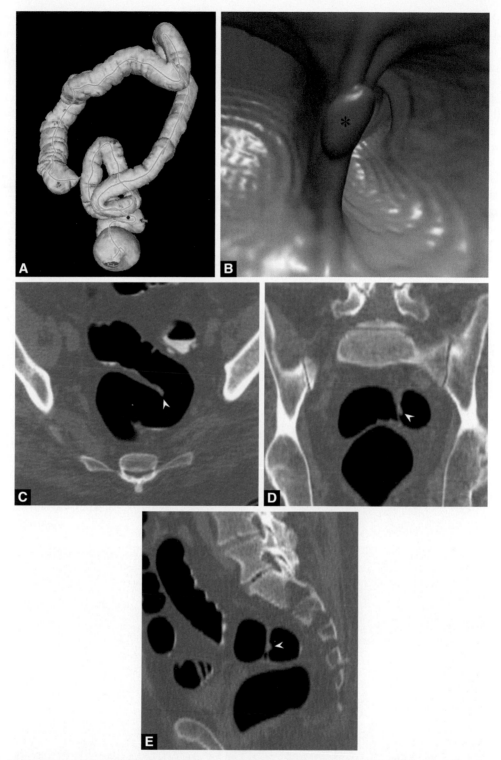

Figure 17-3 Large polyp detected at primary 3D evaluation but missed at primary 2D evaluation. 3D colon map **(A)** with oblique orientation shows the location of a 10-mm rectosigmoid polyp *(red dot bookmark)* that was missed at primary 2D evaluation but identified at primary 3D evaluation. The blue arrow indicates the 3D endoluminal vantage point shown in *B*. The green line on the 3D colon map represents the automated center line for endoluminal navigation. This large polyp was confirmed at same-day optical colonoscopy. 3D endoluminal CTC image **(B)** shows a 10-mm sessile polyp *(asterisk),* which extends off the edge of a fold. The lesion was obvious at real-time 3D fly-through evaluation, was confirmed on secondary 2D correlation, and was given the highest diagnostic confidence score by the interpreting radiologist. 2D transverse CTC image **(C)** with polyp window settings shows the polyp *(arrowhead),* which is difficult to distinguish from the fold it arises from and was missed at primary 2D evaluation. The lesion is somewhat more conspicuous on coronal **(D)** and sagittal **(E)** 2D displays *(arrowheads)* compared with the transverse projection. (From Pickhardt PJ, Lee AD, Taylor AJ, et al. Primary 2D versus primary 3D polyp detection at screening CT colonography. *Am J Roentgenol.* 2007 189;1451-1456.) *(*See associated video clip in DVD.)*

The reason for this difficulty at 2D evaluation is that the spatial relationship of a focal polypoid lesion versus an elongated fold is much harder to appreciate compared with 3D endoluminal evaluation. Confirmation of a polyp on both supine and prone views substantially increases diagnostic confidence because very few lesions of clinical significance will be identifiable on just a single view. Rarely, severe technical limitations such as inadequate preparation or segmental collapse may prevent definitive confirmation of a true lesion on the alternative view.

The major disadvantage to a primary 2D MPR review is that the visual search pattern for polyp detection is both challenging and fatiguing. The lack of conspicuity of soft tissue polyps among the ubiquitous soft tissue folds, which also have a somewhat polypoid appearance on cross-sectional images, is highly problematic. Further-

more, a polyp is only detectable on 2D when viewing the actual slices that contain it, whereas polyps on the 3D endoluminal view are usually visually obvious and often seen well in advance "down the barrel" of the lumen (Fig. 17-4).[9] A primary 2D search therefore demands one's undivided attention because the window of opportunity for polyp detection is so brief. Unfortunately, more than 10,000 2D MPR images must be viewed on average for each advanced neoplasm detected at screening CTC, raising concerns for reader fatigue and eye strain in a high-volume setting. With these shortcomings in mind, how was it that the primary 2D approach dominated the initial decade of CTC (1994-2003)? For one, there were preexisting comfort and skill levels already in place for the 2D approach because it resembled standard CT interpretation. In addition, the 2D MPR display format

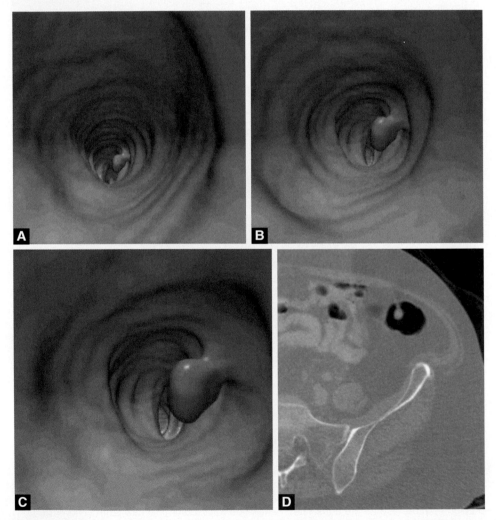

Figure 17-4 **Prolonged polyp visualization on 3D endoluminal fly-through.** 3D endoluminal CTC images **(A-C)** show a 10-mm pedunculated polyp in the descending colon well in advance of reaching the lesion **(A),** which becomes progressively more conspicuous as the endoluminal navigation continues **(B** and **C).** The polyp can be visualized over a relatively long time compared with primary 2D evaluation, allowing for facile detection. 2D transverse CTC image **(D)** confirms the pedunculated polyp, which appears obvious but is only seen on the few slices that actually traverse the lesion. The polyp will generally be visible for a subsecond interval during primary 2D detection, which requires a much more focused and intensive search that is fatiguing and prone to error. *(*See associated video clip in DVD.)*

was already fully mature and, unlike 3D capabilities, has changed very little since. Furthermore, as discussed later, effective and time-efficient primary 3D evaluation tools were not yet widely available. Therefore most CTC software systems were initially based on the paradigm of 2D detection with 3D problem solving.

Primary 3D Polyp Detection

The 3D endoluminal CTC view represents the vantage of a single virtual camera placed in 3D space within the distended colonic lumen. With appropriate thresholding and illumination, the surface-rendered or volume-rendered image display simulates the appearance at optical colonoscopy. Most CTC software systems now provide for at least semiautomated segmentation of the large intestine, with creation of an automated centerline for navigation. A 3D overview map of the segmented colon allows for a clear depiction of the anatomy and precise localization of positive findings (Fig. 17-5). Some workstations also allow for manual user-controlled navigation off the centerline in any direction to better evaluate for potential abnormalities. Primary 3D endoluminal polyp detection usually consists of virtual fly-through evaluation along the centerline, interspersed with focused manual navigation as needed. When potential lesions are identified on 3D evaluation, immediate 2D MPR correlation generally provides definitive evaluation. A bookmark can then be placed on the colon map to identify polyp location and facilitate confirmation on the alternate supine or prone position.

Because polyp conspicuity among the colonic folds on the 3D endoluminal display is greatly enhanced compared with the 2D MPR display (Fig. 17-3), it represents

an ideal polyp detection mode, whereas the source 2D dataset represents the ideal confirmatory step. Simply put, the more sensitive display (3D) should precede the more specific display (2D). Because the 3D search pattern is so much easier, it is much less taxing on the reader than a primary 2D read. In the past, however, most CTC workstations simply did not allow for time-efficient primary 3D evaluation, which represented the main disadvantage of this reading paradigm.[10] Marked differences in both the quality of the endoluminal volume rendering (Fig. 17-6) and the navigational abilities of the different systems were readily apparent.[6] Because of these technical limitations, primary 2D evaluation became the standard CTC reading mode because most investigators were using systems with inadequate primary 3D capability. This preference for primary 2D was readily apparent in the survey results from the faculty at the 3rd and 4th International Symposia on Virtual Colonoscopy, where 24 of 25 CTC experts felt that primary 2D evaluation was sufficient (including 13 experts who believed that secondary 3D problem solving was not even necessary); only one expert believed that primary 3D evaluation was necessary.[11] This strong 2D sentiment was largely a reflection of design limitations in the available technology and is clearly beginning to change toward a stronger reliance on 3D detection. A number of CTC software vendors have already taken notice and have made significant improvements in 3D detection capability. Unfortunately, some systems, in our opinion, still remain incapable of an effective, time-efficient primary 3D read.

The reason that we deviated from the primary 2D reading paradigm early on was that we were using a CTC system specifically developed to allow for an effective primary 3D evaluation.[6] Like most radiologists new to

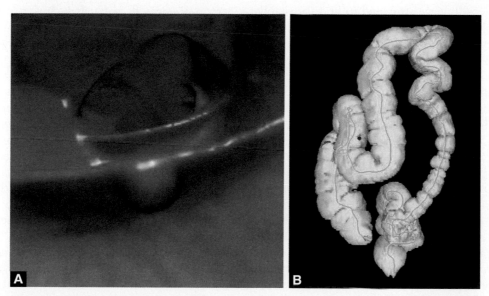

Figure 17-5 3D colon map for polyp localization. 3D endoluminal CTC image **(A)** shows a 6-mm polyp located on the backside of a colonic fold. 3D colon map **(B)** shows the precise anatomic location of the polyp in the proximal transverse colon *(red dot)*. This information is shared with the endoscopist if polypectomy is considered. *(*See associated video clip in DVD.)*

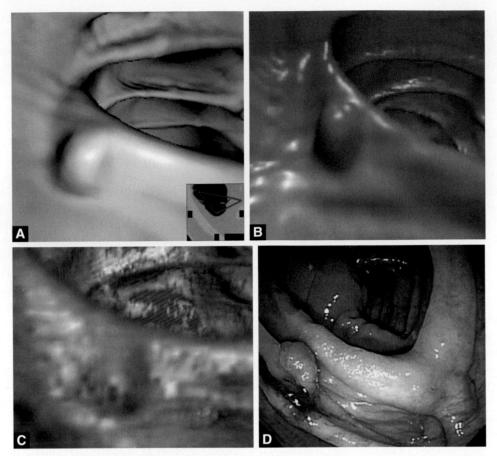

Figure 17-6 Qualitative differences in 3D volume rendering at CTC (in 2002). 3D endoluminal CTC images from three different vendors **(A-C)** show a polyp on a fold captured at the same vantage points. In addition to notable differences in the quality of the volume rendering, the real-time navigational abilities were even more disparate at that time. Considerable improvements in both volume rendering and navigation have since closed the gap somewhat, although the navigational abilities remain noticeably different among the various vendors. Image from same-day optical colonoscopy **(D)** shows the lesion prior to polypectomy.

CTC, we started out as primary 2D readers but soon discovered that polyps that we struggled to find (or simply missed) on 2D MPR were usually obvious on the 3D endoluminal view. Because this process of self-discovery is more convincing than force-fed dogma, and because 2D detection remains an indispensable skill, we require our trainees to attempt initially a primary 2D read, followed by 3D, until they have gained significant experience, which includes missing polyps on the 2D read but finding them on 3D review. With this approach, even the staunchest 2D readers have eventually gravitated toward primary 3D polyp detection.

With the 3D endoluminal display, a tradeoff exists between the visual field of view (FOV) of the virtual camera and the amount of geometric distortion that is introduced (Fig. 17-7). A 90-degree FOV represents the typical default value, for which there is little or no perceived distortion. However, because one-way fly-through (e.g., rectum to cecum) with a 90-degree FOV covers an average of only 75% of the colonic surface, two-way navigation is needed.[12] We have found that increasing the FOV to 120 degrees introduces a small but acceptable amount of distortion yet broadens the surface coverage on one-way fly-through such that polyp detection is not sacrificed.[13,14] At 150-degree FOV, however, the amount of spatial distortion is subjectively too great in our opinion (Fig. 17-7). It is interesting that some polyps will be detected at one-way fly-through at 120 degrees that will not be seen at two-way fly-through at 90 degrees (Fig. 17-8). In addition, the CTC system that we use allows for rapid review of any mucosal patches missed during the initial fly-through, which ensures complete 3D evaluation. As a result, for well-distended cases, comprehensive 3D evaluation can be achieved with one-way fly-through at 120 degrees, decreasing the overall number of supine-prone flights from four to two and significantly reducing the interpretation time. When distention is suboptimal, two-way fly-through at 120 degrees is prudent. Additional 3D tools that facilitate and enhance CTC interpretation are discussed in Chapter 19.

Beyond the standard 3D endoluminal display, alternative 3D viewing modes, such as the virtual dissection and unfolded cube displays, represent further distortions of the CTC dataset and are discussed in greater detail in

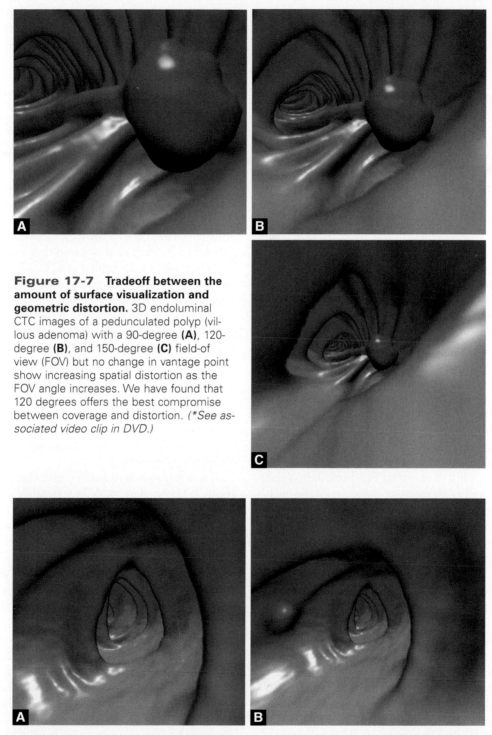

Figure 17-7 Tradeoff between the amount of surface visualization and geometric distortion. 3D endoluminal CTC images of a pedunculated polyp (villous adenoma) with a 90-degree **(A)**, 120-degree **(B)**, and 150-degree **(C)** field-of view (FOV) but no change in vantage point show increasing spatial distortion as the FOV angle increases. We have found that 120 degrees offers the best compromise between coverage and distortion. *(*See associated video clip in DVD.)*

Figure 17-8 Diagnostic value of increasing the 3D endoluminal field-of-view (FOV) angle from 90 to 120 degrees. 3D endoluminal CTC image **(A)** with a 90-degree FOV angle reveals no polyps at bidirectional fly-through along the centerline. 3D endoluminal CTC image **(B)** at the same vantage point as A but with a wider 120-degree FOV angle shows a 7-mm polyp that was not visualized at the 90-degree FOV angle. In this case, unidirectional fly-through at 120 degrees is both more efficient and more effective than bidirectional 90-degree fly-through. *(*See associated video clips in DVD.)*

Chapter 23. These emerging 3D displays are not yet clinically validated for screening but may play an important role in the future. However, it remains to be seen whether the gains in rapid mucosal visualization (leading to shorter interpretation times) are offset by the increased geometric distortion (leading to reduced sensitivity for polyp detection).

RESULTS WITH 2D VERSUS 3D INTERPRETATION

As noted in Chapter 7, one critical distinction that needs to be made clear when critiquing the various CTC performance trials is whether the study population represents a polyp-rich cohort or low-prevalence cohort. For low-prevalence cohorts, further distinction is needed between asymptomatic screening and nonscreening populations. Primary 2D polyp detection has generally fared well in small, polyp-enriched cohorts but cannot seem to maintain an acceptable sensitivity when applied to larger low-prevalence cohorts, where polyp detection is more akin to finding a needle in a haystack. Unfortunately, most of the evidence regarding primary 2D versus primary 3D polyp detection is not from head-to-head comparisons but rather must be indirectly inferred from the larger CTC trials, which did not directly compare the two reader paradigms. Another issue that receives little attention because it is difficult to quantify is the relative "ease" of polyp detection.[6] For example, a given polyp may be detected on both 2D and 3D imaging displays, but one may have to struggle to find it on 2D, whereas it may be obvious without any real effort on 3D. Such a difference will not manifest in the performance results of the trial but nonetheless may have real consequences in terms of diffusion of the technology, reader fatigue, and even job satisfaction. Therefore, although a high sensitivity for primary 2D polyp detection is theoretically possible because the lesions are nearly always detectable, at least in retrospect, this does not imply that primary detection can be achieved in actual practice. This is particularly true when an asymptomatic screening population is studied. By pop-culture analogy, primary 2D polyp detection is essentially a "Where's Waldo?" phenomenon—the finding is generally obvious only after you know where it is.

It is not surprising that the earlier published studies that helped shape the initial reliance on primary 2D interpretation used CTC systems with suboptimal 3D capabilities.[10,15-18] As noted previously, these systems were largely designed based on the primary 2D paradigm and were not suitable for effective primary 3D evaluation. Although other early studies had suggested that a 3D display may offer some interpretive advantage over 2D,[19,20] most radiologists remained firmly entrenched in the primary 2D paradigm.[11] Of the initial four large CTC clinical trials evaluating low-prevalence cohorts, the three trials restricted to a primary 2D approach for polyp detection, including one single-center trial[21] and two multicenter trials,[22,23] fared rather poorly. In comparison, the Department of Defense (DoD) multicenter CTC screening trial used primary 3D polyp detection and showed that CTC sensitivity for clinically relevant polyps was similar to optical colonoscopy.[24,25] The polyp detection performance of these larger trials in a low-prevalence setting is summarized in Table 17-1. The results from two additional CTC screening trials using primary 3D polyp detection demonstrate sensitivity values on par with the DoD trial, providing further support for the 3D approach.[26,27] Although the polyp detection mode represents the most profound protocol difference between the CTC trials with low versus high sensitivity results, another important difference was the use of oral contrast tagging, which also likely had a positive effect on performance but presumably to a lesser degree. A retrospective review of the false-negative results from the 2D trial by Rockey et al. showed that most missed lesions could actually be identified at CTC.[28] In fact, failure to prospectively detect clearly identifiable lesions with primary 2D evaluation accounted for 13 (65%) of the 20 large adenomas and cancers that were missed in that trial. When these readily preventable 2D perceptual errors are eliminated, the CTC sensitivity for large neoplasms in this trial closely matches the results obtained with primary 3D endoluminal polyp detection.[29] Our experience with actual CTC screening using a primary 3D approach in more than 3000 asymptomatic adults has shown a similar detection rate for advanced neoplasia compared with a matched group undergoing optical colonoscopy screening.[30]

A few retrospective studies have directly compared 2D versus 3D polyp detection. In general, it is difficult to draw unifying conclusions from these studies because they are mostly underpowered and the 3D capabilities and formats among the CTC systems have varied greatly. Among the early studies, Beaulieu et al.[20] showed a significant improvement with 3D detection over 2D when evaluating digitally synthesized polyps, whereas Macari et al.[10] showed no difference in sensitivity in a small study that included just one large polyp and only six polyps equal to or greater than 6 mm. More recent studies comparing standard 2D polyp detection against alternative 3D displays, including virtual dissection[31,32] and unfolded cube displays, have not shown a significant difference. These results, however, may simply reflect the geometric distortion introduced by the alternative 3D views (see Chapter 23). Of note, we conducted a large retrospective study whereby a consecutive subset of 730 cases from the DoD screening trial was interpreted with a primary 2D approach by readers with better training and more experience compared with the primary 3D readers from the original trial.[33] The results were striking and are summarized in Table 17-1. Not only was 2D sensitivity significantly lower than what was achieved with primary 3D in the same screening popula-

Table 17-1 ◻ Comparison of Polyp Sensitivity Among Large CTC Trials Evaluating Low-Prevalence Cohorts*

	Pickhardt et al.[33]	Johnson et al.[21†]	Cotton et al.[22]	Rockey et al.[23,28]	Pickhardt et al.[24,25]
Number of patients	730	703	600	614	1233
Primary polyp detection mode	2D	2D	2D	2D	3D
BY-PATIENT SENSITIVITY					
Polyps ≥6 mm	43% (49%)	–	39%	55% (68%)	84% (89%)
Polyps ≥10 mm	63% (81%)	48%	55%	59% (70%)	86% (94%)
BY-POLYP SENSITIVITY					
Polyps ≥6 mm	38% (44%)	43% (47%)	32%	49% (61%)	81% (86%)
Polyps ≥10 mm	60% (75%)	46% (46%)	52%	53% (64%)	84% (92%)

*Sensitivity is for all polyps (i.e., adenomas and nonadenomas), except for percentages in parentheses, which are for adenomas only.
†Percentages represent pooled averages of three readers; some by-patient results were not reported.

tion, but also the results closely mirrored the performance from the three earlier primary 2D trials (Table 17-1), despite the presence of oral contrast tagging and highly skilled readers. This study provides direct evidence of the inferiority of primary 2D interpretation for CTC screening and has further convinced us of the importance of primary 3D polyp detection.

The ACRIN (American College of Radiology Imaging Network) trial protocol 6664, also referred to as the "national CTC screening trial," found only modest gains in sensitivity for 3D detection over 2D, which were not statistically significant.[34] Several reasons likely account for this counterintuitive finding. One important factor was the use of a suboptimal 3D platform (Vitrea, Vital Images) at the majority of the study sites, which effectively reduced the expected 3D performance level.[6] We understand that the 3D polyp detection sensitivity was higher for the few sites that used the Viatronix V3D system. A second factor to consider was the unrealistically long primary 2D interpretation times, which averaged nearly 20 minutes. Polyps, of course, can nearly always be found on a primary 2D search if one is willing to look long and hard enough, but this does not reflect the typical constraints of real-world clinical practice. A third possible factor to consider was that the study was underpowered to show a statistically significant difference in sensitivity. Although 3D sensitivity was generally higher than 2D, it would have taken a much larger cohort to demonstrate "statistical significance."

A few additional issues related to CTC interpretation deserve mention with regard to 2D versus 3D polyp detection: the relative learning curve, study interpretation times, and specificity. It has been well documented that there is a difficult learning curve for primary 2D CTC interpretation.[28,35-39] Perhaps even more disturbing is the fact that even well-trained readers tend to fall off the 2D learning curve, such that experience does not necessarily protect against poor performance. Our experience with primary 3D interpretation, however, appears to be different, at least for the Viatronix V3D system. In our trial, even inexperienced readers in the DoD trial performed well right from the start and performance did not drop off during the course of the study (Fig. 17-9). Judging from the results of the ACRIN trial, this ease of primary 3D learning may not be true for some other CTC systems. Reported interpretation times for primary 2D evaluation have remained relatively constant, whereas primary 3D interpretation times have seen considerable reductions over time, reflecting continued improvements in computer speed and software design. With earlier CTC software versions, primary 3D interpretation times ranged from 20 to 40 minutes or more[10,24] but have since dropped to less than 10 minutes[1,32] With regard to CTC specificity, this reflects the ability of the test to exclude polyps in those without disease. As such, this involves a process of combined 2D/3D problem solving for potential lesions, regardless of the means for initial detection (2D or 3D). Therefore, it is not surprising that the differences in specificity among the various CTC trials are relatively small, including the primary 2D trials with poor sensitivity. The one exception to this is the ACRIN trial, where the relatively poor specificity and positive predictive values are more difficult to explain.

COMBINED STRATEGIES FOR INTEGRATED POLYP DETECTION

It should be clear by now that the "2D versus 3D debate" in CTC has never been about which display or displays to use in general, because both 2D and 3D have

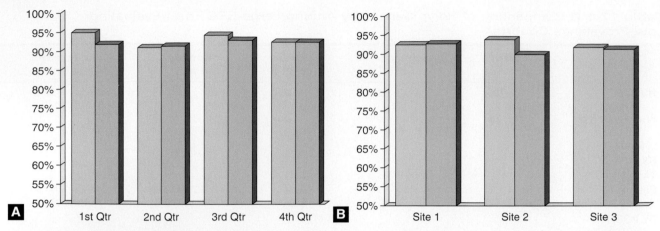

Figure 17-9 **Primary 3D CTC by patient performance for adenomas greater than or equal to 8 mm from the Department of Defense CTC screening trial.** Bar graphs **(A** and **B)** show sensitivity *(green)* and specificity *(blue)* at the 8-mm size threshold according to the temporal quarter **(A)** and by study site **(B)** for the trial. Note the uniform performance characteristics, ranging from 91% to 95% in all cases. The fact that most radiologists in the study were nonacademic and had relatively little prior experience and no formal training suggests that the learning curve with primary 3D polyp detection is much easier compared with the primary 2D approach, at least for the Viatronix V3D system. The ACRIN trial results suggest that the primary 3D learning curve may be more difficult with other CTC systems. (From Pickhardt PJ. Screening CT colonography: How I do it. *Am J Roentgenol.* 2007;189:290-298.)

always been a part of CTC, but rather which display to use for the specific purpose of *polyp detection*. However, even the answer here is not simply "primary 3D," because secondary 2D polyp detection can be an important supplement. It is important to understand that a primary 3D reading approach still retains any residual benefit of secondary 2D polyp detection. The converse is not necessarily true because many who use primary 2D polyp detection either can not or do not perform a complete secondary 3D polyp search. This integrated interpretive approach of 3D/2D polyp detection can maximize performance by capitalizing on the strengths of each display. For the typical CTC screening examination where colonic preparation and distention are generally of good quality, primary 3D usually provides for uncomplicated, comprehensive polyp detection. However, for cases in which either colonic preparation or colonic distention are suboptimal, primary 2D evaluation can assume a more important role in lesion detection (Figs. 17-10 and 17-11), although additional interpretive tools and techniques (e.g., contrast tagging, electronic cleansing, missed region tool, computed-aided detection [CAD], etc.) can also provide further redundancy. The source 2D MPR display can therefore not only serve to confirm suspected polyps detected on 3D, which is its primary mission and provides specificity, but also can provide for secondary polyp detection as needed to supplement overall CTC sensitivity.

One alternative strategy to our integrated primary 3D/2D approach is to combine primary 2D interpretation with computer-aided detection as a second reader (see also Chapter 24). The hope here is that the relatively poor sensitivity for primary 2D interpretation could be raised to a reasonable level by CAD. Although stand-alone CAD sensitivity has been encouraging and generally outperforms typical primary 2D performance, it has fallen short of primary 3D performance levels. For example, the stand-alone by-patient CAD sensitivity for large adenomas in the DoD screening trial was 89%,[40] compared with a sensitivity of 94% by human readers using a primary 3D approach.[24] However, no large studies to date have studied the incremental gain in sensitivity by using CAD to evaluate a low-prevalence screening population. Retrospective studies evaluating polyp-rich cohorts have shown a benefit to adding CAD to a primary 2D read,[41] but sensitivity values are again generally less than primary 3D levels. One small retrospective study of only 20 patients showed that a 2D-CAD approach matched primary 3D sensitivity,[42] but this study was flawed by the use of a suboptimal 3D display, resulting in low sensitivity values for each method.[43] Ultimately, the approach of primary 2D with secondary (or concurrent) CAD falls short simply because it retains the tedious and fatiguing exercise of the primary 2D review. To date, there is no precedent for using CAD as a first reader, which would eliminate the human element of polyp detection. In the end, primary 3D polyp detection, supplemented by secondary 2D detection, appears to be the optimal combined strategy for integrated polyp detection. Whether there is additional benefit to adding CAD to a primary 3D interpretive approach remains to be seen.

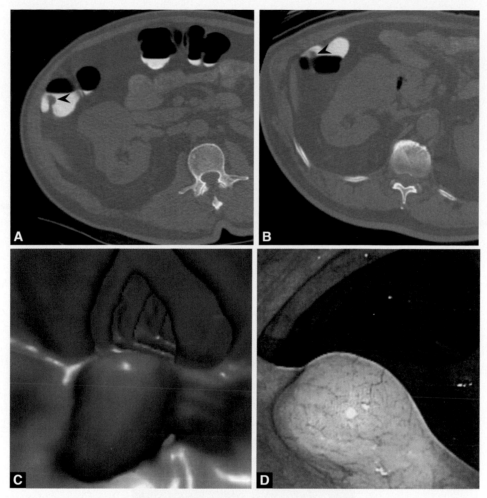

Figure 17-10 **Excessive luminal fluid submerging a large polyp on both supine and prone views.** 2D transverse supine **(A)** and prone **(B)** CTC images show a 12-mm polyp *(arrowheads)* on a fold that is submerged on both views. With fluid tagging, the lesion can be detected on 2D review. With electronic cleansing of the fluid, the lesion can also be detected on 3D review **(C)**. This case was from the DoD trial, when the bowel preparation protocol was not yet refined. With our current preparations, the amount of residual fluid has decreased such that we have essentially never seen a polyp submerged on both views, which is one reason we no longer use electronic fluid cleansing. This large polyp was confirmed at optical colonoscopy **(D)** and proved to be a tubular adenoma.

SUMMARY

There has been considerable confusion and controversy regarding the optimal strategy for polyp detection at CTC. The major approaches include primary 2D and primary 3D strategies. For the reasons and evidence outlined in this chapter, a primary 3D approach represents the most sensitive and effective method for this specific task. It allows for a nontaxing search pattern in which polyps are easily distinguished from colonic folds. Whereas a primary 2D approach could be used in this regard, it remains a mentally challenging method prone to errors, particularly in low polyp–prevalence situations. The 2D evaluation, however, is indispensable once a potential polyp is detected to characterize whether this candidate truly represents a soft tissue polyp. Although the term "primary 3D" is sometimes used to describe our interpretation strategy, it is important to realize that both 2D and 3D displays are both used in the course of detection and characterization.

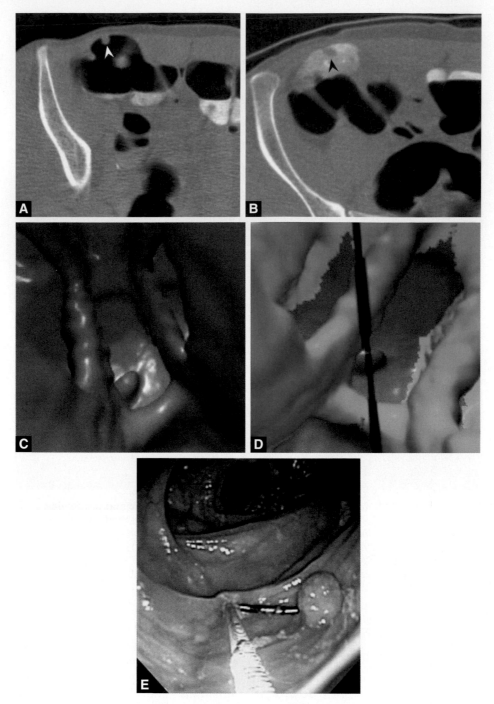

Figure 17-11 **Polyp detection complicated by poor preparation and distention.** 2D transverse supine **(A)** and prone **(B)** CTC images show an 8-mm polyp *(arrowheads)*. On the supine view, suboptimal distention with crowding of the folds obscured the lesion at 3D fly-through along the centerline **(C,** see also video clip), requiring polyp detection on either 2D review **(A)** or with the missed region tool **(D).** The red line in D corresponds to the transverse plane in **A.** On the prone view **(B),** the heterogeneous tagging also obscures the lesion somewhat and precludes effective electronic cleansing for 3D detection. This case was from the low-dose arm of the DoD trial. An 8-mm tubular adenoma was found at optical colonoscopy **(E).** *(*See associated video clip in DVD.)*

REFERENCES

1. Pickhardt PJ. Screening CT colonography: How I do it. *Am J Roentgenol.* 2007;189(2):290-298.
2. Van Dam J, Cotton P, Johnson CD, et al. AGA future trends report: CT colonography. *Gastroenterology.* 2004;127(3):970-984.
3. Bond JH. Progress in refining virtual colonoscopy for colorectal cancer screening. *Gastroenterology.* 2005;129(6):2103-2106.
4. Pickhardt PJ. Virtual colonoscopy. *JAMA.* 2004;292(4):431.
5. Pickhardt PJ, Kim DH. CT colonography (virtual colonoscopy): A practical approach for population screening. *Radiol Clin North Am.* 2007;45(2):361-375.
6. Pickhardt PJ. Three-dimensional endoluminal CT colonography (virtual colonoscopy): Comparison of three commercially available systems. *Am J Roentgenol.* 2003;181(6):1599-1606.

7. Dachman AH, Kuniyoshi JK, Boyle CM, et al. CT colonography with three-dimensional problem solving for detection of colonic polyps. *Am J Roentgenol.* 1998;171(4):989-995.

8. Pickhardt PJ. Differential diagnosis of polypoid lesions seen at CT colonography (virtual colonoscopy). *Radiographics.* 2004;24(6):1535-1556.

9. Lee AD, Pickhardt PJ. Polyp visualization at CT colonography: Comparison of 2D axial and 3D endoluminal displays. Chicago: RSNA Scientific Assembly; 2004.

10. Macari M, Milano A, Lavelle M, Berman P, Megibow AJ. Comparison of time-efficient CT colonography with two- and three-dimensional colonic evaluation for detecting colorectal polyps. *Am J Roentgenol.* 2000;174(6):1543-1549.

11. Barish MA, Soto JA, Ferrucci JT. Consensus on current clinical practice of virtual colonoscopy. *Am J Roentgenol.* 2005;184(3):786-792.

12. Pickhardt PJ, Taylor AJ, Gopal DV. Surface visualization at 3D endoluminal CT colonography: Degree of coverage and implications for polyp detection. *Gastroenterology.* 2006;130(6):1582-1587.

13. Pickhardt PJ, Schumacher S, Kim DH. Polyp detection at 3D endoluminal CT colonography: sensitivity of one-way fly-through at 120° field-of-view angle. *J Comput Assist Tomogr.* 2009 (in press).

14. Schumacher C, Pickhardt PJ, Hinshaw JL, Kim DH. Effect of the field-of-view angle on 3d endoluminal surface coverage at CT colonography. Chicago: RSNA Scientific Assembly; 2007.

15. Fenlon HM, Nunes DP, Schroy PC, Barish MA, Clarke PD, Ferrucci JT. A comparison of virtual and conventional colonoscopy for the detection of colorectal polyps. *N Engl J Med.* 1999;341(20):1496-1503.

16. Yee J, Akerkar GA, Hung RK, Steinauer-Gebauer AM, Wall SD, McQuaid KR. Colorectal neoplasia: Performance characteristics of CT colonography for detection in 300 patients. *Radiology.* 2001;219(3):685-692.

17. Fletcher JG, Johnson CD, Welch TJ, et al. Optimization of CT colonography technique: Prospective trial in 180 patients. *Radiology.* 2000;216(3):704-711.

18. Johnson CD, Toledano AY, Herman BA, et al. Computerized tomographic colonography: Performance evaluation in a retrospective multicenter setting. *Gastroenterology.* 2003;125(3):688-695.

19. McFarland EG, Brink JA, Pilgram TK, et al. Spiral CT colonography: Reader agreement and diagnostic performance with two- and three-dimensional image-display techniques. *Radiology.* 2001;218(2):375-383.

20. Beaulieu CF, Jeffrey RB, Karadi C, Paik DS, Napel S. Display modes for CT colonography—Part II. Blinded comparison of axial CT and virtual endoscopic and panoramic endoscopic volume-rendered studies. *Radiology.* 1999;212(1):203-212.

21. Johnson CD, Harmsen WS, Wilson LA, et al. Prospective blinded evaluation of computed tomographic colonography for screen detection of colorectal polyps. *Gastroenterology.* 2003;125(2):311-319.

22. Cotton PB, Durkalski VL, Benoit PC, et al. Computed tomographic colonography (virtual colonoscopy)—A multicenter comparison with standard colonoscopy for detection of colorectal neoplasia. *JAMA.* 2004;291(14):1713-1719.

23. Rockey DC, Poulson E, Niedzwiecki D, et al. Analysis of air contrast barium enema, computed tomographic colonography, and colonoscopy: Prospective comparison. *Lancet.* 2005;365(9456):305-311.

24. Pickhardt PJ, Choi JR, Hwang I, et al. Computed tomographic virtual colonoscopy to screen for colorectal neoplasia in asymptomatic adults. *N Engl J Med.* 2003;349(23):2191-2200.

25. Pickhardt PJ, Choi JR, Hwang I, Schindler WR. Nonadenomatous polyps at CT colonography: Prevalence, size distribution, and detection rates. *Radiology.* 2004;232(3):784-790.

26. Cash BD, Kim C, Jensen D, et al. Accuracy of computed tomographic colonography for colorectal cancer screening in asymptomatic individuals. *Gastroenterology.* 2007;132(4):A92.

27. Graser A, Stieber P, Nagel D, et al. Comparison of CT colonography, colonoscopy, sigmoidoscopy, and faecal occult blood tests for the detection of advanced adenoma in an average risk population. *Gut.* 2009;58(2):241-248.

28. Doshi T, Rusinak D, Halvorsen RA, Rockey DC, Suzuki K, Dachman AH. CT colonography: False-negative interpretations. *Radiology.* 2007;244(1):165-173.

29. Pickhardt PJ. Missed lesions at primary 2D CT colonography: Further support for 3D polyp detection. *Radiology.* 2008;246:648-649.

30. Kim DH, Pickhardt PJ, Taylor AJ, et al. CT colonography versus colonoscopy for the detection of advanced neoplasia. *N Engl J Med.* 2007;357(14):1403-1412.

31. Johnson CD, Fletcher JG, MacCarty RL, et al. Effect of slice thickness and primary 2D versus 3D virtual dissection on colorectal lesion detection at CT colonography in 452 asymptomatic adults. *Am J Roentgenol.* 2007;189(3):672-680.

32. Kim SH, Lee JM, Eun HW, et al. Two- versus three-dimensional colon evaluation with recently developed virtual dissection software for CT colonography. *Radiology.* 2007;244(3):852-864.

33. Pickhardt PJ, Lee AD, Taylor AJ, et al. Primary 2D versus primary 3D polyp detection at screening CT colonography. *Am J Roentgenol.* 2007;189(6):1451-1456.

34. Johnson CD, Chen MH, Toledano AY, et al. Accuracy of CT colonography for detection of large adenomas and cancers. *N Engl J Med.* 2008;359(12):1207-1217.

35. Gluecker TM, Fletcher JG, Welch TJ, et al. Characterization of lesions missed on interpretation of CT colonography using a 2D search method. *Am J Roentgenol.* 2004;182(4):881-889.

36. Slater A, Taylor SA, Tam E, et al. Reader error during CT colonography: Causes and implications for training. *Eur Radiol.* 2006;16(10):2275-2283.

37. Burling D, Halligan S, Atchley J, et al. CT colonography: Interpretative performance in a non-academic environment. *Clin Radiol.* 2007;62(5):424-429; discussion 30-31.

38. Taylor SA, Halligan S, Burling D, et al. CT colonography: Effect of experience and training on reader performance. *Eur Radiol.* 2004;14(6):1025-1033.

39. Fidler JL, Fletcher JG, Johnson CD, et al. Understanding interpretive errors in radiologists learning computed tomography colonography. *Acad Radiol.* 2004;11(7):750-756.

40. Summers RM, Yao JH, Pickhardt PJ, et al. Computed tomographic virtual colonoscopy computer-aided polyp detection in a screening population. *Gastroenterology.* 2005;129(6):1832-1844.

41. Halligan S, Altman DG, Mallett S, et al. Computed tomographic colonography: Assessment of radiologist performance with and without computer-aided detection. *Gastroenterology.* 2006;131(6):1690-1699.

42. Taylor SA, Halligan S, Slater A, et al. Polyp detection with CT colonography: Primary 3D endoluminal analysis versus primary 2D transverse analysis with computer-assisted reader software. *Radiology.* 2006;239(3):759-767.

43. Pickhardt PJ. Polyp detection at CT colonography: Inadequate primary 3D endoluminal reference standard precludes meaningful comparison. *Radiology.* 2007;244(1):316-317.

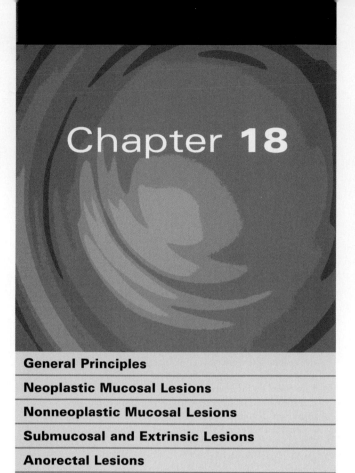

Chapter 18

Polypoid Lesions at CTC: Differential Diagnosis

PERRY J. PICKHARDT, MD

DAVID H. KIM, MD

INTRODUCTION

As discussed in Chapter 1, a colorectal "polyp" may be broadly defined as any luminal growth projecting from the mucosal surface. Although the terms "polyp" and "adenoma" are often used interchangeably, a wide variety of nonadenomatous causes for focal colorectal lesions at CT colonography (CTC) exist (Table 18-1). The primary target lesion for colorectal cancer screening is the "advanced adenoma" because it is believed that detection and removal of all large and/or histologically advanced adenomas would prevent the vast majority of cancers from developing. In addition, emerging evidence suggests that select serrated lesions should also be considered a target. Aside from malignant polyps, frankly invasive adenocarcinoma generally manifests as a large annular or semiannular mass. In addition to these clinically significant epithelial neoplasms, a host of additional lesions and pseudolesions may be encountered that appear polypoid at CTC. There are a variety of useful techniques and observations that increase the specificity of CTC for distinguishing false polyps from true polyps. A subset of "don't touch" lesions can be recognized at CTC and should not be confused for potential neoplasms (Table 18-2). This chapter will focus primarily on illustrating the broad spectrum of neoplastic and non-neoplastic mucosal lesions seen at CTC, with submucosal lesions, "don't touch" lesions, anorectal abnormalities, and other interpretive pitfalls illustrated in other chapters.

GENERAL PRINCIPLES

Colorectal polyps may be categorized at CTC according to size, morphology, location, and internal composition. Unfortunately, although these characteristics may suggest polyp histology, a definite determination at CTC (or optical colonoscopy [OC]) cannot be made short of pathologic analysis. Polyp size has been traditionally characterized by the longest linear dimension, which does not include the stalk of pedunculated lesions. Large polyp size is defined as 10 mm or greater, small size as 6 to 9 mm, and diminutive size as 5 mm or less. Some have referred to small polyps as "medium-sized" or "intermediate-sized" lesions, but we believe that these terms should generally be avoided. Precise polyp measurement at CTC is critical for appropriate patient management and is covered in greater detail in Chapter 19. Although existing endoscopic guidelines for patient management and risk stratification primarily hinge on polyp size and histology, it should be noted that measurement of polyp size at both OC and pathologic evaluation are less accurate than CTC measurement.[1] Going forward, more precise polyp size assessment at CTC may lead to refinements in prevalence and overall clinical significance. Furthermore, polyp volume may ultimately replace linear size as the most relevant parameter.

Table 18-1 ◘ Classification of Polypoid Lesions at CTC

NEOPLASTIC MUCOSAL LESIONS

Adenoma
  Tubular
  Tubulovillous
  Villous
  Serrated
Adenocarcinoma (malignant polyp)

NONNEOPLASTIC MUCOSAL LESIONS

Hyperplastic (nondysplastic serrated) polyp
Normal epithelium ("mucosal" polyp)
Juvenile polyp
Hamartomatous polyp
Inflammatory polyp
Inflammatory pseudopolyp
Prolapsing mucosal polyp
Inverted appendiceal stump
Inverted diverticulum
Gastric heterotopia

SUBMUCOSAL LESIONS (see Chapter 22)

Lipoma
Carcinoid tumor
Lymphoid polyp
Hemangioma
Mesenchymal tumors
Pneumatosis cystoides
Hematoma
Cystic lesions
Extrinsic causes

ANORECTAL LESIONS (see Chapter 20)

Internal hemorrhoids
Hypertrophied anal papilla
Rectal catheter
Solitary rectal ulcer syndrome
Anal condyloma
Anal cancer

POTENTIAL PITFALLS (see Chapter 20)

Adherent stool
Stool-filled diverticulum
Thickened or complex fold
Ileocecal valve
Imaging artifacts
Intraluminal foreign bodies

Table 18-2 ◘ "Don't Touch" Lesions at CTC

Adherent stool
Lipoma
Stool-filled diverticulum
Ileocecal valve
Rectal catheter
Extrinsic impression
Thickened or complex fold
Pneumatosis
Intraluminal foreign bodies
Imaging artifacts

Polyp morphology can be sessile, pedunculated, or flat.[2] Sessile lesions have a broad base of attachment, whereas pedunculated lesions have a connecting stalk between the mucosal surface and polyp head. Flat lesions represent a subset of sessile polyps that have a more plaquelike appearance, definitely have a height less than half their width, and are typically 3 mm or less in height (except for larger flat masses >3 cm). However, clearcut agreement on an exact definition for what constitutes a flat lesion at both CTC and OC has been somewhat elusive. Flat lesions are less conspicuous at CTC evaluation compared with sessile and pedunculated lesions but are still generally detectable with adequate technique unless they are completely flat in nature, which is exceedingly rare.[3,4] In our experience, some suspected flat lesions detected at CTC cannot be found at OC and likely represent false-positive findings. The majority of proven flat lesions detected at CTC that measure 1 to 2 cm in size are hyperplastic, followed by nonaggressive tubular adenomas. Fortunately, the small but aggressive flat adenomas that have been described in East Asian populations, including depressed lesions, seem to be rare in the typical U.S. screening population.[3-6]

Carpet lesions (laterally spreading tumors) are an important subset of large flat polyps because they often represent villous or tubulovillous neoplasms. However, despite their large size (≥3 by definition), these lesions have a relatively low rate of malignancy.[7] The vast majority of carpet lesions are found in the rectum and cecum.[8] Flat and carpet lesions are also covered as potential pitfalls in Chapter 20. Frankly invasive colorectal masses are covered in Chapter 21.

Polyp location is best categorized according to the six named segments: rectum, sigmoid colon, descending colon, transverse colon, ascending colon, and cecum. The hepatic and splenic flexures represent anatomic locations that are easy to recognize at CTC but represent imprecise segments as a result of their arbitrary boundaries with adjacent segments and are also difficult to reliably identify at OC. Therefore, it is probably best to exclude these flexures at segmental localization. At CTC, determination of homogeneous internal soft tissue composition of a polyp is a critical determinant for distinguishing true from false lesions (and lipomas). Oral contrast tagging is extremely useful for excluding residual adherent stool as a potential polyp candidate at CTC.

Generically speaking, the intended target for colorectal cancer screening is the neoplastic polyp, including both benign (adenomatous) and malignant lesions.[9] An emerging secondary target for screening includes select serrated lesions. Ideally, only those lesions with legitimate malignant potential (i.e., advanced neoplasms and select serrated polyps) need to be detected and removed. Unfortunately, diagnostic tests such as CTC and OC are not histology specific. Despite this limitation, large size

(≥10 mm) appears to be a very good surrogate to predict histology to capture these lesions. It remains unclear when and if OC referral is indicated for subcentimeter soft tissue polyps detected at CTC because the vast majority of these lesions will never develop into cancer (see Chapter 2).

Because the imaging appearance of soft tissue polyps does not equate with histology, radiologists interpreting CTC for colorectal cancer screening should be cognizant of both the importance of lesion size and the wide array of entities that can give rise to "lumps and bumps" in the colon. Broad categories of polypoid lesions that will be covered in this chapter include neoplastic mucosal polyps, non-neoplastic mucosal polyps, submucosal lesions, impression from extrinsic structures, and anorectal lesions (Table 18-1). In addition, there are several artifacts and pitfalls unique to CTC that could also be mistaken for true pathology, and a subset of "don't touch" lesions for which an imaging-specific diagnosis is generally possible. In the end, the basic concept behind accurate polyp detection at CTC is straightforward: a true polyp is composed of soft tissue and can be identified at the same location on the supine and prone displays. In actual practice, there are rarely any exceptions to this general rule.

NEOPLASTIC MUCOSAL LESIONS

The great majority of colorectal cancers are believed to develop gradually from benign adenomatous polyps (Table 18-1), with a dwell time measured in years and probably even decades, according to the well-known adenoma–carcinoma sequence (see Chapter 3). Detection and removal of these slow-growing adenomas could potentially prevent the development of the majority of cancers and is the basic rationale behind colorectal screening (see Chapter 5). Tubular adenomas (Figs. 18-1 and 18-2) account for approximately 80% to 85% of all adenomatous polyps. The great majority of tubular adenomas measure less than 10 mm in size (Fig. 18-1). In fact, tubular adenomas account for approximately one third of all diminutive colorectal lesions (≤5 mm) and approximately two thirds of all small

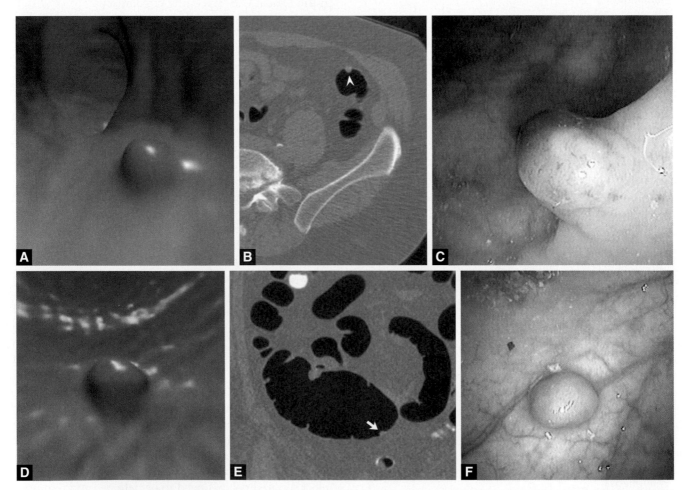

Figure 18-1 **Tubular adenomas (small).** 3D endoluminal **(A)** and 2D transverse **(B)** CTC images show a small 6-mm sessile polyp *(arrowhead)* in the descending colon. The lesion was confirmed and removed at same-day OC **(C)**. 3D endoluminal **(D)** and 2D coronal **(E)** CTC images from a second individual show a 9-mm sessile polyp *(arrow)* in the cecum. This lesion was also confirmed and removed at same-day OC **(F)**.

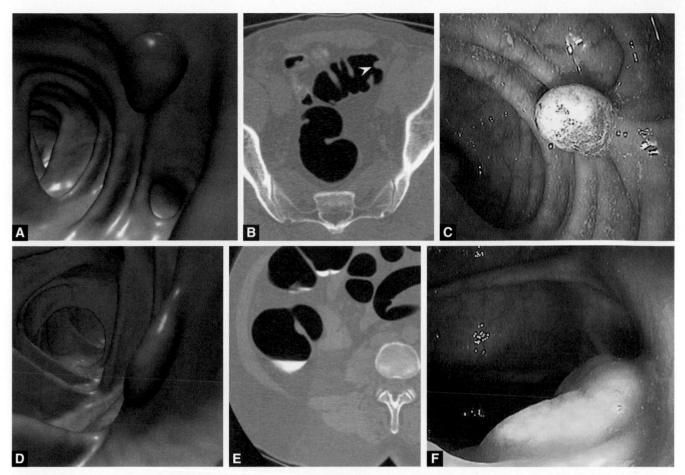

Figure 18-2   Tubular adenomas (large). 3D endoluminal **(A)** and 2D transverse **(B)** CTC images show a 10-mm sessile polyp *(arrowhead)* in the sigmoid colon, adjacent to a diverticulum. The lesion was confirmed and removed at same-day OC **(C)**. 3D endoluminal **(D)** and 2D transverse **(E)** CTC images from a second individual show an elongated 14-mm lesion situated along a fold in the ascending colon. This lesion had a similar morphology at same-day OC for polypectomy **(F)**. Although these adenomas did not demonstrate high-grade dysplasia or a prominent villous component, they are both considered advanced adenomas based on their large size (≥10 mm). (From Pickhardt PJ. CT colonography for population screening: Validation clears the way for clinical implementation. *Nat Clin Pract Oncol.* 2009;6:187-188.) (*See associated video clips in DVD.*)

polyps (6-9 mm).[10] Diminutive polyps are essentially of no practical clinical significance, and as isolated findings their presence or absence should not affect patient management at CTC.[10-12] Evolving natural history data from CTC surveillance (see Chapter 2) suggests that small polyps are generally not of any major clinical importance. However, for the time being, 6- to 9-mm polyps are not considered completely negligible and should be reported at CTC. Most tubular adenomas are sessile in appearance at CTC, with a minority demonstrating either a flat or pedunculated morphology (Fig. 18-1). Tubular adenomas rarely demonstrate high-grade dysplasia. Unless they are large in size (Fig. 18-2), tubular adenomas without significant dysplasia are probably at very low risk for malignant progression.

Tubulovillous adenomas (Figs. 18-3 and 18-4) represent about 10% to 15% of all adenomatous lesions.[13] These neoplasms tend to be larger than tubular adenomas, often 10 mm or greater, and are commonly pedunculated in morphology (Fig. 18-4). In addition, tubulovillous adenomas tend to demonstrate higher degrees of dysplasia at histologic examination (Fig. 18-5). As such, these lesions are a more important target for colorectal screening and cancer prevention. True villous adenomas are relatively uncommon, representing less than 5% of all colorectal neoplasms. These lesions are generally large in size (2-3 cm or more) and tend to have a lobulated appearance at CTC (Fig. 18-6), which corresponds to the frondlike appearance seen at OC. In general, villous adenomas have a greater risk for malignancy. Large carpet lesions often have a prominent villous component, sometimes with foci of high-grade dysplasia (Fig. 18-7).

The concept of the "advanced adenoma" is vitally important because it represents the key target lesion for colorectal screening and prevention.[9,12,14] Advanced adenomas are defined as neoplasms that either measure greater than or equal to 10 mm or demonstrate high-grade dysplasia or a prominent villous component

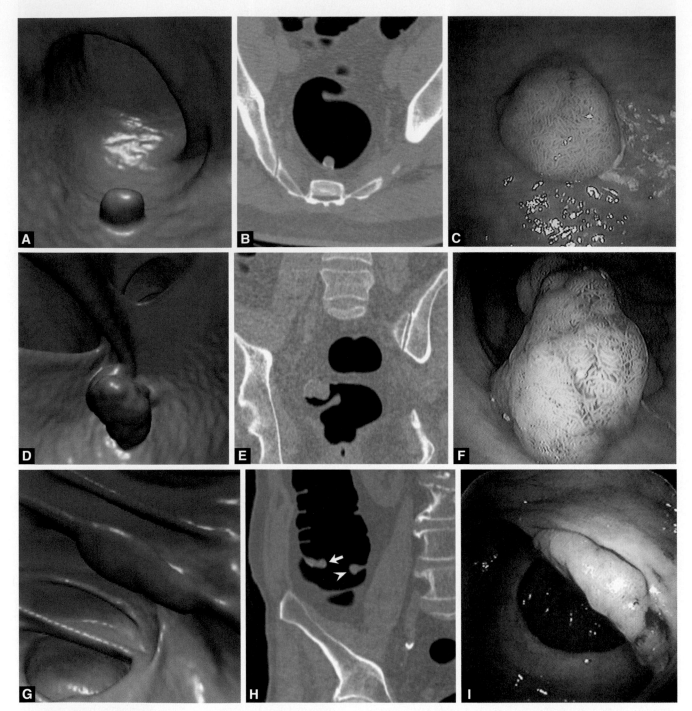

Figure 18-3 **Tubulovillous adenomas (sessile).** 3D endoluminal **(A)** and 2D transverse **(B)** CTC images show a 10-mm sessile polyp in the posterior rectum. The lesion demonstrates a "cerebriform" pit pattern at OC **(C)**, which is characteristic but not diagnostic of adenomatous histology. 3D endoluminal **(D)** and 2D coronal **(E)** CTC images from a second individual show a lobulated 35-mm sessile lesion adjacent to a rectal valve. A cerebriform pit pattern is also seen with this lesion at OC **(F)**. 3D endoluminal **(G)** and 2D coronal **(H)** CTC images show an elongated 35-mm polyp *(arrow)* along a fold in the ascending colon. An additional 17-mm polyp *(arrowhead)* is seen opposite the larger lesion. Both lesions proved to be tubulovillous adenomas after resection at OC **(I)**. *(*See associated video clips on DVD.)*

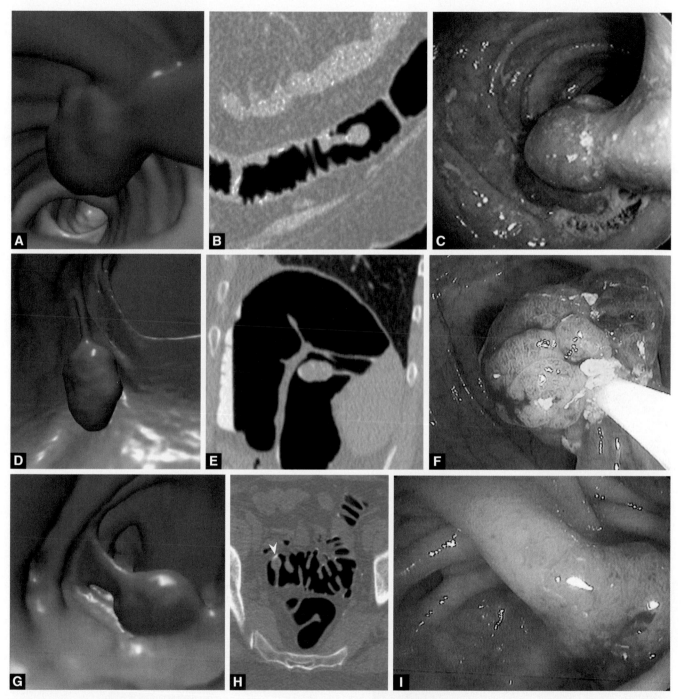

Figure 18-4 **Tubulovillous adenomas (pedunculated).** 3D endoluminal **(A)** and 2D coronal **(B)** CTC images show a pedunculated 23-mm polyp in the sigmoid colon. Note the associated wall thickening in the sigmoid colon related to diverticular disease (myochosis). The pedunculated polyp was removed at same-day OC **(C)**. 3D endoluminal **(D)** and 2D sagittal **(E)** CTC images from a second individual show a large 3-cm pedunculated mass in the descending colon, which was snared at same-day OC **(F)**. 3D endoluminal **(G)** and 2D transverse **(H)** CTC images from a third individual show a pedunculated 17-mm polyp *(arrowhead)* in the sigmoid colon. The fold thickening from diverticulosis makes 2D polyp detection very difficult but does not affect lesion conspicuity on 3D. These findings were confirmed at same-day OC **(I)**. *(*See associated video clips in DVD.)*

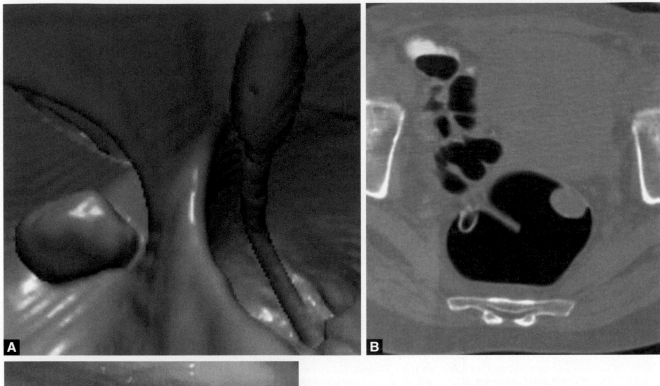

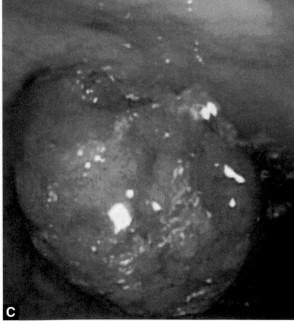

Figure 18-5 Tubulovillous adenoma with high-grade dysplasia. 3D endoluminal **(A)** and 2D transverse **(B)** CTC images from a case from the DoD screening trial show a large sessile 3.5-cm rectal mass, which was confirmed at OC **(C)** and found to contain areas with high-grade dysplasia. The striated appearance of the 3D image relates to the use of 2.5-mm collimation, which was used for most cases in the trial. *(*See associated video clip in DVD.)*

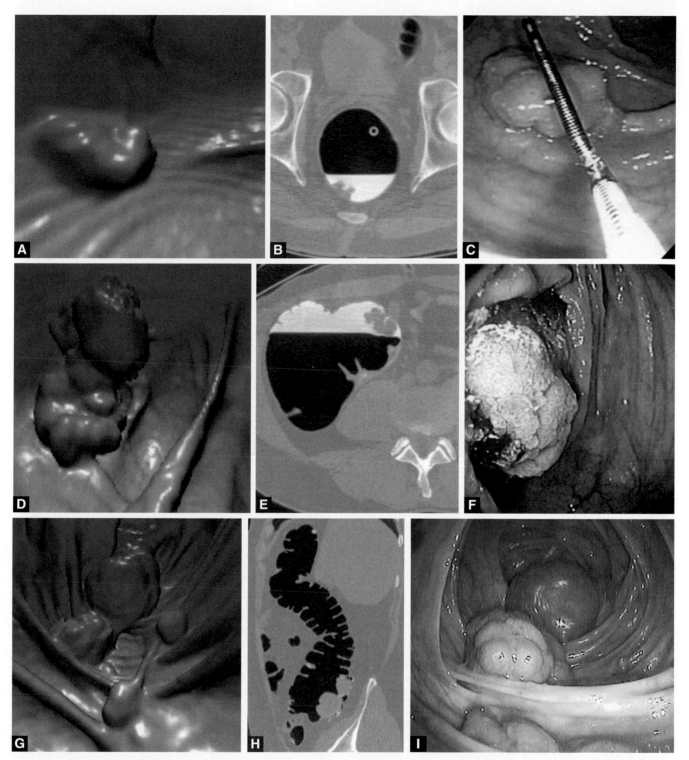

Figure 18-6 Villous adenomas. 3D endoluminal **(A)** and 2D transverse **(B)** CTC images from a case from the DoD screening trial shows a 2.5-cm lobulated rectal lesion, which proved to be a villous adenoma after endoscopic resection **(C).** 3D endoluminal **(D)** and 2D transverse **(E)** CTC images from another DoD case shows a larger 5.5-cm lobulated mass in the cecum, which had a frondlike villous appearance at OC **(F).** In both DoD cases, the degree of residual luminal fluid is considerably greater than what is seen with our current bowel preparation, which is one reason why we no longer use electronic fluid cleansing. 3D endoluminal **(G)** and 2D sagittal **(H)** CTC images from a University of Wisconsin screening case show multiple right-sided polyps and masses measuring up to 4 cm in size. At endoscopy **(I),** all proved to be adenomatous, with the largest masses being pure villous lesions. *(*See associated video clip in DVD.)*

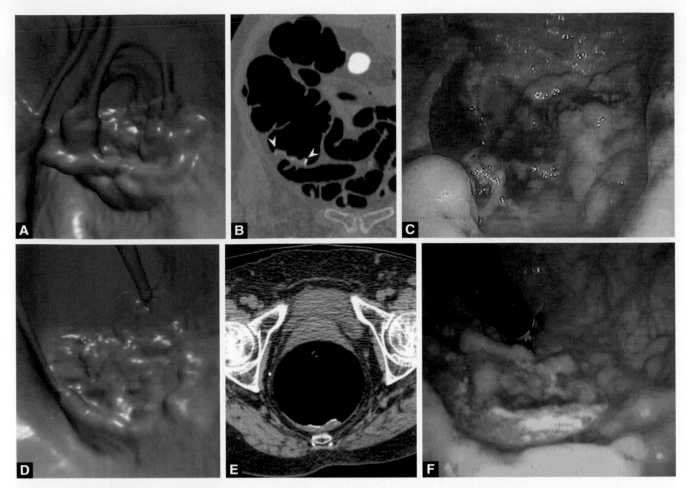

Figure 18-7 **Villous and tubulovillous carpet lesions.** 3D endoluminal **(A)** and 2D coronal **(B)** CTC images show a flat irregular mass near the cecal base *(arrowheads)*, which showed benign tubulovillous histology at both OC biopsy **(C)** and after right hemicolectomy. 3D endoluminal **(D)** and 2D transverse **(E)** CTC images show another flat irregular mass lesion that measured 8 cm in diameter. Benign villous histology was found at endoscopic biopsy **(F)** and after transanal surgical excision. Both cases demonstrate the necessity of operative management for some advanced yet benign carpet lesions. *(*See associated video clips in DVD.)*

(typically 25% or more) on histology. In practice, only 5% to 10% of advanced adenomas measure less than 10 mm, making lesion size the primary inclusion factor.[9,12,14] Therefore, polyp size determination at CTC represents an effective surrogate for advanced neoplasia. Of subcentimeter advanced adenomas, the majority are tubulovillous lesions without high-grade dysplasia.[12,14] Because villous histology is generally believed to be less ominous than high-grade dysplasia, the true clinical significance of subcentimeter tubulovillous adenomas without high-grade dysplasia is unclear. It is likely that the time course for the small percentage of tubulovillous adenomas that ultimately transform to carcinoma is extended and much longer than a similar-sized adenoma with high-grade dysplasia.

Malignant polyps are defined as focal adenomatous polypoid lesions that contain a focus of adenocarcinoma that extends beyond the mucularis mucosae. At CTC, malignant polyps are almost always large in size (Fig. 18-8). In fact, recent data including our own clinical experience

suggest that fewer than 1% of all large polyps measuring 1 to 2 cm in size contain invasive carcinoma.[12,15,16] Malignant polyps represent a relatively small minority of all colorectal adenocarcinomas, which more commonly manifest as frankly invasive masses (see Chapter 21). Malignant polyps, however, represent an early, curable stage of cancer that further strengthens the rationale for screening of asymptomatic adults. With regard to clinical management, the need for surgical treatment following endoscopic resection requires careful consideration.[17,18]

Serrated adenomas represent dysplastic lesions that develop along the "serrated polyp pathway" of colorectal carcinogenesis, which differs from the traditional adenoma–carcinoma sequence.[19] Serrated adenomas are believed to arise from hyperplastic polyps and, as such, represent an alternative route to cancer that may account for about 15% to 20% of all cases. Serrated adenomas are generally easy to detect at CTC evaluation, often presenting as large drooping masses or sessile lesions (Fig. 18-9). Unlike small hyperplastic polyps in the distal

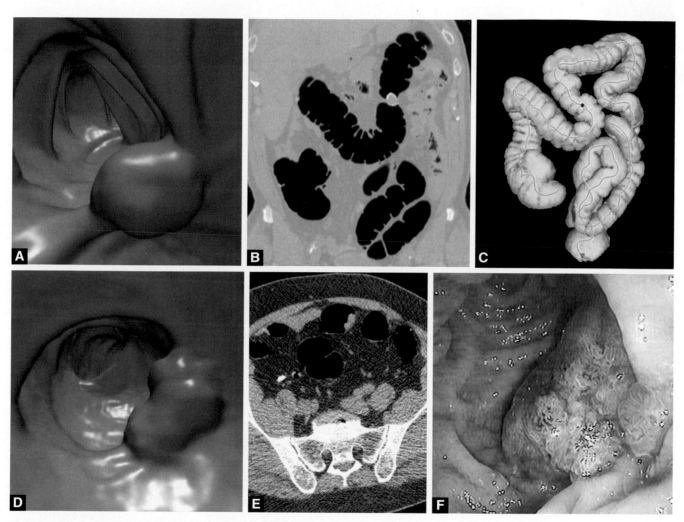

Figure 18-8   Malignant polyps (adenocarcinoma). 3D endoluminal **(A)**, 2D coronal **(B)**, and 3D map **(C)** CTC images show the location *(red dot)* and appearance of a sessile 17-mm polyp, which proved to contain a focus of invasive carcinoma at pathologic evaluation. Note the thin rim of positive oral contrast coating the lesion on 2D. An extended right hemicolectomy was ultimately performed. 3D endoluminal **(D)** and 2D transverse **(E)** CTC images from a second patient show a slightly larger 22-mm polyp in the sigmoid colon that also proved to be malignant after resection at OC **(F)**. A sigmoid colectomy was subsequently performed. Among the first 5000 adults screened by CTC at the University of Wisconsin, these two malignant polyps represent the smallest cancers. *(*See associated video clip in DVD.)*

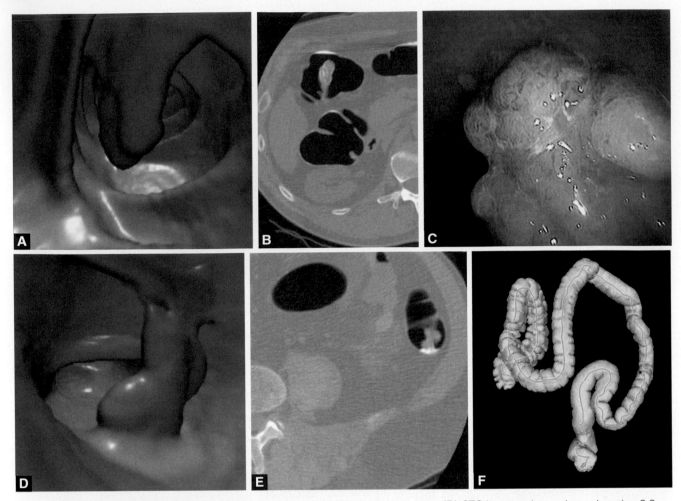

Figure 18-9 **Large serrated adenomas.** 3D endoluminal **(A)** and 2D transverse **(B)** CTC images show a large drooping 3.8-cm lesion in the proximal transverse colon. Note the unusual feature of contrast coating multiple layers or undulations on 2D. The lesion had a soft, lobulated appearance at OC **(C)**, with a mucoid coating that contains the contrast seen at CTC. 3D endoluminal **(D)**, 2D transverse **(E)**, and 3D map **(F)** CTC images show the location *(red dot)* and drooping appearance of another large, lobulated serrated adenoma. *(*See associated video clips on DVD.)*

colon and rectum, most serrated adenomas and large hyperplastic lesions are located in the proximal colon. The serrated polyp pathway for carcinogenesis is discussed in more detail in Chapter 3.

NON-NEOPLASTIC MUCOSAL LESIONS

Unlike the pathologic continuum seen with neoplastic polyps, nonadenomatous mucosal polyps represent a more heterogeneous group of unrelated entities (Table 18-1). Although more than 80% of non-neoplastic mucosal lesions are diminutive and have essentially no malignant potential, non-neoplastic lesions still account for about 40% of polyps greater than or equal to 6 mm in an asymptomatic screening population.[20] Of note, CTC is less sensitive for nonadenomatous lesions compared with adenomas of similar size. In the Department of Defense (DoD) CTC trial, the by-polyp sensitivity for adenomatous and nonadenomatous polyps at the 8-mm size threshold was 93% and 75%, respectively.[20] It appears this phenomenon is largely a result of the fact that nonadenomatous lesions such as hyperplastic polyps more often demonstrate an atypical or flat morphology and also have a tendency to flatten out further with colonic distention at CTC (Fig. 18-10).[21]

Hyperplastic polyps, also referred to as nondysplastic serrated polyps, represent the most common non-neoplastic colorectal polyps (Figs. 18-10 through 18-12). Most hyperplastic polyps are diminutive in size and are located in the distal colon and rectum, whereas larger hyperplastic lesions tend to be more proximal in location. Although fewer than 25% of hyperplastic polyps measure 6 mm or more, they still account for about 75% of all nonadenomatous lesions of potentially significant size in a screening cohort (Fig. 18-11).[20] Many hyperplastic lesions that measure more than 10 mm in diameter have an atypical or bizarre morphology that can make them more difficult to detect, or sometimes even occult, at CTC (Fig. 18-12).[22] In our experience, however, dys-

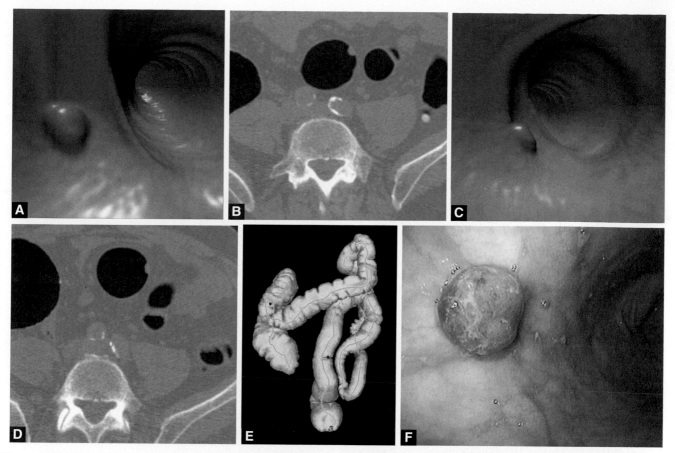

Figure 18-10 **Hyperplastic polyp demonstrating partial flattening with colonic distention.** 3D endoluminal **(A)** and 2D transverse **(B)** CTC images in the prone position show a 8-mm sessile polyp that appears to flatten somewhat on the corresponding supine view **(C** and **D)**. 3D map **(E)** shows the distal sigmoid location of the hyperplastic polyp *(red dot)*. The second bookmark in proximal transverse colon marks the location of the large 3.8-cm serrated adenoma shown in Fig. 18-9. The sigmoid polyp was found at subsequent endoscopy **(F),** as was the proximal lesion (see Fig. 18-9C).

plastic hyperplastic lesions relevant to the serrated polyp pathway may be easier to detect at CTC.

The "mucosal" polyp is the second most frequent non-adenomatous lesion and simply represents normal epithelium in a heaped-up, polypoid, or other recognizable configuration. Compared with hyperplastic polyps, these lesions seldom represent a diagnostic concern at CTC because more than 90% are diminutive in our experience (Fig. 18-13).[20] Detection and removal of these lesions at OC lead to increased costs and potential complications without providing any real clinical benefit (see Fig. 26-14). One exception to the diminutive nature of these non-neoplastic soft tissue lesions is the prolapsing mucosal polyp.[23] Focal prolapse of redundant colonic mucosa, typically associated with sigmoid diverticular disease, can be difficult to distinguish from neoplastic disease at both CTC and OC (see Chapter 20). Another exception is the situation where a large area of mucosa is called "abnormal" at OC, perhaps because of a mild color or texture alteration, but is found to simply represent normal mucosa at pathologic examination. For example, in the

DoD screening trial, an 8-cm area was called a "lesion" at OC but appeared normal at CTC (even in retrospect). At pathologic examination of multiple biopsy specimens, only normal mucosa was seen. This is one reason why it is important to concentrate on lesions with relevant pathology for both CTC and OC comparison trials and for actual clinical practice.

The juvenile polyp is classified as hamartomatous and, as the name implies, is most commonly found between the ages of 1 to 7 years. Although most juvenile polyps regress or slough off, they are occasionally identified in adults. As such, they are usually solitary, pedunculated, and located in the rectosigmoid region (Fig. 18-14).[13] Removal of larger juvenile polyps is indicated because of the risk of bleeding or prolapse. At OC, juvenile polyps may show a cherry-red or mottled appearance. At CTC, we have noticed that some juvenile polyps demonstrate more internal heterogeneity, with areas of decreased attenuation (Fig. 18-14), but a neoplastic polyp cannot be confidently excluded. Hamartomatous polyps can be seen either in isolation or associated polyposis condi-

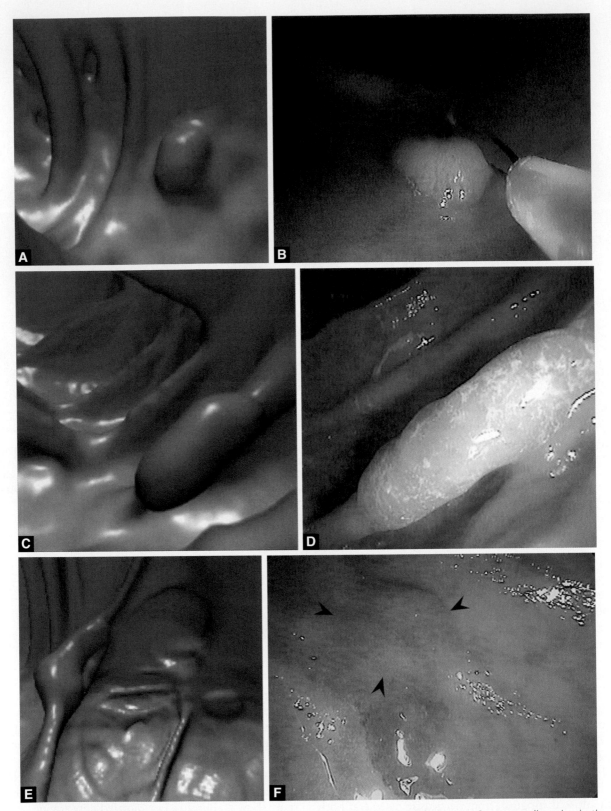

Figure 18-11 **Nondiminutive hyperplastic polyps.** 3D endoluminal CTC image **(A)** shows a 9-mm sessile polyp in the sigmoid colon, in addition to multiple diverticula. The lesion was found at same-day OC **(B)** and proved to be hyperplastic. 3D endoluminal CTC **(C)** and corresponding OC **(D)** images from a second individual show an elongated hyperplastic polyp extending along the edge of a fold in the ascending colon. 3D endoluminal CTC **(E)** and OC **(F)** images from a third individual show a 13-mm flat lesion in the cecum, which was subtle at endoscopy *(arrowheads)*. *(*See associated video clips on DVD.)*

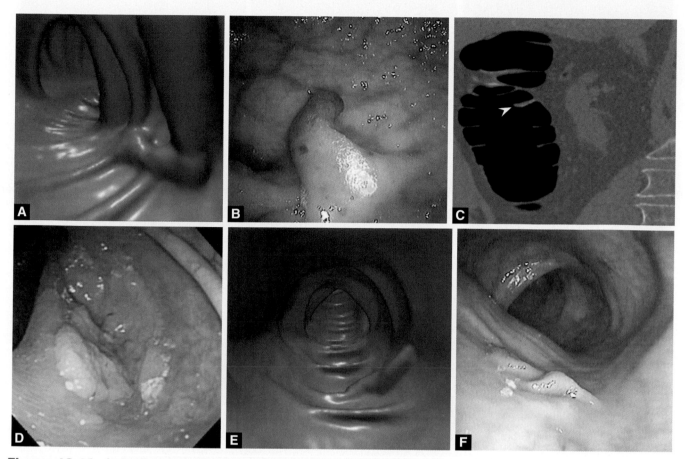

Figure 18-12 **Large hyperplastic polyps with somewhat atypical or unusual morphology.** 3D endoluminal CTC **(A)** and corresponding OC **(B)** images show an elongated lesion that appears to be a stalk without an identifiable polyp head. 2D coronal CTC **(C)** and OC **(D)** images from a second individual show a fold that appears focally thickened *(arrowhead)* as a result of a flat hyperplastic lesion. 3D endoluminal CTC **(E)** and OC **(F)** images show another large flat lesion from a third individual. *(*See associated video clips on DVD.)*

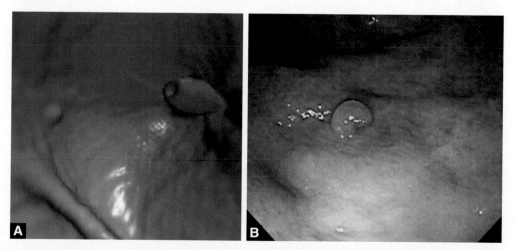

Figure 18-13 **Diminutive mucosal polyp.** 3D endoluminal CTC **(A)** and corresponding OC **(B)** images show a tiny 3-mm lesion that simply proved to be normal mucosa at histologic examination. We would not report such lesions in isolation but may mention them in the setting of other nondiminutive lesions. (From Pickhardt PJ, Choi JR, Hwang I, Schindler WR. Nonadenomatous polyps at CT colonography: Prevalence, size distribution, and detection rates. *Radiology.* 2004;232:784-790.)

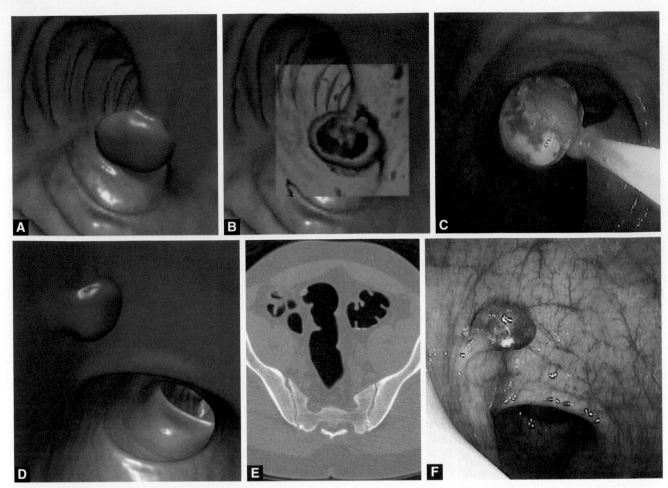

Figure 18-14 **Sporadic juvenile polyps in adults.** 3D endoluminal CTC images without **(A)** and with **(B)** translucency rendering show a large 15-mm polyp in the transverse colon, which proved to be an isolated juvenile-type polyp after resection at OC **(C).** The stalk of this pedunculated polyp was evident on other CTC projections (not shown). The translucency appearance of juvenile polyps can be more heterogeneous, with less uniform red compared with neoplastic polyps. However, this feature is not reliable enough to be diagnostic, and polypectomy is probably indicated anyway for a juvenile polyp of this size, given the risk for bleeding. 3D endoluminal **(D)** and 2D transverse **(E)** CTC images from a second individual show a 11-mm lesion in the sigmoid colon. At 3D CTC and OC **(F),** a short stalk can be appreciated. Both cases were asymptomatic screening individuals. (*See associated video clips in DVD.)*

tions, such as Peutz-Jegher syndrome or Cowden's disease (Fig. 18-15).

Inflammatory polyps are occasionally seen as an isolated finding in adults (Fig. 18-16). Some are believed to be formed by local extrusion of mucosa from peristaltic forces and may demonstrate a pale fibrinous cap at OC. Inflammatory pseudopolyps can be seen in the setting of severe acute inflammatory bowel disease (ulcerative colitis and Crohn's disease), representing islands of inflamed mucosa surrounded by areas of denuded epithelium (Fig. 18-17). Unlike diagnostic CT evaluation of the abdomen and pelvis, CTC has a very limited role in the setting of acute inflammatory bowel disease because of the risk of perforation. Inflammatory pseudopolyps should not be confused with postinflammatory polyps, which are seen in the chronic regenerative phase of inflammatory bowel disease (Fig. 18-18).

One final non-neoplastic soft tissue lesion to consider is the inverted appendiceal stump from prior appendectomy with stump inversion technique. The specific location and correlation with prior surgical history should suggest the diagnosis, but confident exclusion of a mucosal neoplasm is not always possible (see Chapter 20).[24]

SUBMUCOSAL AND EXTRINSIC LESIONS

A wide variety of submucosal lesions, including both intramural and extramural entities, can elevate the overlying colonic mucosa and produce a smooth, broad-based polypoid appearance (Table 18-1). Although most intramural submucosal lesions will have a nonspecific soft tissue appearance at CTC, there are some characteristic entities, such as lipomas and pneumatosis, that can be specifically

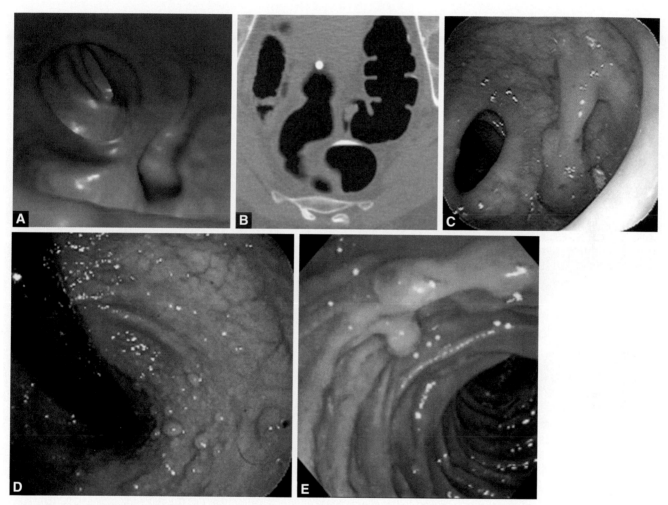

Figure 18-15 Hamartomatous polyps. 3D endoluminal **(A)** and 2D transverse **(B)** CTC images in an asymptomatic screening individual show a 15-mm pedunculated polyp in the sigmoid colon, which proved to be a hamartoma after polypectomy at OC **(C)**. OC images from patients with Cowden's disease **(D)** and Peutz-Jegher syndrome **(E)** show multiple colonic hamartomas. (D and E from Pickhardt PJ. Differential diagnosis of polypoid lesions seen at CT colonography (virtual colonoscopy). *Radiographics.* 2004;24:1535-1559.) *(*See associated video clip in DVD.)*

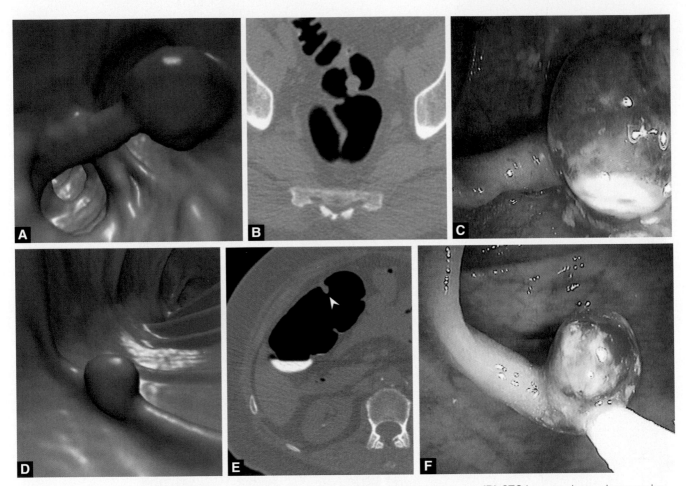

Figure 18-16   Sporadic inflammatory polyps. 3D endoluminal **(A)** and 2D transverse **(B)** CTC images show a large pedunculated polyp in the sigmoid colon, which proved to be inflammatory after polypectomy at OC **(C)**. 3D endoluminal CTC **(D)**, 2D transverse CTC **(E),** and OC **(F)** images show a 10-mm inflammatory polyp *(arrowhead)* at the hepatic flexure. *(*See associated video clip in DVD.)*

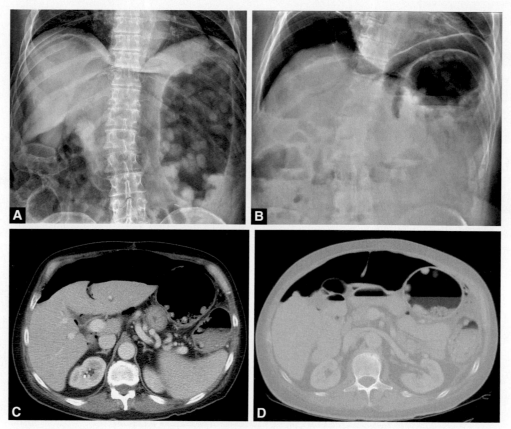

Figure 18-17   **Inflammatory pseudopolyps in acute ulcerative colitis (with perforation).** Supine **(A)** and upright **(B)** frontal abdominal radiographs show massive pneumoperitoneum, which manifests on the supine view as lucency over the liver and Rigler's sign (gas outlining both sides of the bowel wall). Multiple polypoid lesions project over the distended left colon. Contrast-enhanced CT images with soft tissue **(C)** and polyp **(D)** windows redemonstrate the pneumoperitoneum and colonic polypoid lesions, which represent inflammatory pseudopolyps in the setting of fulminant ulcerative colitis with frank perforation.

identified at CTC. These two entities both belong to the group of "don't touch" lesions that will be discussed later. Submucosal lesions are covered in detail in Chapter 22.

ANORECTAL LESIONS

Entities peculiar to the anorectum are illustrated as pitfalls in Chapter 20 but deserve specific mention here (Table 18-1), in part because further evaluation of a CTC finding in this region may only require digital rectal examination or anoscopy and not full endoscopic examination. Although incidental abnormalities in the anorectal region are not rare, they are generally benign and usually do not require intervention or therapy. Location is the key to recognition at CTC evaluation. In particular, internal hemorrhoids are a relatively frequent finding and represent dilated vascular channels above the dentate line. When advanced or thrombosed, internal hemorrhoids may appear masslike at CTC. The soft tissue fullness from internal hemorrhoids often appears prominent on transverse 2D images but is less masslike on other 2D planes and 3D endoluminal views. Hypertrophied anal papilla represents focal fibrous prominence of tissue at the dentate line, usu-

ally in response to chronic irritation.[13] Most anal papillae measure 5 to 6 mm or less but they can rarely attain a larger size. The key to recognition of an anal papilla is its constant anatomic location at the anorectal junction, virtually always abutting the rectal catheter at its lowest visualized point. Low-lying rectal adenomas will almost always show at least some separation from the anorectal junction.

The rectal catheter is a constant finding in the anorectal region. Although its tip may appear polypoid at 3D CTC, or cause extrinsic impression on an adjacent rectal fold, it should always be easily recognized for what it is. The rectal catheter can potentially obscure or distort a significant polyp,[25] especially with the use of retention balloons or large-caliber tubes. In general, we prefer a small-caliber catheter whenever possible. The poorly understood solitary rectal ulcer syndrome, despite its name, will manifest as a polypoid lesion and not an ulcer in about 25% of cases.[13] Anal warts, or condylomata acuminata, represent a sexually transmitted disease caused by the human papillomavirus and may have an endorectal component. A more aggressive form can be seen in patients who are immunocompromised, particularly those with acquired immunodeficiency syndrome (AIDS). Approximately 80% of cancers

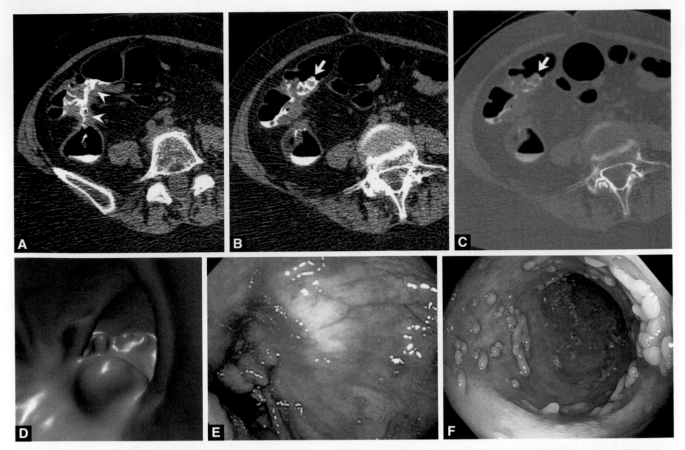

Figure 18-18 **Postinflammatory polyps in longstanding Crohn's colitis.** 2D CTC images with soft tissue (**A** and **B**) and polyp (**C**) windows performed for prior incomplete OC as a result of high-grade right-sided colonic stricture shows colonic wall thickening, colocolic fistula *(arrowheads),* and multiple polypoid lesions *(arrows)* associated with the colonic stricture. Images from 3D endoluminal CTC (**D**) and the incomplete OC study (**E**) show the postinflammatory polyps at the distal aspect of the benign stricture. OC image (**F**) from a patient with longstanding ulcerative colitis shows multiple postinflammatory polyps with a characteristic filiform appearance.

of the anal canal are squamous cell carcinomas, with the rest representing adenocarcinomas. Although CTC may detect some anal cancers (See Fig. 20-95), the examination is not designed to effectively evaluate this region. Therefore, the digital rectal examination should remain as a standard component of the adult health maintenance physical.

POTENTIAL PITFALLS

A variety of false lesions can mimic true polyps at CTC (Table 18-1), many of which can be recognized as "don't touch" lesions. Chief among these are residual adherent stool, impacted diverticula, thickened folds, the ileocecal valve, and imaging artifacts. These pitfalls are covered in detail in Chapter 20.

"DON'T TOUCH" LESIONS AT CTC

There are a host of lesions and pseudolesions encountered at CTC that can simulate true pathology but, with proper training and experience, can almost always be recognized as a "don't touch" lesion. These entities are listed in Table 18-2 and are covered in more detail in Chapters 20 and 22.

CONCLUSION

Polypoid lesions seen at CTC can result from a wide variety of causes beyond colorectal neoplasms, which are the intended focus of screening. In general, non-neoplastic mucosal-based polyps cannot be reliably distinguished from adenomatous polyps. Perhaps future advances in colorectal imaging may one day allow for noninvasive distinction between these entities, which would be valuable given their disparate clinical implications. Although non-neoplastic lesions such as hyperplastic and "mucosal" polyps dominate at diminutive polyp sizes, they are much less common at the larger polyp sizes that are clinically relevant. Recognition of the alternative pathway to cancer via serrated polyps does not diminish the potential of CTC screening because polyp size remains the critical determinant. For many of the nonmucosal entities discussed herein, there a variety of useful techniques and observations that allow for distinguishing false polyps from true polyps at CTC. Additional tools will likely be introduced in the future to increase specificity even further. A subset of polypoid entities that we have labeled "don't touch" lesions should generally be recognized as such at CTC and left alone. As CTC for primary colorectal screening makes the transition from scientific validation to widespread clinical implementation, it will be important for radiologists to be aware of the wide array of potential causes of polypoid lesions that may be encountered.

REFERENCES

1. Park SH, Choi EK, Lee SS, et al. Polyp measurement reliability, accuracy, and discrepancy: Optical colonoscopy versus CT colonography with pig colonic specimens. *Radiology.* 2007;244(1):157-164.
2. Zalis ME, Barish MA, Choi JR, et al. CT colonography reporting and data system: A consensus proposal. *Radiology.* 2005;236(1):3-9.
3. Pickhardt PJ, Nugent PA, Choi JR, Schindler WR. Flat colorectal lesions in asymptomatic adults: Implications for screening with CT virtual colonoscopy. *Am J Roentgenol.* 2004;183(5):1343-1347.
4. Pickhardt PJ, Levin B, Bond JH. Screening for nonpolypoid colorectal neoplasms. *JAMA.* 2008;299(23):2743; author reply 2744.
5. O'Brien M J, Winawer SJ, Zauber AG, et al. Flat adenomas in the National Polyp Study: Is there increased risk for high-grade dysplasia initially or during surveillance? *Clin Gastroenterol Hepatol.* 2004;2(10):905-911.
6. Pickhardt PJ, Choi JR, Nugent PA, Hwang I, Schindler WR. Flat lesions at virtual and optical colonoscopy: Prevalence, histology, and sensitivity for detection in an asymptomatic screening population. *Am J Roentgenol.* 2004;182(4):74-75.
7. Tanaka S, Haruma K, Oka S, et al. Clinicopathologic features and endoscopic treatment of superficially spreading colorectal neoplasms larger than 20 mm. *Gastrointest Endosc.* 2001;54(1):62-66.
8. Rubesin S, Saul S, Laufer I, Levine M. Carpet lesions of the colon. *Radiographics.* 1985;5(4):537-552.
9. Winawer SJ, Zauber AG. The advanced adenoma as the primary target of screening. *Gastrointest Endosc Clin N Am.* 2002;12(1):1-9, v.
10. Pickhardt PJ, Choi JR, Hwang I, et al. Computed tomographic virtual colonoscopy to screen for colorectal neoplasia in asymptomatic adults. *N Engl J Med.* 2003;349(23):2191-2200.
11. Bond JH. Clinical relevance of the small colorectal polyp. *Endoscopy.* 2001;33(5):454-457.
12. Kim DH, Pickhardt PJ, Taylor AJ, et al. CT colonography versus colonoscopy for the detection of advanced neoplasia. *N Engl J Med.* 2007;357(14):1403-1412.
13. Pickhardt PJ. Differential diagnosis of polypoid lesions seen at CT colonography (virtual colonoscopy). *Radiographics.* 2004;24(6):1535-1556.
14. Kim DH, Pickhardt PJ, Taylor AJ. Characteristics of advanced adenomas detected at CT colonographic screening: Implications for appropriate polyp size thresholds for polypectomy versus surveillance. *Am J Roentgenol.* 2007;188(4):940-944.
15. Odom SR, Duffy SD, Barone JE, Ghevariya V, McClane SJ. The rate of adenocarcinoma in endoscopically removed colorectal polyps. *Am Surg.* 2005;71(12):1024-1026.
16. Yoo TW, Park DI, Kim YH, et al. Clinical significance of small colorectal adenoma less than 10mm: The KASID study. *Hepatogastroenterology.* 2007;54(74):418-421.
17. Hassan C, Zullo A, Winn S, et al. The colorectal malignant polyp: Scoping a dilemma. *Digest Liver Dis.* 2007;39(1):92-100.
18. Hassan C, Zullo A, Risio M, Rossini FP, Morini S. Histologic risk factors and clinical outcome in colorectal malignant polyp: A pooled-data analysis. *Dis Colon Rectum.* 2005;48(8):1588-1596.
19. O'Brien MJ. Hyperplastic and serrated polyps of the colorectum. *Gastroenterol Clin North Am.* 2007;36(4):947-968.
20. Pickhardt PJ, Choi JR, Hwang I, Schindler WR. Nonadenomatous polyps at CT colonography: Prevalence, size distribution, and detection rates. *Radiology.* 2004;232(3):784-790.
21. Waye JD, Bilotta JJ. Rectal hyperplastic polyps—Now you see them, now you don't—A differential point. *Am J Gastroenterol.* 1990;85(12):1557-1559.
22. MacCarty RL, Johnson CD, Fletcher JG, Wilson LA. Occult colorectal polyps on CT colonography: Implications for surveillance. *Am J Roentgenol.* 2006;186(5):1380-1383.
23. Tendler DA, Aboudola S, Zacks JF, O'Brien MJ, Kelly CP. Prolapsing mucosal polyps: an underrecognized form of colonic polyp—A clinicopathological study of 15 cases. *Am J Gastroenterol.* 2002;97(2):370-376.
24. Prout TM, Taylor AJ, Pickhardt PJ. Inverted appendiceal stumps simulating large pedunculated polyps on screening CT colonography. *Am J Roentgenol.* 2006;186(2):535-538.
25. Pickhardt PJ, Choi JR. Adenomatous polyp obscured by small-caliber rectal catheter at low-dose CT colonography: A rare diagnostic pitfall. *Am J Roentgenol.* 2005;184(5):1581-1583.

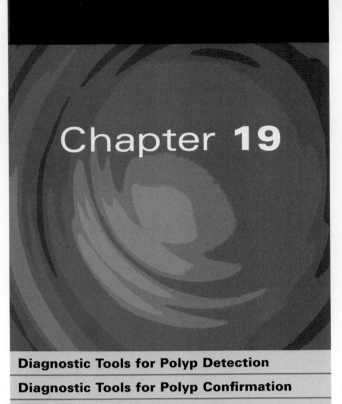

Chapter **19**

Diagnostic Tools for CTC Interpretation

DAVID H. KIM, MD
PERRY J. PICKHARDT, MD

INTRODUCTION

CT colonography (CTC) interpretation using a combined three-dimensional/two-dimensional (3D/2D) approach requires a specific set of diagnostic tools to facilitate this strategy. The software viewing platform should provide these tools to maximize the advantages of this interpretation algorithm. These tools allow ease of manipulation and localization within a specific environment and seamless transition between 3D and 2D views. Specific functions such as polyp measurement and attenuation determination should be implemented without difficulty. In addition, advanced postprocessing tools such as electronic fluid cleansing or computer-aided detection (CAD) may help some readers. This chapter explores the available tools necessary to facilitate CTC interpretation. Some of these tools are demonstrated in the instructional video on the DVD. Without such tools, the clinically proven 3D/2D combined approach cannot be effectively undertaken and polyp detection would likely suffer.

DIAGNOSTIC TOOLS FOR POLYP DETECTION

As stated in previous chapters, the search pattern used for polyp detection using a primary 3D approach is a more effective and easily applied strategy than a primary 2D approach. However, a set of specific tools is needed to facilitate this task of detecting potential polyps with a primary 3D approach. These tools allow the user to easily segment out the colorectum to create the 3D model and fly-through. Diagnostic tools such as automated centerline navigation allow the reader to devote complete attention to the detection of polyps, whereas functions such as mucosal coverage tracking provide important feedback to the reader. Increased field of view (FOV) at endoluminal fly-through or alternative 3D displays may be helpful by allowing increased speed of interpretation and increased surface visualization.

Colonic Segmentation: 3D Map and Centerline

A necessary diagnostic tool is colonic segmentation and centerline generation. The colorectum must be easily segmented out from the body, and a 3D model must be created (Fig. 19-1). Although a complete air column defining the colon is present for a number of cases, there is a substantial fraction where the colon is fragmented as a result of incomplete distention of a segment or a column of fluid in a portion of the colon. In these cases, the segments must be connected together to complete a fly-through. In addition, air or CO_2 may reflux into loops of small bowel and even the stomach. These areas must be excluded from the colon map that is created (Fig. 19-2). Correct segmentation of the large intestine with subsequent generation of a centerline along its entire length is a requirement for the primary 3D interpretive approach. This allows for automated navigation along the centerline and ultimately in a highly sensitive, time-efficient fly-through. With automated centerline navigation, the reader is able to de-

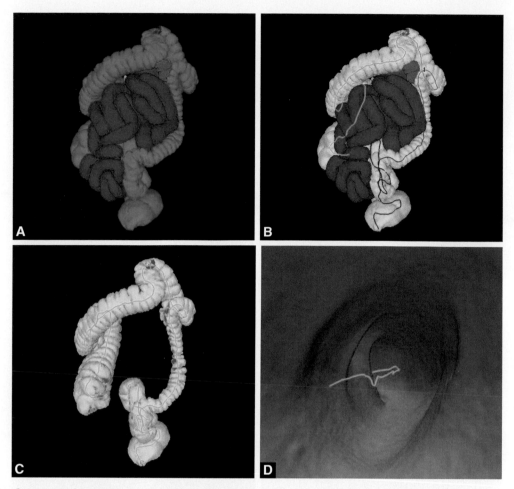

Figure 19-1 Segmentation and creation of the 3D model. Initial automated 3D map **(A)** prior to the final segmentation step demonstrates multiple tubular gas-filled segments. The process of selecting **(B)** and segmenting out the colorectum **(C)** from the small bowel for the endoluminal fly-through should be an easy task to accomplish. Note the red-green line represents the generated centerline on the 3D map, which is also demonstrated on the 3D endoluminal view **(D).** Automated guided fly-through along this centerline is a requisite for time-efficient, sensitive 3D evaluation.

vote complete attention to polyp detection and not on navigating the various turns of the colon. It is equally important, however, that the generated colonic model allows for a fully interactive 3D environment. When a potential polyp is detected during the automated fly-through, the reader can disengage from the centerline and manually navigate around the polyp for full assessment. Stepping though a set of predetermined 3D images is not acceptable and precludes full evaluation. Once a potential polyp is detected, bookmarking is an integral tool that allows a reader to create a list of potential polyps that need to be further evaluated (Fig. 19-3). Ultimately, the bookmarks can be whittled down to the true polyps after appropriate characterization.

The centerline also allows precise distance measurements from the anorectal junction (if there are not confounding segments of collapse or fluid columns markedly altering measurements). In our opinion, these distances are more helpful in determining the total

length of the colon as opposed to documenting specific polyp locations. Polyp locations are better reported by placement in one of the six named segments (e.g., cecum, ascending, transverse, descending, sigmoid, and rectum) as opposed to a distance measurement from the anorectal junction. Although this centerline measurement is accurate, it does not directly correlate with the distance from the anal verge measured at colonoscopy and thus may cause confusion if reported out. Colonoscopic measurements may be only half the distance of the CTC centerline measurements of the colon because of telescoping of the bowel over the endoscope. For example, a polyp seen at a 120 cm centerline measurement from the anorectal junction at CTC may be seen at 60 cm at colonoscopy. The centerline measurement is more useful for assessing total colonic length. We consider a measurement of colonic length greater than 200 cm at CTC to be elongated, and it correlates with increased frequency of incomplete colo-

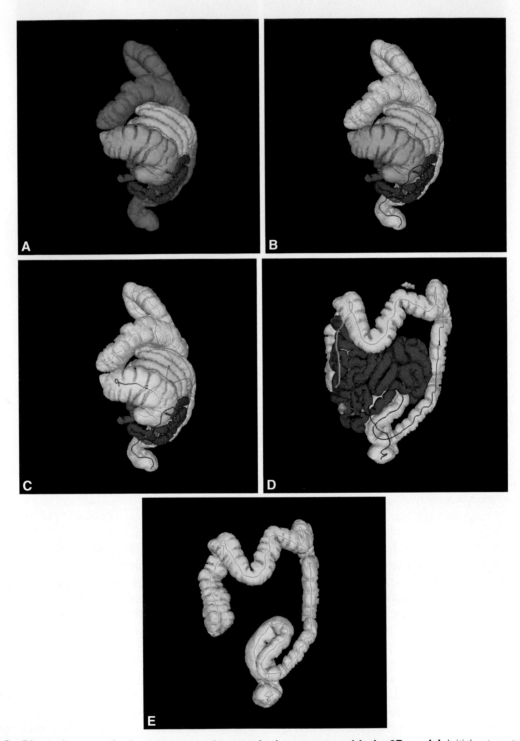

Figure 19-2 Discontinuous colonic segments and extracolonic segments with the 3D model. Initial automated 3D map **(A)** demonstrates discontinuous colonic segments *(right colon demarcated in blue and the remainder of the colon in green)* that need to be connected to complete the 3D model. In this case, the discontinuity is due to a hairpin turn of fluid filling the lumen at the hepatic flexure. Stitching together the colon **(B** and **C)** should be easily accomplished. Exclusion of extracolonic segments from a second case *(small bowel in red and blue; stomach in yellow;* **D)** should also be easy to undertake, resulting in the final 3D colonic model **(E).**

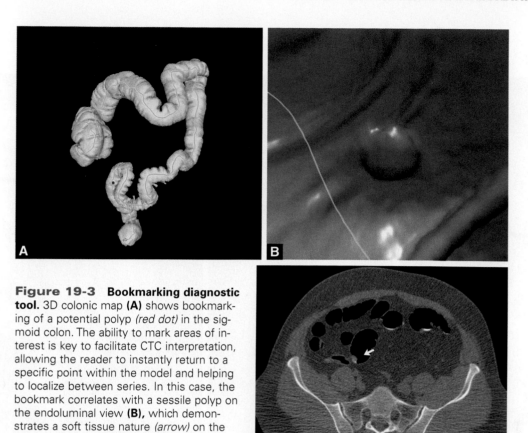

Figure 19-3 Bookmarking diagnostic tool. 3D colonic map **(A)** shows bookmarking of a potential polyp *(red dot)* in the sigmoid colon. The ability to mark areas of interest is key to facilitate CTC interpretation, allowing the reader to instantly return to a specific point within the model and helping to localize between series. In this case, the bookmark correlates with a sessile polyp on the endoluminal view **(B),** which demonstrates a soft tissue nature *(arrow)* on the 2D transverse view **(C).** A 7-mm tubular adenoma was removed at colonoscopy.

noscopy (Fig. 19-4).[1] Such information is potentially helpful for patients screened by CTC, where positive results needing colonoscopy in redundant colons may need additional measures to ensure success, such as a different endoscope or an operator with greater skill.

Tracking 3D Mucosal Coverage

Accurate tracking of colonic mucosal coverage at 3D is an important function of an endoluminal CTC viewing system (Figs. 19-5 through 19-8). Such tracking tools give important feedback to the reader during the detection phase of the interpretation. A software platform should allow for a continuous update of the visualized endoluminal surface. Typically, this is reported as a percent of visualized surface voxels in relation to the total endoluminal surface. On average, a unidirectional fly-through displays approximately 75% of the colonic mucosal surface when the FOV is set at 90 degrees (Figs. 19-5 and 19-6).[2] This amount of mucosal coverage at CTC is increased by nearly 20% with the addition of the fly-through in the opposite direction and can be further increased by review of the remaining patches of nonvisualized mucosa. This "missed patch" tool allows a reader to quickly click though these areas (Figs. 19-5 and 19-7). Typically, this adds only 20 to

30 seconds to the interpretation.[2] In practice, patches less than 300 mm^2 are ignored because significant polyps are very unlikely to be wholly contained within this small area of nonvisualized mucosa. Using this tool increases the amount of mucosa seen to 98% but only rarely uncovers polyps not seen during centerline navigation (Fig. 19-8). Color coding directly on the 3D view is very helpful to assess whether an area has been examined or not (Figs. 19-6 through 19-8).

Tracking mucosal coverage allows a reader to gauge that the examination was adequately evaluated by excluding the possibility that large areas of colonic mucosa remain unviewed. Contrast this to the case of optical colonoscopy, where visualization of the colonic mucosa is done mainly during withdrawal of the endoscope after cecal intubation. CTC would suggest that such an approach would leave nearly one fourth of the mucosa unexamined, correlating with the single retrograde CTC fly-though from rectum to cecum. Obviously, the situations do not completely equate because folds may be effaced somewhat at OC to increase mucosal visualization and retroflexion of the scope is possible. However, the potential implications from decreased coverage at OC may account for the increase in OC miss rates for large polyps from 6% at tandem colonoscopic studies to 12%

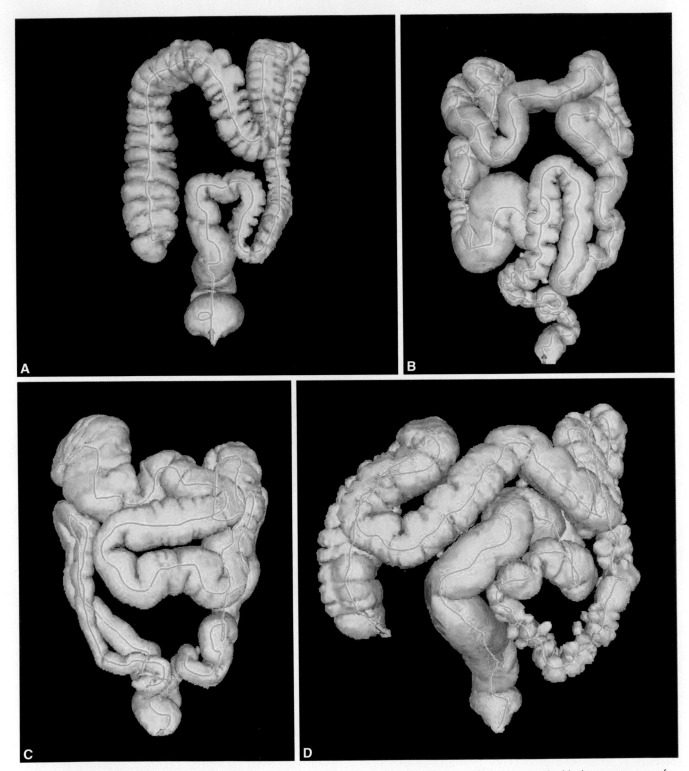

Figure 19-4   Colonic length and the 3D map. 3D colon map of a normal length colon **(A)** is compared with the appearance of the large intestine in three patients sent to CTC following incomplete colonoscopy **(B-D).** Note the increased length and tortuosity of the colon in the patients with incomplete OC. The 3D colon map is useful at depicting overall colonic anatomy and for documenting the location of abnormalities along its length.

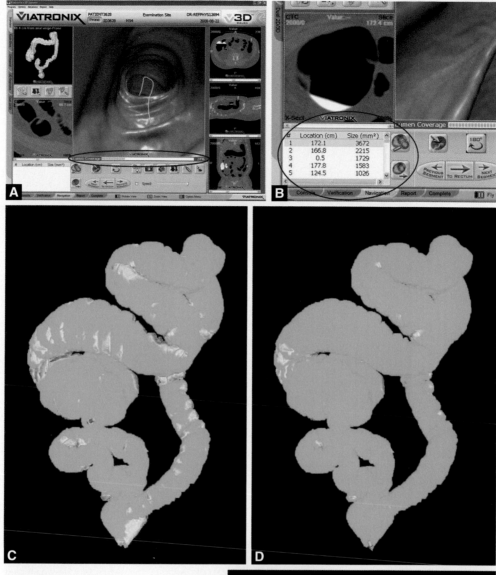

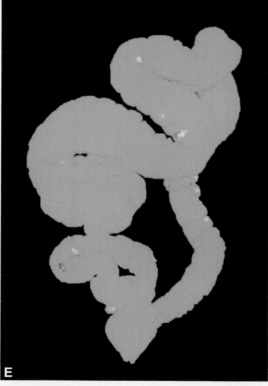

Figure 19-5 Tracking of mucosal coverage. Navigation pane **(A)** from the Viatronix V3D colon platform shows the percentage of visualized mucosa *(red oval)* on a continually updating basis. Such knowledge is important to provide feed-back to the reader so that large areas of colon are not missed. Magnified view **(B)** of the navigation pane mucosa shows the missed patch tool *(red oval),* which can be used following endoluminal fly-through to visualize the patches not seen during 3D centerline navigation. 3D map with color coding shows the visualized mucosa (painted as green; 70% coverage in this case) at unidirectional retrograde fly-through with a 90-degree FOV **(C),** the amount seen after bidirectional fly-though **(D,** 95% coverage in this case) and after use of the missed patch tool **(E).** Typically, 98% to 99% of the mucosa is visualized after use of the missed patch tool.

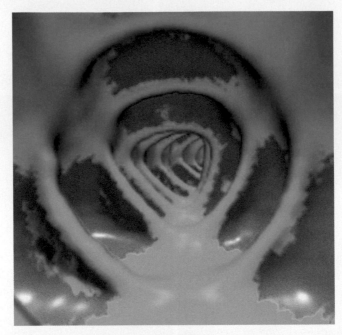

Figure 19-6 Colonic surface seen at unidirectional fly-through. 3D endoluminal view (90-degree FOV), with the paint function on depicts the areas not seen following unidirectional fly-through from the rectum to the cecum. The green areas are the portions of the visualized colon, and the unpainted orange areas represent the areas not seen. Typically, about 25% of the mucosa is not seen with a unidirectional fly-through with a 90-degree FOV, but this can increase with underdistention and crowding of haustra. Note that these areas correspond to the backsides of the colonic folds that may not be fully evaluated at optical colonoscopy.

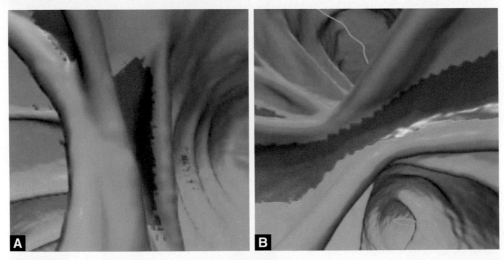

Figure 19-7 Missed patch tool. Use of the missed patch tool is helpful to evaluate areas not seen during the standard endoluminal fly-throughs. 3D endoluminal view **(A)** generated from clicking through the missed patches shows a typical unpainted orange area deep between two crowded haustra at the inner turn of a flexure. Similar unseen area is identified with the missed patch tool in a second patient **(B).** Note that these areas can be difficult to assess at colonoscopy.

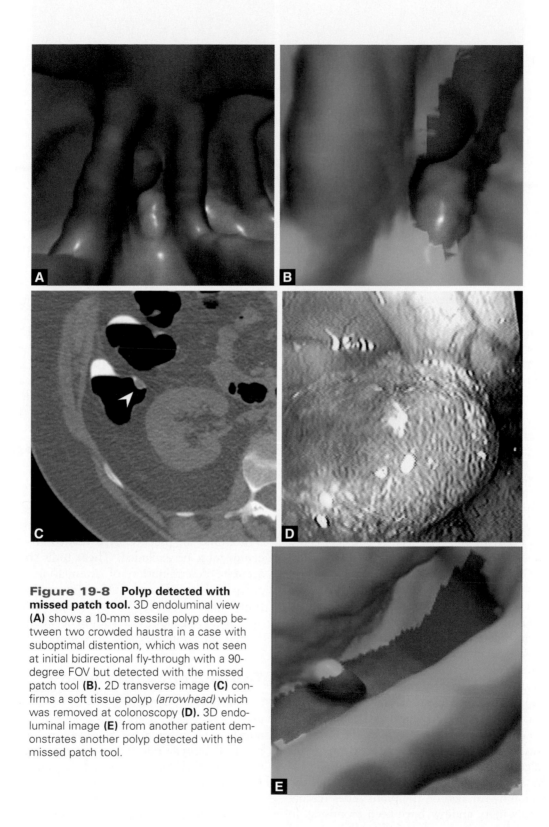

Figure 19-8   Polyp detected with missed patch tool. 3D endoluminal view **(A)** shows a 10-mm sessile polyp deep between two crowded haustra in a case with suboptimal distention, which was not seen at initial bidirectional fly-through with a 90-degree FOV but detected with the missed patch tool **(B)**. 2D transverse image **(C)** confirms a soft tissue polyp *(arrowhead)* which was removed at colonoscopy **(D)**. 3D endoluminal image **(E)** from another patient demonstrates another polyp detected with the missed patch tool.

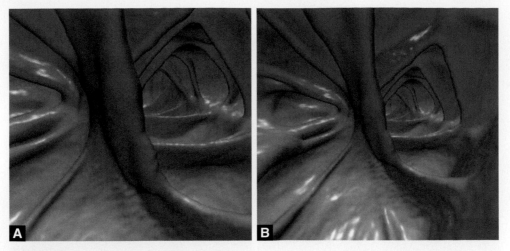

Figure 19-9   90-degree versus 120-degree FOV angle. 3D endoluminal view **(A)** at 90-degree FOV depicts the ileocecal valve in the center of the image. Note the increased coverage with a 120-degree FOV **(B)** where more of the cecal apex *(lefthand side of image)* and ascending colon *(righthand side)* is seen. Increased coverage, however, is at the expense of mild distortion at the periphery of the image.

when CTC is used as the reference standard.[3,4] In addition, tracking mucosal coverage at CTC allows an individual to easily resume an interrupted interpretation. This tool allows a reader to quickly determine what has already been evaluated and what remains for completion, as opposed to restarting the interrupted evaluation from the beginning.

Expanded FOV and Alternative 3D Displays

Expanded field of view (FOV) is a diagnostic tool that increases the amount of mucosal coverage with the purpose of decreasing time of interpretation related to an endoluminal fly-through. Traditionally, the default FOV angle for endoluminal CTC fly-through has been 90 degrees in both the vertical and horizontal planes or 127 degrees on the diagonal plane. Such an FOV angle allows for evaluation without any distortion. However, bidirectional fly-throughs are required for complete colonic coverage. An expanded FOV angle of 120 degrees increases mucosal coverage with the tradeoff of introducing distortion into the image. This expanded FOV essentially flattens and peels back the folds, allowing for increased visualization with the potential of decreasing the total number of fly-throughs from four to two (Fig. 19-9). With a unidirectional fly-though, nearly 90% of the mucosa is seen on average with a 120-degree FOV angle, increasing to 98%-99% with a bidirection approach.[5] Such coverage has led to the investigation of interpretation algorithms where a single fly-though is completed for the supine series (rectum to cecum) and the opposite direction fly-through on the prone series (cecum to rectum). Preliminary findings have been promising. In one study, 104 polyps initially identified on bidirectional fly-through at 90 degrees were all detectable with unidirectional at 120-degree evaluation on either the retrograde

supine or antegrade prone fly-through, with 83% of the polyps seen on both views.[5]

Similarly, the purpose of alternative 3D displays such as the perspective filet and unfolded cube views is to decrease interpretation times (see Chapter 23). Although mucosal coverage is increased, distortion and the introduction of artifacts are also increased, creating important potential pitfalls.

DIAGNOSTIC TOOLS FOR POLYP CONFIRMATION

A set of diagnostic tools is needed to allow easy application of strategies for polyp confirmation. Once a potential polyp is detected, it needs to be further characterized and all pseudopolyps related to stool or other causes must be excluded. These tools should allow for accurate determination of attenuation of a potential polyp in both 3D and 2D environments and seamless transition between the 3D views and the 2D source images, including facile localization between a point on the 3D model, 2D images, and 3D colonic map.

Translucency Rendering

Translucency rendering is a 3D diagnostic tool that gives attenuation information regarding the internal matrix of an interrogated 3D structure.[6] There is an element of transparency to look deep to the rendered surface combined with a color-coded attenuation map (Fig. 19-10). This tool allows for quick assessment of a polypoid structure at 3D (i.e., does it appear to have a soft tissue attenuation core possibly representing a true polyp or a dense contrast-impregnated or airy center suggesting stool?). Without such a tool, interpretation may become tedious if, for example, the colon is poorly cleansed (Fig.

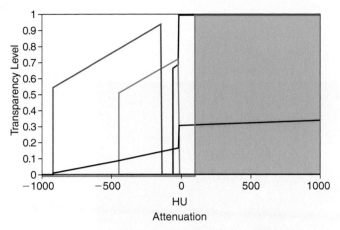

Figure 19-10 Translucency function at CTC. Graph depicting various color assignments and level of transparency *(black line)* as a function of attenuation (in Hounsfield units) for translucency rendering. Transparency level of 1 is opaque, whereas level of 0 is transparent. Blue, green, red, and white (pictured as gray on the graph) assignments correspond to increasing attenuation values. Red color assignment is centered at soft tissue attenuation levels. Above a threshold of 200 HU, the color assignment of white is made for tagged stool. (From Pickhardt PJ. Translucency rendering in 3D endoluminal CT colonography: A useful tool for increasing polyp specificity and decreasing interpretation time. *Am J Roentgenol.* 2004;183(2):429-436.)

19-11). This tool helps to decrease interpretation times by reducing the need to consult the 2D source images to determine attenuation characteristics for every polypoid lesion seen on 3D.

The color coding is arbitrary. The predominant system in use utilizes red for soft tissue attenuation values, white for very high attenuation values (threshold set higher than 200 HU),[6] blue for very negative values such as air, and green for negative values in the fat attenuation range (Fig. 19-10). Application of the translucency function aids in polyp characterization, although ultimate confirmation at the 2D level is needed in most cases. The classic appearance of a soft tissue polyp is a solid red central core surrounded by concentric rings of green to shades of blue (Fig. 19-12). Tagged stool will present with white signal architecture where tagging agents have substantially raised the internal attenuation (Fig. 19-13). Untagged stool may have a range of appearances from a homogenous red soft tissue appearance indistinguishable from a true polyp to heterogenous lesions containing green and blue signals suggestive of fat and air (Fig. 19-14). Finally, colonic lipomas present with a homogeneous green center related to their fatty nature (Fig. 19-15).

Translucency is particularly helpful in the evaluation of the ileocecal valve (Fig. 19-16) because it is a lobulated structure with varied appearances. The application of translucency on the valve is often helpful where lobulated or focal projections that code purely green simply represent an innocuous lipoma or lipomatous component, whereas a focal red collection in an area of lobulation may represent a soft tissue polyp on the valve. In the latter case, further evaluation is warranted on the 2D images.

Although translucency is a helpful diagnostic tool to suggest the attenuation characteristics of polyp candidates at 3D, there are important pitfalls related to its use to be aware of, which are described in detail in Chapter 20. It is important to remember that ultimate determination of attenuation and polyp characterization is undertaken with the 2D source images.

Attenuation Tools at 2D

Attenuation assessment of a suspected polyp is a core task at 2D. Demonstration of internal homogenous soft tissue attenuation fulfills a critical criterion of a true polyp (the other major criterion is a fixed position with respect to the colon wall). Although translucency rendering at 3D can suggest the soft tissue nature of a polyp candidate, the evaluation on the 2D source image determines whether it truly is a soft tissue polyp. Diagnostic tools to allow this assessment are typically present with basic level PACS functionality. These tools include application of various window width and level settings, and ROI (region of interest) measurements to the 2D images. The standard polyp window/level setting is 2000/0 HU. It allows a reader to differentiate soft tissue and fat without obscuring small soft tissue polyps (Fig. 19-17). Choosing an abdominal soft tissue setting (e.g., window/level of 350/40 HU) may be helpful in some instances to confirm the soft tissue nature of a polyp but may accentuate artifactual heterogeneity related to the low-dose technique (see Chapter 20). ROI measurements allow for specific Hounsfield unit determination of a suspected polyp, but in general only a qualitative comparison against the psoas muscle or other internal standard is needed. Other basic 2D tools such as pan and zoom functions, multiplanar reformation (MPR) evaluation, and stack-mode cine viewing are required to adequately evaluate the 2D source data.

Tools for Localizing Between Different Displays

Besides soft tissue attenuation determination, the ability to localize a structure or point on different displays—whether between 2D and 3D environments or between supine or prone positions—is a necessity. Confirming a potential lesion on different positions allows the reader to determine whether a soft tissue structure is fixed in position within the colon (and thus a potential polyp) or is mobile (and thus stool). Diagnostic tools should allow a reader to easily undertake this task. Although all transitions between the various series are important, the most important one from a primary 3D interpretive approach

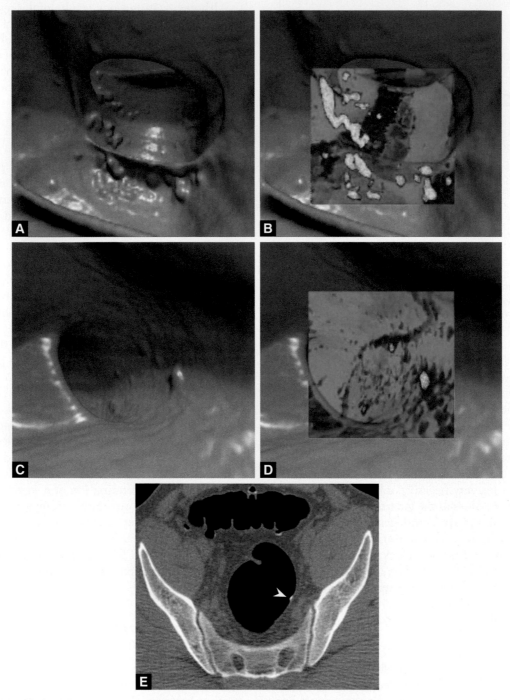

Figure 19-11 Residual stool and translucency rendering. Translucency rendering can be helpful to suggest the attenuation characteristics of polypoid structures at 3D. 3D endoluminal view **(A)** shows multiple polypoid lesions. Translucency **(B)** can quickly demonstrate that this simply represents retained tagged stool in a somewhat poorly cleansed colon. 3D endoluminal image in another patient **(C)** shows a potential small polyp. However, translucency **(D)** quickly suggests a pseudopolyp related to tagged stool, which is easily confirmed on the transverse 2D image **(E,** *arrowhead*).

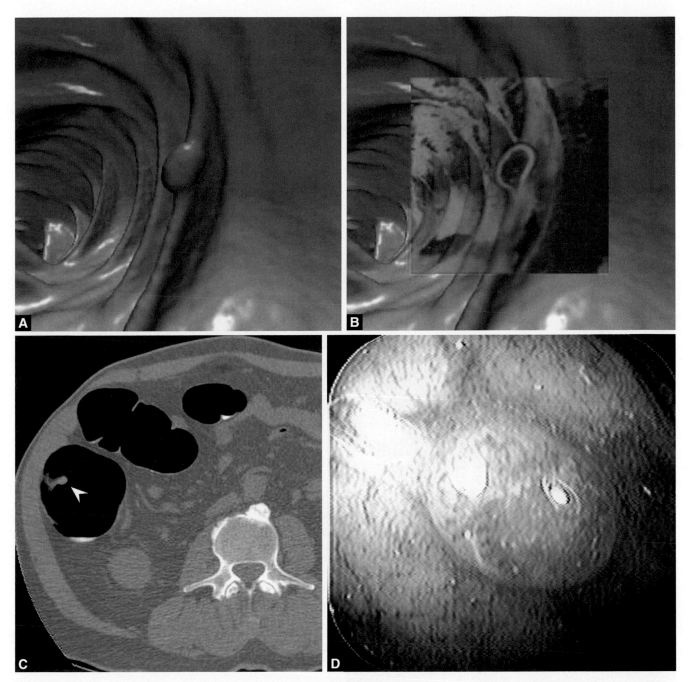

Figure 19-12   Soft tissue polyp with translucency rendering. 3D endoluminal image **(A)** shows a sessile polyp projecting off a colonic fold in the ascending colon. Application of translucency rendering **(B)** depicts the color signature of a soft tissue polyp with a red signal core surrounded by a green to blue halo. 2D transverse image **(C)** confirms a soft tissue lesion (*arrowhead*). A 9-mm tubular adenoma was removed at colonoscopy **(D)**.

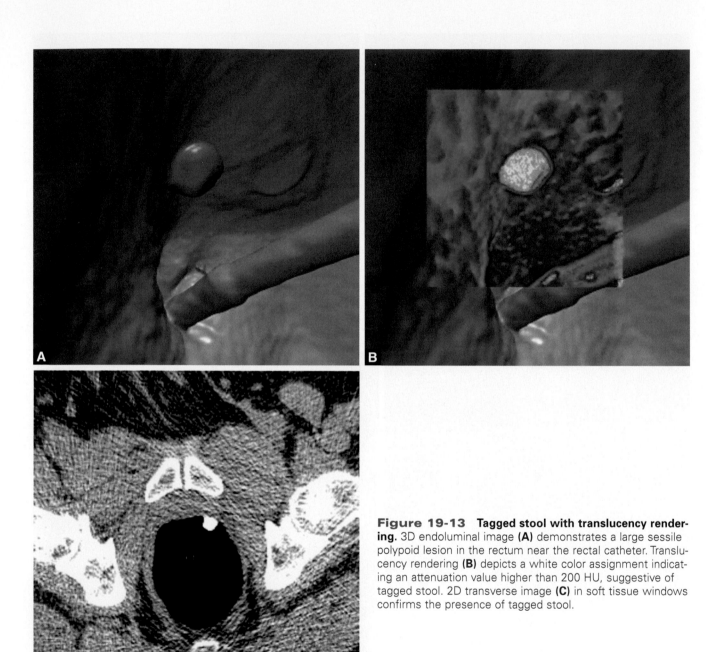

Figure 19-13 Tagged stool with translucency rendering. 3D endoluminal image **(A)** demonstrates a large sessile polypoid lesion in the rectum near the rectal catheter. Translucency rendering **(B)** depicts a white color assignment indicating an attenuation value higher than 200 HU, suggestive of tagged stool. 2D transverse image **(C)** in soft tissue windows confirms the presence of tagged stool.

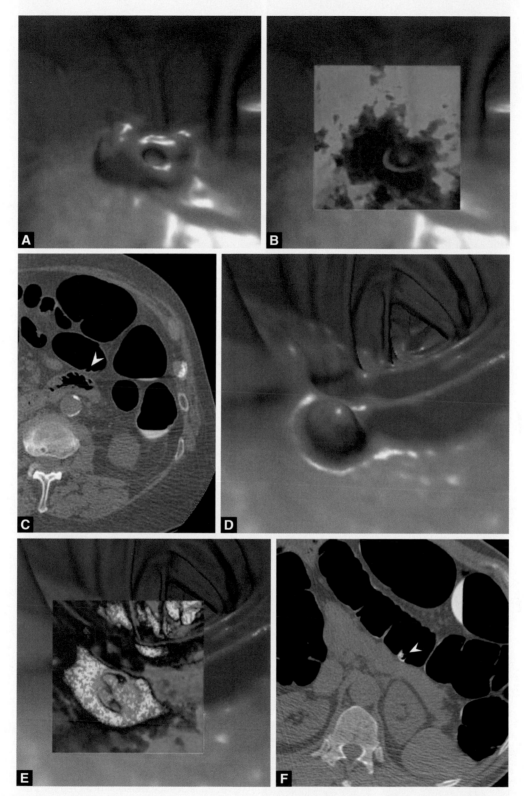

Figure 19-14   Untagged stool at translucency. Untagged stool can have a variety of appearances. 3D endoluminal image **(A)** shows an unusually shaped polypoid structure in the colon. Translucency **(B)** demonstrates red signal consistent with attenuation values in the soft tissue range but also an internal region of lower attenuation that is incompatible with a true polyp. Untagged stool with an air bubble is confirmed at 2D (**C,** *arrowhead*). In addition, there was movement of this polyp candidate between supine and prone positions consistent with stool (not shown). 3D endoluminal view **(D)** in another patient demonstrate a large polypoid structure, which represents poorly tagged stool that contains air and fat densities giving a blue and green appearance **(E)** sitting within a pool of tagged fluid. 2D transverse view **(F)** in the decubitus position confirms the translucency findings *(arrowhead).* Adherent stool is almost always well tagged with our contrast regimen, whereas mobile stool is sometimes untagged but never a diagnostic dilemma.

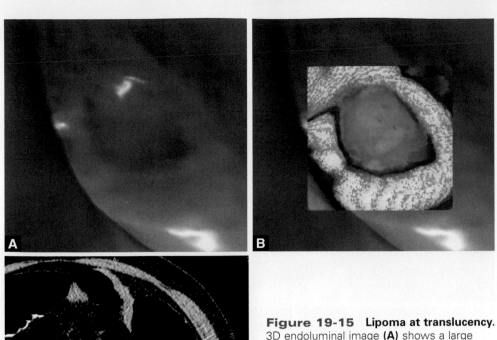

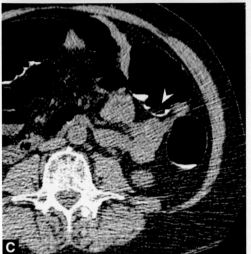

Figure 19-15 Lipoma at translucency.
3D endoluminal image **(A)** shows a large broad-based sessile polyp in the distal transverse colon. Translucency rendering **(B)** depicts the characteristic appearance of a lipoma with a green core. This lipoma is seen partially submerged in a tagged fluid pool *(white areas)*. 2D transverse image **(C)** in soft tissue windows confirms the lipoma *(arrowhead)* within the tagged fluid pool.

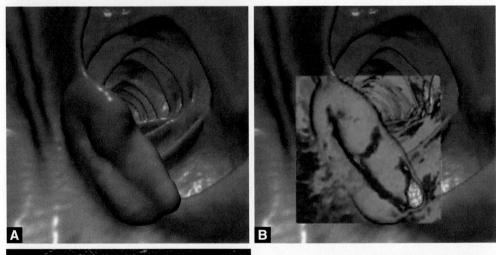

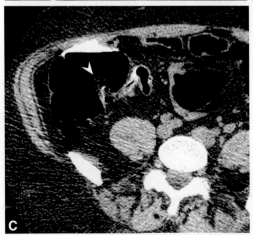

Figure 19-16 Lipomatous ileocecal valve. The ileocecal valve is often lobulated with focal projections. 3D endoluminal view **(A)** shows a potential polyp projecting off the valve. Translucency **(B)** depicts a green signature throughout the ileocecal valve including the focal projection consistent with a lipomatous valve. Note the value of translucency application on the valve. 2D transverse image **(C)** in soft tissue windows confirms the fatty nature of the valve and the focal projection *(arrowhead)*. If there had been red color assignment corresponding to the focal projection, suspicion for a true polyp protruding off the valve should be raised and appropriate 2D evaluation then should be undertaken.

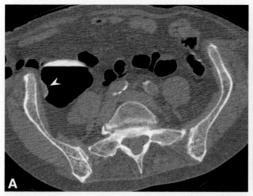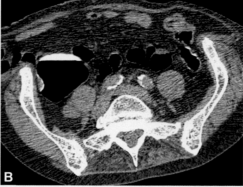

Figure 19-17 **Window width and level settings.** 2D tools include basic functions such as the ability to quickly change window and level settings. 2D transverse image **(A)** in polyp window setting shows a sessile polyp *(arrowhead)* in the cecum. The same image **(B)** in soft tissue window setting allows for increased distinction between soft tissue, positive oral contrast, and fat but at the expense of increased heterogeneity, which may cause incorrect assignment of the polyp as poorly tagged stool. This lesion was a tubulovillous adenoma. The use of soft tissue settings may also obscure small polyps.

involves localizing the position of a detected polyp on 3D within the 2D image (Fig. 19-18). If the diagnostic tool set does not allow a reader to easily implement this task, it is difficult to use a primary 3D approach. Unfortunately, the majority of CTC workstations have difficulty with this process because they were built for a primary 2D detection paradigm. Thus, they do well at localizing the 3D location of a detected 2D polyp candidate but often cannot do the reverse task well.

DIAGNOSTIC TOOLS FOR POLYP MEASUREMENT

Once a true polyp is confirmed, accurate measurement is a key task because subsequent management decisions are primarily based on size. Diagnostic tools should allow accurate measurements to be obtained for both 3D and 2D MPR displays. Currently, linear measurements are the accepted convention, although automated volume measurements may eventually replace linear measurements in the future.

Manual Measurement of Linear Size

Measurement tools must be present on the CTC viewing platform to allow for accurate sizing of a polyp. Measurements should be easily accomplished in both the 3D and 2D realms. In addition, the orientation of the orthogonal 2D images in relation to the polyp seen on the 3D views must be easily ascertained to allow correct "weighting" of the 2D measurements (Fig. 19-19). The "optimized" orthogonal 2D view used for measurement can undersize the true length of the polyp because the long axis may not orient perfectly along one of the orthogonal views. Therefore, 2D measurements represent a lower limit of polyp size, ranging from underestimation up to true size—but not an overestimate.

Accurate measurement at 3D requires that the polyp is positioned so that it is viewed "head-on" and not "down the barrel" of the colonic lumen. Consequently, the reader must be able to independently maneuver within the 3D environment. Again, stepping through preset views is not acceptable. Once in proper 3D endoluminal position, care must be taken to place the electronic calipers at the edges of the polyps without inclusion of the polyp shadow or penumbra. Viewing the polyp at an angle down the length of the colon is likely to result in erroneous measurements. Several measurements obtained at the correct viewing angles and in both the supine and prone series help to increase accuracy. In actual practice, this is truly important only when the polyp resides near a critical threshold (e.g., between a diminutive 5-mm lesion and a small 6-mm polyp or between the small/large dividing point at 9-10 mm). It is important to note that 3D measurements can falsely overestimate the size of a polyp if there is a substantial coating of contrast. In these cases, appropriate "downsizing" of the polyp based on the 2D views is needed (Fig. 19-20). Alternatively, a polyp that is partially submerged in residual luminal fluid can be undersized on the 3D view. The 2D display will also provide a better measurement in this scenario.

Accurate measurement at 2D requires viewing in the orthogonal plane that most closely aligns with the long axis of polyp (if sessile) or polyp head (if pedunculated). Tools should allow the images to be magnified, and electronic calipers should be placed at the edge of the polyp on this "optimized" 2D view. The degree to which the long axis of the polyp aligns to the 2D orthogonal view determines whether the measurement is equivalent or underestimates the corresponding 3D measurement (Fig. 19-19). For example, if the 3D measurement of a polyp was 20 mm but the optimized 2D measurement was only 15 mm, it would be important to note that the optimized 2D slice imaged obliquely to the polyp long axis. This would suggest that the polyp is closer to 20 mm than 15 mm. Most but not all phantom and in vivo studies

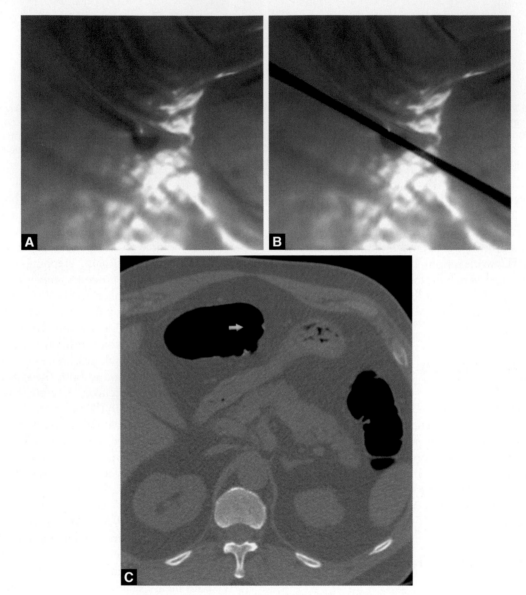

Figure 19-18 **Localization of 3D polypoid lesion on the 2D display.** Diagnostic tools should allow quick, easy performance of this task; otherwise, a primary 3D interpretation strategy will be severely hampered. 3D endoluminal image **(A)** demonstrates a small polypoid lesion in the transverse colon. The ability to ascertain the 2D correlate confidently and quickly is paramount. The V3D colon platform undertakes this task by displaying a red line corresponding to the slice level and orientation of the slice on the 3D image **(B)** as the reader scrolls through the 2D images. Once the red line intersects the polyp, the level of the 2D transverse slice is determined. The arrow points to the direction of the viewed 3D image to allow for identification of the 3D finding on the 2D image **(C).**

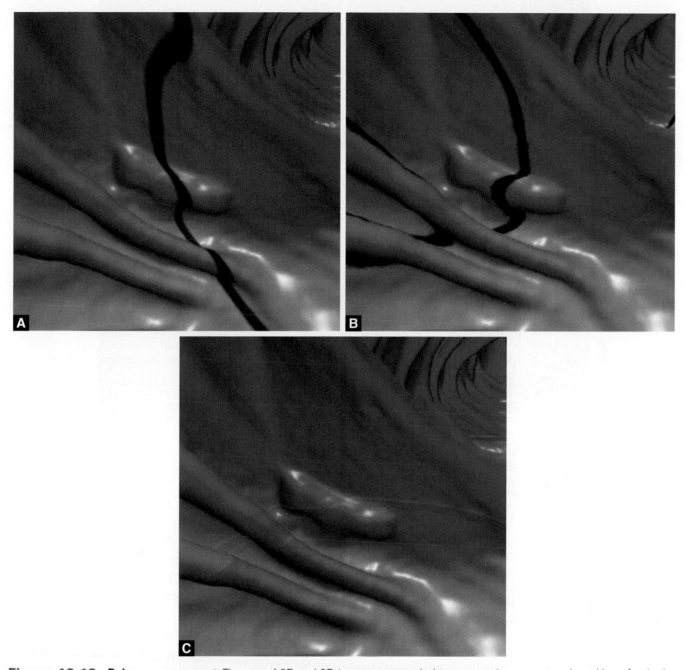

Figure 19-19   Polyp measurement. The use of 3D and 2D images are needed to accurately measure polyps. Use of only the orthogonal 2D images will systematically undersize polyps because the long axis of a polyp will not always match one of the standard orthogonal views. For example, if measurement of the polyp in this case was done on the 2D orthogonal series, it would be grossly undersized. 3D endoluminal views **(A-C)** of this polyp nicely demonstrate the reason. The transverse slice **(A,** *red line*) and coronal slice **(B,** *blue line*) cut through the short axis of the polyp. However, even the "optimized" orthogonal view of the sagittal orientation **(C,** *green line*) undersizes the polyp where it is obliquely measured. For this particular case, the measurement at 3D would be more accurate.

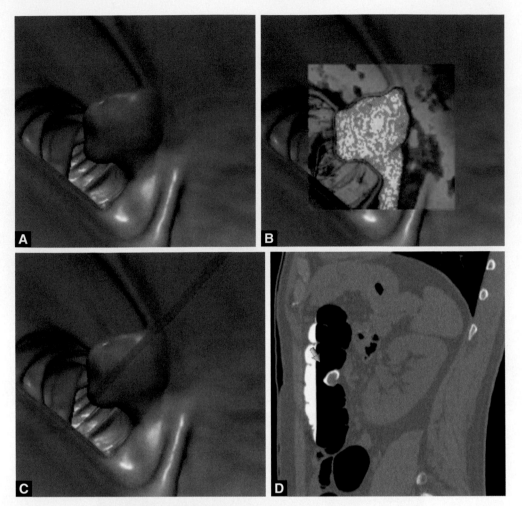

Figure 19-20 Downsizing 3D measurement as a result of contrast coat. 3D endoluminal view **(A)** shows a large polyp. Translucency **(B)**, however, suggests a contrast coat. Measurement at 3D would thus artificially increase the polyp size. The green line on the 3D view **(C)** demarcating the optimal 2D orientation shows that the long axis of the contrast-covered polyp parallels well the sagittal orthogonal view. Measurement excluding the contrast on the 2D sagittal view **(D)** would be the most accurate measurement for this case. *(*See associated video clip in DVD.)*

have shown that the 3D measurements are more accurate than the 2D measurements overall.[7,8]

In practice, both sets of measurements (with appropriate 2D "weighting") are needed to increase precision and accuracy. That is, both 2D and 3D polyp measurements need to be considered to gain a sense of the true size of a polyp. To reiterate, this is truly important only when the size of a polyp is at a critical boundary (e.g., between 5 and 6 mm or 9 and 10 mm). Ultimately, volume measurements may substitute longest linear measurements. Particularly for the issue of surveillance of small unresected polyps, volume measurements better depict small incremental changes.[9] For subcentimeter polyps that closely approximate hemispheric volumes of the same diameter, a 1-mm-diameter change in a hemispheric polyp results in a relative change of 31% to 53% in volume but only 11% to 18% in linear size (a roughly 3:1 ratio). Automated or semiautomated segmentation and volume measurements may eventually play a larger role in assessing interval change in small polyps under CTC surveillance (Fig. 19-21).

ADVANCED APPLICATIONS AND DIAGNOSTIC TOOLS

Electronic Fluid Cleansing (Digital Subtraction)

The electronic fluid cleansing diagnostic tool may help in some reading paradigms. This software programming process electronically subtracts the high-density residual tagged colonic fluid to digitally "cleanse" the colon. Some systems accomplish this task by use of a segmentation ray technique to address the partial volume averaging effects that occur at specific interfaces between air, fluid, and bowel wall. After addressing these interfaces, the tagged material is subsequently subtracted by simple thresholding.[10] The primary purpose of digital subtraction is to uncover soft tissue polyps hidden within the colonic pool (Fig. 19-22). If not undertaken, a polyp would be obscured on that particular 3D fly-though view. It is important to remember, however, that the polyp would likely be seen on the complementary fly-through

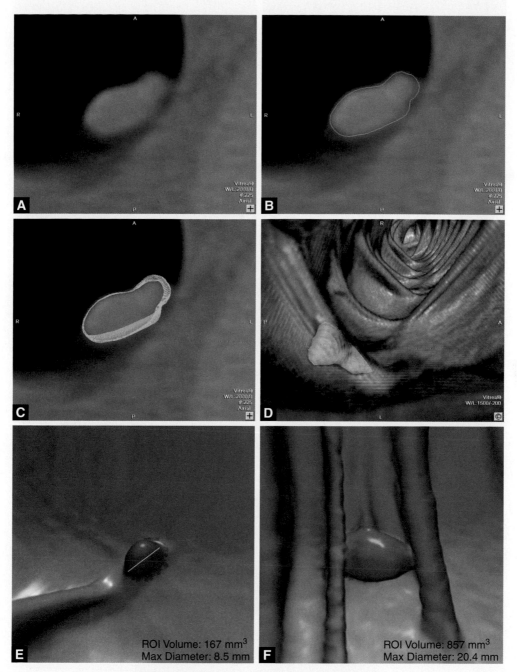

ROI Volume: 167 mm³
Max Diameter: 8.5 mm

ROI Volume: 857 mm³
Max Diameter: 20.4 mm

Figure 19-21 **Volume measurement tools.** Ultimately, volume measurements may be the most sensitive and accurate way to assess for interval change. 2D transverse images **(A-C)** show manual segmentation of a polyp for semiautomated volume calculation. 2D transverse image **(A)** of a tubulovillous adenoma is seen in the ascending colon prior to segmentation. The border for segmentation can be manually drawn by a mouse-driven stylus on each image the polyp is seen **(B)**. The volume is subsequently calculated **(C)**. Endoluminal image **(D)** shows the lesion segmentation on 3D. In the future, more automated segmentation and volume measurements will be needed to allow quick and easy assessment. 3D endoluminal images **(E** and **F)** in two different patients show automated processes on the Viatronix V3D Colon platform where the polyp is segmented out and painted in purple with longest linear dimension and volume determined. Manual efforts involved are related to adjusting segmentation boundaries as needed. (Figs. A-D from Pickhardt PJ, Lehman VT, Winter TC, Taylor AJ. Polyp volume versus linear size measurements at CT colonography: Implications for noninvasive surveillance of unresected colorectal lesions. *Am J Roentgenol.* 2006;186(6):1605-1610.)

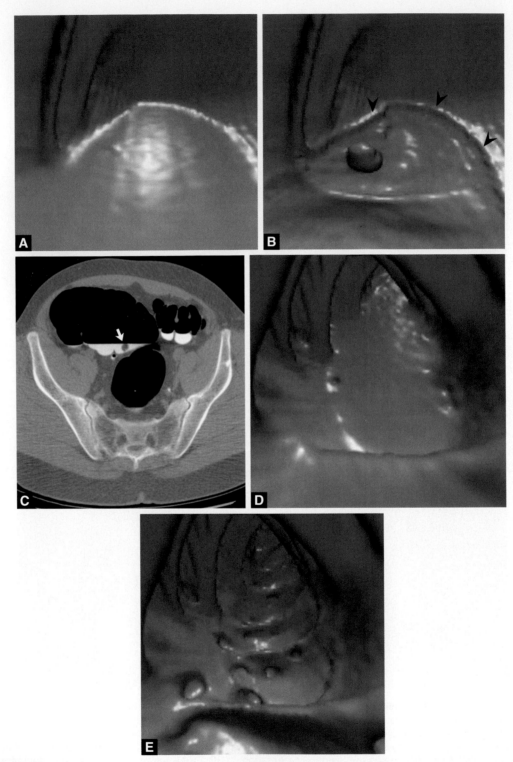

Figure 19-22 Electronic cleansing. 3D endoluminal view **(A)** demonstrates the surface of a residual colonic pool. Electronic subtraction techniques **(B)** can allow removal of the tagged fluid to allow visualization of a submerged polyp. Note the "bathtub ring" artifact *(arrowheads)* on this postprocessed image. Although such processes may be helpful for some readers, remember that the submerged polyp *(arrowhead)* would be seen on the 2D series **(C)** and also very likely seen on the opposite position fly-through as a result of the shifting of fluid. Note that digital subtraction is neither necessary nor indicated on the 2D display for polyp detection. 3D endoluminal view **(D)** in another patient reveals scattered diverticula hidden in the residual colonic pool following electronic cleansing **(E)**. *(*See associated video clip in DVD.)*

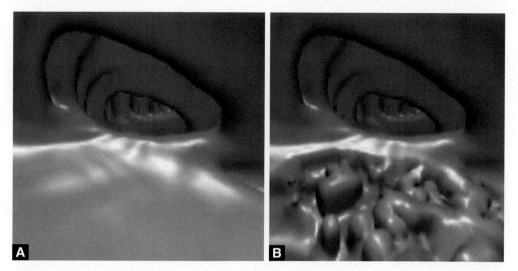

Figure 19-23 **Artifact related to electronic cleansing.** 3D endoluminal view before **(A)** and after **(B)** electronic cleansing results in bizarre polypoid structures that represent subtraction artifacts. This is the downside of electronic cleansing where this post-processing of the data leads to another level of artifacts that could potentially decrease sensitivity and specificity. (From Pickhardt PJ, Choi JHR. Electronic cleansing and stool tagging in CT colonography: Advantages and pitfalls with primary three-dimensional evaluation. *Am J Roentgenol.* 2003;181(3):799-805.)

as the fluid would shift away on that series and also would be apparent on both 2D series. It is also critical to keep the 2D images untainted by digital subtraction because any artifacts created by electronic cleansing on 3D need to be compared against the unsubtracted source images.

Unfortunately, electronic fluid cleansing creates a number of artifacts that interfere with time-efficient 3D fly-through evaluation. In addition to a bathtub ring artifact (which is not too distracting), incomplete subtraction can cause bizarre polypoid structures in place of a smooth fluid pool (Fig. 19-23). Untagged stool and trapped air bubbles within the colonic pool and air–fluid interface artifacts often cause pseudopolyps that require additional investigation time to exclude a true soft tissue polyp (see Chapter 20).

In our opinion, electronic fluid cleansing clearly is not beneficial to the overall interpretation and probably should not be used, unless completely devoid of artifacts. Early in our experience we did use it, but the artifacts that were created caused more problems than solutions. It also required readers to decrease the speed of the fly-through to decipher the artifacts, and it required additional 2D correlation for a number of pseudolesions. The redundancy of our interpretative technique allows polyps that are submerged on one view to be detected on one of the many other views, and the lack of subtraction allows more time-efficient interpretation of the endoluminal views.

Computer-Aided Detection/ Diagnosis

Another advanced diagnostic tool is computer-aided detection/diagnosis (CAD). Like digital subtraction, CAD is not intrinsically required for full functionality of a CTC operating platform. CAD modules use software algorithms to detect specific patterns within the CT dataset to point out a potential polyp (Fig. 19-24). Whether this tool is ultimately beneficial for effective interpretation in clinical practice remains to be seen. It does hold the potential to help some readers achieve appropriate diagnostic sensitivity. Whether this is at the expense of decreased specificity or whether there is a true improvement in overall performance remains largely unknown. CAD is explored in greater detail in Chapter 24.

SUMMARY

The integrated 3D/2D interpretative strategy requires a CTC operating platform with a defined set of diagnostic tools. These tools allow specific tasks to be easily accomplished in both the 3D and 2D environments and allow for seamless transition between the two. If these tools and functionality are not present, the interpretive algorithm cannot be efficiently applied and the effectiveness of this approach diminishes.

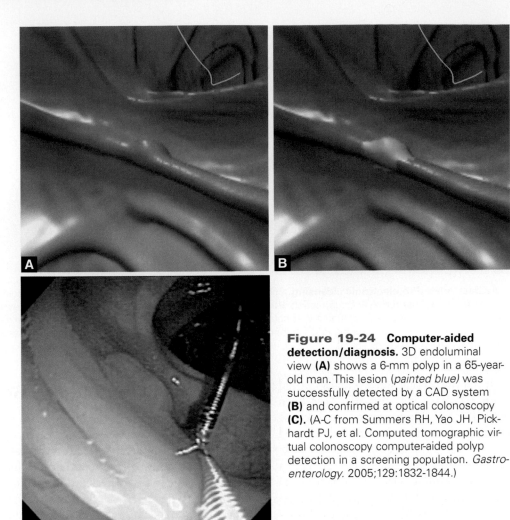

Figure 19-24 Computer-aided detection/diagnosis. 3D endoluminal view **(A)** shows a 6-mm polyp in a 65-year-old man. This lesion (*painted blue*) was successfully detected by a CAD system **(B)** and confirmed at optical colonoscopy **(C).** (A-C from Summers RH, Yao JH, Pickhardt PJ, et al. Computed tomographic virtual colonoscopy computer-aided polyp detection in a screening population. *Gastroenterology.* 2005;129:1832-1844.)

REFERENCES

1. Hanson ME, Pickhardt PJ, Kim DH, Pfau PR. Anatomic factors predictive of incomplete colonoscopy based on findings at CT colonography. *Am J Roentgenol.* 2007;189(4):774-779.

2. Pickhardt PJ, Taylor AJ, Gopal DV. Surface visualization at 3D endoluminal CT colonography: Degree of coverage and implications for polyp detection. *Gastroenterology.* 2006;130(6):1582-1587.

3. Rex DK, Cutler CS, Lemmel GT, et al. Colonoscopic miss rates of adenomas determined by back-to-back colonoscopies. *Gastroenterology.* 1997;112(1):24-28.

4. Pickhardt PJ, Nugent PA, Mysliwiec PA, Choi JR, Schindler WR. Location of adenomas missed by optical colonoscopy. *Ann Intern Med.* 2004;141(5):352-359.

5. Pickhardt PJ, Schumacher C, Kim DH. Polyp detection at 3D endoluminal CT colonography: Sensitivity of one-way flythrough at 120-degree field-of-view angle. *J Comp Assist Tomog.* 2009 [in press].

6. Pickhardt PJ. Translucency rendering in 3D endoluminal CT colonography: A useful tool for increasing polyp specificity and decreasing interpretation time. *Am J Roentgenol.* 2004;183 (2):429-436.

7. Pickhardt PJ, Lee AD, McFarland EG, Taylor AJ. Linear polyp measurement at CT colonography: In vitro and in vivo comparison of two-dimensional and three-dimensional displays. *Radiology.* 2005;236(3):872-878.

8. Yeshwant SC, Summers RM, Yao JH, Brickman DS, Choi JR, Pickhardt PJ. Polyps: Linear and volumetric measurement at CT colonography. *Radiology.* 2006;241(3):802-811.

9. Pickhardt PJ, Lehman VT, Winter TC, Taylor AJ. Polyp volume versus linear size measurements at CT colonography: Implications for noninvasive surveillance of unresected colorectal lesions. *Am J Roentgenol.* 2006;186(6):1605-1610.

10. Pickhardt PJ, Choi JHR. Electronic cleansing and stool tagging in CT colonography: Advantages and pitfalls with primary three-dimensional evaluation. *Am J Roentgenol.* 2003;181(3):799-805.

Potential Pitfalls at CTC Interpretation

PERRY J. PICKHARDT, MD
DAVID H. KIM, MD

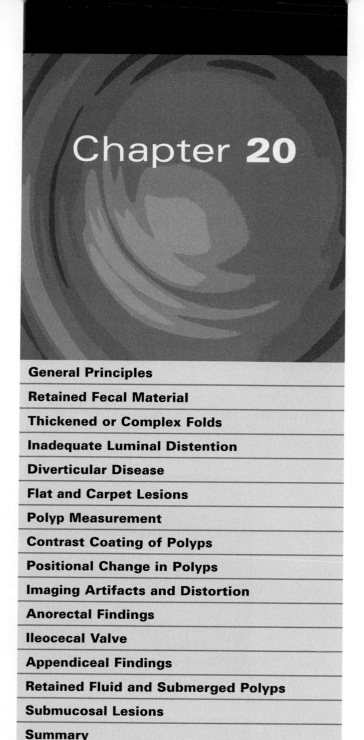

Chapter **20**

INTRODUCTION

There are a number of interpretive pitfalls at CT colonography (CTC) evaluation that need to be recognized and handled appropriately. The most critical step in learning to avoid these diagnostic traps is simply to be aware of their existence. With a little experience, most of these potential pitfalls will be easily recognized. This chapter will largely serve as an imaging atlas for demonstrating the appearance of these pitfalls, including tips and pointers on how to effectively handle them. In addition, many of the illustrated cases will have an associated video clip in the accompanying DVD, which is indicated by the "(video clip)" designation within the figure captions.

GENERAL PRINCIPLES

Some interpretive pitfalls at CTC, such as prominent folds and shifting of pedunculated polyps, present more of a problem on two-dimensional (2D) evaluation, whereas other pitfalls, such as submucosal lesions and stool-filled diverticula, are more of an issue on 3D evaluation. However, after biphasic assessment including both 2D and 3D evaluation, most of these pitfalls are easily recognized because of the complementary nature of these two imaging displays.

The long list of potential pitfalls at CTC covered herein may appear daunting at first glance, but these individual items can be rearranged into a just a handful of major categories. First, there are potential prep-related pitfalls, including retained stool, contrast coating of polyps, and submerged polyps. Second are the important pitfalls that largely result from sigmoid diverticular disease (albeit not exclusively), such as incomplete luminal distention and thickened folds. Additional pitfalls that are specific to diverticular disease include stool-filled diverticula and mucosal prolapse.

Third are potential pitfalls related to inherent morphologic characteristics of polyps, including flat lesions, carpet lesions, shifting of pedunculated polyps, and appropriate polyp measurement. Fourth are specific anatomic locations and structures that comprise a subset of potential pitfalls, including the anorectal region, the ileocecal valve, and the appendix. Finally, imaging-related artifacts and submucosal lesions comprise additional pitfall groups. The specific order in which individual pitfalls are discussed is intended to roughly reflect their relative difficulty, frequency, or perceived importance, in descending order.

RETAINED FECAL MATERIAL

Even with the use of a cathartic preparation, residual stool remains a major diagnostic challenge for CTC interpretation. Although laxatives generally clear out the major bulk of fecal volume, it is the smaller adherent debris that can cause problems by closely mimicking the appearance of soft tissue polyps (Fig. 20-1). Unlike larger collections of stool, adherent fecal material that mimics polyps often will not contain characteristic foci of air density. Large and/or formed stool balls are more of a nuisance at CTC and generally not an interpretive challenge because they are more easily recognized by their mottled low-density composition (Fig. 20-2) or clearly mobile nature (Fig. 20-3). However, bulky stool can also superficially resemble the appearance of large villous lesions on 3D (Fig. 20-4). The presence of a squared, faceted, or polygonal appearance is almost pathognomonic for retained stool but is infrequently seen and therefore is not an effective discriminator (Fig. 20-5).

Oral contrast tagging, particularly with CT-grade barium sulfate (2% w/v), is highly effective for internally labeling nonspecific residual adherent stool (Figs. 20-6 and 20-7), allowing for easy distinction from true polyps.[1,2] Translucency rendering can rapidly demonstrate internal tagging of fecal material at primary 3D evaluation (Figs. 20-6 and 20-7), but the 2D display provides the most definitive assessment in equivocal cases. Some CTC systems (e.g., Viatronix V3D) allow for manual marking of tagged stool during rapid 2D review to avoid the need for repeated interrogation at 3D evaluation (Fig. 20-8). Ionic iodinated water-soluble contrast agents (diatrizoate), although indispensable for fluid tagging and secondary catharsis, may not provide adequate internal tagging of solid debris if used in isolation without barium. We believe that a laxative preparation that includes a dual tagging regimen of dilute barium followed by diatrizoate is necessary to achieve an acceptable level of accuracy for screening, as shown repeatedly in the major clinical trials (see Chapter 7).

In some cases, areas of the colonic surface will be studded with adherent residual stool, despite the use of a cathartic preparation. With the use of a dual contrast tagging regimen, this is usually limited to the cecum and

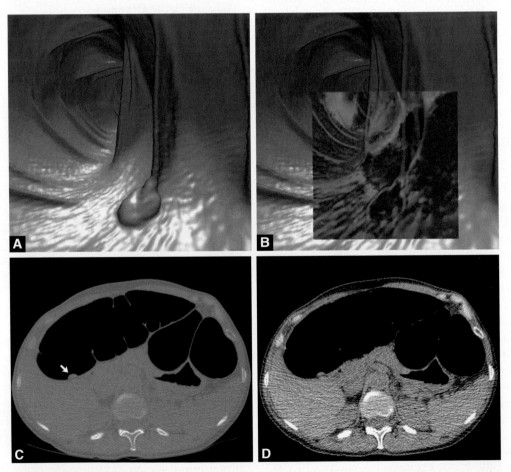

Figure 20-1 **Untagged stool mimicking a soft tissue polyp.** 3D endoluminal CTC image **(A)** shows a polypoid lesion near the hepatic flexure, which demonstrates a predominately red translucency pattern **(B)** suggestive of soft tissue. These findings are confirmed on 2D with polyp **(C)** and soft tissue **(D)** window settings *(arrow)*. Note, however, that oral contrast tagging was not used and that this "lesion" fell to the dependent wall of the prone position (not shown), consistent with untagged stool. With stool tagging, this issue is avoided, thereby saving time and improving interpretation. *(*See associated video clip on DVD.)*

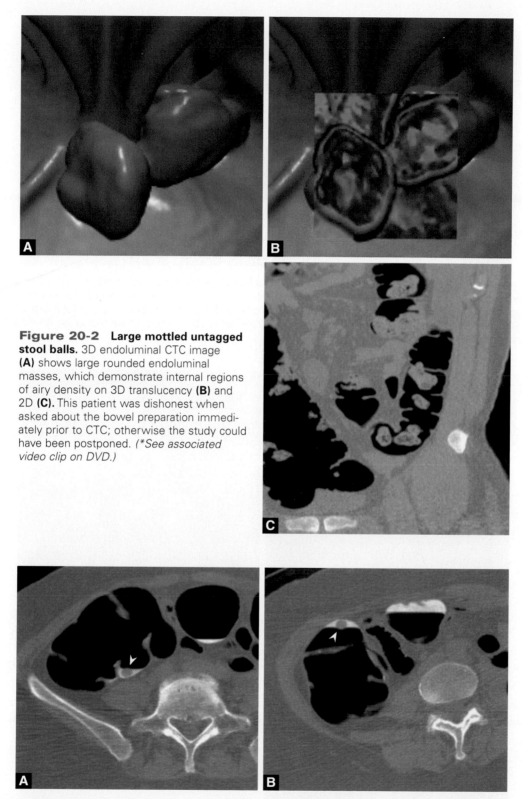

Figure 20-2   Large mottled untagged stool balls. 3D endoluminal CTC image **(A)** shows large rounded endoluminal masses, which demonstrate internal regions of airy density on 3D translucency **(B)** and 2D **(C).** This patient was dishonest when asked about the bowel preparation immediately prior to CTC; otherwise the study could have been postponed. *(*See associated video clip on DVD.)*

Figure 20-3   Mobile stool. Supine **(A)** and prone **(B)** transverse 2D CTC images show a rounded lesion *(arrowheads)* that shifts dependently with the luminal fluid. The homogeneous soft tissue density is atypical for untagged stool and could have mimicked a true polyp if adherent. Fortunately, untagged adherent stool demonstrating soft tissue density is extremely rare with our bowel prep strategy.

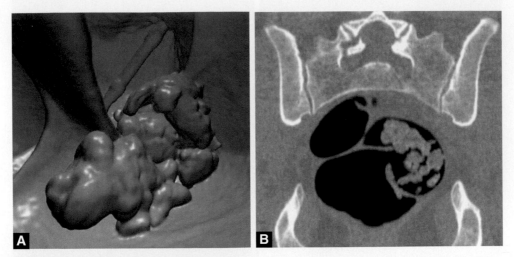

Figure 20-4   Bulky residual stool superficially resembling a large villous tumor. 3D endoluminal CTC image **(A)** shows an irregular lobulated "mass" in the rectum, which simulates a large, frondlike villous tumor. Note rectal catheter in the background. On 2D with polyp windowing **(B),** the typical heterogeneous composition characteristic of untagged stool is present but less obvious than usual. Although such stool should never be confused for true pathology after complete evaluation, this issue is completely avoided with combined catharsis and contrast tagging.

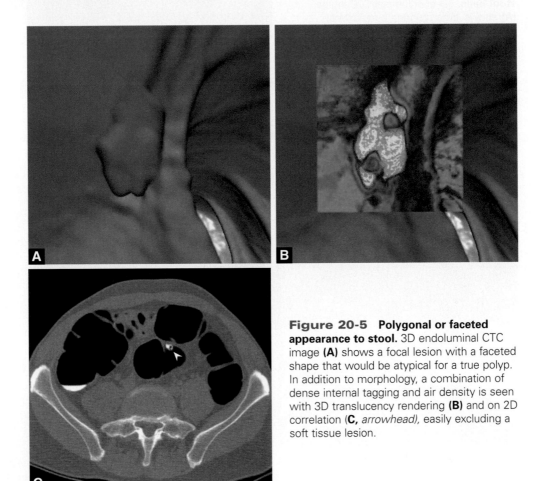

Figure 20-5   Polygonal or faceted appearance to stool. 3D endoluminal CTC image **(A)** shows a focal lesion with a faceted shape that would be atypical for a true polyp. In addition to morphology, a combination of dense internal tagging and air density is seen with 3D translucency rendering **(B)** and on 2D correlation **(C,** *arrowhead),* easily excluding a soft tissue lesion.

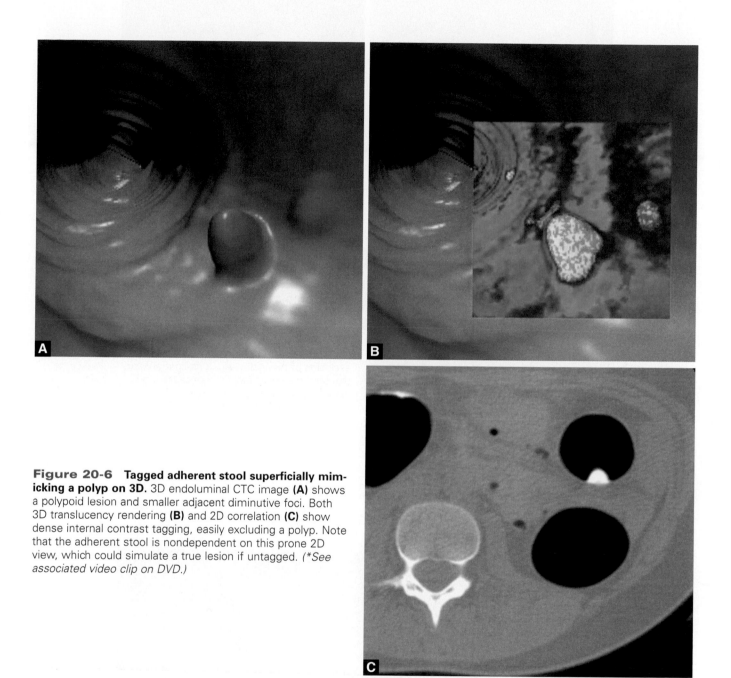

Figure 20-6   Tagged adherent stool superficially mim-icking a polyp on 3D. 3D endoluminal CTC image **(A)** shows a polypoid lesion and smaller adjacent diminutive foci. Both 3D translucency rendering **(B)** and 2D correlation **(C)** show dense internal contrast tagging, easily excluding a polyp. Note that the adherent stool is nondependent on this prone 2D view, which could simulate a true lesion if untagged. (*See associated video clip on DVD.)

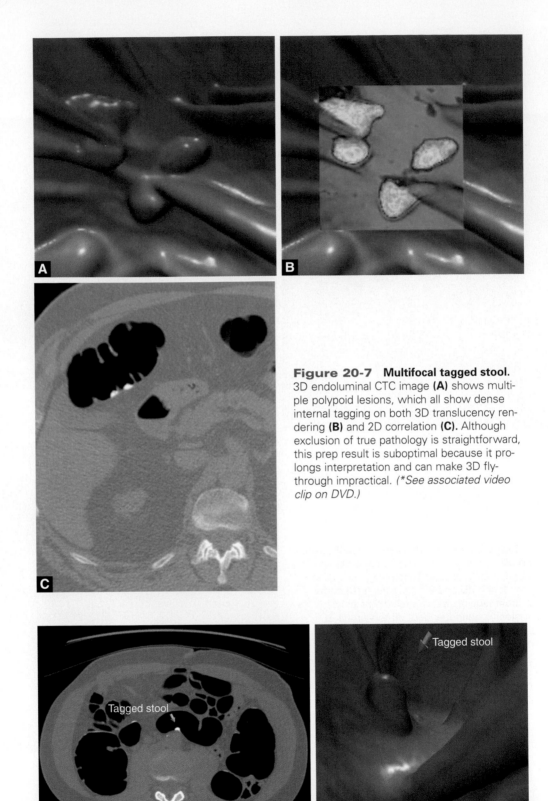

Figure 20-7   Multifocal tagged stool.
3D endoluminal CTC image **(A)** shows multiple polypoid lesions, which all show dense internal tagging on both 3D translucency rendering **(B)** and 2D correlation **(C)**. Although exclusion of true pathology is straightforward, this prep result is suboptimal because it prolongs interpretation and can make 3D flythrough impractical. *(*See associated video clip on DVD.)*

Figure 20-8   Labeling of stool at 2D CTC interpretation. If tagged adherent stool is identified on rapid 2D review **(A)** preceding the 3D evaluation, a label can be placed on the 2D images *(red arrow with text)* that will appear at 3D endoluminal fly-through **(B)**, avoiding the need for further interrogation. *(*See associated video clip on DVD.)*

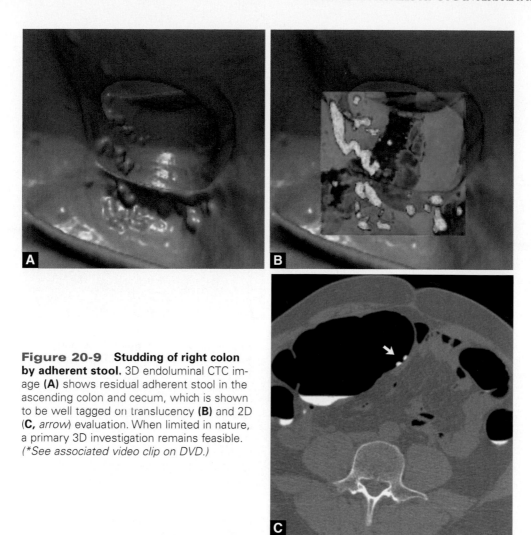

Figure 20-9   Studding of right colon by adherent stool. 3D endoluminal CTC image **(A)** shows residual adherent stool in the ascending colon and cecum, which is shown to be well tagged on translucency **(B)** and 2D **(C,** *arrow)* evaluation. When limited in nature, a primary 3D investigation remains feasible. *(*See associated video clip on DVD.)*

proximal ascending colon (Fig. 20-9). If extensive, the irregularity and polyposis-like appearance at 3D evaluation will effectively reduce the interpretation to just a primary 2D polyp search for the affected region, with all its inherent shortcomings (see Chapter 17). This tends to occur more with the denser 40% w/v preparations (Fig. 20-10) and/or when the water-soluble diatrizoate is not taken (Fig. 20-11). In our experience, a false-positive interpretation because of residual stool is extremely rare with our current cathartic preparation with dual contrast tagging (Figs. 20-12 and 20-13). However, untagged stool continues to be a major issue with same-day completion CTC following incomplete OC when tagging is not used and also will likely be a vexing problem for some noncathartic CTC approaches,[3] especially if it precludes primary 3D evaluation.

Beyond residual fecal material, other intraluminal debris will sometimes mimic polyps. Most notably, ingested pills and capsules have a striking resemblance to polyps on the 3D endoluminal display (Fig. 20-14). Fortunately, the internal attenuation of these foreign bodies is almost always incompatible with a soft tissue lesion

(Fig. 20-15). Furthermore, these foreign bodies are rarely adherent and therefore fall to the dependent surface with positional changes (Fig. 20-16). The only real pitfall here is to distinguish free dependent movement of luminal debris from positional change of a pedunculated polyp at 2D evaluation, which is fortunately obvious on the 3D endoluminal view (see later). Undigested or partially digested food particles, such as vegetable matter, may occasionally give rise to focal polypoid lesions (Fig. 20-17). Such cases can be challenging when adherent and similar to soft tissue in attenuation but are encountered only rarely with our bowel preparation.

THICKENED OR COMPLEX FOLDS

Diffuse, segmental fold thickening is a common feature of sigmoid diverticulosis. At 2D evaluation, the appearance of diverticular fold thickening can be striking (Figs. 20-18 and 20-19), especially when associated with suboptimal distention, making the search for polyps extremely difficult. However, as long as the lumen is at least partially distended, primary 3D evaluation provides an

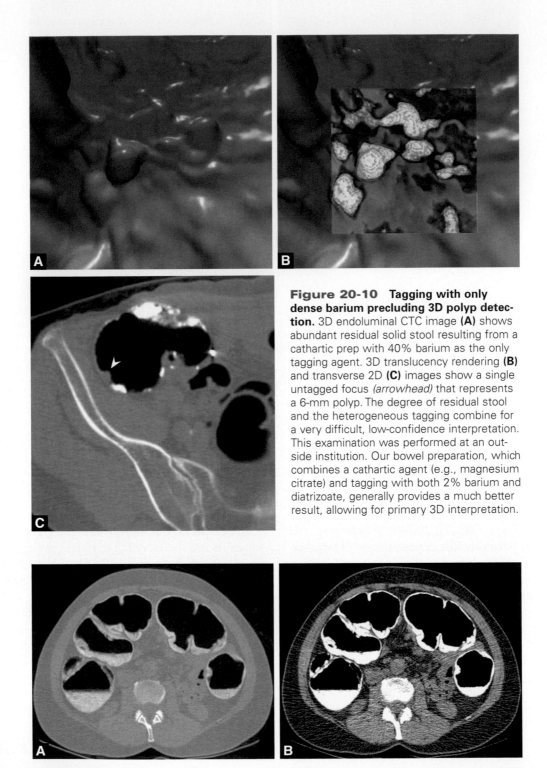

Figure 20-10 **Tagging with only dense barium precluding 3D polyp detection.** 3D endoluminal CTC image **(A)** shows abundant residual solid stool resulting from a cathartic prep with 40% barium as the only tagging agent. 3D translucency rendering **(B)** and transverse 2D **(C)** images show a single untagged focus *(arrowhead)* that represents a 6-mm polyp. The degree of residual stool and the heterogeneous tagging combine for a very difficult, low-confidence interpretation. This examination was performed at an outside institution. Our bowel preparation, which combines a cathartic agent (e.g., magnesium citrate) and tagging with both 2% barium and diatrizoate, generally provides a much better result, allowing for primary 3D interpretation.

Figure 20-11 **Barium-only tagging result.** Transverse 2D CTC images with polyp **(A)** and soft tissue **(B)** windowing show a thick rind of partially tagged residual material coating the entire colonic surface. The patient did not take the iodinated water-soluble contrast (diatrizoate). We almost never see this appearance with the use of diatrizoate, which tends to wash the colonic walls free of stool.

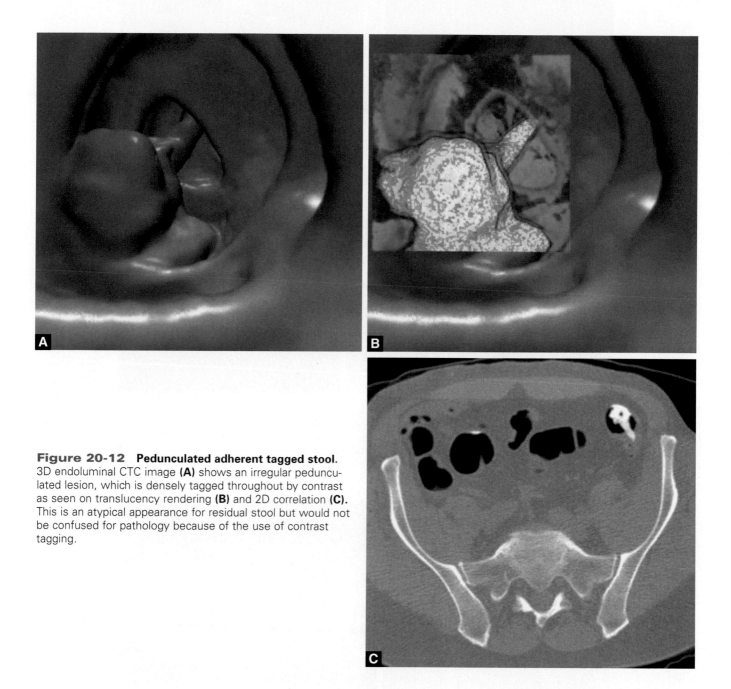

Figure 20-12   Pedunculated adherent tagged stool.
3D endoluminal CTC image **(A)** shows an irregular pedunculated lesion, which is densely tagged throughout by contrast
as seen on translucency rendering **(B)** and 2D correlation **(C)**.
This is an atypical appearance for residual stool but would not
be confused for pathology because of the use of contrast
tagging.

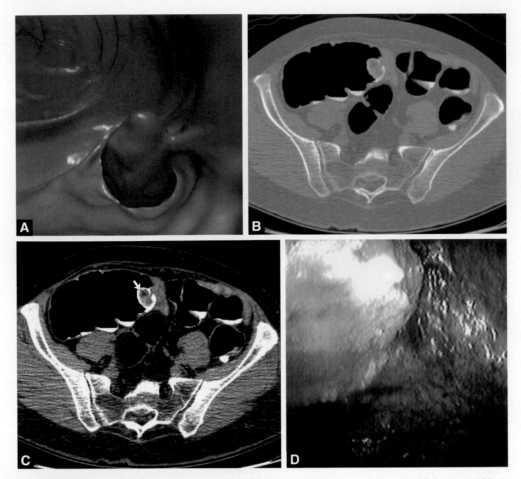

Figure 20-13 **Unusual false-positive result related to untagged stool.** 3D endoluminal CTC image **(A)** shows an irregular masslike lesion in the cecum, which fails to demonstrate internal tagging. On 2D images with polyp windowing **(B),** only subtle internal heterogeneity is seen. However, with soft tissue windowing **(C),** an area of low attenuation incompatible with soft tissue becomes more apparent *(arrow).* Unfortunately, this lesion was mistaken for potential pathology and sent to OC **(D),** where a large adherent stool ball was verified. With our current CTC approach, residual stool is a very rare cause of false-positive interpretation.

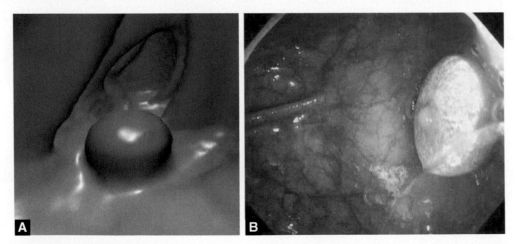

Figure 20-14 **Retained oral medication.** 3D endoluminal CTC image **(A)** shows a smooth polypoid object that represents a retained pill or capsule. OC image from another individual **(B)** shows a similar finding. Mobility and/or lack of internal soft tissue attenuation make for an easy distinction from true polyps.

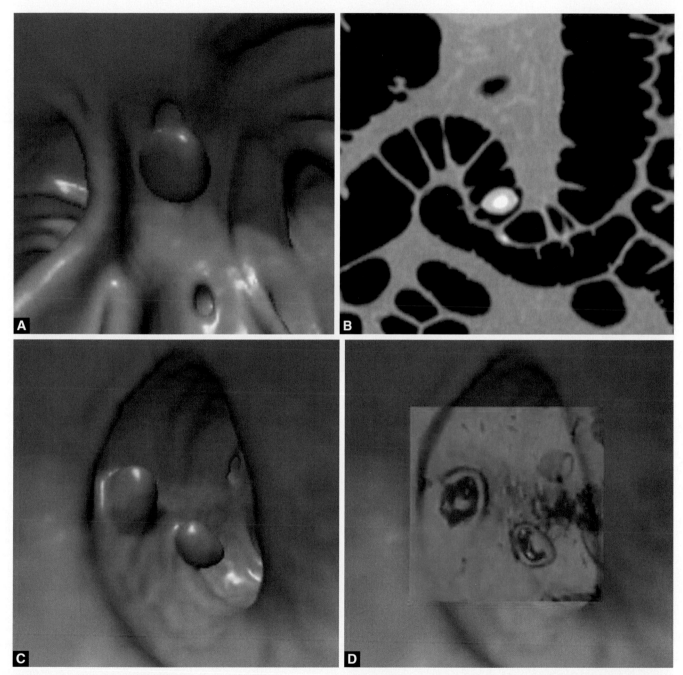

Figure 20-15 Internal attenuation of retained pills and capsules. 3D endoluminal **(A)** and coronal 2D **(B)** CTC images show a pill adjacent to a diverticulum that demonstrates internal high attenuation (relative to soft tissue). 3D endoluminal views without **(C)** and with **(D)** translucency rendering from a second individual show two polypoid lesions with foci of internal low attenuation (relative to soft tissue). In both cases, true polyps are easily excluded, even if the retained foreign bodies are adherent.

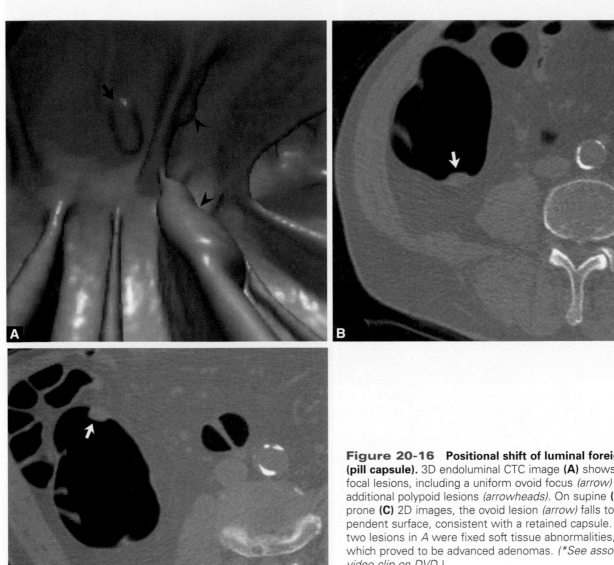

Figure 20-16   Positional shift of luminal foreign body (pill capsule). 3D endoluminal CTC image **(A)** shows several focal lesions, including a uniform ovoid focus *(arrow)* and two additional polypoid lesions *(arrowheads)*. On supine **(B)** and prone **(C)** 2D images, the ovoid lesion *(arrow)* falls to the dependent surface, consistent with a retained capsule. The other two lesions in *A* were fixed soft tissue abnormalities, both of which proved to be advanced adenomas. *(*See associated video clip on DVD.)*

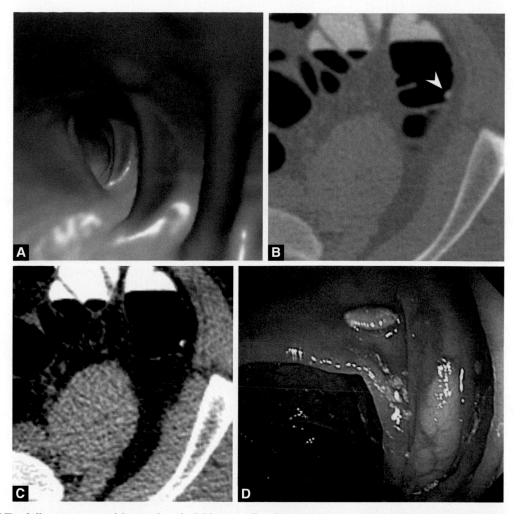

Figure 20-17 **Adherent vegetable seeds mimicking small polyps.** 3D endoluminal CTC image **(A)** shows a small polypoid lesion measuring 5 to 6 mm in size. Transverse 2D CTC images with polyp **(B)** and soft tissue **(C)** window settings show that the lesion *(arrowhead)* is slightly higher than soft tissue in attenuation. Other similar foci were seen, all of which proved to be retained vegetable seeds at OC **(D).** If these were the only findings at CTC, OC referral would not be indicated.

Figure 20-18 **Sigmoid diverticular fold thickening (myochosis).** Transverse 2D CTC image shows diffuse sigmoid wall thickening and luminal narrowing, which causes the thickened folds to crowd together. Scattered diverticula are present but the striking (and challenging) feature of sigmoid diverticulosis is the fold thickening and luminal narrowing. The key to effective CTC interpretation is to distend the lumen just enough to allow for 3D endoluminal fly-through. A stool ball is incidentally noted within a tagged fluid pool in the rectum.

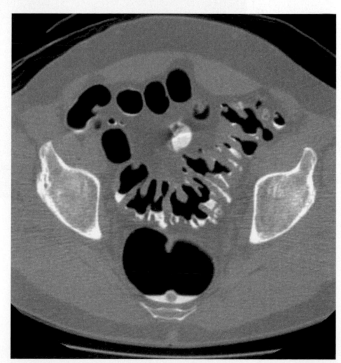

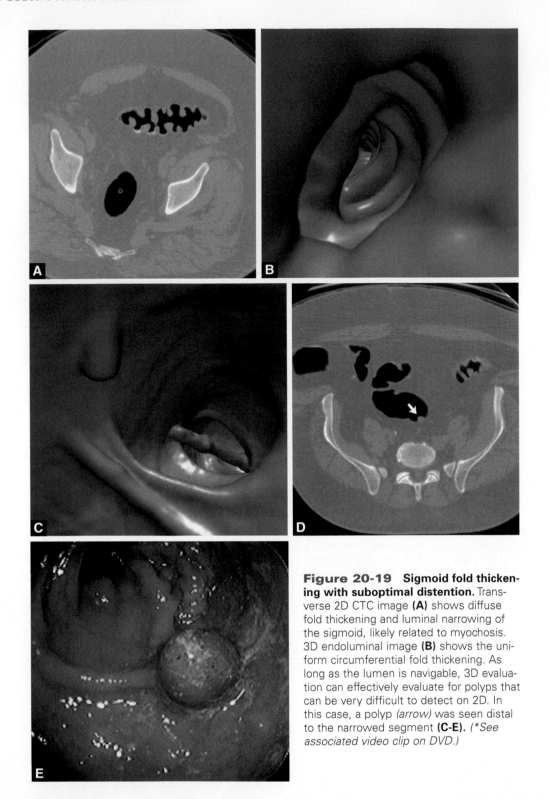

Figure 20-19 Sigmoid fold thickening with suboptimal distention. Transverse 2D CTC image **(A)** shows diffuse fold thickening and luminal narrowing of the sigmoid, likely related to myochosis. 3D endoluminal image **(B)** shows the uniform circumferential fold thickening. As long as the lumen is navigable, 3D evaluation can effectively evaluate for polyps that can be very difficult to detect on 2D. In this case, a polyp *(arrow)* was seen distal to the narrowed segment **(C-E).** *(*See associated video clip on DVD.)*

easy search pattern because the elongated circumferential nature of the thickened folds is readily apparent (Fig. 20-20). In fact, even the presence of advanced diverticular disease does not significantly affect the diagnostic performance of primary 3D polyp detection at CTC.[4]

An isolated thickened fold can present a diagnostic challenge at CTC but rarely if ever represents significant pathology if smooth and uniform appearing on 3D (Fig. 20-21).[1] Thickened but otherwise normal–appearing folds may be confirmed at OC, and even biopsied, but typically yield only normal mucosa. Even for cases where a thickened fold has a focal bulbous appearance, colonoscopic biopsy will generally be negative (Fig. 20-22). Unlike diverticular disease, where fold thickening tends

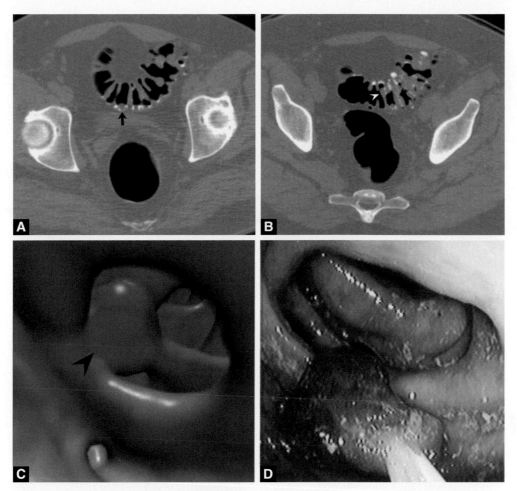

Figure 20-20 **Pedunculated polyp within underdistended sigmoid diverticulosis.** Supine **(A)** and prone **(B)** 2D CTC images show extensive sigmoid diverticulosis, which makes polyp detection very difficult on 2D. A pedunculated polyp is present that is lying in the fluid pool on supine *(arrow)* and mimics a fold on prone *(arrowhead)*. On 3D **(C),** however, there is enough luminal distention to allow for easy polyp detection because the lesion *(arrowhead)* is conspicuous against the circumferential folds. A 1.2-cm tubular adenoma was removed at OC **(D).** (From Sanford MS, Pickhardt PJ. Diagnostic performance of primary 3-dimensional computed tomography colonography in the setting of colonic diverticular disease. *Clin Gastroenterol Hepatol.* 2006;4:1039-1047.) *(*See associated video clip on DVD.)*

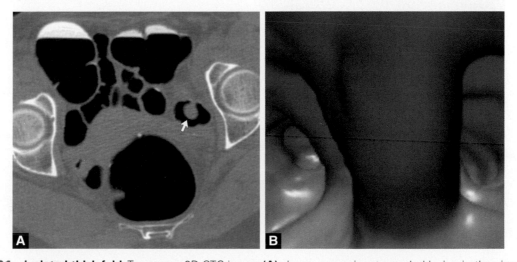

Figure 20-21 **Isolated thick fold.** Transverse 2D CTC image **(A)** shows a prominent rounded lesion in the sigmoid *(arrow).* The corresponding 3D endoluminal image **(B)** shows only a broad but uniform fold located at the inner turn of a flexure. Thick folds can appear polypoid on 2D, but the elongated nature of the fold is obvious on 3D. For folds that are smooth and uniform in appearance, OC referral is not indicated.

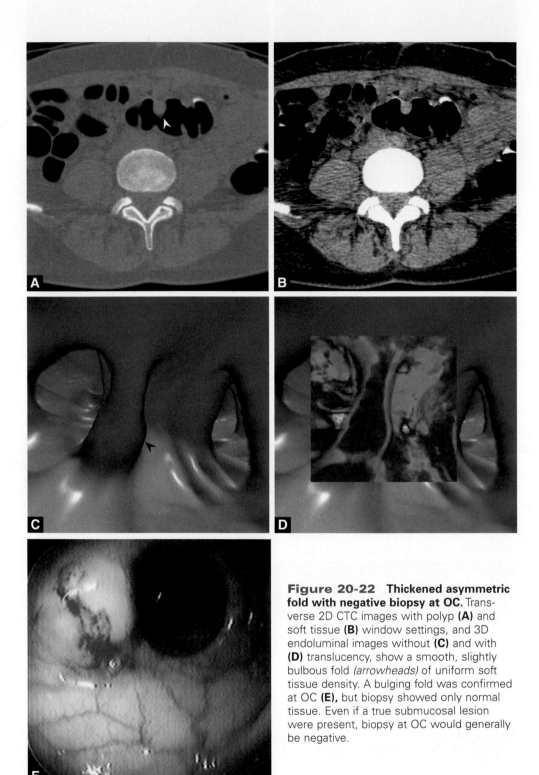

Figure 20-22 Thickened asymmetric fold with negative biopsy at OC. Transverse 2D CTC images with polyp **(A)** and soft tissue **(B)** window settings, and 3D endoluminal images without **(C)** and with **(D)** translucency, show a smooth, slightly bulbous fold *(arrowheads)* of uniform soft tissue density. A bulging fold was confirmed at OC **(E),** but biopsy showed only normal tissue. Even if a true submucosal lesion were present, biopsy at OC would generally be negative.

to be more segmental in distribution, isolated prominent folds are usually seen at a flexure point along the inner curvature or where a relative twist occurs, or where multiple folds converge together. Redundant colonic segments with mesenteric laxity can result in subclinical twisting or torsion that can be difficult to work out on 2D but is more easily recognized on 3D evaluation (Figs. 20-23 and 20-24). Similarly, a convergence of two folds is much easier to appreciate on 3D (Fig. 20-25). In general, the smooth, uniform, and elongated nature of a prominent fold or convergence of folds will be readily apparent on the 3D endoluminal view. Without the associated features of a lobulated contour or a focal polypoid lesion on a fold at 3D evaluation, we have found that the diagnostic yield of sending these thick folds on to OC is too low to justify. Therefore, based on our extensive experience with CTC–OC correlation, we no longer send uniformly thickened folds for evaluation at OC.

Occasionally, a hyperplastic or even an adenomatous polyp will manifest as a focally thickened fold at CTC but there is usually some fusiform asymmetry on 3D (Fig.

20-26) or contrast coating on 2D (Fig. 20-27) to suggest a true lesion. Such findings may be difficult to confirm at OC, particularly if right-sided (Fig. 20-26). Distinguishing an innocuous focally prominent noncircumferential fold as shown above from a saddle-shaped or semi-annular invasive cancer is typically straightforward, assuming luminal distention is adequate. However, even when distention is poor, the smooth and uniform appearance of segmental collapse is different from a fixed, malignant mass. In general, colonic folds will diffusely thicken in a dynamic, uniform fashion as segmental distention decreases (Fig. 20-25). Similarly, distinguishing focal spasm of an interhaustral fold from an annular constricting mass or pathologic stricture is another important task. The smooth, thin, and uniform doughnut-shaped appearance of spasm (Figs. 20-28 and 20-29) is in stark contrast to an irregular, shouldered apple-core malignancy, which will also demonstrates a substantial longitudinal component that focal spasm does not (see Chapter 21). Furthermore, spasm is often transient and may not persist on all views, which allows for easy recognition of this pitfall (Fig. 20-29).

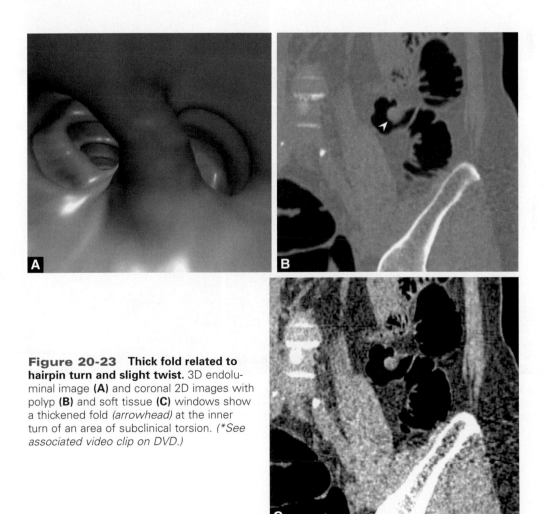

Figure 20-23 **Thick fold related to hairpin turn and slight twist.** 3D endoluminal image **(A)** and coronal 2D images with polyp **(B)** and soft tissue **(C)** windows show a thickened fold *(arrowhead)* at the inner turn of an area of subclinical torsion. *(*See associated video clip on DVD.)*

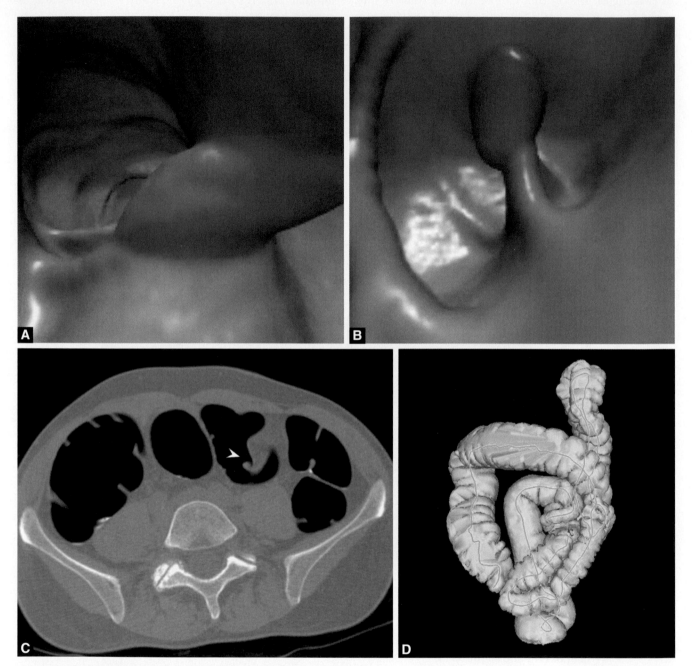

Figure 20-24 **Thick fold related to subclinical torsion.** 3D endoluminal **(A** and **B)** and transverse 2D **(C)** images show a thickened fold *(arrowhead)* related to an area of twisting, which can be best appreciated on the interactive 3D map **(D,** *blue arrow).* A pseudopolyp appearance can be seen at the area of torsion on 3D **(B).**

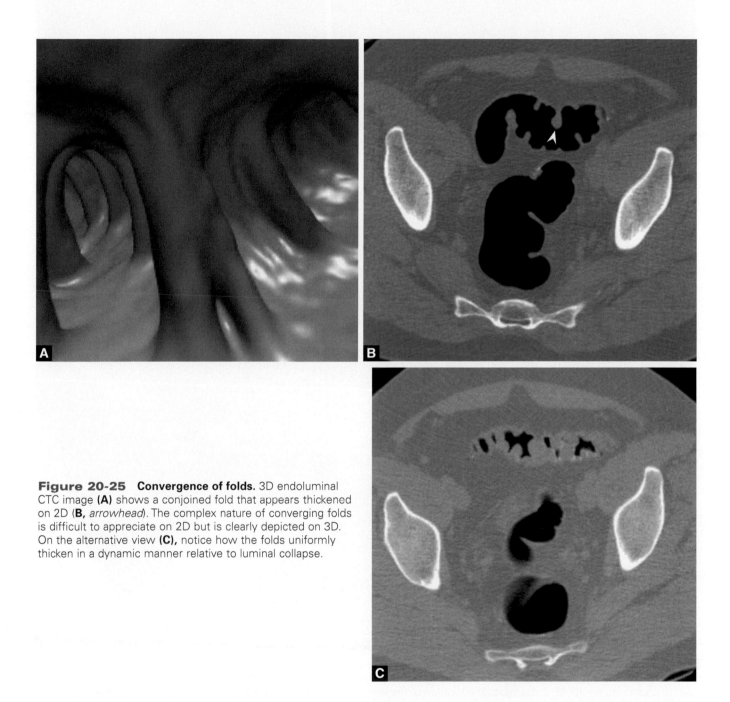

Figure 20-25 Convergence of folds. 3D endoluminal CTC image **(A)** shows a conjoined fold that appears thickened on 2D **(B,** *arrowhead*). The complex nature of converging folds is difficult to appreciate on 2D but is clearly depicted on 3D. On the alternative view **(C),** notice how the folds uniformly thicken in a dynamic manner relative to luminal collapse.

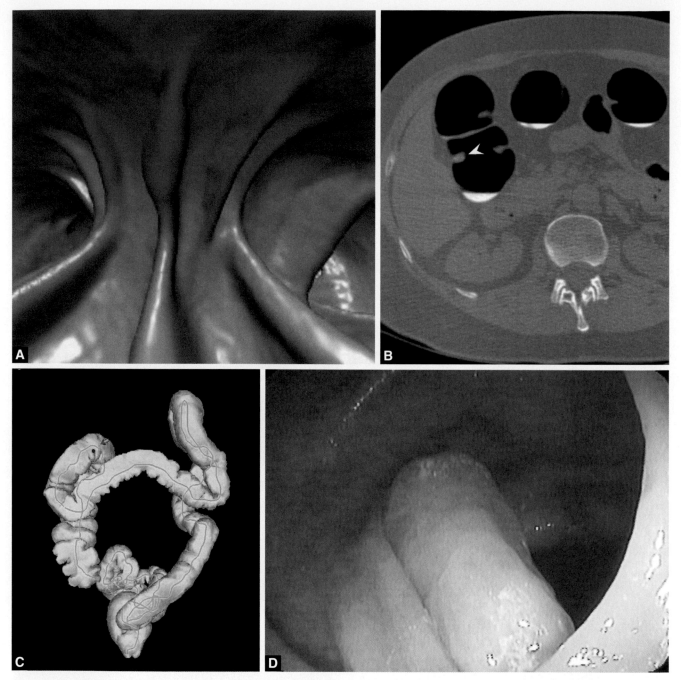

Figure 20-26 **Flat hyperplastic polyp on a fold missed at initial OC referral.** 3D endoluminal CTC image **(A)** shows mild fusiform thickening of a fold in the hepatic flexure region. The asymmetric nature, which is more concerning for a true lesion, is difficult to appreciate on 2D **(B,** *arrowhead*). The location of the lesion is depicted by the red dot on the 3D colon map **(C).** No lesion was found at same-day OC, perhaps related to its right-sided location. However, after the abnormality was noted again at followup CTC, a repeat OC examination found the lesion **(D),** which proved to be a flat 14-mm hyperplastic polyp. *(*See associated video clip on DVD.)*

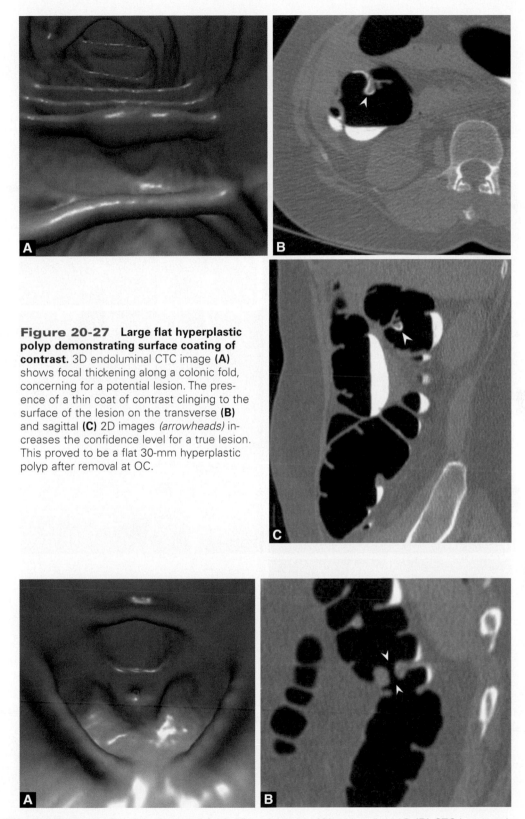

Figure 20-27 Large flat hyperplastic polyp demonstrating surface coating of contrast. 3D endoluminal CTC image **(A)** shows focal thickening along a colonic fold, concerning for a potential lesion. The presence of a thin coat of contrast clinging to the surface of the lesion on the transverse **(B)** and sagittal **(C)** 2D images *(arrowheads)* increases the confidence level for a true lesion. This proved to be a flat 30-mm hyperplastic polyp after removal at OC.

Figure 20-28 Focal spasm of an interhaustral fold. 3D endoluminal **(A)** and sagittal 2D **(B)** CTC images show the characteristic appearance of focal spasm of an interhaustral fold as a narrowed uniform ring *(arrowheads)*. Note the lack of irregularity or shouldering to suggest an annular mass.

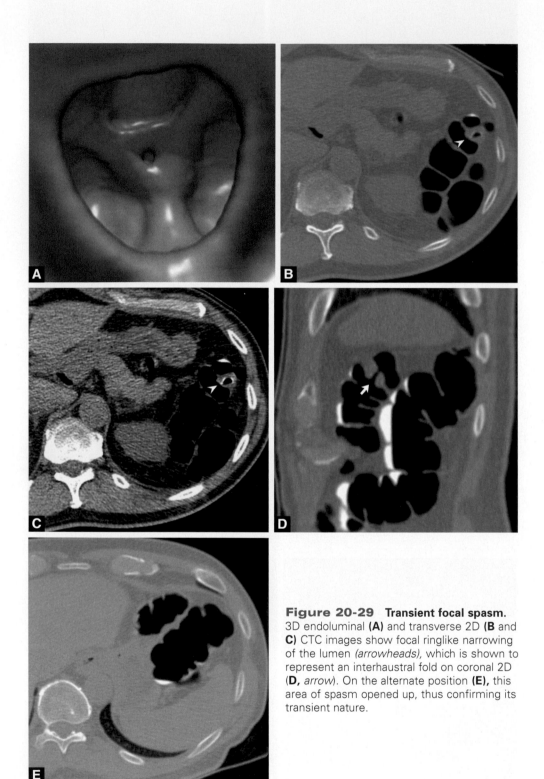

Figure 20-29 Transient focal spasm.
3D endoluminal **(A)** and transverse 2D **(B** and **C)** CTC images show focal ringlike narrowing of the lumen *(arrowheads),* which is shown to represent an interhaustral fold on coronal 2D **(D,** *arrow).* On the alternate position **(E),** this area of spasm opened up, thus confirming its transient nature.

INADEQUATE LUMINAL DISTENTION

Inadequate luminal distention or frank collapse affects both 2D and 3D evaluation at CTC. In terms of colonic distention, the minimum requirement for a diagnostic evaluation is to have all segments adequately distended on at least one view. Fortunately, the complementary nature of supine and prone positioning allows for a diagnostic evaluation in the majority of cases with full segmental collapse (Figs. 20-30 and 20-31). Most series with partial but suboptimal distention are "readable" but require more intense scrutiny compared with cases in which excellent distention is achieved. Dynamic luminal collapse and thickening of the colonic wall in cases of underdistention can degrade the quality of both the 2D and 3D displays (Fig. 20-32). Within the right colon, underdistention can affect polyp detection be-

cause of the encroaching interhaustral folds (Fig. 20-33). Fortunately, the right colon is typically well distended in the great majority of cases, particularly when automated CO_2 is used, which may help to explain the difference in CRC detection between CTC and OC.[5]

For cases in which focal collapse persists at the same point on both supine and prone displays, a decubitus view will usually allow for diagnostic assessment. Because the sigmoid colon accounts for the vast majority of such cases, usually related to diverticular disease, a right lateral decubitus view is typically performed (Fig. 20-34). This assessment for adequate left-sided distention during CTC examination must be made on the 2D reconstructions at the console because the scout view is unreliable for this region of colon (Fig. 20-35). We have not found spasmolytics to be necessary because less than 1% of cases will have a persistent area of luminal collapse in our experience. Furthermore, glucagon is not reliably effec-

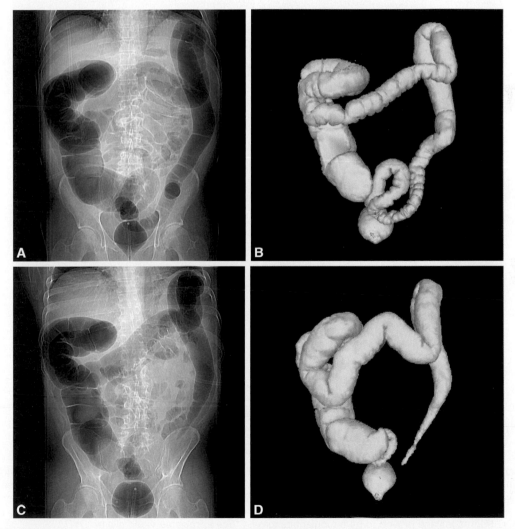

Figure 20-30 **Segmental collapse on one view but overall diagnostic examination.** Supine scout **(A)** and 3D colon map **(B)** for CTC show excellent distention, whereas the scout **(C)** and map **(D)** for the prone position show narrowing and collapse in the sigmoid region. Although optimal distention on both views is desired, this examination is nonetheless diagnostic and a decubitus view is not necessary.

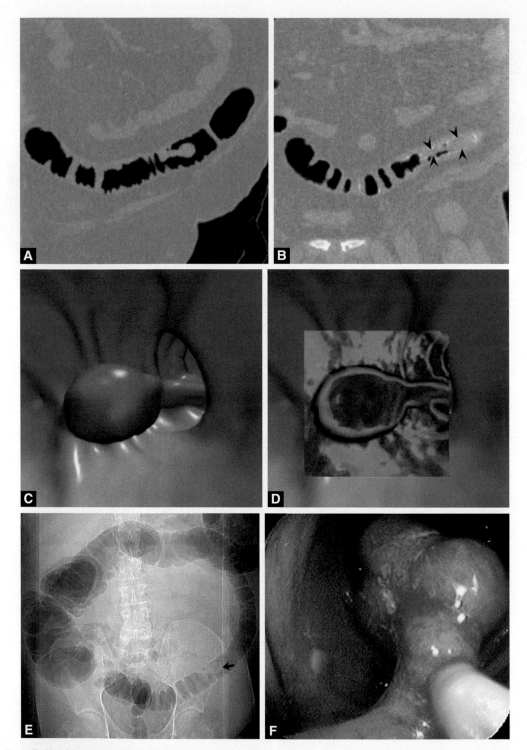

Figure 20-31 **Polyp in segmental collapse.** Supine coronal 2D CTC image **(A)** shows an obvious pedunculated polyp in the sigmoid colon, in addition to diffuse wall thickening from myochosis. On the prone coronal image **(B),** this spastic segment has partially collapsed around the polyp *(arrowheads)*. Although detection on prone would be difficult, this less optimal view is needed only for polyp confirmation—not detection. This 23-mm pedunculated polyp is also demonstrated on 3D **(C** and **D),** scout **(E,** *arrow*), and OC **(F)** images and proved to be a tubular adenoma. *(*See associated video clip on DVD.)*

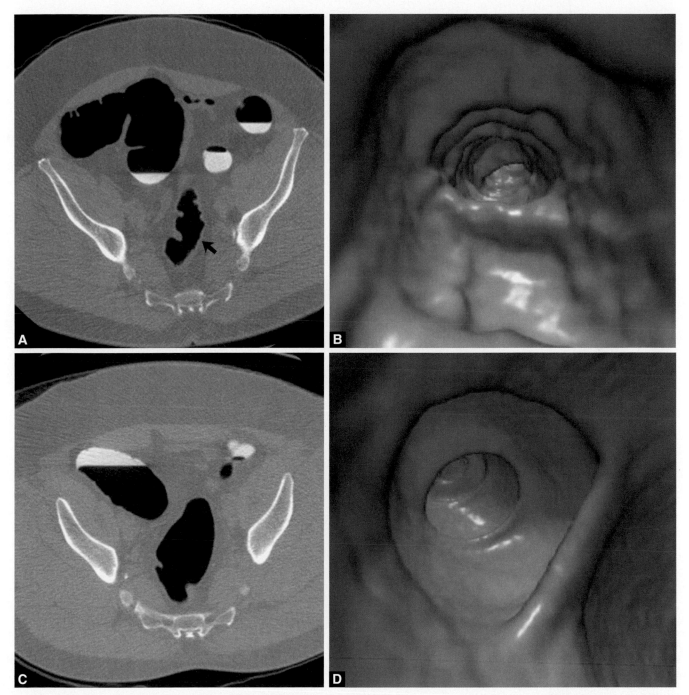

Figure 20-32 The effect of suboptimal distention on 2D and 3D CTC displays. Suboptimal distention affects both 2D and 3D displays. In this case, note how underdistention of the rectosigmoid region on supine degrades not only the 2D image (**A**, *arrow*), but also the 3D display (**B**). In comparison, note the excellent distention of this area on prone positioning (**C** and **D**), making both 2D and 3D evaluation easier. **B** and **D** are taken from the same 3D endoluminal vantage point.

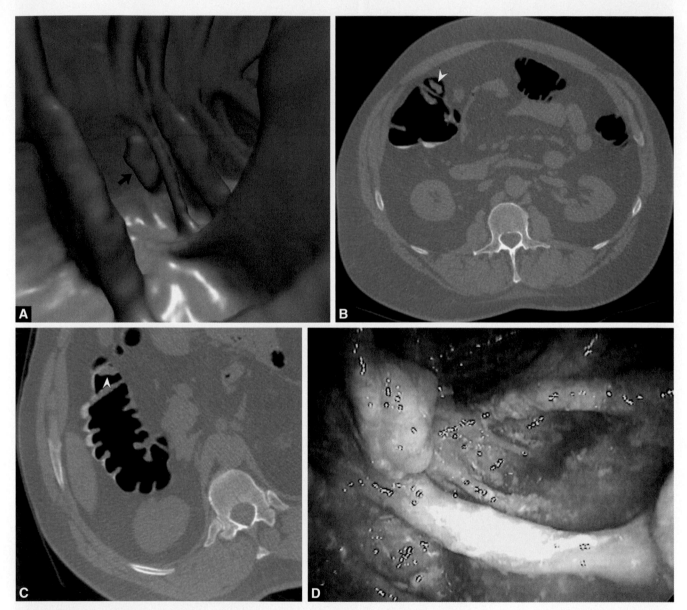

Figure 20-33 **Right-sided polyp detection made challenging by underdistention.** 3D endoluminal CTC image **(A)** shows an elongated 22-mm polyp *(arrow).* The lesion can be confirmed on both supine **(B)** and decubitus **(C)** 2D images *(arrowheads),* although the thickened adjacent folds make the evaluation more difficult. More important, the luminal narrowing caused by the thickened folds may obscure the lesion at 3D navigation along the centerline (as shown on video clip). The lesion was confirmed at OC **(D)** and proved to be a tubulovillous adenoma. Note the thick appearance of the folds at OC as well. *(*See associated video clip on DVD.)*

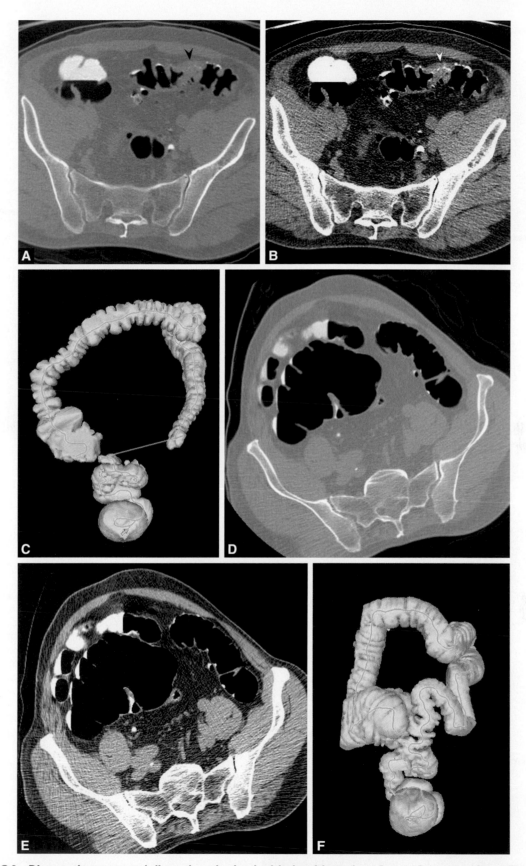

Figure 20-34 **Diagnostic segmental distention obtained with decubitus view.** Prone 2D images **(A** and **B)** and 3D colon map **(C)** show segmental spasm *(arrowheads)* of the diverticular sigmoid, which had persisted from the supine position (not shown). On right-lateral decubitus positioning **(D-F),** this spastic segment relaxes and fully distends, allowing for diagnostic evaluation. In cases of sigmoid spasm, the right-lateral decubitus view often provides the best evaluation, excluding a true stricture and sparing the patient of the need for sigmoidoscopy. We do not use glucagon in this or any other setting.

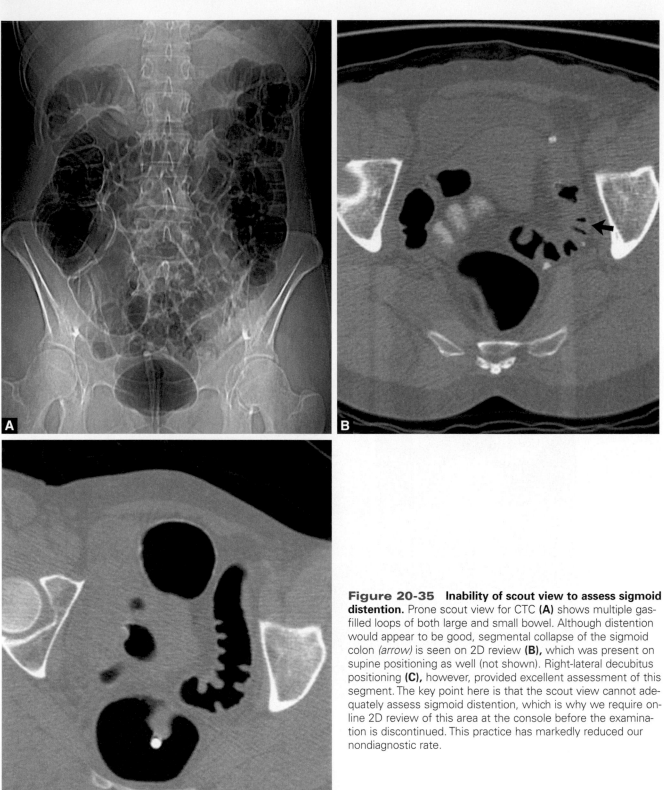

Figure 20-35 **Inability of scout view to assess sigmoid distention.** Prone scout view for CTC **(A)** shows multiple gas-filled loops of both large and small bowel. Although distention would appear to be good, segmental collapse of the sigmoid colon *(arrow)* is seen on 2D review **(B),** which was present on supine positioning as well (not shown). Right-lateral decubitus positioning **(C),** however, provided excellent assessment of this segment. The key point here is that the scout view cannot adequately assess sigmoid distention, which is why we require on-line 2D review of this area at the console before the examination is discontinued. This practice has markedly reduced our nondiagnostic rate.

tive (Fig. 20-36) and a number of these difficult cases will actually represent fixed pathologic strictures (Fig. 20-37). For cases of truly incomplete evaluation in the sigmoid or descending colon, unsedated same-day flexible sigmoidoscopy may be performed to complete the screening evaluation. The region of nondiagnostic evaluation from focal collapse typically accounts for just a tiny fraction of the total colonic length. Because lesions require detection on just one view, confirmation is often possible on the alternative view even in cases of inadequate distention on that view (Fig. 20-38).

Automated low-pressure CO_2 delivery provides for adequate distention on a more consistent basis than manual room air insufflation.[6] However, the lower pressures and increased resorption with the CO_2 technique can also result in partial collapse, particularly in the transverse colon in the prone position (Fig. 20-39) and rectosigmoid region in the supine position (Fig. 20-40). Collapse of the transverse colon on prone positioning can be alleviated somewhat by placing pillow support under the thorax. However, in extreme cases of morbid obesity in which CO_2 distention cannot overcome extracolonic pressures, decubitus positioning and even conversion to

manual room air may be necessary (Fig. 20-41). Appropriate caution should be given when converting to staff-controlled manual room air insufflation because this bypasses the built-in safety mechanisms with regard to luminal pressures. There are two rare pitfalls to recognize in the setting of poor distention. One is inguinal herniation of the sigmoid colon, which could lead to perforation if vigorous staff-controlled room air insufflation is performed (Fig. 20-42).[7] The other rare pitfall leading to inadequate distention (in women) is inadvertent vaginal insertion of the rectal catheter (Fig. 20-43).

DIVERTICULAR DISEASE

Colonic diverticular disease is endemic in Western populations, largely related to dietary factors.[8] The prevalence of diverticular disease has increased significantly throughout the past century.[9] Moderate or extensive colonic diverticular disease is seen at CTC in about 50% of all screening adults, heavily favoring the sigmoid colon, followed by the descending colon.[4] The pathologic features are characterized by myochosis, with elastin deposition, thickening of the circular smooth muscle, shorten-

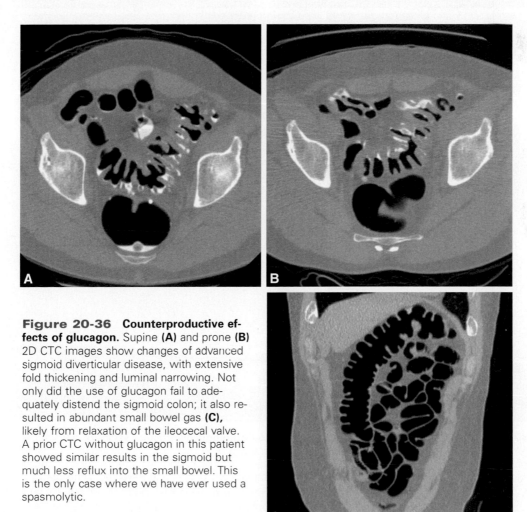

Figure 20-36 Counterproductive effects of glucagon. Supine **(A)** and prone **(B)** 2D CTC images show changes of advanced sigmoid diverticular disease, with extensive fold thickening and luminal narrowing. Not only did the use of glucagon fail to adequately distend the sigmoid colon; it also resulted in abundant small bowel gas **(C),** likely from relaxation of the ileocecal valve. A prior CTC without glucagon in this patient showed similar results in the sigmoid but much less reflux into the small bowel. This is the only case where we have ever used a spasmolytic.

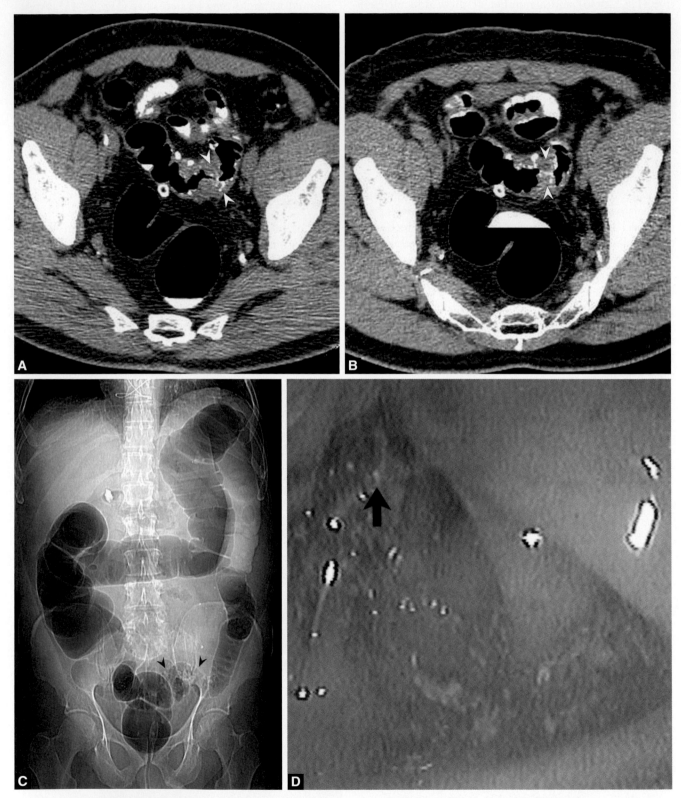

Figure 20-37 **Nondiagnostic sigmoid distention related to pathologic diverticular stricture.** Supine **(A)** and prone **(B)** 2D images show focal irregular sigmoid wall thickening and high-grade luminal narrowing *(arrowheads)* associated with diverticular changes. The changes persist on both views. Note how the CTC scout **(C)** fails to demonstrate this area of nondistention *(arrowheads)*. At flexible sigmoidoscopy **(D),** this area of benign narrowing *(arrow)* could not be traversed, consistent with a diverticular stricture. (From Pickhardt PJ, Kim DH. CT colonography (virtual colonoscopy): A practical approach for population screening. *Radiol Clin North Am.* 2007;45:361-375.)

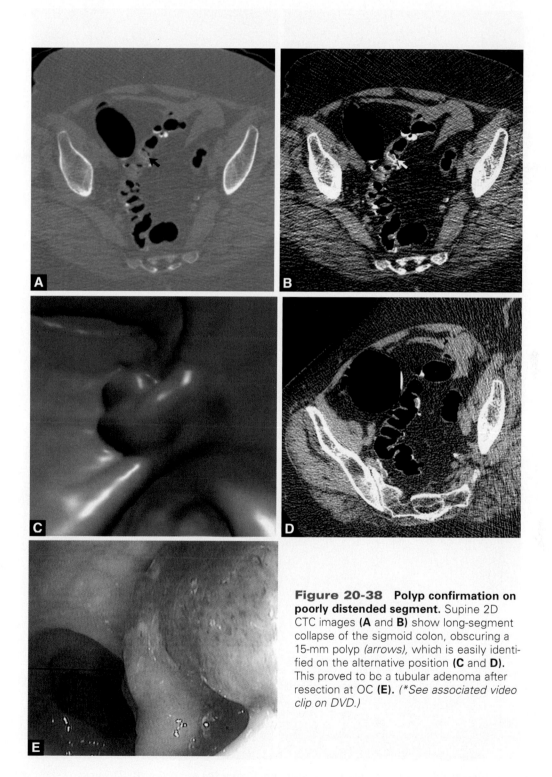

Figure 20-38   Polyp confirmation on poorly distended segment. Supine 2D CTC images (**A** and **B**) show long-segment collapse of the sigmoid colon, obscuring a 15-mm polyp *(arrows),* which is easily identified on the alternative position (**C** and **D**). This proved to be a tubular adenoma after resection at OC (**E**). *(*See associated video clip on DVD.)*

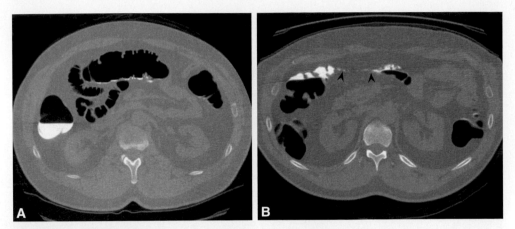

Figure 20-39 Compression of transverse colon with prone positioning. Supine **(A)** and prone **(B)** CTC images show long-segment compression of the transverse colon *(arrowheads)* on prone positioning. This segment is well distended, however, on the supine view.

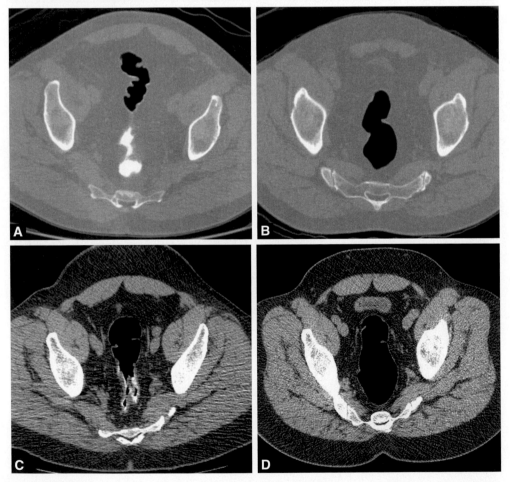

Figure 20-40 Rectosigmoid collapse on supine positioning. Supine **(A)** and prone **(B)** CTC images show collapse of the rectosigmoid region on supine, with excellent distention on prone. A similar phenomenon is seen in a second individual **(C** and **D).**

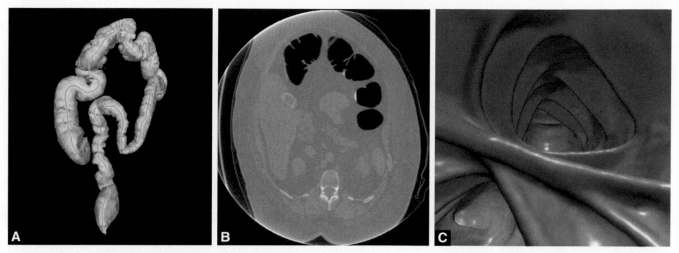

Figure 20-41 Bilateral decubitus technique for morbid obesity. Decubitus 3D colon map **(A)**, transverse 2D image **(B)**, and endoluminal 3D image **(C)** from a patient who is morbidly obese (5 feet tall, 330 pounds) show diagnostic quality despite the physical challenges. The alternative decubitus view was equally diagnostic. These examinations may need to be performed on a large-bore scanner.

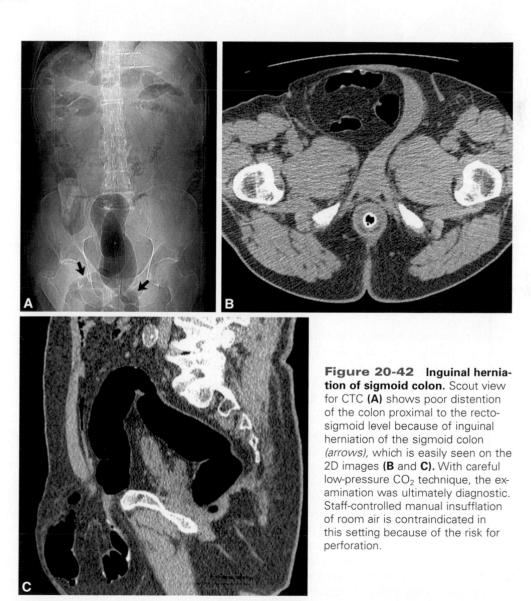

Figure 20-42 Inguinal herniation of sigmoid colon. Scout view for CTC **(A)** shows poor distention of the colon proximal to the recto-sigmoid level because of inguinal herniation of the sigmoid colon *(arrows)*, which is easily seen on the 2D images **(B** and **C)**. With careful low-pressure CO_2 technique, the examination was ultimately diagnostic. Staff-controlled manual insufflation of room air is contraindicated in this setting because of the risk for perforation.

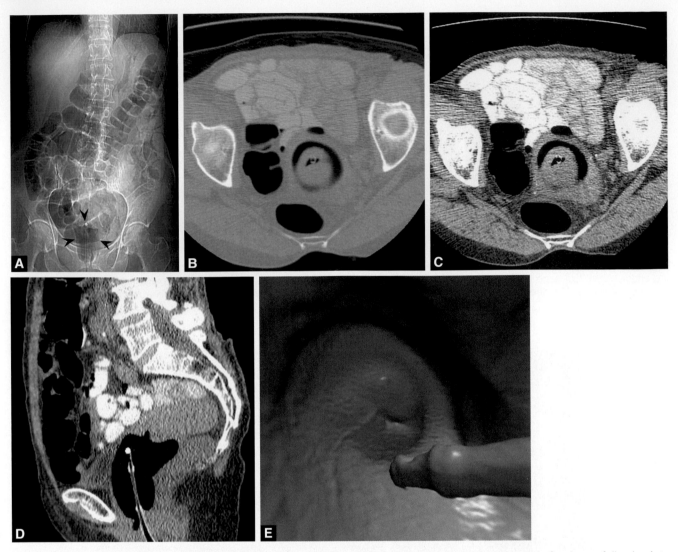

Figure 20-43   Inadvertent vaginal insertion of rectal catheter. Scout view **(A)** for CTC performed after hours following late-afternoon incomplete OC shows inadequate colonic distention. The column of gas overlying the catheter *(arrowheads)* does not represent the rectum but the vagina. Transverse 2D **(B** and **C),** sagittal 2D **(D),** and 3D **(E)** CTC images directly demonstrate the vaginal positioning of the catheter, with air surrounding the uterine cervix.

ing of the tenia, decreased compliance, and luminal narrowing. From these pathologic features, and from the high prevalence of this disease, it should come as no surprise that diverticular disease represents the leading cause of nondiagnostic segmental evaluation at CTC. In fact, it is fairly uncommon not to encounter at least one case of advanced diverticular disease each day on our CTC screening service (Fig. 20-44). Fortunately, our methods for colonic preparation and distention usually allow for good diagnostic evaluation.

Unlike barium enema examination, the diverticula themselves cause little problem at CTC interpretation. However, there are a number of other potential pitfalls at CTC related to diverticular disease. The two most important challenges—fold thickening and inadequate luminal distention—have already been covered in this chapter. These factors can make polyp detection very

challenging, especially on the 2D view (Figs. 20-45 and 20-46). Stool-filled diverticula and mucosal prolapse represent additional pitfalls in the setting of diverticular disease. Impacted diverticula, which are filled with inspissated stool, often bulge or prolapse slightly into the colonic lumen, creating a polypoid appearance on the 3D endoluminal view (Figs. 20-47 and 20-48). Exclusion of a true polyp on the 2D display (or 3D translucency rendering) is straightforward, and such "lesions" are merely a nuisance and never a diagnostic dilemma. Frankly inverted diverticula are rare but represent a related potential pitfall. Prolapsing mucosal polyps represent redundant colonic mucosa in the setting of sigmoid diverticular disease (Fig. 20-49). These non-neoplastic lesions can be symptomatic and may be difficult to differentiate from neoplastic disease (Fig. 20-50).[10]

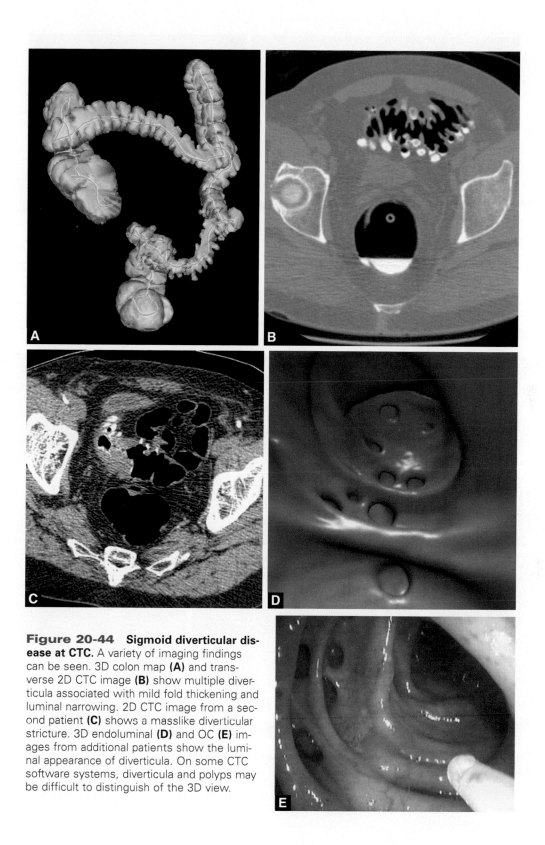

Figure 20-44 Sigmoid diverticular disease at CTC. A variety of imaging findings can be seen. 3D colon map **(A)** and transverse 2D CTC image **(B)** show multiple diverticula associated with mild fold thickening and luminal narrowing. 2D CTC image from a second patient **(C)** shows a masslike diverticular stricture. 3D endoluminal **(D)** and OC **(E)** images from additional patients show the luminal appearance of diverticula. On some CTC software systems, diverticula and polyps may be difficult to distinguish of the 3D view.

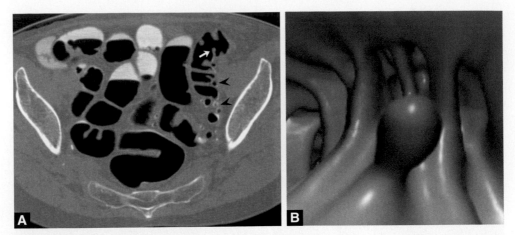

Figure 20-45 Small sigmoid polyp in segment with diverticulosis. Transverse 2D CTC image **(A)** shows changes of moderate sigmoid diverticulosis *(arrowheads)*. In addition, a foldlike structure *(arrow)* actually represents a small pedunculated polyp, which is obvious at 3D endoluminal fly-through **(B)**. In general, polyp detection in diverticular segments is much easier on 3D. (From Sanford MS, Pickhardt PJ. Diagnostic performance of primary 3-dimensional computed tomography colonography in the setting of colonic diverticular disease. *Clin Gastroenterol Hepatol.* 2006;4:1039-1047.) *(*See associated video clip on DVD.)*

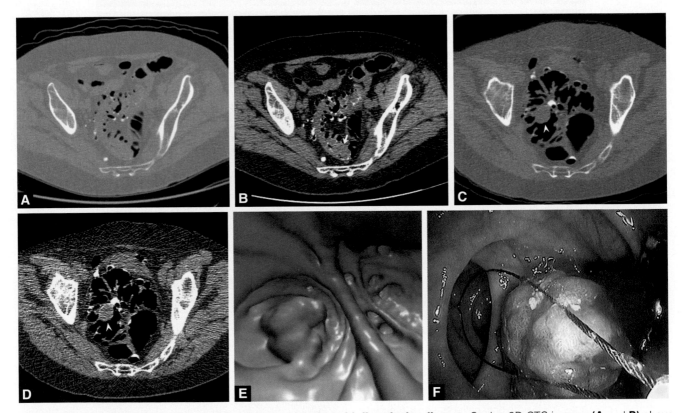

Figure 20-46 Polypoid mass partially obscured by sigmoid diverticular disease. Supine 2D CTC images **(A** and **B)** show long segment spasm or collapse of the sigmoid colon, which demonstrates changes of diverticulosis. Prone 2D **(C** and **D)** and 3D **(E)** images show improved distention, uncovering a large 40-mm mass *(arrowheads)*, which can be seen only in retrospect on supine **(B,** *arrow)* and is all that is needed for confirmation. This large mass was removed in a piecemeal fashion at OC **(F)** and proved to be a benign tubular adenoma without high-grade dysplasia. This reinforces the fact that even large polyps are often benign (yet likely still premalignant).

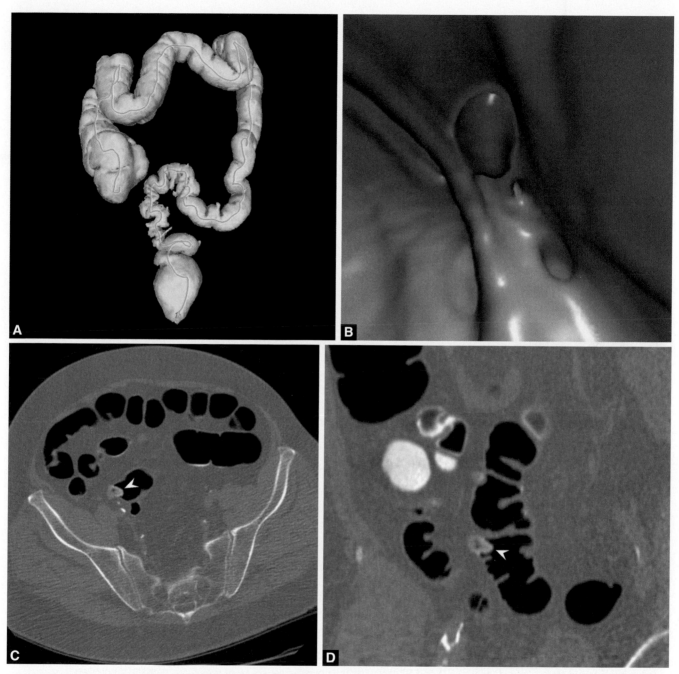

Figure 20-47 **Impacted diverticulum.** 3D colon map **(A)** shows changes of moderate sigmoid diverticular disease. 3D endoluminal image **(B)** shows a polypoid lesion adjacent to sigmoid diverticula. 2D correlation **(C** and **D)** clearly shows that the "polyp" is actually a stool-filled diverticulum *(arrowheads)*. Although the 2D correlation adds time to the primary 3D search pattern, impacted diverticula do not represent a diagnostic dilemma. *(*See associated video clip on DVD.)*

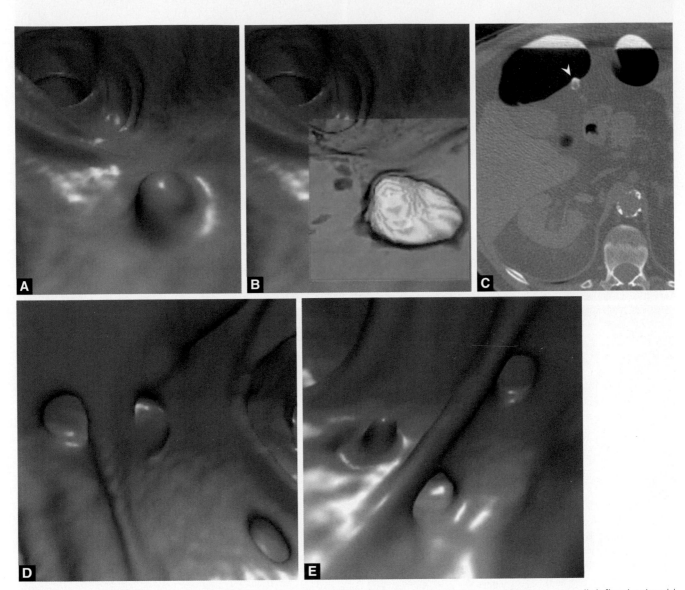

Figure 20-48 **Other cases of stool-filled diverticula at CTC.** 3D endoluminal CTC image **(A)** shows a well-defined polypoid lesion near the hepatic flexure. Translucency rendering **(B)** shows that the lesion "blooms" with a white color signature, indicating a tip-of-the-iceberg effect from an impacted diverticulum, which is also easily confirmed with 2D correlation (**C,** *arrowhead*). 3D endoluminal images from other individuals **(D** and **E)** show multiple diverticula, some of which are partially stool-filled.

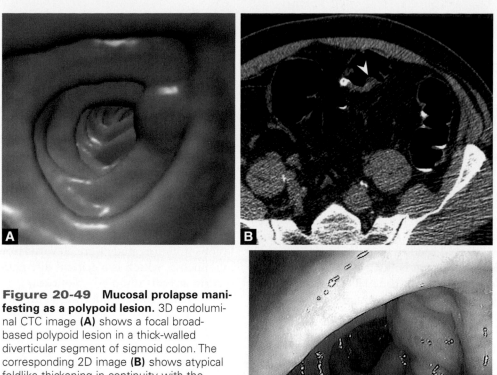

Figure 20-49 **Mucosal prolapse manifesting as a polypoid lesion.** 3D endoluminal CTC image **(A)** shows a focal broadbased polypoid lesion in a thick-walled diverticular segment of sigmoid colon. The corresponding 2D image **(B)** shows atypical foldlike thickening in continuity with the polyp *(arrowhead)*. At OC **(C),** similar findings were seen, related to mucosal prolapse in the setting of sigmoid diverticular disease.

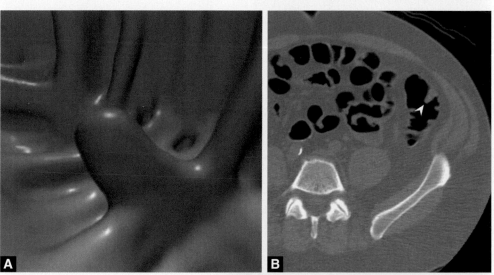

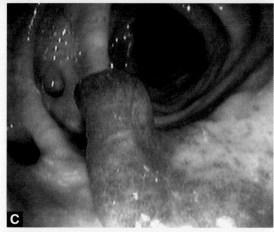

Figure 20-50 **Tubular adenoma mimicking mucosal prolapse at OC.** 3D endoluminal **(A)** and transverse 2D **(B)** CTC images show a polypoid lesion *(arrowhead)* in the sigmoid, associated with diverticular changes. This sessile lesion is somewhat atypical given its tall appearance. At OC **(C),** this lesion was felt to simply represent mucosal prolapse. Biopsy, however, revealed a tubular adenoma.

FLAT AND CARPET LESIONS

Flat lesions represent a subset of sessile polyps that, as the name implies, have a "nonpolypoid" plaquelike morphology, with a height that is generally well under half the width. For flat polyps less than 3 cm in size, lesion elevation above the mucosal surface is typically 3 mm or less (Figs. 20-51 through 20-55).[11] Categorization of larger masses that are generally flat or plaquelike in morphology but taller than 3 mm appears to be less uniform. The term "carpet lesion," also referred to as a laterally or superficially spreading tumor, applies to an important subset of flat lesions that tend to be quite large (≥3 cm) in cross-sectional area but not bulky.[12] Carpet lesions will be considered in more detail at the end of this section.

Both the prevalence and clinical significance of flat colonic lesions have been the source of recent debate. However, unlike other parts of the world,[13] there is little evidence to suggest they represent a major problem in the U.S. screening population. A single center Veterans Administration (VA) study suggested that nonpolypoid lesions may be more common in the United States, and more histologically ominous, than previously thought.[14] However, a closer look at this work reveals that the conclusions are not supported by the findings.[15] First of all, a clear distinction must be made between the *relatively flat* lesions described in this study (defined as elevated lesions with a height less than half the diameter) and *completely flat* or *depressed lesions*. The authors noted that "completely flat lesions are exceedingly rare" and were presumably absent in this study. Depressed lesions comprised less than 1% of all colorectal lesions (18 of 2770), only 4 of which were seen at screening. Therefore, nearly all nonpolypoid lesions from this study were elevated from the surrounding mucosa, which is a critical distinction favoring detection at both standard colonoscopy and CT colonography. In addition, the authors combined "carcinoma in situ," which is more appropriately termed "high-grade dysplasia," with invasive cancers. This is an unfortunate and misleading way to report histology, especially because the majority of nonpolypoid "cancers" in this study (11 of 15) were actually noninvasive advanced adenomas. It is unclear if any depressed cancers were

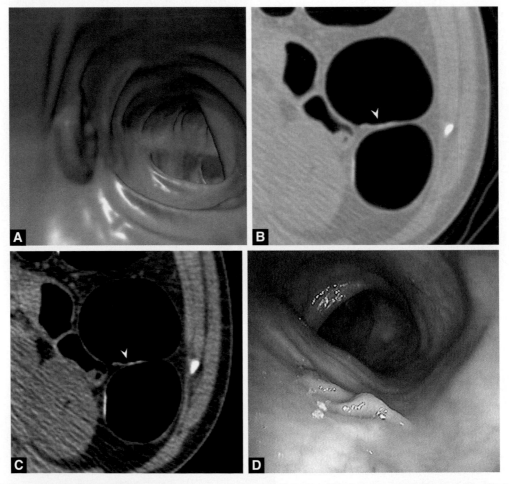

Figure 20-51 **Large flat hyperplastic polyp.** 3D endoluminal CTC image **(A)** shows a large flat lesion in the transverse colon, which is subtle *(arrowheads)* but confirmed at both 2D CTC **(B and C)** and subsequent OC **(D)**. This flat lesion proved to be hyperplastic. *(*See associated video clip on DVD.)*

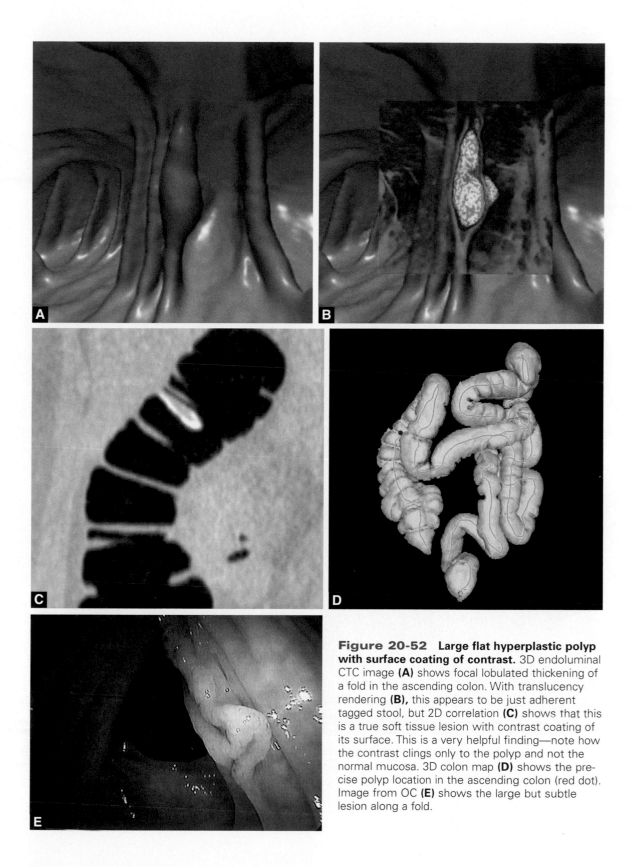

Figure 20-52 Large flat hyperplastic polyp with surface coating of contrast. 3D endoluminal CTC image **(A)** shows focal lobulated thickening of a fold in the ascending colon. With translucency rendering **(B),** this appears to be just adherent tagged stool, but 2D correlation **(C)** shows that this is a true soft tissue lesion with contrast coating of its surface. This is a very helpful finding—note how the contrast clings only to the polyp and not the normal mucosa. 3D colon map **(D)** shows the precise polyp location in the ascending colon (red dot). Image from OC **(E)** shows the large but subtle lesion along a fold.

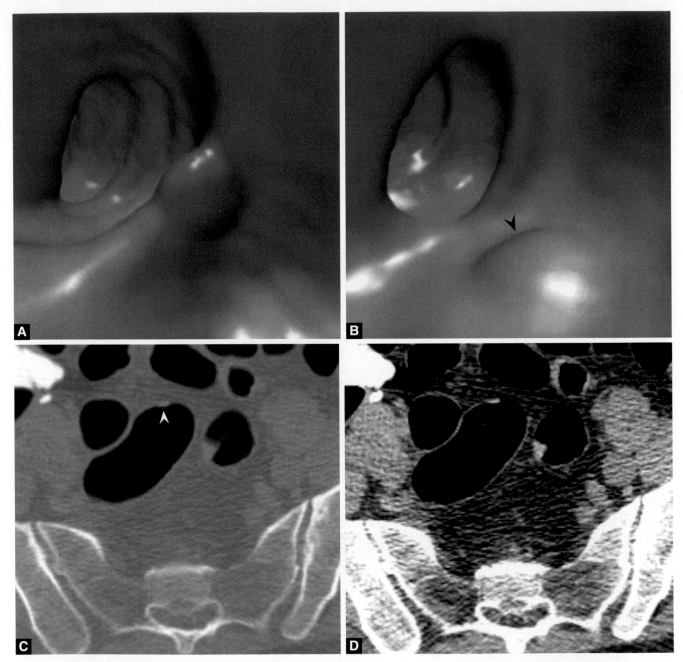

Figure 20-53 Flattening of small hyperplastic polyp at CTC. Supine 3D endoluminal CTC image **(A)** shows a 7-mm sessile lesion on a fold. On prone imaging **(B-D),** the lesion appears to have moved off the fold and flattened out *(arrowheads)*, possibly related to increased luminal distention.

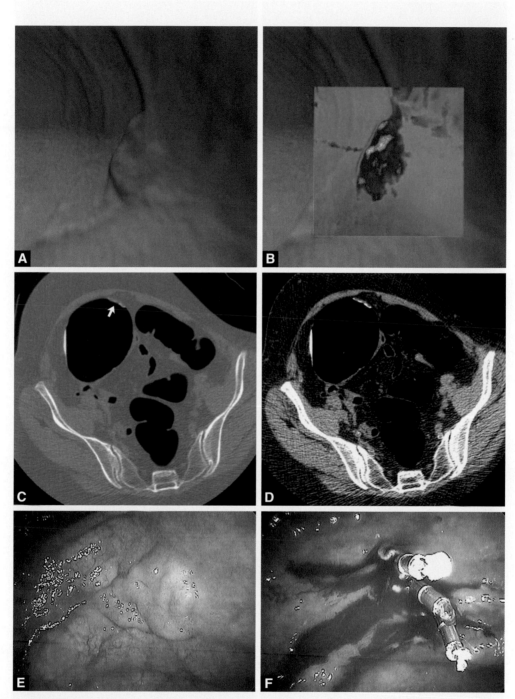

Figure 20-54 **Large flat tubulovillous adenoma.** 3D endoluminal **(A** and **B)** and decubitus 2D **(C** and **D)** CTC images show a large 24-mm cecal lesion with a plaquelike appearance *(arrow)*. A thin rim of contrast coats the surface of this soft tissue lesion. At OC **(E),** the lesion was successfully removed, despite some bleeding requiring the use of vascular clips **(F),** and proved to be a tubulovillous adenoma. *(*See associated video clip on DVD.)*

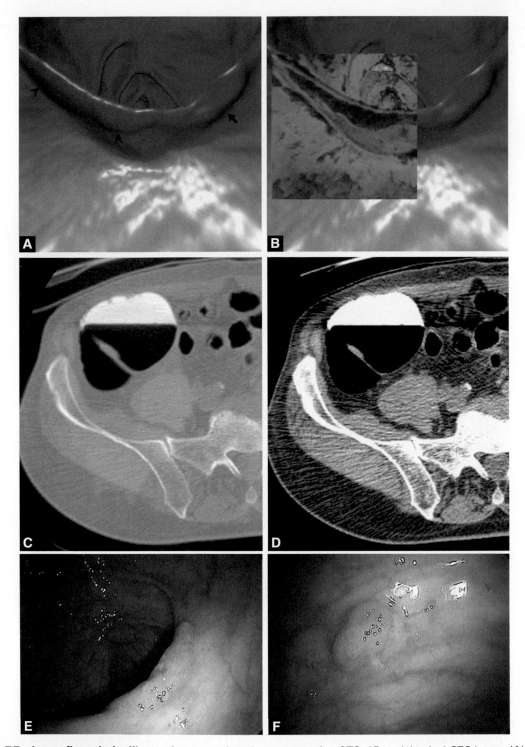

Figure 20-55 Large flat tubulovillous adenoma missed at prospective CTC. 3D endoluminal CTC image **(A)** from the cecal apex shows subtle thickening *(arrowheads)* along the ileocecal fold, adjacent to the valve *(arrow)*. Soft tissue is suggested by 3D translucency **(B)** and confirmed on 2D correlation **(C** and **D)**. This lesion was not prospectively called, but a sessile polyp was identified. At OC, the subtle flat lesion along the fold was identified **(E)**, as was the sessile polyp that was called at CTC **(F)**.

detected at screening, with only 2 cases among the entire cohort. The average size of advanced nonpolypoid lesions was relatively large (1.6 cm) and similar in size to their polypoid counterparts (1.9 cm), which also bodes well for standard colonoscopic detection—whether optical or virtual—because these lesions are important to detect. Finally, the generalizability of this VA cohort to general screening populations is uncertain.

Data from the National Polyp Study show that flat adenomas were less likely to harbor high-grade dysplasia compared with sessile and pedunculated adenomas.[16] In addition, patients with flat adenomas were not found to be at greater risk for advanced adenomas at subsequent surveillance colonoscopy. Furthermore, if aggressive flat lesions in this trial had somehow been missed (e.g., from not using high-magnification chromoendoscopic technique), more incident cancers should have developed over the course of longitudinal evaluation.[17] In fact, the relative frequency of flat adenomas in the National Polyp Study was similar to that reported when narrow band imaging or chromoendoscopic techniques are used.[16] Therefore, there appears to be no justification for using these more time-consuming endoscopic techniques for screening in the United States.

Our own experience with 125 flat lesions measuring ≥6 mm detected at CTC screening has also demonstrated a nonaggressive picture.[18] Of 92 flat lesions less than 3 cm in size evaluated at subsequent OC, 23 (25.0%) were neoplastic, 5 (5.4%) were histologically advanced, and none were malignant. In comparison, polypoid lesions measuring less than 3 cm were much more likely to be neoplastic (60.3%; 363 of 602), histologically advanced (12.1%; 73 of 602), and malignant (0.5%; 3 of 602). None of the 9 flat lesions seen only at colonoscopy (i.e., CTC false negatives) were histologically advanced and only 2 were neoplastic (tubular adenomas). All 10 carpet lesions (i.e., laterally spreading tumors ≥3 cm in size) were neoplastic and 9 were histo-

logically advanced. These findings indicate that flat lesions less than 3 cm in size are not a major concern compared with polypoid lesions of similar size and that large carpet lesions represent the subset of polyps with flat morphology of most interest.

Although flat lesions are less conspicuous and therefore more challenging to initially detect at CTC, the sensitivity of combined 3D–2D polyp detection appears to be satisfactory (Fig. 20-51 through 20-55).[19] Phantom and clinical studies have shown that 3D improves the sensitivity for detecting flat lesions.[13,20] In our recent clinical experience, more large flat advanced adenomas were detected at primary CTC screening compared with primary OC screening.[21] It is interesting to note that histologically advanced or depressed small flat lesions appear to be exceedingly rare in our screening population. In fact, the majority of flat lesions detected (or missed) at CTC are hyperplastic (Figs. 20-51 through 20-53).[22,23] The relative increase in flat versus polypoid hyperplastic lesions likely results in part from their tendency to flatten out when the colonic lumen is distended,[24] which should generally be the case for CTC (Fig. 20-53). In the Mayo Clinic experience, the great majority of occult polyps at CTC (i.e., missed lesions that could not be identified even retrospectively) were flat hyperplastic polyps ranging in size from 6 mm to 2.1 cm.[25] This mirrors our own clinical experience with occult lesions at CTC, which are very uncommon.[23] Retained adherent stool can often mimic a flat polyp, making contrast tagging critical for confidently distinguishing between the two (Fig. 20-56). Given these collective findings, we believe that flat lesions are important to be aware of but do not represent a significant drawback to widespread CTC screening.

Carpet lesions are an important subset of flat lesions that, despite their large surface area, can be relatively subtle on CTC because of the relative lack of tumor bulk (Figs. 20-57 through 20-59). These lesions have a strong predilection for the rectum and cecum.[26] Despite their

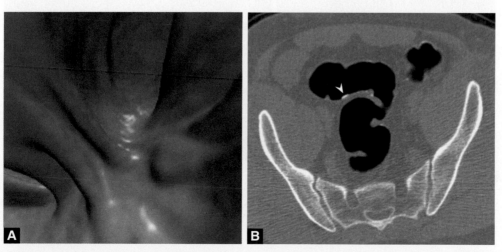

Figure 20-56 **Tagged adherent stool mimicking flat lesion at 3D CTC.** 3D endoluminal **(A)** and transverse 2D **(B)** CTC images show a subtle flat lesion *(arrowhead)* that clearly represents adherent tagged stool at 2D.

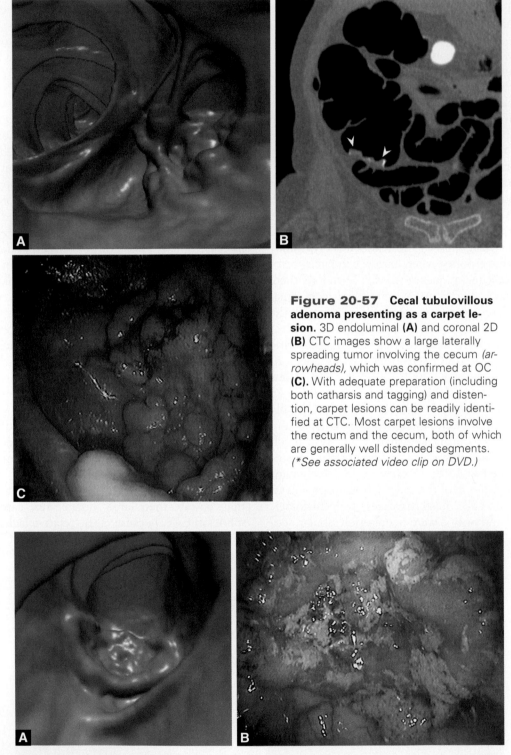

Figure 20-57 Cecal tubulovillous adenoma presenting as a carpet lesion. 3D endoluminal **(A)** and coronal 2D **(B)** CTC images show a large laterally spreading tumor involving the cecum *(arrowheads)*, which was confirmed at OC **(C).** With adequate preparation (including both catharsis and tagging) and distention, carpet lesions can be readily identified at CTC. Most carpet lesions involve the rectum and the cecum, both of which are generally well distended segments. *(*See associated video clip on DVD.)*

Figure 20-58 Carpet lesion (tubulovillous adenoma) with central depression. 3D endoluminal CTC **(A)** and OC **(B)** images show a laterally spreading tumor with rolled-up edges and a central depression. This tumor demonstrated high-grade dysplasia but not invasive cancer at pathology. Depressed lesions are rarely seen in our patient population. *(*See associated video clip on DVD.)*

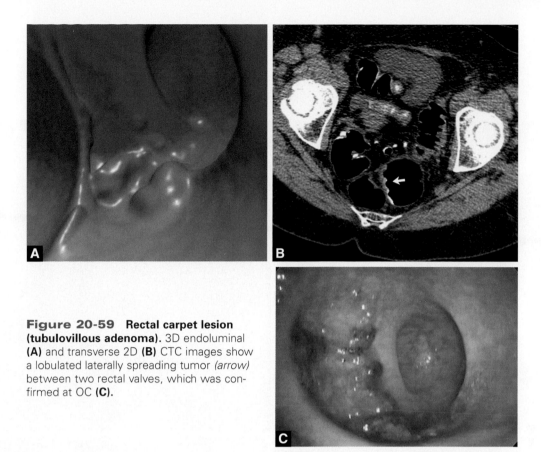

Figure 20-59 Rectal carpet lesion (tubulovillous adenoma). 3D endoluminal **(A)** and transverse 2D **(B)** CTC images show a lobulated laterally spreading tumor *(arrow)* between two rectal valves, which was confirmed at OC **(C)**.

large linear size, they have a relatively low rate of malignancy but frequently demonstrate villous features, with or without high-grade dysplasia.[12,26] Although classic carpet lesions are less conspicuous than sessile or pedunculated polyps, and may even have a central depression (Fig. 50-58), they are nonetheless detectable at CTC because of fixed fold distortion or edges with a rolled-up or polypoid appearance (Figs. 20-57 through 20-59). Optimal preparation and distention, and a hybrid 3D–2D detection strategy, allow for confident detection of carpet lesions. In some cases, endoscopic mucosal resection can serve as the definitive treatment, whereas others will require more aggressive surgery.[12]

POLYP MEASUREMENT

Polyp size measurement at CTC was largely covered in the preceding chapter but is also included here as a potential pitfall because of the ample opportunity for incorrect size assessment, which could lead to inappropriate patient management. 2D measurement of polyps should be carried out on the wider "polyp" window setting (i.e., 2000 HU wide window centered at 0 HU) because the lesion will be undersized on the soft tissue window setting (Fig. 20-60). 2D polyp size will also be artifactually decreased for lesions submerged under densely opacified fluid (Fig. 20-60). It is important to recognize that 2D polyp measurement on the

standard orthogonal views (i.e., transverse, coronal, and sagittal) will undersize lesions whenever the long axis of the polyp does not align perfectly with an orthogonal plane.[27] Therefore, despite its name, the "optimized" orthogonal 2D measurement can definitely underestimate polyp size (Fig. 20-61). This is a more relevant issue for lesions with an irregular or elongated morphology. Polyp measurement on the 3D endoluminal view can also be fraught with error if care is not taken to optimize the vantage point (i.e., directly over polyp and not "down the barrel"). In addition, incorrect caliper placement, partially submerged polyps, and thick contrast coating of polyps can all lead to erroneous 3D measurement. Oversizing diminutive and small polyps on 3D is a common pitfall that can lead to overaggressive management if not carefully correlated with the 2D polyp size. Over time, one learns to appreciate lesions that are diminutive in size without the need to formally measure each one (Fig. 20-62).

In the end, for all suspected polyps in the 5- to 6-mm range or greater, we recommend performing a careful combined 2D and 3D assessment of polyp size. For most polyps, the 2D and 3D measurements will be within 1 mm of each other. Unless the lesion is at or near a critical size threshold (i.e., 6 mm and 10 mm), the final reported size is not problematic. However, if the lesion is bordering a critical size threshold or there is a relatively large discrepancy between the 2D and 3D assessment,

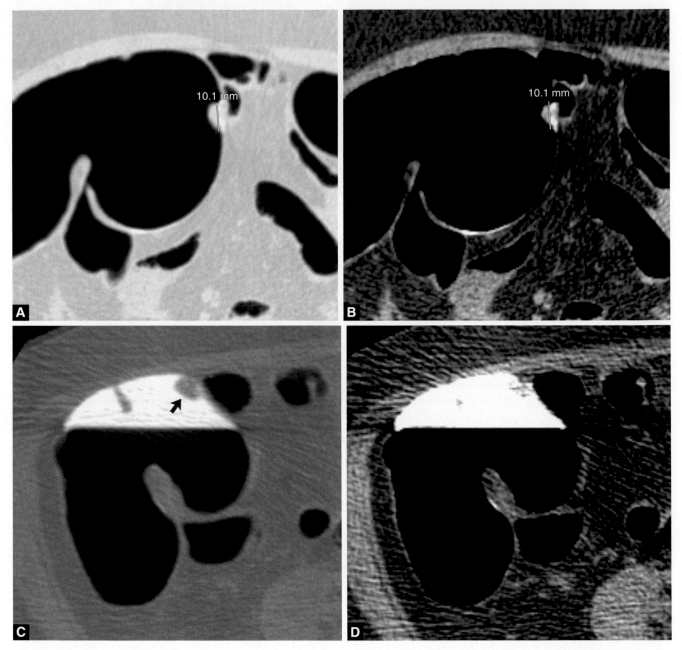

Figure 20-60 Apparent decrease in polyp size on soft tissue window setting. Supine transverse 2D CTC image **(A)** with polyp window setting (2000/0) shows a 10-mm sessile polyp in the cecum *(calipers)*. On a soft tissue window setting **(B,** 350/40), the polyp appears to decrease in size to less than 10-mm. Polyp measurement on soft tissue windows could lead to inappropriate management. On the prone 2D CTC images **(C** and **D),** the polyp *(arrow)* is submerged under densely opacified fluid, which accentuates artifactual decreases in polyp size. Note how the lesion is barely perceptible on the soft tissue window setting **(D).**

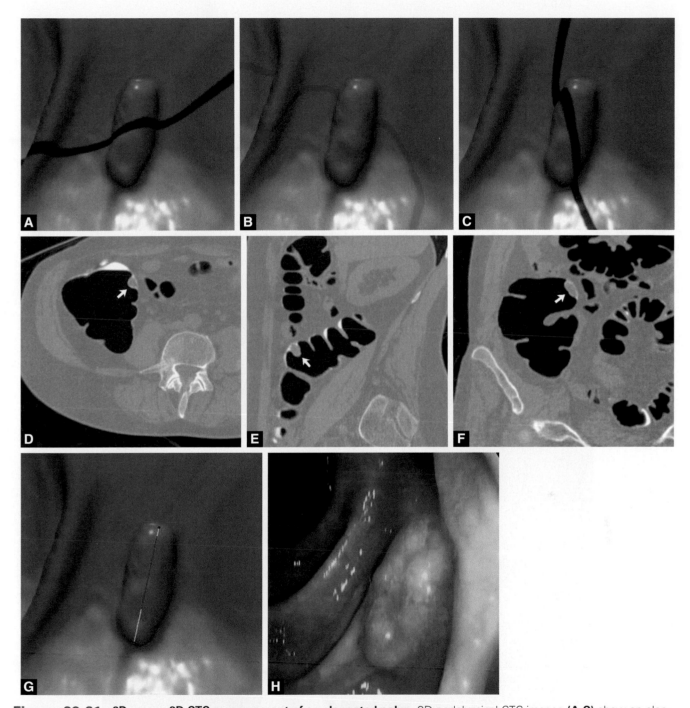

Figure 20-61   2D versus 3D CTC measurement of an elongated polyp. 3D endoluminal CTC images **(A-C)** show an elongated polyp with the transverse **(A)**, sagittal **(B)**, and coronal **(C)** 2D planes as colored lines through the polyp, corresponding to the 2D images **(D-F,** *arrows*). Even with the "optimized" coronal 2D measurement **(C** and **F)**, the polyp is significantly undersized, whereas the 3D measurement **(G)** corresponds to the actual long axis of the polyp and correlated best with OC **(H)**.

Illustration continued on following page

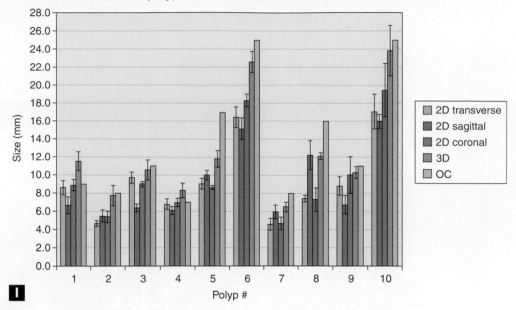

2D versus 3D polyp measurement: *In vivo* clinical cases

Legend:
- 2D transverse
- 2D sagittal
- 2D coronal
- 3D
- OC

X-axis: Polyp #
Y-axis: Size (mm)

I

Figure 20-61 (Continued) **2D versus 3D CTC measurement of an elongated polyp.** Bar graph **(I)** shows the comparison of 2D and 3D polyp measurement at CTC with OC polyp measurement in 10 clinical cases. Note how the agreement is best between the 3D CTC and OC measurements, whereas 2D CTC tended to undersize polyps—sometimes considerably. (From Pickhardt PJ, Lee AD, McFarland EG, Taylor AJ. Linear polyp measurement at CT colonography: In vitro and in vivo comparison of two-dimensional and three-dimensional displays. *Radiology.* 2005;236:872-878.)

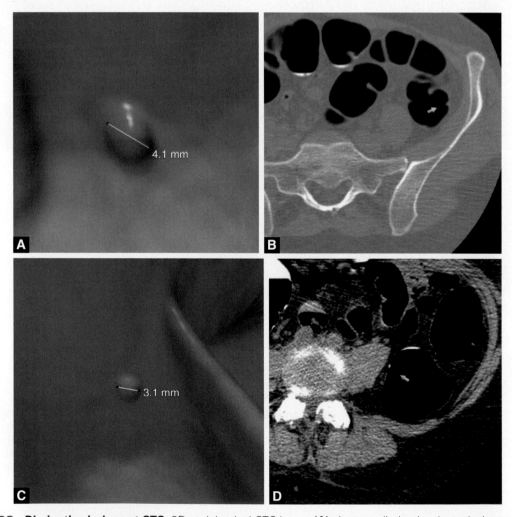

Figure 20-62 **Diminutive lesions at CTC.** 3D endoluminal CTC image **(A)** shows a diminutive 4-mm lesion, which appears to be composed of soft tissue at 2D correlation **(B,** *arrow*). Most diminutive lesions **(C),** however, will represent residual adherent stool, which will often demonstrate internal contrast tagging **(D,** *arrow*). Regardless of whether these lesions are true polyps or pseudolesions, they should not be reported in isolation at CTC. Therefore, it behooves the reader to become familiar with the appearance of lesions in the 5- to 6-mm range, which generally require further interrogation.

then a judgment call by the reader is necessary to determine the most appropriate size to report. We only report size to the nearest millimeter, avoiding the use of submillimeter reporting even though it is provided by most systems. It should be recognized that CTC is the most accurate diagnostic tool available for polyp measurement, followed by OC with use of a calibrated probe. Visual estimation at OC is less accurate, and postpolypectomy and pathology measurements are the least accurate of all.[28,29] Polyp volume assessment, and automated linear and volume measurements, could play important roles in the future.[30-33]

CONTRAST COATING OF POLYPS

One potential pitfall that has actually become a useful interpretive asset for us is the tendency for true soft tissue polyps to demonstrate a thin surface coating of adherent positive oral contrast (Figs. 20-63 and 20-64).[34] It is interesting that this contrast etching is typically seen only with true polyps and not with the surrounding normal colonic mucosa or adherent stool. On 2D, contrast coating of polyps is easy to distinguish from internal tagging of stool, which is an extremely important distinction. In effect, this thin surface coating of contrast serves as a beacon for polyp detection, for which computer-aided detection (CAD) systems could also take advantage. One notable pitfall is the fact that coated polyps can mimic tagged stool on the 3D translucency view because the underlying red soft tissue signature can be obscured by the shell of white contrast (Fig. 20-64). In addition, this contrast coat could lead to oversizing of a polyp measured at 3D, as mentioned earlier.

POSITIONAL CHANGE IN POLYPS

The potential for relative positional shifting of polyps between views is a widely recognized 2D pitfall. The primary concern, of course, is that such a lesion could

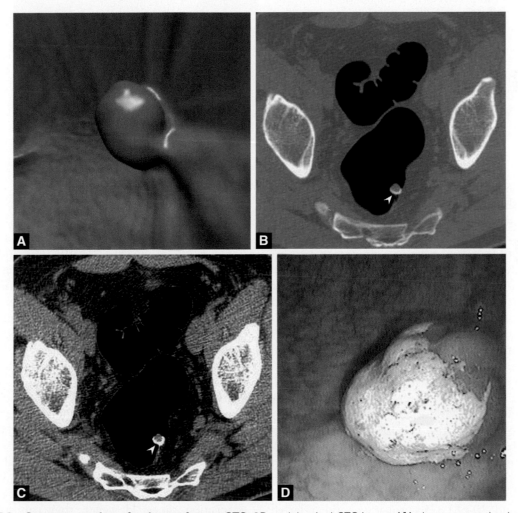

Figure 20-63 **Contrast coating of polyp surface at CTC.** 3D endoluminal CTC image **(A)** shows a rectal polyp, which demonstrates a partial coating of its surface on 2D CTC **(B** and **C,** *arrowheads*) and at subsequent OC **(D).** Note how this film layer only clings to the polyp and not the surrounding normal mucosa, an observation that acts as a beacon for polyp detection. (From Pickhardt PJ. Screening CT colonography: How I do it. *Am J Roentgenol.* 2007;189:290-298.)

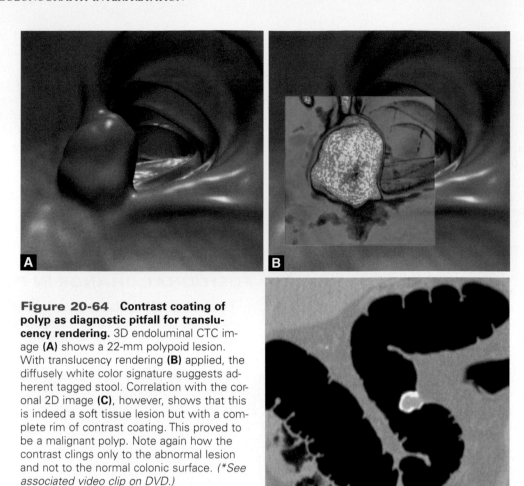

Figure 20-64 Contrast coating of polyp as diagnostic pitfall for translucency rendering. 3D endoluminal CTC image **(A)** shows a 22-mm polypoid lesion. With translucency rendering **(B)** applied, the diffusely white color signature suggests adherent tagged stool. Correlation with the coronal 2D image **(C)**, however, shows that this is indeed a soft tissue lesion but with a complete rim of contrast coating. This proved to be a malignant polyp. Note again how the contrast clings only to the abnormal lesion and not to the normal colonic surface. *(*See associated video clip on DVD.)*

be mistaken for mobile stool. The most typical scenario is dependent shifting of a pedunculated polyp on a relatively long stalk (Fig. 20-65). On primary 3D evaluation, however, the connecting stalk is almost always readily apparent, but it may be less obvious in rare instances (Fig. 20-66). Regardless, the uniform soft tissue attenuation of the polyp head on 2D, even if the stalk is not immediately recognized, should be a tipoff. In addition to shifting of pedunculated lesions, it has also been recognized that sessile lesions can significantly change in their relative orientation between supine and prone relative to rotation or twisting of the colon.[35,36] This tends to occur more with the intraperitoneal colonic segments, which can rotate somewhat on their mesenteric attachment, and in cases with a mobile cecum (Fig. 20-67). To address this issue of relative rotation, a tenia-based system for circumferential localization has been proposed but is still experimental.[37] As an anecdote, we have also noticed that polyp location relative to colonic folds is not a truly fixed relationship (Figs. 20-53 and 20-68). This suggests some relative mobility of the overlying mucosa relative to the deeper intramural layers.

IMAGING ARTIFACTS AND DISTORTION

There are a wide variety of potential artifacts related to CT scanning, image reconstruction, and postprocessing that can result in interpretive challenges. Most radiologists with extensive experience in CT interpretation, including advanced visualization techniques, will be adept at handling these imaging artifacts. The larger concern stems from potential interpretation by nonradiologists with minimal CTC training and little or no familiarity with either general CT interpretation or the basic physics of medical imaging. Although CAD has been advanced as a saving crutch for this group to maintain an adequate sensitivity for polyp detection, this does not address the issue of poor specificity leading to an unacceptable false-positive rate.

Respiratory and other motion-related artifacts are much less common with multidetector CT (MDCT) scanners having 16 or more channels because of shorter acquisition times. However, they can still occur and result in distortion on the 3D endoluminal view (Fig. 20-69). Localized motion artifact seems to occur more

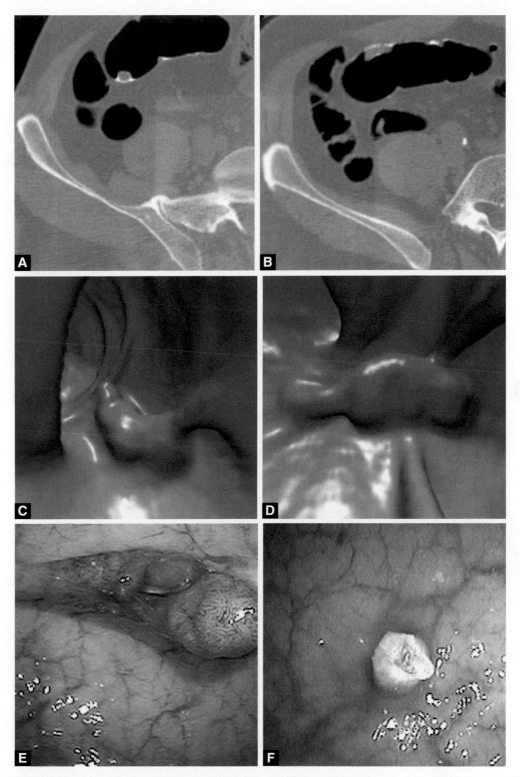

Figure 20-65 Dependent positional shifting of pedunculated polyp. Supine **(A)** and prone **(B)** transverse 2D CTC images show a lesion of homogeneous soft tissue density that falls to the dependent wall on each position. The reason for this shift is obvious on the corresponding 3D endoluminal images **(C** and **D),** where a pedunculated polyp is seen that hinges around the stalk. On 2D, the key to diagnosis is recognition of the site of stalk attachment, which remains fixed relative to the colon. The polyp was found **(E)** and removed **(F)** at OC, clearly showing the site of stalk attachment to the wall.

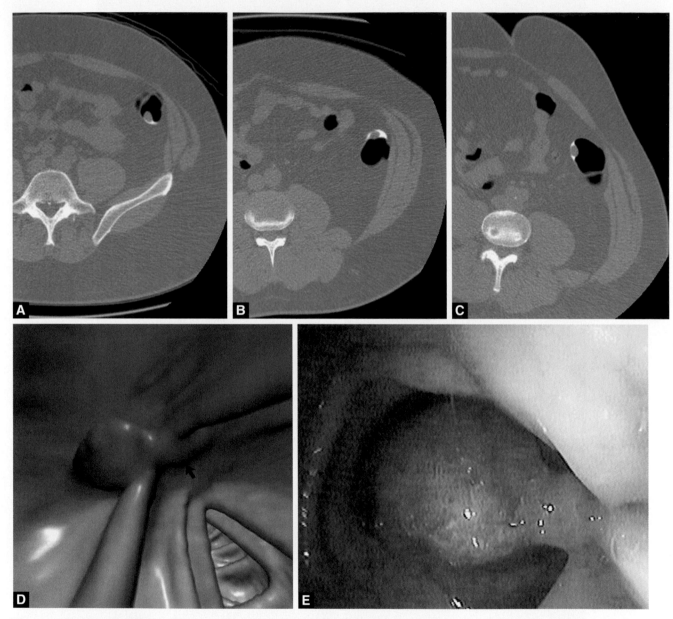

Figure 20-66   Positional shift of polyp with subtle stalk. Supine **(A),** prone **(B),** and decubitus **(C)** transverse 2D images show a polypoid lesion that lies dependently on all three views. The stalk of this pedunculated polyp was much less obvious, even on 3D **(D)** where the stalk *(arrow)* was seen to curl over a fold. A pedunculated polyp with a short stalk was confirmed at OC for polypectomy **(E).**

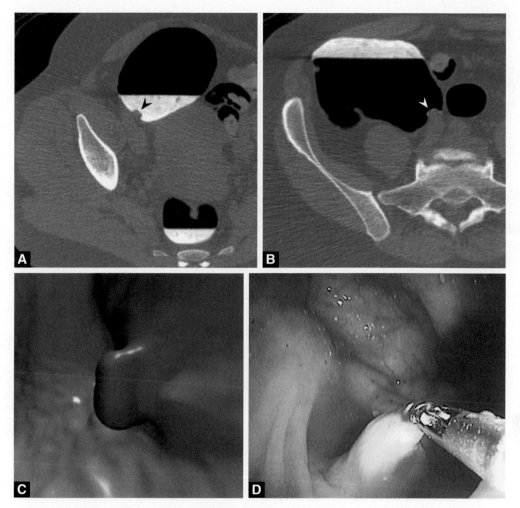

Figure 20-67 **Cecal rotation shifting relative position of polypoid lesion (inverted appendiceal stump).** Supine **(A)** and prone **(B)** transverse 2D CTC images, and 3D image **(C)**, show an atypical squared-off soft tissue lesion *(arrowheads)* that moves from a lateral position on supine to a more medial position on prone. The relative position of the ileocecal valve also shifted in a similar manner (not shown). In such cases, it is critical to recognize the fixed location of a lesion relative to colonic anatomy, despite the change relative to the extracolonic environment. This lesion was located at or near the expected position of the appendix and proved to be an inverted stump at OC **(D).**

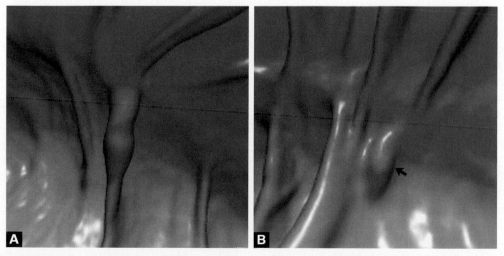

Figure 20-68 **Apparent positional change of polyp relative to adjacent fold.** Supine 3D endoluminal image **(A)** shows a lobulated polyp situated along the edge of a colonic fold. On the prone 3D image **(B),** the lesion *(arrow)* appears to have moved off the fold, which is largely effaced.

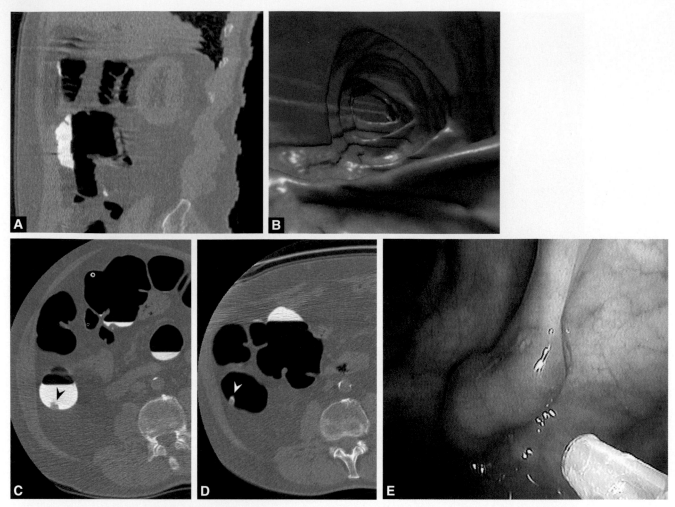

Figure 20-69 **Severe motion artifact related to involuntary shaking.** Sagittal 2D **(A)** and 3D endoluminal **(B)** CTC images show exaggerated stairstep artifacts relating to violent uncontrollable shaking. The supine **(C)** and prone **(D)** transverse images, which correspond to the plane of acquisition, show significantly less distortion. Despite the motion artifact, a 20-mm polyp was identified *(arrowheads)*, which proved to be hyperplastic after resection at OC **(E)**. A number of left-sided diminutive lesions were also seen at CTC and confirmed at subsequent OC (not shown). This represents an extreme example of motion artifact.

often in the left upper quadrant near the splenic flexure region (Fig. 20-70). On single-detector or multidetector CT scanners with four or fewer channels, stairstep artifacts were a common finding at CTC. Stairstep artifacts present only on the reconstructed 2D images (coronal or sagittal) and the 3D endoluminal images, manifesting as evenly spaced ridges or rings (Fig. 20-71).[38] These artifacts are easily identified and generally are just an annoyance. Stairstep artifacts are minimized or absent on 16-detector row (or higher) scanners with contiguous or overlapping 1.25-mm source.

Because of the inherent characteristics of the soft tissue–air interface at CTC, substantial dose reduction compared with standard abdominal CT imaging is possible. However, at very low doses, image noise from quantum mottle can become an important issue, especially with the use of thin collimation in patients who are obese. With a fixed mA low-dose technique, image noise is accentuated inferiorly because of the bony pelvis (Fig. 20-72). We have found that dose modulation is a more efficient strategy that limits such artifacts by increasing tube current only to the desired level and no more (see Chapter 14). Image noise is more apparent on soft tissue window settings compared with the wider polyp window (Fig. 20-72 and Fig. 20-73), which can markedly limit extracolonic evaluation (see Chapter 27). On the 3D endoluminal view, image noise from low-dose technique manifests with diffusely mottled surface irregularity that can approach a cobblestone-like appearance in extreme cases (Fig. 20-72). It is critical not to mistake the image noise within a true polyp or mass on 2D soft tissue windowing or 3D translucency rendering as low-attenuation heterogeneity from stool or fat (Figs. 20-73 and 20-74). Another pitfall related to soft tissue windowing is that some polyps may be completely obscured within heavily tagged fluid, which is why the wider polyp

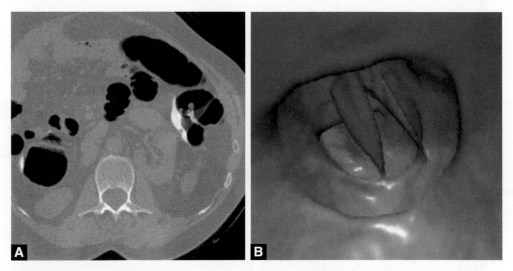

Figure 20-70 **Focal motion artifact.** Transverse 2D CTC image **(A)** shows focal motion artifact in the descending colon, which gives rise to a nonanatomic endoluminal artifact at 3D **(B).** No other motion was present in the remainder of the colon.

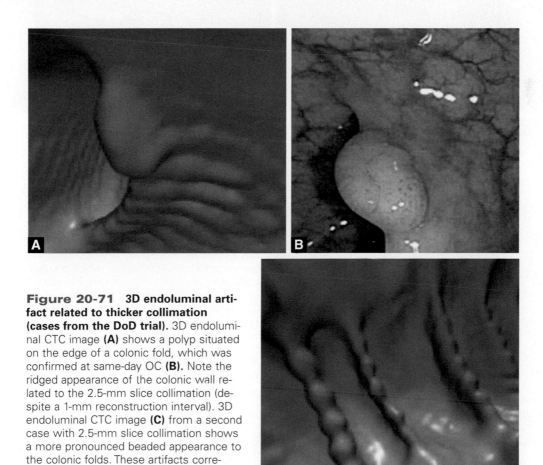

Figure 20-71 **3D endoluminal artifact related to thicker collimation (cases from the DoD trial).** 3D endoluminal CTC image **(A)** shows a polyp situated on the edge of a colonic fold, which was confirmed at same-day OC **(B).** Note the ridged appearance of the colonic wall related to the 2.5-mm slice collimation (despite a 1-mm reconstruction interval). 3D endoluminal CTC image **(C)** from a second case with 2.5-mm slice collimation shows a more pronounced beaded appearance to the colonic folds. These artifacts correspond to the orientation of the plane of scanning. With 1.25-mm collimation, these artifacts are largely absent.

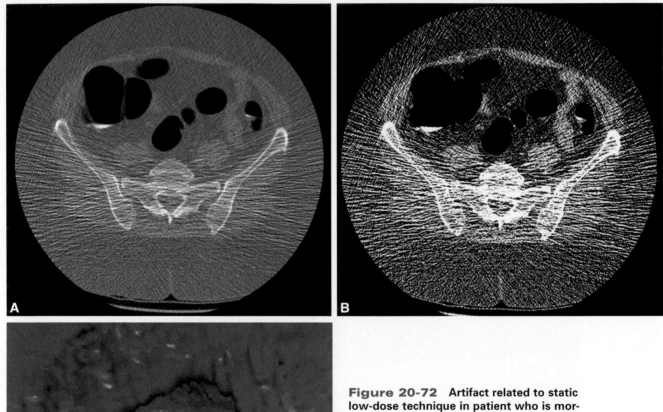

Figure 20-72 Artifact related to static low-dose technique in patient who is morbidly obese. Transverse 2D CTC images with polyp **(A)** and soft tissue **(B)** window settings, obtained with static low-dose technique (25 mAs) in a patient who is obese, demonstrate significant noise, which is especially pronounced on the soft tissue window setting. Note, however, that the soft tissue–air interface would probably still allow for detection of large lesions. Corresponding 3D view **(C)** shows the effect of image noise on the endoluminal projection. We now use dose modulation to prevent this level of image artifact. (*See associated video clip on DVD.)

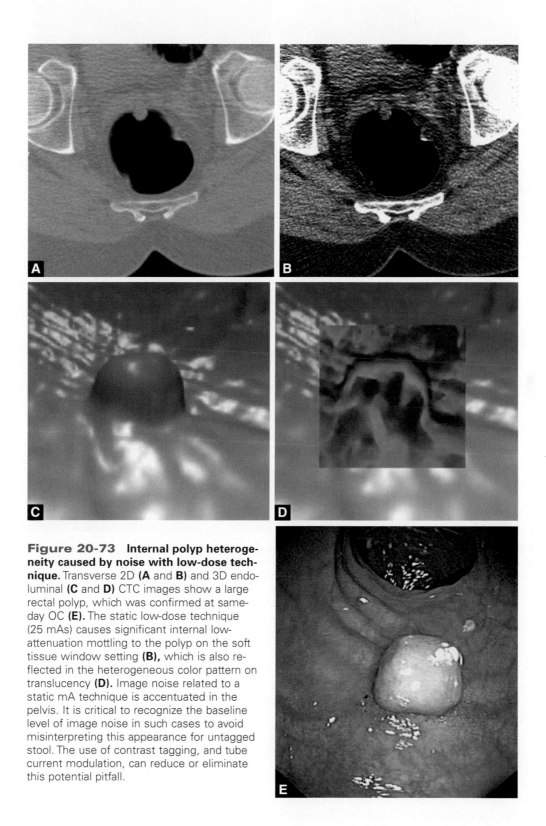

Figure 20-73 Internal polyp heterogeneity caused by noise with low-dose technique. Transverse 2D (**A** and **B**) and 3D endoluminal (**C** and **D**) CTC images show a large rectal polyp, which was confirmed at same-day OC (**E**). The static low-dose technique (25 mAs) causes significant internal low-attenuation mottling to the polyp on the soft tissue window setting (**B**), which is also reflected in the heterogeneous color pattern on translucency (**D**). Image noise related to a static mA technique is accentuated in the pelvis. It is critical to recognize the baseline level of image noise in such cases to avoid misinterpreting this appearance for untagged stool. The use of contrast tagging, and tube current modulation, can reduce or eliminate this potential pitfall.

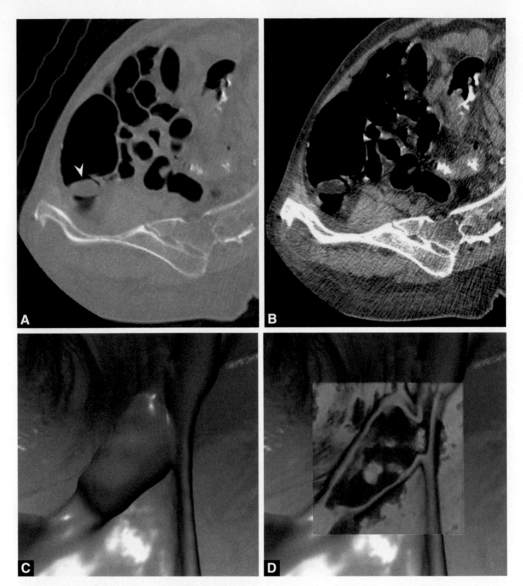

Figure 20-74 **Low-dose technique causing soft tissue mass to mimic lipoma or untagged stool.** Decubitus 2D **(A** and **B)** and 3D endoluminal **(C** and **D)** CTC images show an elongated cecal mass *(arrowhead)*. On the soft tissue window setting **(B)** and 3D translucency rendering **(D)**, internal areas of fat attenuation are suggested, related to accentuated quantum mottle and beam hardening. However, this lesion proved to be malignant (adenocarcinoma).

window should be used for initial detection and evaluation (Fig. 20-75). Beam-hardening artifacts related to metallic objects such as spinal hardware or hip prostheses are accentuated by low-dose CTC technique, but lesion detection on polyp windowing is usually still possible (Figs. 20-76 and 20-77).

A number of important artifacts result from postprocessing of the MDCT source data. Chief among these are the geometric distortions that are introduced in creating nonstandard 3D displays, such as the 360-degree virtual dissection view. The primary motivation for developing these alternative views is to reduce the time needed to visualize the entire luminal surface. However, geometric distortion is the unavoidable tradeoff, which can compromise polyp recognition, even if the lesion is "visualized" (Fig. 20-78). Polyp size is also difficult to judge on

the 360-degree virtual dissection view because information on relative size is lost (Fig. 20-79). These alternative 3D displays are discussed in more detail in Chapter 23. We prefer a milder form of distortion that simply consists of widening the field-of-view angle to 120 degrees but maintains the more familiar 3D endoluminal view. By decreasing the number of fly-throughs from four down to two for well-distended cases, we achieve the goal of decreased interpretation time without introducing troublesome spatial distortion (see Chapter 23).

Another important source of postprocessing artifacts is digital fluid subtraction or "electronic cleansing" of tagged luminal fluid (Fig. 20-80).[2] Because of volume averaging effects at the interfaces between luminal gas, tagged fluid, and the colonic wall, pseudopolyps are a common result of the digital subtraction process

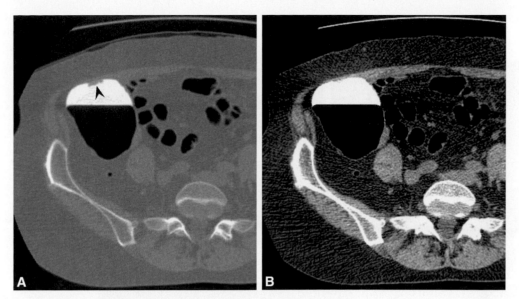

Figure 20-75 Flat lesion obscured by opacified fluid on soft tissue windowing. Transverse 2D CTC image with polyp windowing **(A)** shows a flat cecal polyp *(arrowhead),* which is submerged under opacified fluid but nonetheless detectable. On the soft tissue window setting **(B),** however, the lesion is virtually obscured by the dense surrounding fluid. This windowing phenomenon is also the reason why 2D lesion measurement must take place on the wider polyp window setting.

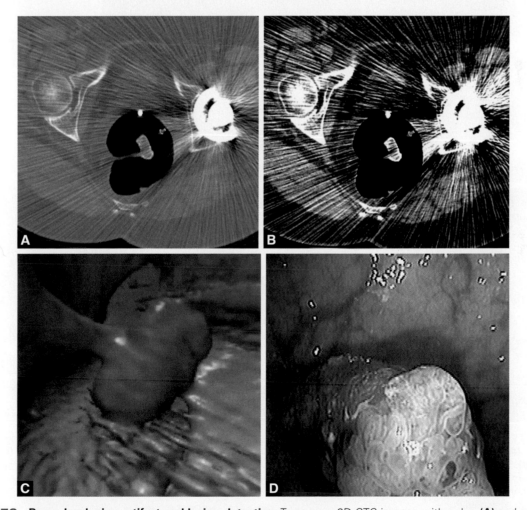

Figure 20-76 Beam-hardening artifact and lesion detection. Transverse 2D CTC images with polyp **(A)** and soft tissue **(B)** window settings show significant beam-hardening artifact related to the metallic left hip prosthesis. Nonetheless, a 3-cm rectal mass is apparent *(blue arrows),* demonstrating a characteristic rim of contrast coating. The streak artifact, which is especially pronounced on the soft tissue window setting **(B),** also appears on the 3D endoluminal view **(C)** but does not preclude lesion detection. This mass proved to be a villous adenoma after resection at OC **(D).** *(*See associated video clip on DVD.)*

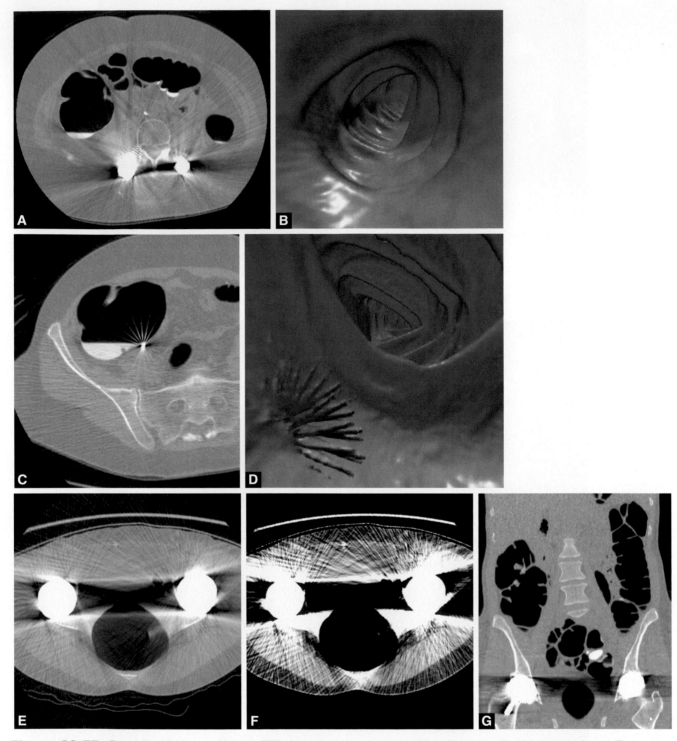

Figure 20-77   Beam-hardening artifact at CTC. Several cases of streak artifact from metallic objects are shown. Transverse 2D CTC image **(A)** from the first case shows artifact related to spinal hardware, which has relatively little effect on the 3D endoluminal image **(B).** Transverse 2D **(C)** and 3D endoluminal **(D)** images from a second case show focal streak artifact related to a metallic clip from prior appendectomy. 2D transverse **(E** and **F)** and coronal **(G)** images from a third case show extensive beam-hardening artifact related to bilateral hip replacements. Note on the coronal view **(G)** how the artifact is essentially limited to the transverse plane of acquisition.

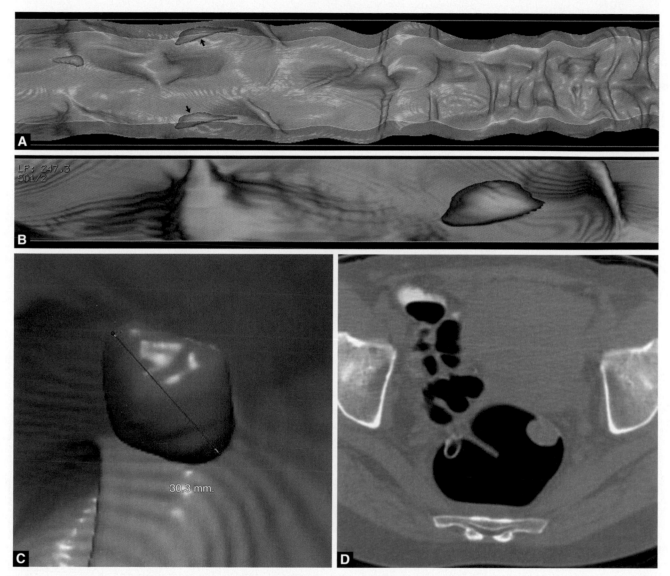

Figure 20-78   Spatial distortion on the 360-degree 3D virtual dissection display. Image from 3D virtual dissection **(A)** with full 360-degree display (plus overlap) shows a tear-dropped shaped abnormality *(arrows),* which appears more masslike on the older 120-degree strip **(B).** On the standard 3D endoluminal **(C)** and transverse 2D **(D)** views, an obvious 3-cm mass is seen, which proved to be a tubulovillous adenoma with high-grade dysplasia. *(*See associated video clip on DVD.)*

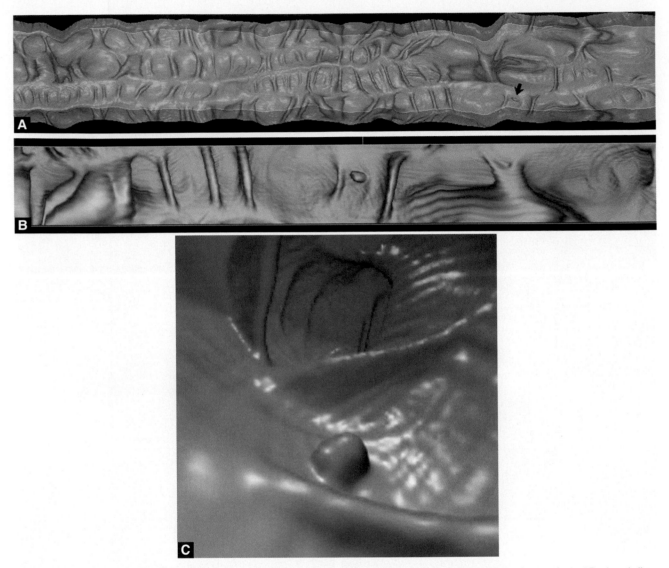

Figure 20-79 **Difficulty assessing polyp size on the 360-degree 3D virtual dissection view.** Image from 3D virtual dissection **(A)** with 360-degree display shows a tiny-appearing polypoid lesion *(arrow)*, which appears larger on the older 120-degree strip **(B)** and standard endoluminal view **(C).** This polyp measured 8 mm at both CTC and OC. The small polyp size on the 360-degree dissection view relates to the fact that the colonic circumference is normalized to fit the strip. Therefore, lesions in the more capacious right colon will appear relatively smaller, whereas lesions in a narrow sigmoid segment will appear much larger. The inability to gauge polyp size is a significant drawback of this display because relevant lesions could be dismissed as diminutive. *(*See associated video clip on DVD.)*

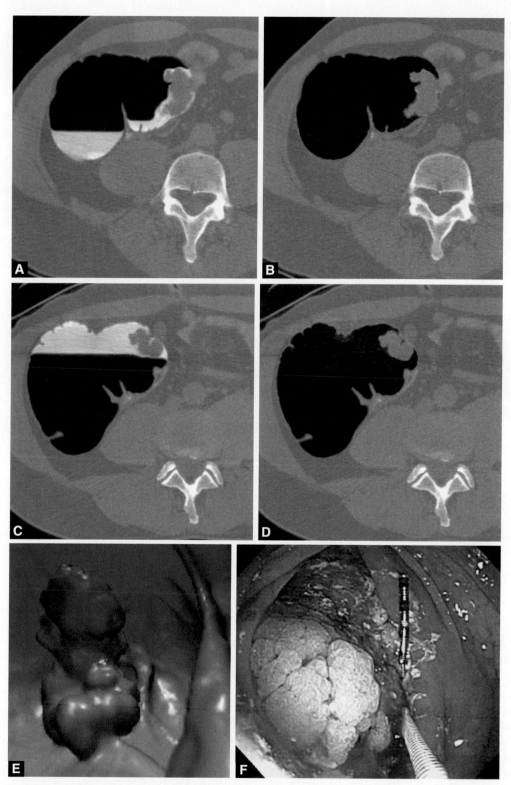

Figure 20-80 **Electronic cleansing (digital fluid subtraction) at CTC.** Supine and prone 2D CTC images **(A-D)** demonstrate the appearance without electronic fluid subtraction **(A** and **C)** and with subtraction **(B** and **D)**. Note how 2D lesion detection is not improved with fluid cleansing, which only introduces artifacts that could negatively affect the evaluation. Therefore, the 2D displays should never be subjected to electronic cleansing. Electronic cleansing can uncover submerged lesions on the 3D display **(E)**. However, with our current preparation, the amount of opacified fluid is minimized and almost never overlaps between the supine and prone positions. This lobulated lesion proved to be a tubulovillous adenoma after resection at OC **(F)**.

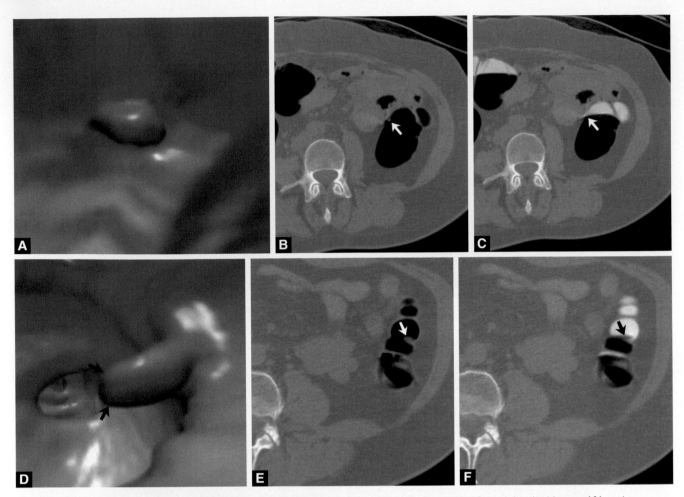

Figure 20-81 Pseudopolyps created by electronic cleansing artifact (DoD case). 3D endoluminal image **(A)** and transverse 2D image **(B)** with electronic fluid cleansing show a polypoid lesion *(arrow)*. However, without subtraction **(C)**, no lesion is seen *(arrow)*. The polypoid "lesion" on both 2D and 3D was created by partial volume effects where the air–fluid meniscus contacts the bowel wall. 3D endoluminal image **(D)** from a second case shows another polypoid lesion *(arrows)*, which has a correlate on the subtracted 2D image **(E)** but is again shown to be simply a subtraction artifact on the uncleansed source image **(F)**. Without the true unadulterated 2D source images, a polyp may be incorrectly called if only the subtracted 2D images are used for confirmation of 3D findings. (From Pickhardt PJ, Choi JR. Electronic cleansing and stool tagging in CT colonography: Advantages and pitfalls encountered with primary three-dimensional evaluation. *Am J Roentgenol.* 2003;181:799-805.)

(Fig. 20-81). Submerged semisolid stool that approaches soft tissue density can appear polypoid as well (Fig. 20-82). Even air bubbles in a fluid-filled lumen can appear polypoid after digital subtraction (Fig. 20-83). Interrogating these pseudopolyps will not only increase interpretation time; it also has the potential to decrease specificity if such lesions are mistaken for true pathology. With our current bowel preparation, the fluid level almost never overlaps between supine and prone positioning.[39] Therefore, primary 3D evaluation without digital fluid extraction generally covers the entire luminal surface, and navigation is much faster without the vexing artifacts. As such, we have not used this tool since the conclusion of the Department of Defense (DoD) trial in 2003. At the very least, digital subtraction should never be applied on the 2D display because any polypoid artifacts present on the 3D display are re-created on a subtracted 2D image, leading to an erroneous interpretation

(Figs. 20-80 and 20-81). Furthermore, true lesions are detectable on 2D within tagged fluid pools without subtraction. One final pitfall we have noticed with electronic fluid cleansing is that the centerline, which is virtually infallible when digital subtraction is not used, can burrow through a colonic wall and bypass segments of the colon (Fig. 20-84). Presumably, digital fluid subtraction techniques will continue to improve and the various artifacts will be minimized or eliminated. At that point, we may reconsider using this tool in clinical practice.

ANORECTAL FINDINGS

A number of findings specific to the anorectum deserve attention because they are relatively common and can mimic neoplastic disease.[1] However, if appropriately recognized, most incidental findings will not require further evaluation. For those that do, correlation with digital rec-

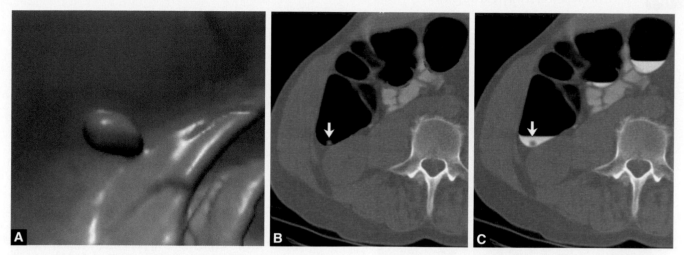

Figure 20-82 **Pseudopolyp from subtraction around submerged stool (DoD case).** 3D endoluminal image **(A)** and 2D image **(B)** with electronic fluid cleansing show a polypoid lesion *(arrow)* at the dependent wall. 2D image without electronic cleansing **(C)** shows that this "lesion" was submerged untagged stool *(arrow),* which was mobile and remained within the fluid pool on the prone images (not shown). With electronic cleansing, such lesions must be investigated at 3D evaluation, whereas mobile submerged debris is never visualized at 3D fly-through without cleansing (our preference). (From Pickhardt PJ, Choi JR. Electronic cleansing and stool tagging in CT colonography: Advantages and pitfalls encountered with primary three-dimensional evaluation. *Am J Roentgenol.* 2003;181:799-805.)

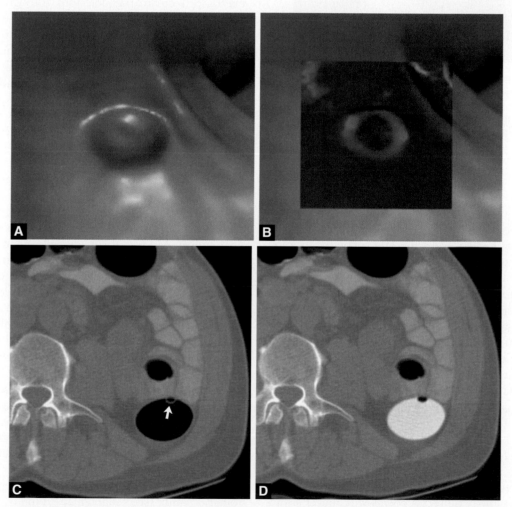

Figure 20-83 **Pseudopolyp from cleansing artifact created by air bubble (DoD case).** 3D endoluminal images **(A** and **B)** and 2D image **(C)** with electronic fluid cleansing show a polypoid lesion on 3D, which is seen to be composed of air centrally on 2D **(C,** *arrow).* This air density is also reflected by the dark blue–black color pattern at 3D translucency **(B).** On the uncleansed 2D source image **(D),** this "lesion" is shown to represent volume averaging related to a trapped air bubble in an otherwise fluid-filled lumen. We almost never see this much residual fluid with our current prep regimen. Although such a finding would never be confused for a true polyp, it does add time to the overall interpretation.

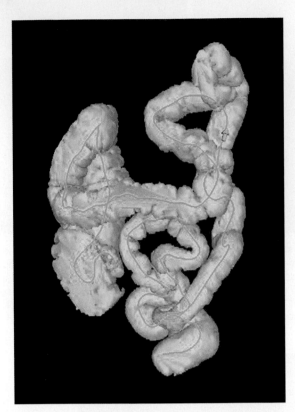

Figure 20-84 **Incorrect centerline for endoluminal navigation because of electronic fluid cleansing.** 3D colon map shows that the automated green centerline has incorrectly excluded the splenic flexure, which is related to electronic cleansing that causes artificial thinning of the colon wall. This error is not seen when electronic cleansing is turned off, although this approach will also lead to more discrete colonic segments as fluid-filled turns must be jumped.

tal examination or anoscopy may be all that is needed, sparing the patient full endoscopic examination with sedation. As with the ileocecal valve and appendix, location is the first key to recognition of anorectal-specific pathology. The three entities that probably cause the most trouble at CTC interpretation are hypertrophied anal papillae, internal hemorrhoids, and the rectal balloon catheter. Each of these will be considered in turn.

Hypertrophied anal papillae represent focal fibrous thickenings at the dentate line and often have a polypoid appearance. Simply put, anal papillae are essentially skin tags that project internally, usually in response to chronic irritation or anal fissuring. Most anal papillae measure 5 to 6 mm or less (Fig. 20-85), but they rarely can attain a larger size and become pedunculated (Fig. 20-86). The key to recognition for a typical anal papilla is its constant anatomic location at the anorectal junction, virtually always abutting the rectal catheter at its lowest visualized point. In comparison, low-lying rectal polyps will almost always show at least some separation from the anorectal junction (Fig. 20-87). However, rare pedunculated anal papillae can be mistaken for true rectal polyps if the connection to the anorectal junction is obscured (Fig. 20-88).

Internal hemorrhoids are a relatively common finding and represent dilated vascular channels above the dentate line. Internal hemorrhoids may present with bleeding or prolapse. When advanced or thrombosed, internal hemorrhoids may appear polypoid or masslike at CTC (Figs. 20-89 and 20-90). Circumferential involvement around the rectal catheter is often seen in prominent cases (Fig. 20-90). The soft tissue fullness from internal hemorrhoids often appears prominent on transverse 2D images but is often less masslike on other 2D planes or the 3D endoluminal view and may change with patient position (Fig. 20-91). Rectal varices, which are associated with portal hypertension, are occasionally seen at CTC, but their serpiginous appearance should not be confused for neoplastic disease (see Chapter 22).

The rectal catheter is a constant finding in the anorectal region at CTC. The catheter tip may itself appear polypoid at 3D or cause extrinsic impression on an adjacent rectal fold (Fig. 20-92). In addition, the balloon, which is nearly invisible except for the mass effect it exerts, can create pseudolesions through contact with fluid or the rectal wall (Fig. 20-93). These pitfalls, however, should be easily recognized, even by a novice reader. The real issue with the rectal catheter at CTC is that it can potentially obscure or distort a significant lesion, especially with the use of large-caliber catheters with large retention cuffs. In general, we prefer a small-caliber catheter with a small (20-30 cc) retention balloon, but even these can partially obscure or distort significant lesions (Fig. 20-94).[40] A challenge for CAD systems is to avoid marking the rectal catheter as a positive "hit" because this unnecessarily increases interpretation time.

A variety of other anorectal pathology is much less commonly encountered.[1] Of greatest concern perhaps is anal cancer. Most anal cancers are squamous cell carcinomas, followed by adenocarcinoma. Because the anal canal is not well evaluated at CTC, detection of anal cancer requires either a prominent endorectal component (Fig. 20-95), or detection during catheter placement or digital rectal examination. Digital rectal examination, however, is generally not a formal component of CTC, especially because the CTC technologist may place the catheter. Anal warts, or condylomata acuminata, represent a sexually transmitted disease caused by the human papillomavirus and may have an endorectal component (Fig. 20-96). A more aggressive form can be seen in patients who are immunocompromised, particularly those with acquired immunodeficiency syndrome (AIDS). Retrorectal cystic hamartoma is perhaps the most commonly encountered presacral lesion in asymptomatic adults (see Chapter 22). Finally, a spectrum of entities loosely related to mucosal prolapse includes solitary rectal ulcer syndrome, colitis cystica profunda, and inflammatory cloacogenic polyps. These diseases may be incidentally detected or present with symptoms such as

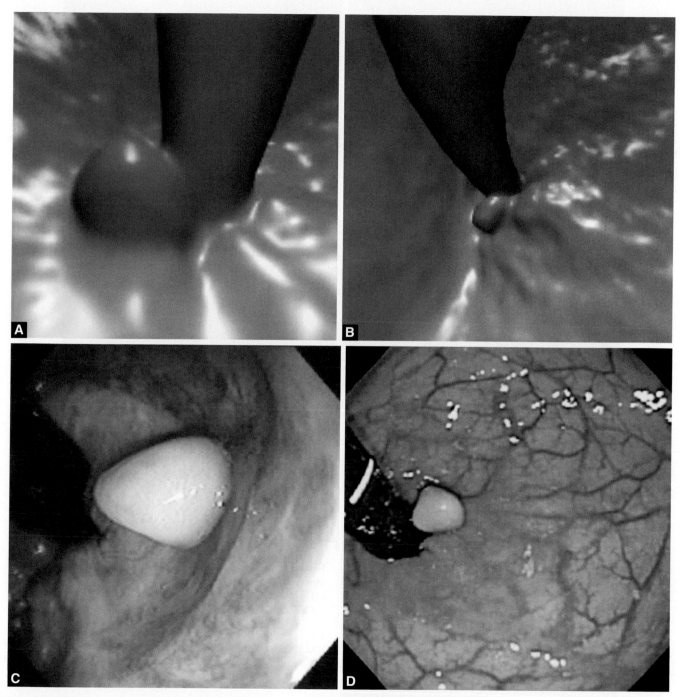

Figure 20-85   Small hypertrophied anal papillae. 3D endoluminal CTC (**A** and **B**) and OC (**C** and **D**) images from four different individuals show the typical endoluminal appearance of hypertrophied anal papillae. These lesions are characteristically located at the anorectal junction, tucked up against the rectal catheter, and tend to measure 5 to 6 mm in maximal size. As an isolated finding, these should not trigger endoscopic referral.

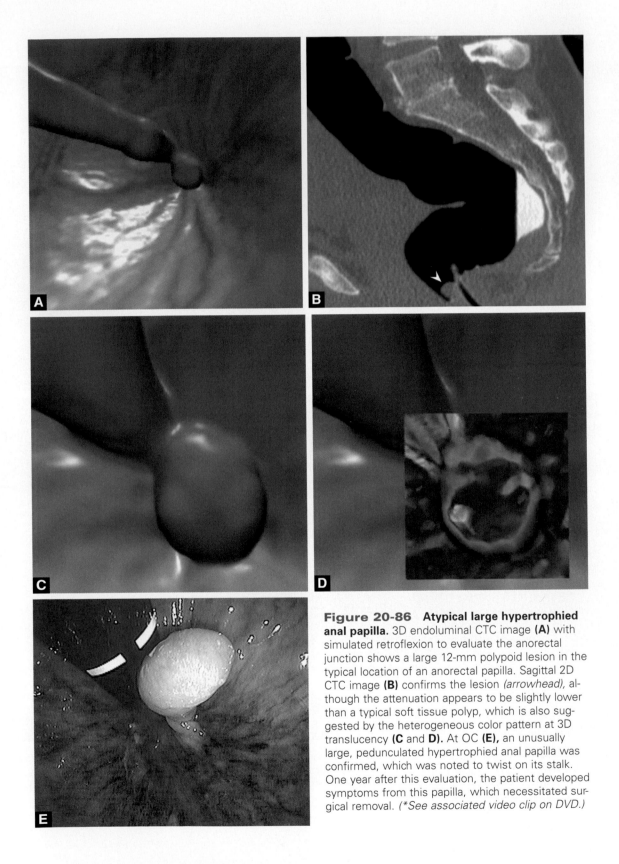

Figure 20-86 Atypical large hypertrophied anal papilla. 3D endoluminal CTC image **(A)** with simulated retroflexion to evaluate the anorectal junction shows a large 12-mm polypoid lesion in the typical location of an anorectal papilla. Sagittal 2D CTC image **(B)** confirms the lesion *(arrowhead)*, although the attenuation appears to be slightly lower than a typical soft tissue polyp, which is also suggested by the heterogeneous color pattern at 3D translucency **(C** and **D). At OC (E),** an unusually large, pedunculated hypertrophied anal papilla was confirmed, which was noted to twist on its stalk. One year after this evaluation, the patient developed symptoms from this papilla, which necessitated surgical removal. *(*See associated video clip on DVD.)*

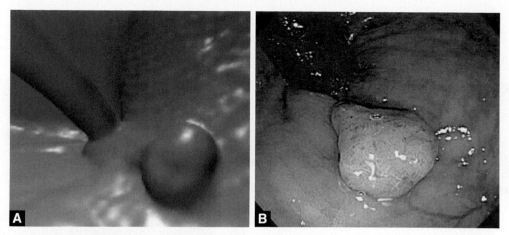

Figure 20-87   Low-lying rectal polyp (tubular adenoma). 3D endoluminal CTC image **(A)** shows a large polyp in the distal rectum, which is slightly removed from the anorectal junction—a key finding to distinguish this from an anal papilla or internal hemorrhoid. The lesion was confirmed at same-day OC **(B)**. *(*See associated video clip on DVD.)*

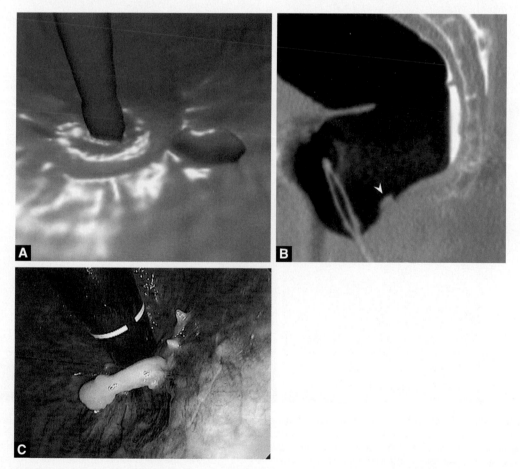

Figure 20-88   Balloon from rectal catheter obscures anal connection of pedunculated papilla. 3D endoluminal **(A)** and sagittal 2D **(B)** CTC images show a small polyp *(arrowhead)* that appears to be removed from the anorectal junction, similar to Fig. 20-87. However, at OC **(C)** a small pedunculated anal papilla was found. The stalk of the papilla was compressed by the rectal balloon at CTC, so the connection to the anorectal junction was not appreciated. This is an unusual case but serves as a reminder that the rectal catheter and balloon can occasionally obscure relevant findings. The artifact on the 2D image is related to a metallic hip prosthesis.

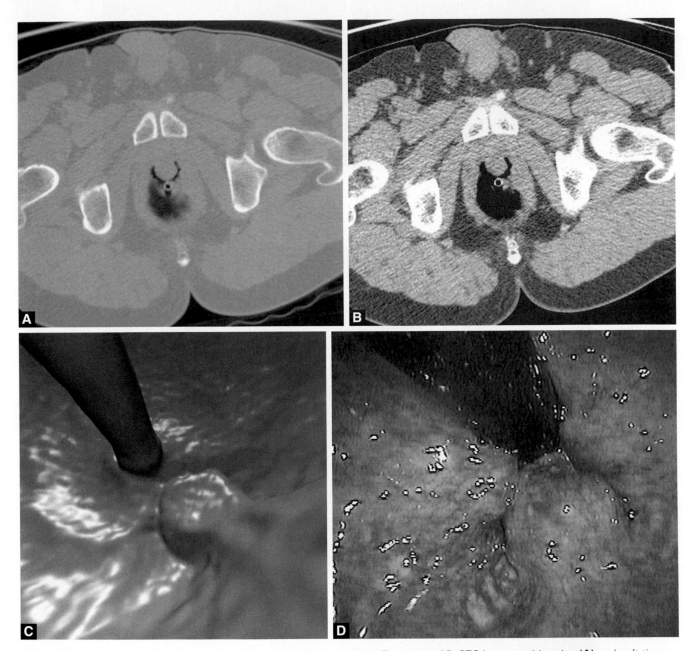

Figure 20-89 Internal hemorrhoids with polypoid appearance. Transverse 2D CTC images with polyp **(A)** and soft tissue **(B)** window settings show a polypoid soft tissue lesion immediately anterior to the rectal catheter. On the 3D endoluminal image **(C),** the lesion appears less prominent and is partially compressed by the rectal balloon. At OC **(D),** which was performed for positive findings elsewhere in the colon, internal hemorrhoids were seen. In general, the transverse projection at CTC accentuates the appearance of internal hemorrhoids, which are usually less impressive on the remaining 2D MPR and 3D endoluminal views.

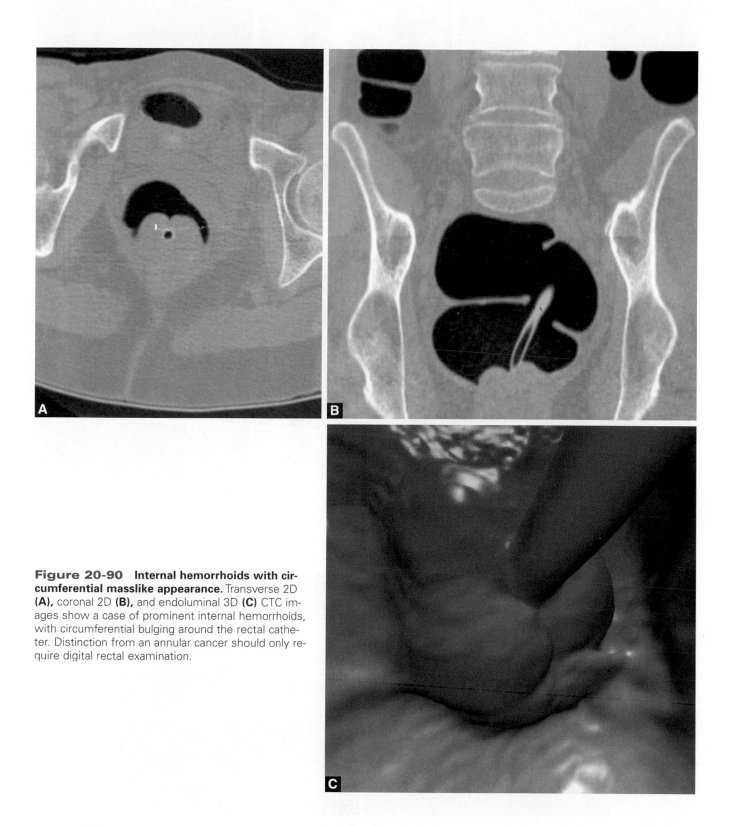

Figure 20-90   Internal hemorrhoids with circumferential masslike appearance. Transverse 2D **(A)**, coronal 2D **(B)**, and endoluminal 3D **(C)** CTC images show a case of prominent internal hemorrhoids, with circumferential bulging around the rectal catheter. Distinction from an annular cancer should only require digital rectal examination.

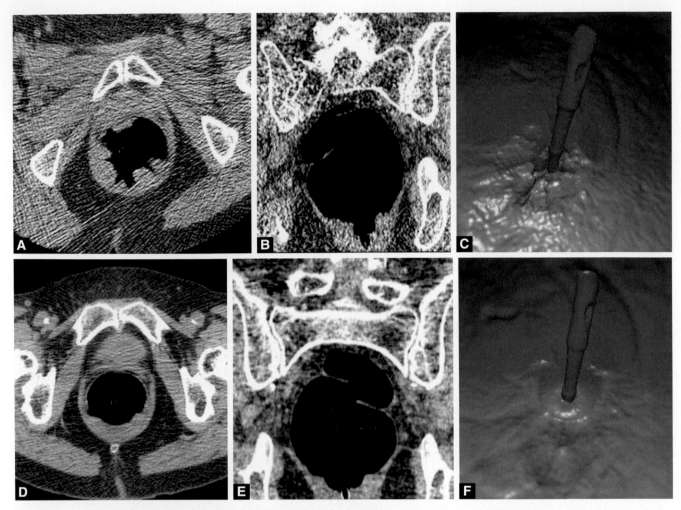

Figure 20-91 **Change in hemorrhoid appearance with position.** Decubitus transverse 2D **(A),** coronal 2D **(B),** and endoluminal 3D **(C)** CTC images show an irregular lobulated appearance to internal hemorrhoids, which largely efface on the corresponding supine views **(D-F).** Such positional changes are reassuring for hemorrhoids over a scirrhous mass.

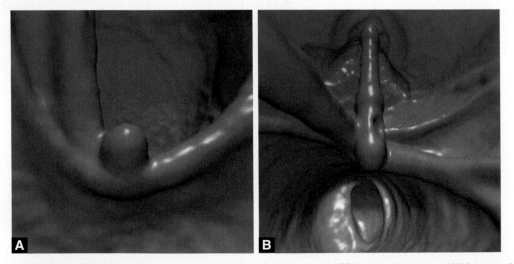

Figure 20-92 **Tip of rectal catheter transiently simulating a polyp at 3D CTC.** 3D endoluminal CTC image **(A)** shows a polypoid lesion on a rectal fold, which is easily dismissed as the tip of the rectal catheter **(B)** as the fly-through continues. *(*See associated video clip on DVD.)*

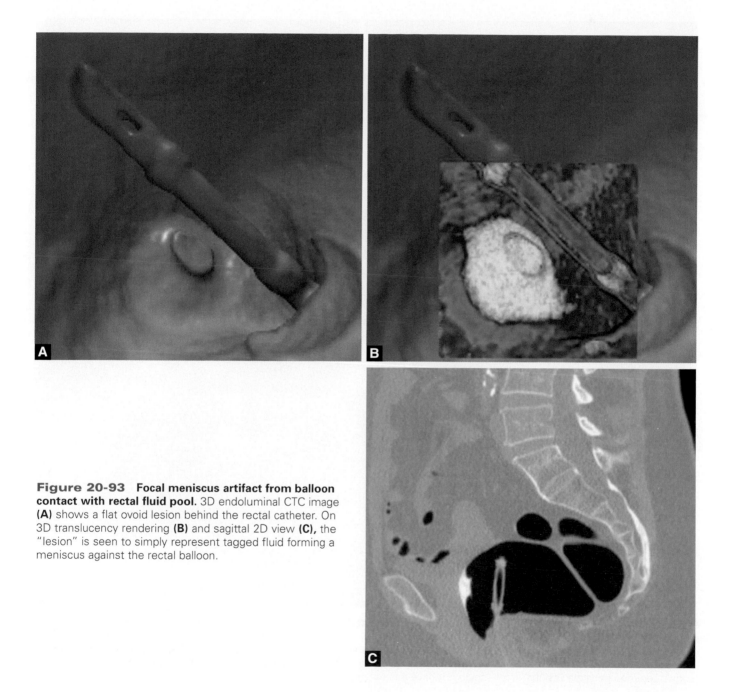

Figure 20-93 **Focal meniscus artifact from balloon contact with rectal fluid pool.** 3D endoluminal CTC image **(A)** shows a flat ovoid lesion behind the rectal catheter. On 3D translucency rendering **(B)** and sagittal 2D view **(C)**, the "lesion" is seen to simply represent tagged fluid forming a meniscus against the rectal balloon.

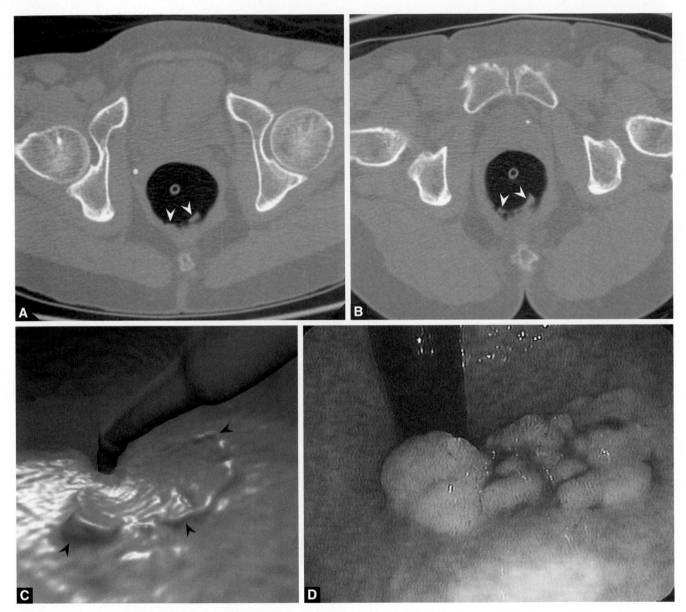

Figure 20-94 **Low rectal carpet lesion partially compressed by rectal balloon.** Supine **(A)** and prone **(B)** transverse 2D images show odd soft tissue projections *(arrowheads)* that appear to be partially compressed by the rectal balloon. The 3D endoluminal view **(C)** also demonstrates the balloon compression of this soft tissue abnormality *(arrowheads),* which proved to be a tubulovillous adenoma at OC **(D).** This is a difficult case but such soft tissue abnormalities must be taken seriously with our contrast tagging regimen because residual stool should not have this untagged appearance.

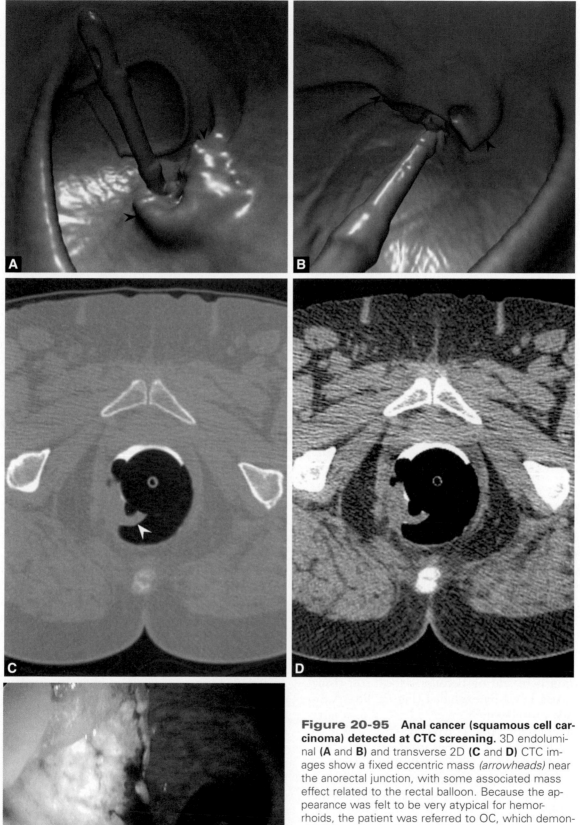

Figure 20-95   Anal cancer (squamous cell carcinoma) detected at CTC screening. 3D endoluminal **(A** and **B)** and transverse 2D **(C** and **D)** CTC images show a fixed eccentric mass *(arrowheads)* near the anorectal junction, with some associated mass effect related to the rectal balloon. Because the appearance was felt to be very atypical for hemorrhoids, the patient was referred to OC, which demonstrated an ulcerated mass **(E)** that proved to be squamous cell carcinoma arising from the anal canal. *(*See associated video clip on DVD.)*

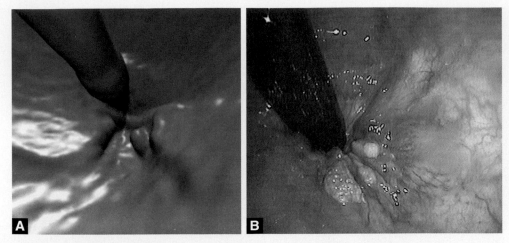

Figure 20-96 **Anal condyloma.** 3D endoluminal CTC image **(A)** shows mild irregularity at the anorectal junction, which proved to be a small anal condyloma at OC **(B),** which was performed primarily for positive findings elsewhere in the colon.

hematochezia, tenesmus, and rectal pain. The poorly understood solitary rectal ulcer syndrome, despite its name, can manifest with a polypoid appearance and not an ulcer in about 25% of cases. Other entities that can involve radiologic assessment include perianal fistula and retained rectal foreign bodies.

ILEOCECAL VALVE

Confident assessment of the ileocecal valve at CTC seems to be a concern for many novice readers.[41] The valve itself is easy to identify given its constant anatomic location relative to the cecum and terminal ileum. However, there is a relatively wide range of normal appearances to the ileocecal valve, ranging from a bulbous papillary or polypoid appearance to a more labial appearance (Figs. 20-97). The overall morphology of the valve is much easier to appreciate on the 3D endoluminal view compared with 2D projections, where it is much more difficult to exclude a superimposed polyp. It is good practice to specifically interrogate the ileocecal valve in each case, assessing both its morphology and composition. A diffusely fatty valve or focal fatty projection on 3D translucency rendering or 2D evaluation is reassuring because a focal soft tissue abnormality can be easily excluded (Fig. 20-98). A focal soft tissue protuberance on or adjacent to a fatty valve is suspicious for a true polyp (Fig. 20-99). A mass involving or replacing the valve itself can present a more challenging problem (Fig. 20-100). The ileocecal valve is a relatively common location to see a drip of contrast, which can superficially mimic a polyp on the 3D display (Fig. 20-101). With time and experience, however, recognizing the range of normal and knowing when to suspect an abnormality eventually become easier tasks. As with the rectal catheter, CAD systems should strive to avoid marking the normal ileocecal valve to streamline interpretation.[42]

One additional related pitfall to be aware of is what we refer to as a "pseudovalve" lesion. This is a large right-sided polyp or mass that bears a resemblance to an ileocecal valve and could potentially be misinterpreted to represent this normal structure. The keys for recognition are location and multiplicity; as long as positive identification of the real valve is always made, any other finding cannot be the valve and therefore represents something else. The superficial resemblance of some right-sided cancers and large advanced adenomas to the ileocecal valve at CTC can be striking (Figs. 20-102 and 20-103).

APPENDICEAL FINDINGS

As with the ileocecal valve, the vermiform appendix represents another anatomic landmark that can give rise to a number of unique findings at CTC interpretation, most notably false polyps and appendiceal neoplasms. As part of our general intake form, we obtain a surgical history on all patients scheduling a CTC examination. Knowledge of prior appendectomy is useful because an inverted appendiceal stump can closely mimic a true cecal polyp at CTC and even at OC (Figs. 20-67 and 20-104).[43] Keys to recognition of an inverted appendiceal stump include a polypoid lesion at the expected location of the appendiceal orifice and history of prior (often remote) appendectomy. These stumps can closely mimic large pedunculated polyps, for which polypectomy would otherwise be indicated. In some cases, confident distinction between stump and true polyp is not possible and endoscopic evaluation is unavoidable (Fig. 20-105). In patients without a history of appendectomy, partial invagination or, rarely, complete intussusception may give rise to an intraluminal polypoid lesion. In these cases, continuity of the remainder of the appendix in its expected location prevents misdiagnosis. The appendiceal orifice is usually easily identified at CTC,

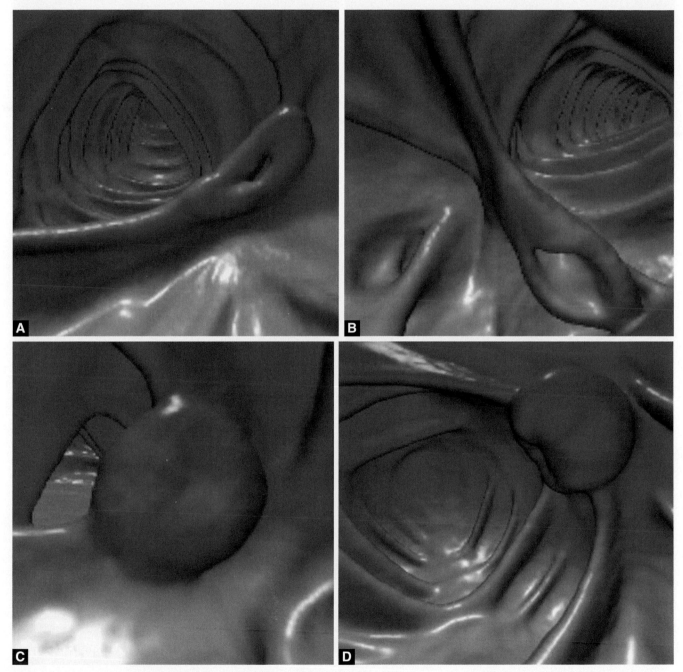

Figure 20-97   Varied appearances of the normal ileocecal valve. 3D endoluminal CTC images **(A-D)** from four different individuals show normal ileocecal valves, ranging from a labial to polypoid morphology. The ileocecal valve should be identified and inspected during every CTC interpretation.

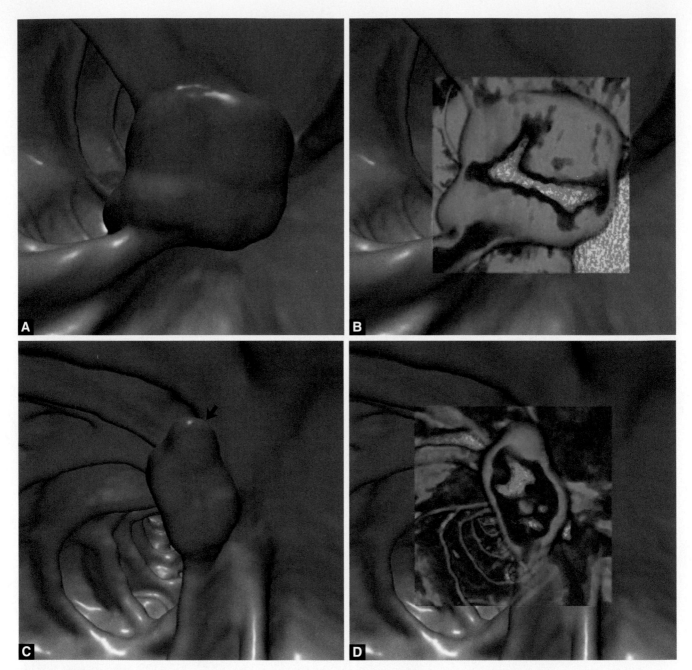

Figure 20-98   Translucency rendering for evaluating the ileocecal valve. 3D endoluminal CTC images **(A-D)** from two individuals show the utility of translucency rendering for quickly and confidently clearing a potentially suspicious ileocecal valve. The first case demonstrates a very prominent amorphous valve **(A),** but translucency rendering **(B)** shows only lipomatous change throughout the valve, indicated by the green color. The second case demonstrates a polypoid projection off the valve **(C,** *arrow),* which is shown to represent a lipoma *(in green)* projecting off the valve on translucency **(D).** The valve is otherwise composed of soft tissue attenuation *(red).* Although 2D correlation can show similar findings to translucency, it tends to be a more difficult task with a lower confidence level.

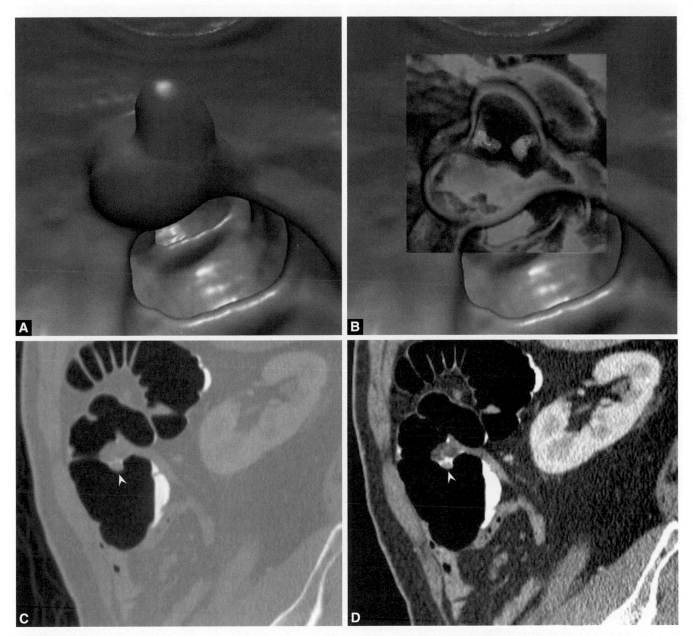

Figure 20-99 **Soft tissue polyp on the ileocecal valve.** 3D endoluminal CTC image **(A)** shows a prominent polypoid projection off the valve, which demonstrates a red soft tissue color signature on translucency rendering **(B)**. The soft tissue nature *(arrowheads)* can be confirmed on the sagittal 2D images **(C** and **D)**. Note that this study was performed with IV contrast.

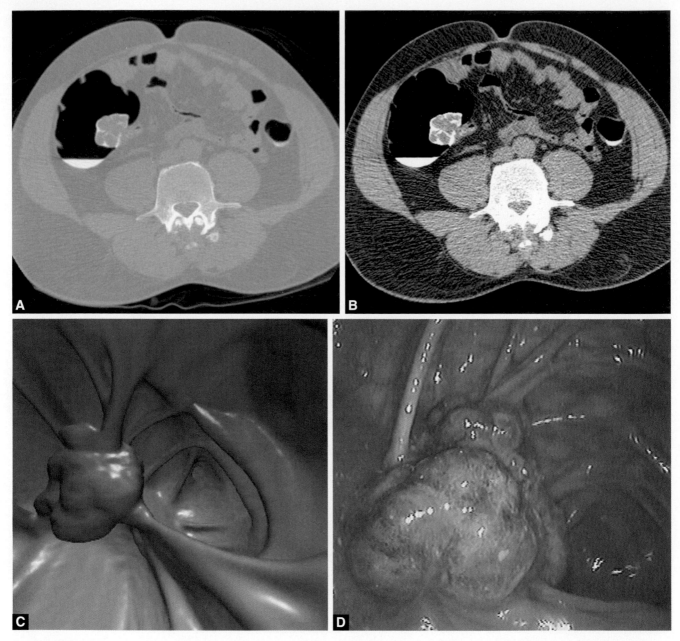

Figure 20-100 **Large tubulovillous adenoma involving the ileocecal valve.** Transverse 2D CTC images with polyp **(A)** and soft tissue **(B)** window settings show a multilobulated mass occupying the expected location of the ileocecal valve. Note the distinct contrast etching outlining the surfaces of the lesion. 3D endoluminal **(C)** and OC **(D)** images show the mass, which involved the ileocecal valve. (*See associated video clip on DVD.*)

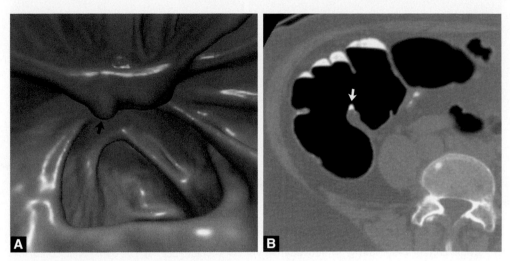

Figure 20-101 **Drip off the ileocecal valve simulating a polyp on 3D.** 3D endoluminal CTC image **(A)** shows a polypoid projection off the ileocecal valve *(arrow),* which corresponds to a drip of contrast at prone 2D correlation **(B,** *arrow).* Translucency rendering can also make the distinction from a true polyp.

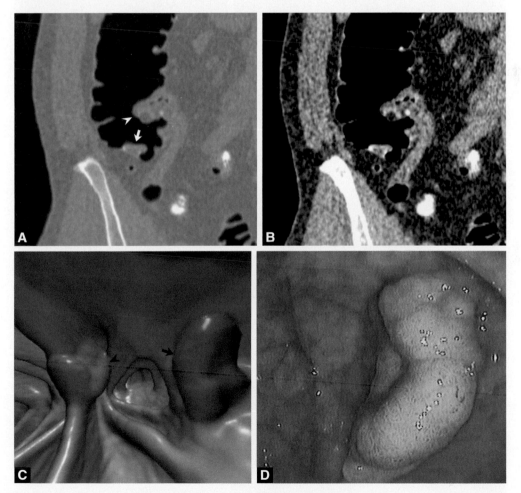

Figure 20-102 **Cecal polyp (tubulovillous adenoma) as a "pseudovalve."** Coronal 2D CTC images with polyp **(A)** and soft tissue **(B)** window settings, and the 3D endoluminal view **(C),** show a cecal soft tissue lesion *(arrows)* separate from the ileocecal valve *(arrowheads).* At OC **(D),** the cecal lesion bears a superficial resemblance to an ileocecal valve. *(*See associated video clip on DVD).*

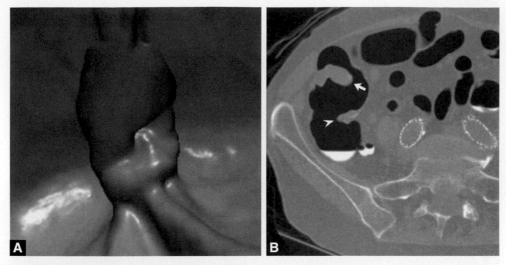

Figure 20-103 **Cecal cancer resembling an ileocecal valve.** 3D endoluminal **(A)** and transverse 2D **(B)** CTC images show a cecal mass *(arrow)* that resembles the appearance of a large ileocecal valve. However, the normal valve itself *(arrowhead)* is clearly identified along the opposite cecal wall.

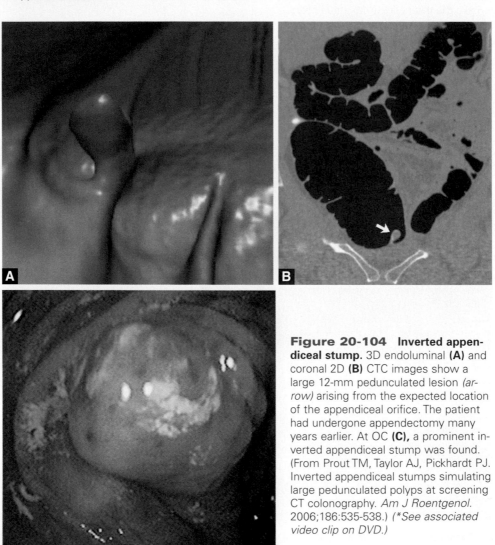

Figure 20-104 **Inverted appendiceal stump.** 3D endoluminal **(A)** and coronal 2D **(B)** CTC images show a large 12-mm pedunculated lesion *(arrow)* arising from the expected location of the appendiceal orifice. The patient had undergone appendectomy many years earlier. At OC **(C),** a prominent inverted appendiceal stump was found. (From Prout TM, Taylor AJ, Pickhardt PJ. Inverted appendiceal stumps simulating large pedunculated polyps at screening CT colonography. *Am J Roentgenol.* 2006;186:535-538.) *(*See associated video clip on DVD.)*

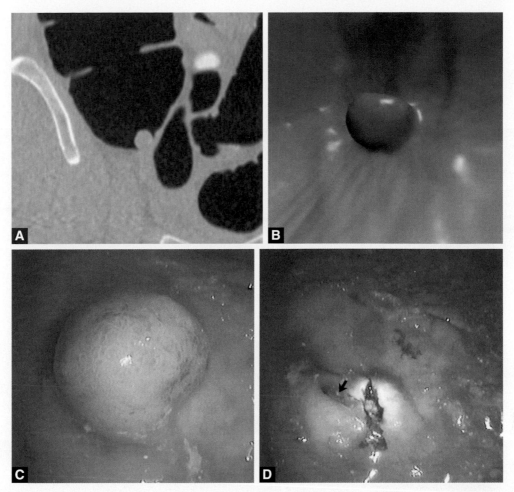

Figure 20-105 **True polyp (tubulovillous adenoma) overlying the appendiceal orifice.** Coronal 2D **(A)** and 3D endoluminal **(B)** CTC images show a 15-mm polyp at the expected location of the appendiceal orifice. Images at OC before **(C)** and after **(D)** polypectomy show the appendiceal orifice *(arrow)*, which was obscured by the lesion.

allowing for detection of true polyps that are adjacent to but separate from the appendix (Fig. 20-106)

The most common primary tumor of the appendix to present as an incidental imaging finding in adults is a benign mucinous adenoma, which manifests as a mucocele from cystic dilatation of the appendix.[44,45] In most cases, OC confirmation of a CTC-detected appendiceal mucocele is not necessary and may even be negative or lead to confusion, given the extraluminal nature of appendiceal tumors (Fig. 20-107). Surgery is indicated for appendiceal mucoceles because almost all lesions are neoplastic and considered at least potentially malignant. CTC represents an ideal study for both detection and preoperative assessment of these tumors. Carcinoid tumors of the appendix are more common at pathologic examination than mucinous neoplasms, but these are typically subcentimeter in size and rarely identified at imaging.[44] Primary appendiceal neoplasms are covered in more detail in Chapter 22.

As an interesting aside, the appendix is nearly always identifiable at 2D CTC evaluation, unless it is surgically absent. Furthermore, with our current protocol for co-

lonic preparation and distention, the appendiceal lumen will almost always fill with air and/or oral contrast. This fact could potentially be of some value in cases where chronic or intermittent appendicitis is questioned. In addition, we have noticed a normal variant of a very long appendix (i.e., >10 cm in length) in roughly 10% of adults undergoing CTC screening (Fig. 20-108).

RETAINED FLUID AND SUBMERGED POLYPS

Residual luminal fluid, if untagged, can obscure even large polyps and masses when submerged. Early on, some advocated for the routine use of intravenous contrast to help identify submerged lesions,[46] but we have found it much simpler, safer, faster, cheaper, and probably more effective to "enhance" the surrounding fluid instead.[47] It is important to note that iodinated contrast agents tag luminal fluid more homogeneously than barium preparations.[48] We believe that both barium and iodinated contrasts agents are probably needed in tandem for adequate tagging of both solid and liquid residuals, respec-

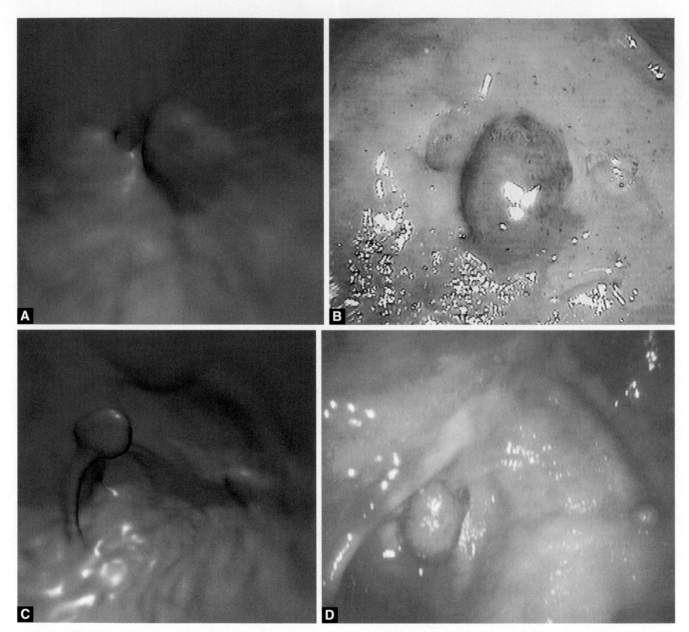

Figure 20-106 **Polyps near the appendiceal orifice at CTC.** Typically, polyps near the appendiceal orifice will not obscure its identification. 3D endoluminal CTC and OC images from two different cases show a hyperplastic polyp adjacent to the orifice **(A** and **B)** and a tubulovillous adenoma adjacent to the orifice **(C** and **D)**. In the second case, a diminutive adenoma is also seen laterally at both CTC and OC.

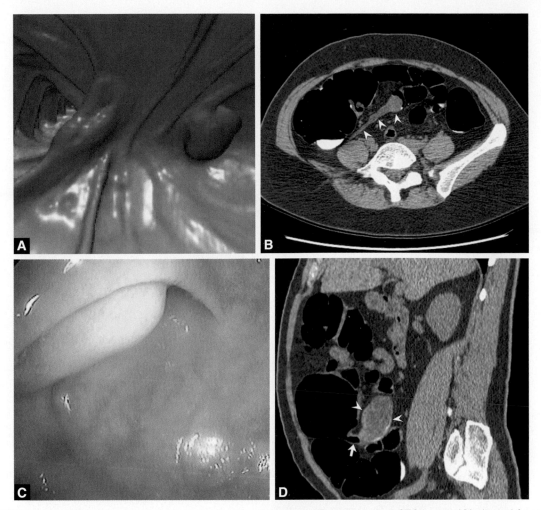

Figure 20-107 **Appendiceal mucoceles from mucinous adenomas.** 3D endoluminal CTC image **(A)** viewed from the cecal apex shows a large polypoid lesion at the expected location of the appendiceal orifice. Note the normal-appearing ileocecal valve. Curved reformatted transverse 2D image **(B)** shows that the polypoid lesion is in continuity with a dilated appendix *(arrowheads)*. At OC **(C)**, the appearance was assumed to represent postappendectomy changes (the surgical history was not correlated). Subsequent surgery confirmed a mucocele from mucinous adenoma of the appendix. Sagittal 2D CTC image **(D)** from a second patient shows a classic mucocele of the appendix *(arrowheads)*, with sparing of the base of the appendix *(arrow)*. (*See associated video clip on DVD.*)

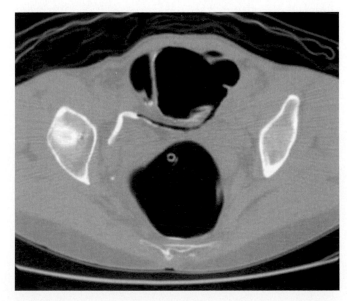

Figure 20-108 **Long appendix as a common normal variant at CTC screening.** Curved reformatted 2D CTC image shows an appendix that measured more than 12 cm in length. At CTC, the normal appendix will almost always fill with gas and/or contrast material.

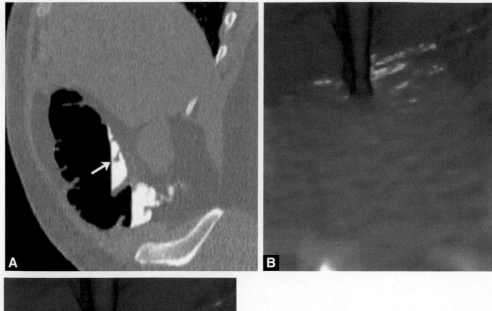

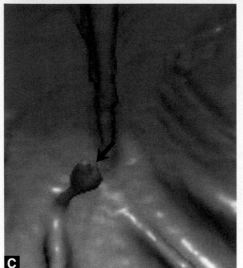

Figure 20-109 Polyp submerged in tagged fluid. Sagittal 2D CTC image **(A)** shows a small pedunculated polyp *(arrow)* that is completely covered by opacified fluid in this position. 3D endoluminal image without electronic cleansing **(B)** shows the surface of the luminal fluid but, with electronic fluid cleansing **(C),** the polyp is visualized *(arrow).* In truth, the lesion could be seen on 3D without fluid cleansing on the complementary prone position (not shown), which is typically the case. (From Pickhardt PJ, Choi JR. Electronic cleansing and stool tagging in CT colonography: advantages and pitfalls encountered with primary three-dimensional evaluation. *Am J Roentgenol.* 2003;181:799-805.)

tively.[47] Although in the past we performed electronic cleansing on the tagged fluid prior to CTC interpretation, we discontinued this practice in 2003. With our current bowel preparation, it is nearly impossible to have a significant polyp completely submerged under fluid on both supine and prone views.[39] Even with older iterations of the prep, which resulted in greater volumes of residual fluid, polyp submersion on both views was an exceedingly rare event (see Chapter 17). However, even in such rare cases, significant polyps were detectable on both 2D views and could also be uncovered by electronic cleansing (Fig. 20-109). Currently, we prefer to concentrate on the opacified fluid on 2D evaluation and not use electronic cleansing because the volume of residual fluid is generally so low. The most common scenario in which we still may encounter larger volumes of residual luminal fluid is in the setting of same-day tagging following failed OC. In these cases, total or partial submersion of polyps is possible (Fig. 20-110). We currently administer 30 mL of diatrizoate by mouth as soon

as the patient has adequately recovered from sedation following incomplete OC, and we wait up to 2 hours prior to scanning. A better approach might be to give diatrizoate as part of the standard prep the evening before planned OC, which would allow for a reduction in the amount of cathartic needed and also provide fluid tagging for CTC in the event of an incomplete OC examination. Occasionally, a drop of tagged fluid will mimic a polyp on 3D (Fig. 20-111), but this pitfall is easily dismissed after assessment of internal density.

SUBMUCOSAL LESIONS

By its broadest definition, a "submucosal" location includes any finding deep to the mucosal surface, including both intramural (Fig. 20-112) and extrinsic lesions (Fig. 20-113). Evaluation of submucosal lesions at CTC is covered in much greater detail in Chapter 22. Fortunately, only a subset of all lesions arising deep in the colonic surface might potentially be confused for a

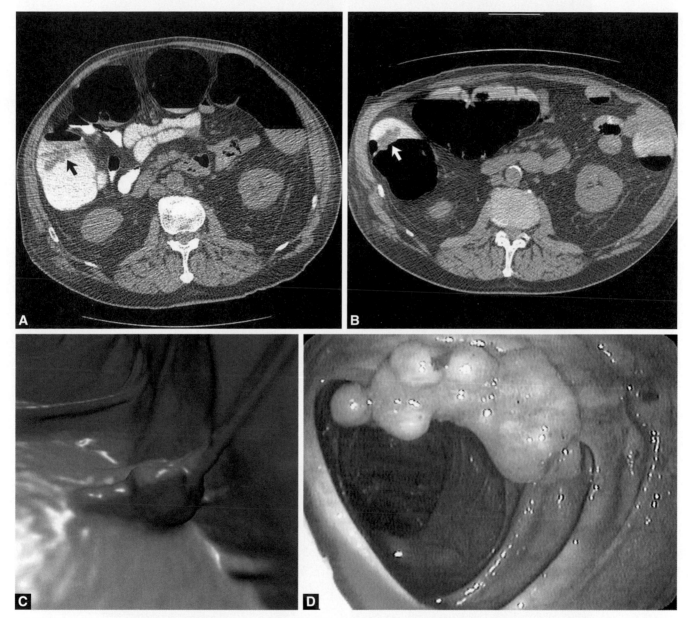

Figure 20-110 Near-total submersion of polyp at CTC following aborted OC. Supine **(A)** and prone **(B)** transverse CTC images show a 4-cm soft tissue mass *(arrows)* growing along a fold in the ascending colon, which is almost completely submerged under opacified fluid on both positions. The lesion is partially visualized on the prone 3D endoluminal fly-through without fluid cleansing **(C)**. This degree of residual fluid is not seen with our current CTC bowel preparation but is commonly seen with same-day tagging following incomplete OC, as was the case here. At subsequent OC **(D)**, the mass was confirmed and proved to be a large tubular adenoma.

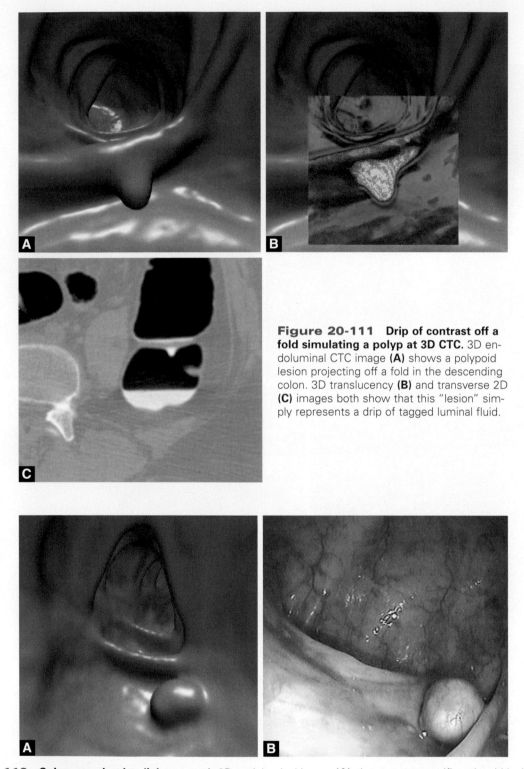

Figure 20-111 Drip of contrast off a fold simulating a polyp at 3D CTC. 3D endoluminal CTC image **(A)** shows a polypoid lesion projecting off a fold in the descending colon. 3D translucency **(B)** and transverse 2D **(C)** images both show that this "lesion" simply represents a drip of tagged luminal fluid.

Figure 20-112 Submucosal polyp (leiomyoma). 3D endoluminal image **(A)** shows a nonspecific polypoid lesion, which was confirmed and partially removed at same-day OC **(B).** At pathology, a submucosal leiomyoma was diagnosed. *(*See associated video clip on DVD.)*

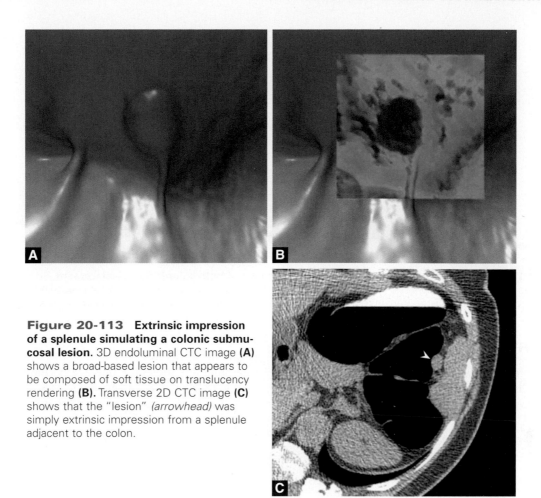

Figure 20-113 Extrinsic impression of a splenule simulating a colonic submucosal lesion. 3D endoluminal CTC image **(A)** shows a broad-based lesion that appears to be composed of soft tissue on translucency rendering **(B)**. Transverse 2D CTC image **(C)** shows that the "lesion" *(arrowhead)* was simply extrinsic impression from a splenule adjacent to the colon.

mucosal-based soft tissue polyp or mass at CTC. Neoplastic intramural submucosal lesions that can mimic a mucosal lesion include carcinoid tumor, lymphoma, hemangioma, hematogenous metastases, and mesenchymal tumors (e.g., leiomyoma) that do not demonstrate an exoenteric component.[49] Non-neoplastic submucosal lesions that manifest as polypoid lesions of soft tissue attenuation include lymphoid polyps and venous blebs.[50] Extrinsic or submucosal entities that may mimic primary CRC include endometriosis, peritoneal carcinomatosis, and hemangiomatosis. Other entities such as colonic lipomas, pneumatosis cystoides coli, and extrinsic impression from extracolonic structures may appear polypoid or masslike at 3D endoluminal CTC evaluation, but 2D correlation provides definitive evidence to the contrary (Fig. 20-113). The same cannot be said for strictly luminal examinations such as OC (Fig. 20-114). The presence of inwardly displaced but uninterrupted folds at 3D endoluminal CTC strongly suggests extrinsic impression (Fig. 20-115).

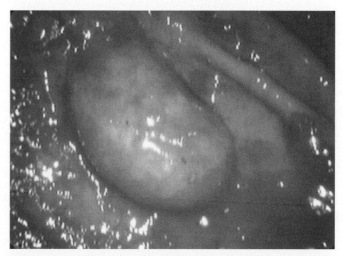

Figure 20-114 Subserosal uterine fibroid mimicking a colonic submucosal lesion. OC image shows a smooth, ovoid lesion that was concerning for an intramural submucosal colonic mass. Subsequent CTC (not shown) demonstrated that this finding was a result of extrinsic impression from an exophytic uterine fibroid.

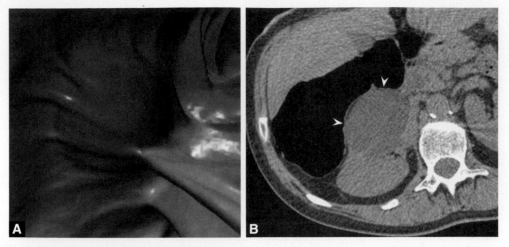

Figure 20-115 **Extrinsic impression from an exophytic renal cyst with colonic fold displacement.** 3D endoluminal CTC image **(A)** shows a broad-based impression that displaces but does not efface the colonic folds, which suggests an extracolonic process. At 2D correlation **(B),** a large benign renal cyst is seen to be the cause of the luminal bulge *(arrowheads).*

SUMMARY

In this chapter, we have presented an extensive array of potential pitfalls at CTC interpretation. More important, we have tried to identify those pitfalls that can be avoided altogether and those that cannot always be avoided but should be recognized to prevent mismanagement. In actual practice, the true challenges may come from cases in which more than one pitfall intersects on the same case. Fortunately, the built-in redundancy of 2D and 3D CTC interpretation allows for ample opportunity for lesion detection in most cases. With proper attention to technique, including patient preparation, colonic distention, and scanning protocol, in addition to a combined 2D–3D interpretive strategy, the vast majority of these potential pitfalls can be handled appropriately.

REFERENCES

1. Pickhardt PJ. Differential diagnosis of polypoid lesions seen at CT colonography (virtual colonoscopy). *Radiographics.* 2004;24(6): 1535-1556.
2. Pickhardt PJ, Choi JHR. Electronic cleansing and stool tagging in CT colonography: Advantages and pitfalls with primary three-dimensional evaluation. *Am J Roentgenol.* 2003;181(3):799-7805.
3. Pickhardt PJ. Colonic preparation for computed tomographic colonography: Understanding the relative advantages and disadvantages of a noncathartic approach. *Mayo Clin Proc.* 2007;82 (6):659-661.
4. Sanford MF, Pickhardt PJ. Diagnostic performance of primary 3-dimensional computed tomography colonography in the setting of colonic diverticular disease. *Clin Gastroenterol Hepatol.* 2006; 4(8):1039-1047.
5. Baxter NN, Goldwasser MA, Paszat LF, Saskin R, Urbach DR, Rabeneck L. Association of colonoscopy and death from colorectal cancer. *Ann Intern Med.* 2009;150(1):1-8.
6. Shinners TJ, Pickhardt PJ, Taylor AJ, Jones DA, Olsen CH. Patient-controlled room air insufflation versus automated carbon dioxide delivery for CT colonography. *Am J Roentgenol.* 2006;186(6):1491-1496.
7. Sosna J, Blachar A, Amitai M, et al. Colonic perforation at CT colonography: Assessment of risk in a multicenter large cohort. *Radiology.* 2006;239(2):457-463.
8. Painter NS, Truelove SC, Ardran GM, Tuckey M. Segmentation and localization of intraluminal pressures in human colon with special reference to pathogenesis of colonic diverticula. *Gastroenterology.* 1965;49(2):169-177.
9. Painter NS, Burkitt DP. Diverticular disease of colon—Deficiency disease of Western civilization. *Br Med J.* 1971;2(5759):450-454.

10. Tendler DA, Aboudola S, Zacks JF, O'Brien MJ, Kelly CP. Prolapsing mucosal polyps: an underrecognized form of colonic polyp—A clinicopathological study of 15 cases. *Am J Gastroenterol.* 2002;97(2):370-376.
11. Zalis ME, Barish MA, Choi JR, et al. CT colonography reporting and data system: A consensus proposal. *Radiology.* 2005;236(1):3-9.
12. Tanaka S, Haruma K, Oka S, et al. Clinicopathologic features and endoscopic treatment of superficially spreading colorectal neoplasms larger than 20 mm. *Gastrointest Endosc.* 2001;54(1):62-66.
13. Park SH, Lee SS, Choi EK, et al. Flat colorectal neoplasms: Definition, importance, and visualization on CT colonography. *Am J Roentgenol.* 2007;188(4):953-959.
14. Soetikno RM, Kaltenbach T, Rouse RV, et al. Prevalence of nonpolypoid (flat and depressed) colorectal neoplasms in asymptomatic and symptomatic adults. *JAMA.* 2008;299(9):1027-1035.
15. Pickhardt PJ, Levin B, Bond JH. Screening for nonpolypoid colorectal neoplasms. *JAMA.* 2008;299(23):2743; author reply 2744.
16. O'Brien M J, Winawer SJ, Zauber AG, et al. Flat adenomas in the National Polyp Study: is there increased risk for high-grade dysplasia initially or during surveillance? *Clin Gastroenterol Hepatol.* 2004;2(10):905-911.
17. Pickhardt PJ. High-magnification chromoscopic colonoscopy: Caution needs to be exercised before changing screening policy—Reply. *Am J Roentgenol.* 2006;186(2):577-578.
18. Robbins J, Pickhardt PJ, Kim DH. Flat (nonpolypoid) lesions detected at CT colonography. Maui, HI: Annual Meeting for the Society of Gastrointestinal Radiologists; 2009.
19. Pickhardt PJ, Choi JR, Nugent PA, Hwang I, Schindler WR. Flat lesions at virtual and optical colonoscopy: Prevalence, histology, and sensitivity for detection in an asymptomatic screening population. *Am J Roentgenol.* 2004;182(4):74-75.

20. Mang TG, Schaefer-Prokop C, Maier A, Schober E, Lechner G, Prokop M. Detectability of small and flat polyps in MDCT Colonography using 2D and 3D imaging tools: Results from a phantom study. *Am J Roentgenol.* 2005;185(6):1582-1589.

21. Kim DH, Pickhardt PJ, Taylor AJ, et al. CT colonography versus colonoscopy for the detection of advanced neoplasia. *N Engl J Med.* 2007;357(14):1403-1412.

22. Fidler JL, Johnson CD, MacCarty RL, Welch TJ, Hara AK, Harmsen WS. Detection of flat lesions in the colon with CT colonography. *Abdom Imag.* 2002;27(3):292-300.

23. Pickhardt PJ, Choi JR, Hwang I, Schindler WR. Nonadenomatous polyps at CT colonography: Prevalence, size distribution, and detection rates. *Radiology.* 2004;232(3):784-790.

24. Waye JD, Bilotta JJ. Rectal hyperplastic polyps—Now you see them, now you don't—A differential point. *Am J Gastroenterol.* 1990;85(12):1557-1559.

25. MacCarty RL, Johnson CD, Fletcher JG, Wilson LA. Occult colorectal polyps on CT colonography: Implications for surveillance. *Am J Roentgenol.* 2006;186(5):1380-1383.

26. Rubesin S, Saul S, Laufer I, Levine M. Carpet lesions of the colon. *Radiographics.* 1985;5(4):537-552.

27. Pickhardt PJ, Lee AD, McFarland EG, Taylor AJ. Linear polyp measurement at CT colonography: In vitro and in vivo comparison of two-dimensional and three-dimensional displays. *Radiology.* 2005;236(3):872-878.

28. Park SH, Choi EK, Lee SS, et al. Polyp measurement reliability, accuracy, and discrepancy: Optical colonoscopy versus CT colonography with pig colonic specimens. *Radiology.* 2007;244(1):157-164.

29. Barancin C, Pickhardt PJ, Kim DH, et al. Prospective blinded study of polyp size on CT colonography and various endoscopic measures. *Gastrointest Endosc.* 2008;67(5):AB305.

30. Yeshwant SC, Summers RM, Yao JH, Brickman DS, Choi JR, Pickhardt PJ. Polyps: Linear and volumetric measurement at CT colonography. *Radiology.* 2006;241(3):802-811.

31. Pickhardt PJ, Lehman VT, Winter TC, Taylor AJ. Polyp volume versus linear size measurements at CT colonography: Implications for noninvasive surveillance of unresected colorectal lesions. *Am J Roentgenol.* 2006;186(6):1605-1610.

32. Burling D, Halligan S, Roddie ME, et al. Computed tomography colonography: automated diameter and volume measurement of colonic polyps compared with a manual technique—In vitro study. *J Comput Assist Tomogr.* 2005;29(3):387-393.

33. Blake ME, Soto JA, Hayes RA, Ferrucci JT. Automated volumetry at CT colonography: A phantom study. *Acad Radiol.* 2005;12(5):608-613.

34. O'Connor SD, Summers RM, Choi JR, Pickhardt PJ. Oral contrast adherence to polyps on CT colonography. *J Comput Assist Tomogr.* 2006;30(1):51-57.

35. Laks S, Macari M, Bini EJ. Positional change in colon polyps at CT colonography. *Radiology.* 2004;231(3):761-766.

36. Chen JC, Dachman AH. Cecal mobility: A potential pitfall of CT colonography. *Am J Roentgenol.* 2006;186(4):1086-1089.

37. Huang A, Roy DA, Summers RM, et al. Teniae coli-based circumferential localization system for CT colonography: Feasibility study. *Radiology.* 2007;243(2):551-560.

38. Mang T, Maier A, Plank C, Mueller-Mang C, Herold C, Schima W. Pitfalls in multi detector row CT colonography: A systematic approach. *Radiographics.* 2007;27(2):431-454.

39. Pickhardt P, Kim D, Taylor A, Husain S. Complementary shifting of luminal fluid between supine and prone positioning at CT colonography: Implications for 3D mucosal coverage. Boston: 8th International VC Symposium; 2007.

40. Pickhardt PJ, Choi JR. Adenomatous polyp obscured by small-caliber rectal catheter at low-dose CT colonography: A rare diagnostic pitfall. *Am J Roentgenol.* 2005;184(5):1581-1583.

41. Iafrate F, Rengo M, Ferrari R, Paolantonio P, Celestre M, Laghi A. Spectrum of normal findings, anatomic variants and pathology of ileocecal valve: CT colonography appearances and endoscopic correlation. *Abdom Imag.* 2007;32(5):589-595.

42. O'Connor SD, Summers RM, Yao JH, Pickhardt PJ, Choi JR. CT Colonography with computer-aided polyp detection: Volume and attenuation thresholds to reduce false-positive findings owing to the ileocecal valve. *Radiology.* 2006;241(2):426-432.

43. Prout TM, Taylor AJ, Pickhardt PJ. Inverted appendiceal stumps simulating large pedunculated polyps on screening CT colonography. *Am J Roentgenol.* 2006;186(2):535-538.

44. Pickhardt PJ, Levy AD, Rohrmann CA, Kende AI. Primary neoplasms of the appendix: Radiologic spectrum of disease with pathologic correlation. *Radiographics.* 2003;23(3):645-662.

45. Pickhardt PJ, Kim DH, Taylor AJ, Gopal DV, Weber SM, Heise CP. Extracolonic tumors of the gastrointestinal tract detected incidentally at screening CT colonography. *Dis Colon Rectum.* 2007;50(1):56-63.

46. Morrin MM, Farrell RJ, Kruskal JB, Reynolds K, McGee JB, Raptopoulos V. Utility of intravenously administered contrast material at CT colonography. *Radiology.* 2000;217(3):765-771.

47. Pickhardt PJ. Screening CT colonography: How I do it. *Am J Roentgenol.* 2007;189(2):290-298.

48. Zalis ME, Perumpillichira JJ, Magee C, Kohlberg G, Hahn PF. Tagging-based, electronically cleansed CT colonography: Evaluation of patient comfort and image readability. *Radiology.* 2006;239(1):149-159.

49. Pickhardt PJ, Kim DH, Menias CO, Gopal DV, Arluk GM, Heise CP. Evaluation of submucosal lesions of the large intestine: Part 1. Neoplasms. *Radiographics.* 2007;27(6):1681-1692.

50. Pickhardt PJ, Kim DH, Menias CO, Gopal DV, Arluk GM, Heise CP. Evaluation of submucosal lesions of the large intestine: Part 2. Nonneoplastic causes. *Radiographics.* 2007;27(6):1693-1703.

Chapter 21

Evaluation for Invasive Cancer at CTC

PERRY J. PICKHARDT, MD

DAVID H. KIM, MD

GENERAL PRINCIPLES

Invasive colorectal cancer (CRC) is defined by the extension of malignant cells beyond the muscularis mucosae layer of the colonic or rectal wall. As such, invasive cancer does not include either "carcinoma in situ," which is more properly referred to as high-grade dysplasia, or intramucosal carcinoma. In practice, the great majority of invasive CRC will manifest as a relatively bulky mass lesion at the time of diagnosis, with a small percentage manifesting as a large malignant polyp (Figs. 21-1 through 21-3). Anecdotal cases of small subcentimeter cancers certainly exist but are rare, especially at screening. In general, symptomatic cancers tend to be large annular constricting, bulky, and/or ulcerated mass lesions (Fig. 21-1), whereas silent asymptomatic cancers are more likely to be semiannular, eccentric, or polypoid in morphology (Figs. 21-2 and 21-3). Unlike the highly technique-dependent diagnostic performance of CT colonography (CTC) for detecting benign colorectal polyps (see Chapter 17), the reported sensitivity of CTC for detecting CRC has been uniformly high from its inception at around 96% or more.[1] This high sensitivity reflects the fact that invasive cancer tends to be readily detectable at primary two-dimensional (2D) evaluation (Figs. 21-1 and 21-2), which was the predominate search pattern in the earlier phases of CTC investigation. Even before the advent of CTC in the mid-1990s, the utility

of a CT pneumocolon technique was demonstrated for cancer detection in symptomatic patients.[2,3]

In the absence of bowel preparation and colonic distention, we have found that the accuracy of routine nontargeted CT (without colonography technique) in evaluating for CRC is decent but considerably less than CTC because of both false-negative and false-positive results related to luminal collapse and residual untagged stool (Fig. 21-4). In a retrospective study of routine intravenous (IV) contrast-enhanced CT scans in an enriched cohort consisting of a 29% CRC rate, we found a mean sensitivity and specificity for CRC detection of 72% and 84%, respectively, with an area under the ROC curve (AUC) ranging from 0.775 to 0.857.[4] Although these numbers are respectable given the lack of any colonography-specific technique, the performance is clearly well below what is readily achievable at CTC. Therefore, if confident exclusion of CRC is desired, CTC technique is indicated, although noncathartic approaches may be suitable for elderly and/or debilitated symptomatic cohorts. One exception to pursuing colonography technique is with patients presenting acutely with high-grade large bowel obstruction, for whom CT without any bowel preparation or colonic distention represents the diagnostic study of choice (Fig. 21-5).

In the setting of known or highly suspected CRC, diagnostic CTC with IV contrast can provide comprehensive preoperative evaluation, including precise assessment and localization of the primary tumor, evaluation for synchronous colorectal lesions, and detection of metastatic disease (Fig. 21-6). When an unsuspected invasive cancer is found at noncontrast CTC, metastatic disease may be detectable but an IV contrast CT study is still generally indicated for proper metastatic staging (Fig. 21-7). Currently, imaging does not play a definitive role in the assessment of local and regional staging of colon cancer (generally, this is determined at surgical resection with

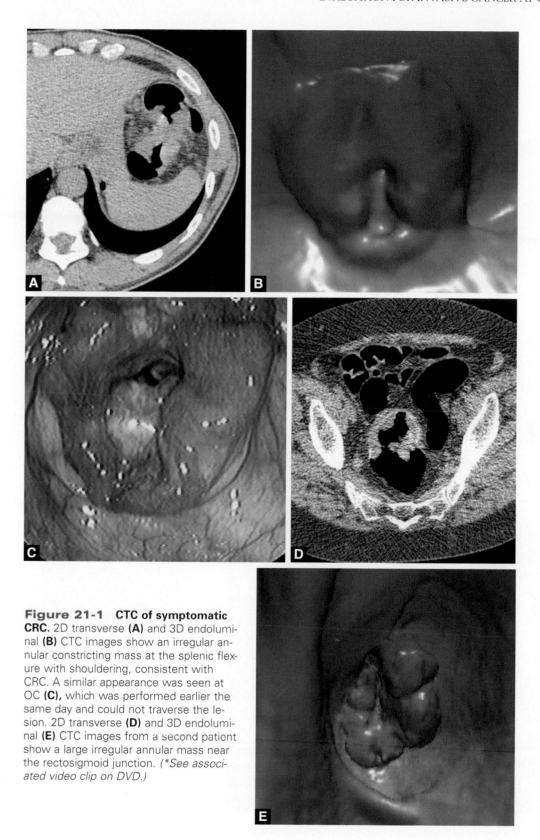

Figure 21-1   CTC of symptomatic CRC. 2D transverse **(A)** and 3D endoluminal **(B)** CTC images show an irregular annular constricting mass at the splenic flexure with shouldering, consistent with CRC. A similar appearance was seen at OC **(C)**, which was performed earlier the same day and could not traverse the lesion. 2D transverse **(D)** and 3D endoluminal **(E)** CTC images from a second patient show a large irregular annular mass near the rectosigmoid junction. (*See associated video clip on DVD.)

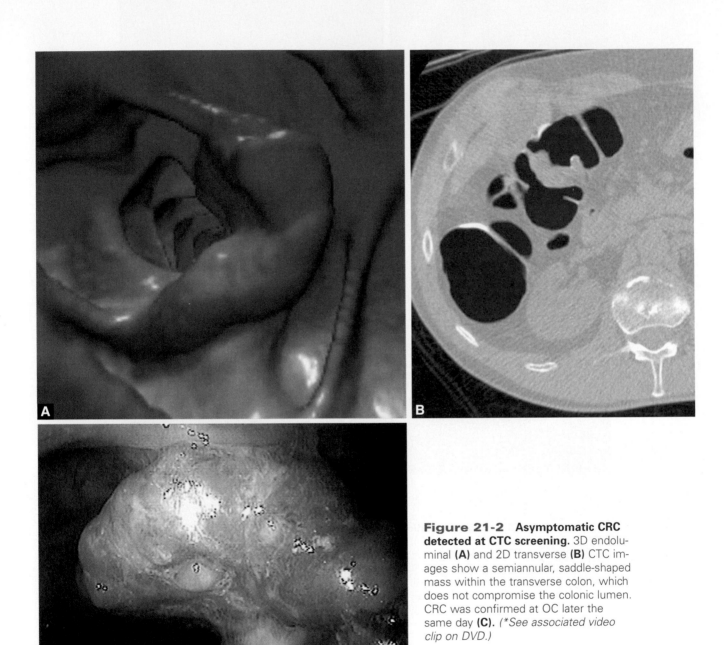

Figure 21-2 Asymptomatic CRC detected at CTC screening. 3D endoluminal **(A)** and 2D transverse **(B)** CTC images show a semiannular, saddle-shaped mass within the transverse colon, which does not compromise the colonic lumen. CRC was confirmed at OC later the same day **(C)**. (*See associated video clip on DVD.)

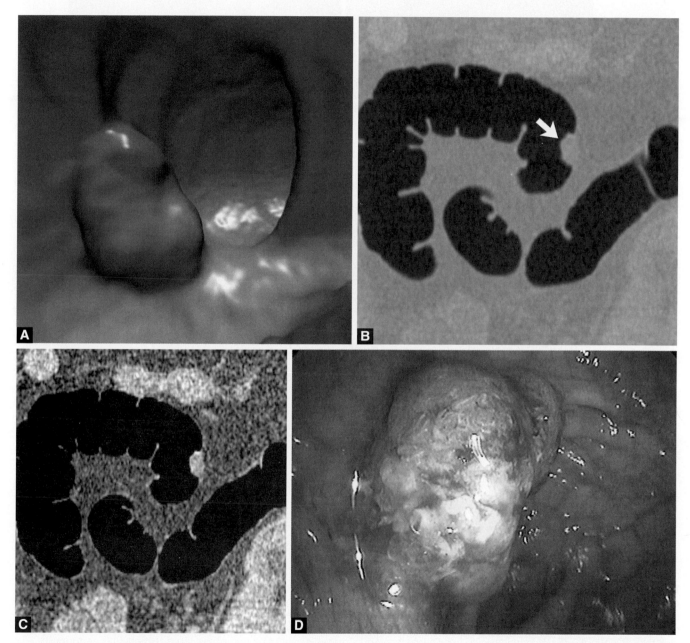

Figure 21-3   Malignant polyp detected at CTC screening. 3D endoluminal CTC image **(A)** shows a 22-mm polypoid lesion in the sigmoid colon, which is confirmed on 2D coronal images with soft tissue **(B)** and polyp **(C)** windows *(arrow)*. The lesion was confirmed at same-day OC **(D)** and proved to have a focus of invasive adenocarcinoma at pathologic evaluation. *(*See associated video clips on DVD.)*

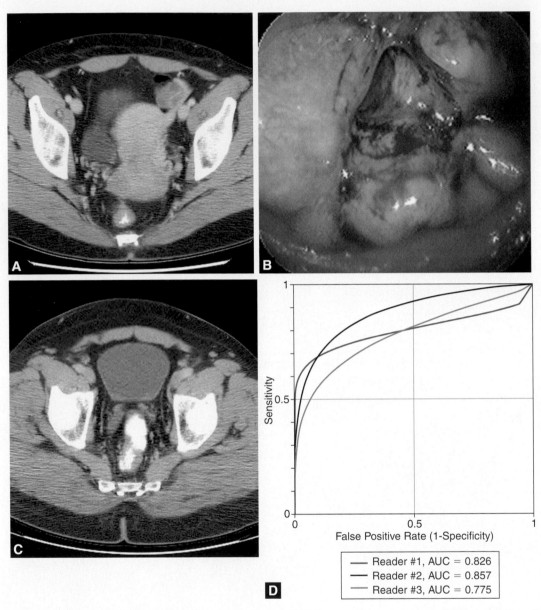

Figure 21-4 **False-negative and false-positive interpretations for CRC at routine nontargeted CT evaluation.** Contrast-enhanced CT scan **(A)** performed without colonography technique shows rectal wall thickening, which was interpreted as collapse and not cancer by all three readers in a retrospective research study. However, an annular rectal cancer was present at OC **(B)**, indicating a false-negative CT interpretation. Routine contrast-enhanced CT from a second patient **(C)** shows irregular and eccentric wall thickening in the rectosigmoid region, which was scored as probable cancer by two of the three readers. OC performed 1 month later was normal. ROC curve for CRC detection by the three readers **(D)** shows slight variations but no significant differences in performance.

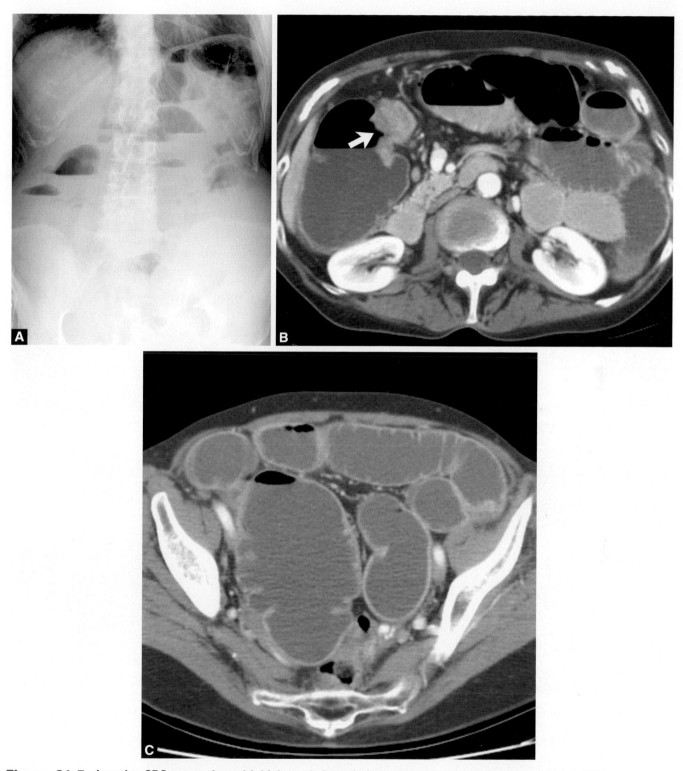

Figure 21-5 **Invasive CRC presenting with high-grade bowel obstruction.** Upright abdominal radiograph **(A)** in a symptomatic patient shows multiple dilated bowel loops with air-fluid levels. Images from contrast-enhanced CT **(B** and **C)** show a large mass at the hepatic flexure *(arrow)* causing high-grade obstruction. Colonography technique would be unnecessary and inappropriate in this clinical setting.

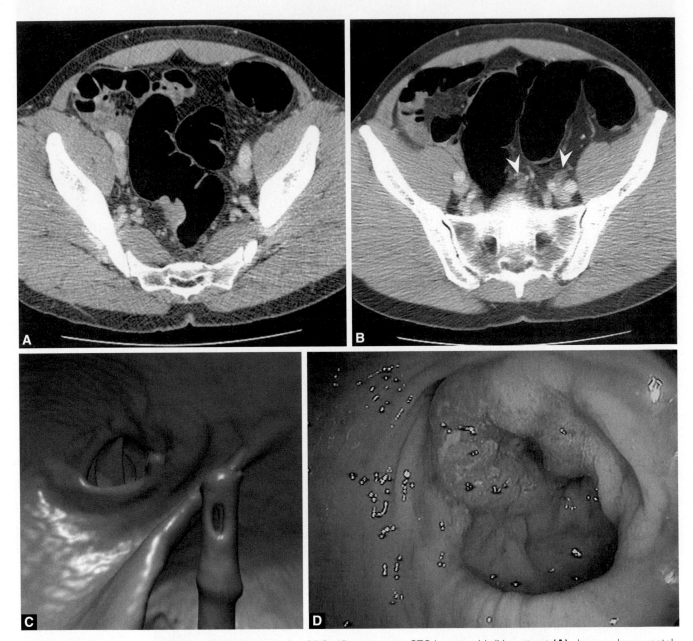

Figure 21-6 **Diagnostic CTC with IV contrast for CRC.** 2D transverse CTC image with IV contrast **(A)** shows a large rectal mass. A more cephalad image **(B)** shows slightly prominent rounded lymph nodes *(arrowheads)*. 3D CTC **(C)** and OC **(D)** images show the primary tumor from the endoluminal perspective. Four of 17 lymph nodes were positive at low anterior resection.

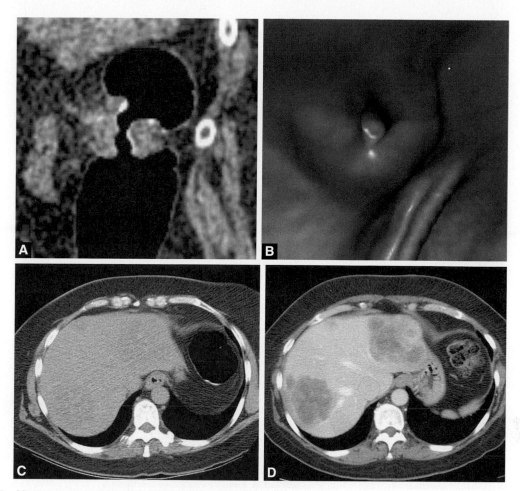

Figure 21-7 **Unsuspected metastatic CRC detected at CTC screening.** 2D coronal **(A)** and 3D endoluminal **(B)** CTC images in an asymptomatic 55-year-old woman show an annular constricting mass in the descending colon. Subtle but large hepatic metastases are apparent on the low-dose unenhanced CTC images **(C)** but are much better demonstrated on a subsequent diagnostic CT with IV contrast **(D)**. *(*See associated video clip on DVD.)*

pathologic staging), but it is the mainstay for determination of distant malignant disease. Rectal cancer represents an exception to this practice where imaging in the form of rectal magnetic resonance (MR) or transrectal ultrasound (US) is being increasingly used for preoperative local and regional staging of the tumor to assess the need for neoadjuvant chemoradiation (see Chapter 4). We are currently investigating the use of CT proctography (virtual proctoscopy) to allow accurate local staging and to assess the response of rectal cancer to neoadjuvant therapy by evaluating the change in tumor volume (Fig. 21-8). As will be discussed later in this chapter, the different clinical scenarios where CRC may be encountered at CTC include the diagnostic evaluation of symptomatic patients, detection of unsuspected cancer at asymptomatic screening, and referral from incomplete optical colonoscopy (OC) related to either an occlusive CRC or another cause. The CTC appearance of CRC will depend in part on the clinical scenario. In addition, there are a number of mimics that can resemble the appearance at CTC. The specific CTC protocol used, particularly the type of bowel preparation, the use of IV contrast, and the interpretive approach, will all be influenced by the specific indication that leads to the CTC examination itself.

The malignant potential of an adenomatous polyp directly correlates with its size, histologic subtype, and degree of dysplasia. Fortunately, invasive CRC is encountered in less than 1% of asymptomatic adults undergoing screening—about 1 every 500 adults in our experience.[5] Malignant polyps are relatively rare but can appear similar to large advanced adenomas (Fig. 21-3). Unlike the classic 5% to 10% rate of malignancy reported in older series involving high-risk cohorts,[6,7] less than 1% of large polyps will be malignant in a true screening population.[5] The more typical mass-forming invasive adenocarcinoma will manifest with either an eccentric saddlelike appearance (Fig. 21-2) or as an annular constricting ("apple core" or "napkin ring") lesion (Fig. 21-1). Unlike polypoid lesions, which are more easily detected on the 3D endoluminal display, invasive cancers form masses that are also readily identified on the 2D images, which allow for mural and extramural evaluation.

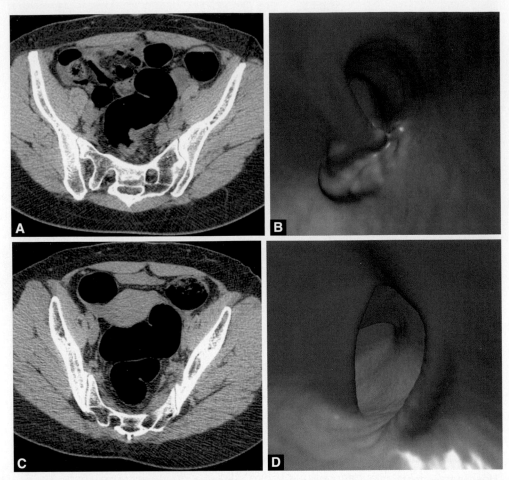

Figure 21-8 **CT proctography (virtual proctoscopy) for assessing response of rectal cancer to neoadjuvant therapy.** 2D transverse **(A)** and 3D endoluminal **(B)** images from CT proctography show an eccentric irregular rectal mass consistent with primary adenocarcinoma, which was proven at biopsy. Similar images following neoadjuvant chemoradiation therapy **(C** and **D)** show a complete response. Carcinoma was not indentified on pathologic examination of the low anterior resection specimen, and all nodes were negative.

CRC EVALUATION IN SYMPTOMATIC PATIENTS

The primary goals and target lesions of interest at CTC evaluation depend on the specific clinical indication, which also determines which specific techniques ought to be used. For screening of asymptomatic adults, the primary goal is cancer prevention through detection of important benign precursors, with the advanced adenoma representing the optimal target lesion. Because CTC technique and interpretation in this setting are designed to optimize polyp detection, invasive mass lesions (CRC) will also be readily detectable. However, if the clinical indication for performing CTC is to "rule out cancer" in a symptomatic elderly or frail patient, then both the technique and interpretive approach may be modified because detection of benign polyps is no longer a primary concern. For this group of patients, we often find it useful to use a noncathartic bowel preparation with oral contrast tagging and to perform a diagnostic

CTC with IV contrast. The use of IV contrast serves not only to stage any CRC that is found, but also to better evaluate extracolonic structures for other significant pathology.[8] Regardless of the specific technique that is used, this can be a challenging group of patients compared with the asymptomatic screening population. In some cases, one must be willing to accept a level of study quality that would be suboptimal for polyp detection, keeping in mind that the target of cancer is much more forgiving.

For patients presenting with a more acute large bowel obstruction, bowel preparation or distention will not only be unnecessary but is generally contraindicated. In such cases, routine diagnostic CT with IV contrast allows for rapid and effective evaluation (Fig. 21-5). Similarly, if the clinical concern is primarily acute diverticulitis (versus perforated CRC), CTC is contraindicated and a diagnostic CT with IV contrast is the more appropriate test (Fig. 21-9). A followup OC (or CTC) generally should be performed following treatment and resolu-

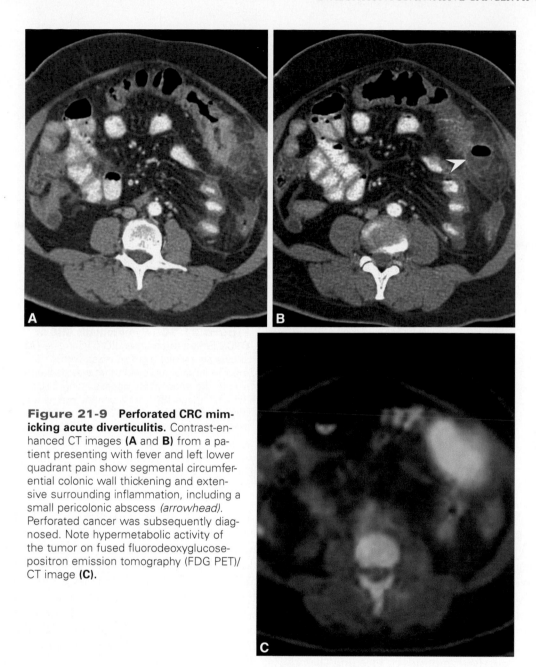

Figure 21-9 Perforated CRC mimicking acute diverticulitis. Contrast-enhanced CT images **(A** and **B)** from a patient presenting with fever and left lower quadrant pain show segmental circumferential colonic wall thickening and extensive surrounding inflammation, including a small pericolonic abscess *(arrowhead)*. Perforated cancer was subsequently diagnosed. Note hypermetabolic activity of the tumor on fused fluorodeoxyglucose-positron emission tomography (FDG PET)/CT image **(C)**.

tion of diverticulitis to exclude the unlikely possibility of a perforated cancer masquerading as diverticulitis. With more subacute or chronic clinical presentations, CTC technique is often warranted. When CRC is the main clinical question, modification in the interpretive approach may include more emphasis on primary 2D evaluation, given its proven efficacy for this target lesion. However, whenever possible, we would still urge the use of both primary 3D and 2D evaluations, unless the degree of residual stool or luminal collapse precludes effective 3D evaluation. For more borderline cases, where symptoms are relatively vague and not particularly alarming, the addition of IV contrast can be reserved as a selective case-by-case decision.

Differing goals and target lesions among cancer screening programs may even be evident at the international level. For example, whereas the emphasis of CRC screening in the United States is focused primarily on prevention through detection and removal of advanced adenomas,[9] the National Health System (NHS) in the United Kingdom has chosen not to pursue CRC prevention but instead has largely targeted CRC detection in symptomatic patients.[10] The rationale behind this policy in the United Kingdom is that limited resources do not allow for primary colorectal screening with the structural examinations (whether by OC, CTC, or barium enema [BE]) and that fecal occult blood test (FOBT) screening will presumably detect

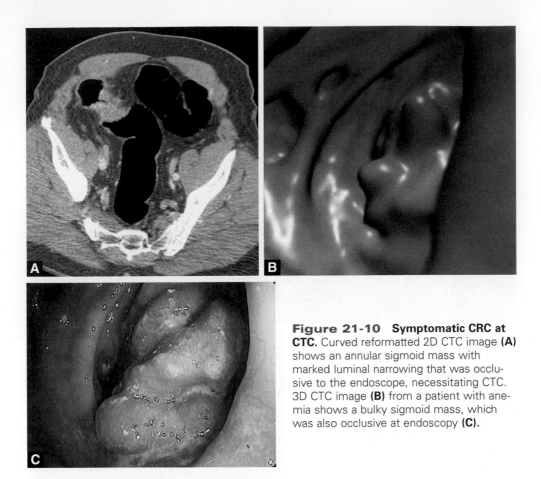

Figure 21-10 Symptomatic CRC at CTC. Curved reformatted 2D CTC image **(A)** shows an annular sigmoid mass with marked luminal narrowing that was occlusive to the endoscope, necessitating CTC. 3D CTC image **(B)** from a patient with anemia shows a bulky sigmoid mass, which was also occlusive at endoscopy **(C)**.

most bleeding cancers at a curable stage. With this approach, CTC could still represent an effective intermediary between a positive FOBT result and OC because the great majority of positive FOBT results will be falsely positive for cancer. A large randomized trial evaluating CRC detection with OC, CTC, and BE was recently completed in the United Kingdom.

The imaging appearance of symptomatic CRC at CTC often reflects the fact that the tumor has presented with obstructive symptoms or bleeding (i.e., the lesions tend to be either annular constricting with marked luminal narrowing or bulky and/or ulcerated masses; Fig. 21-1 and 21-10). These findings of the primary tumor are analogous to the old familiar features of symptomatic cancer at BE evaluation (Fig. 21-11). On finding CRC at CTC, one must resist the "satisfaction of search" phenomenon and remain vigilant for synchronous lesions, including both additional cancers and large polyps (Fig. 21-12). In addition, a thorough search for metastatic disease is performed, including lymphatic, hematogenous, and peritoneal routes of spread. If IV contrast was not administered for the CTC study, an additional standard diagnostic CT with IV contrast will generally be indicated for assessment of distant metastatic disease.

Beyond CRC-related disease, a careful search for extracolonic pathology is also warranted because a number of these cases will present with nonspecific abdominal complaints. In this symptomatic cohort, the ability of CTC to provide both colorectal and extracolonic assessment is a great benefit over the purely colorectal examinations such as endoscopy and BE. In one study of 400 elderly patients with abdominal symptoms concerning for lower gastrointestinal pathology, 49 (12%) were found to have at least one cancer at CTC, including 29 cases of CRC and 23 extracolonic malignancies.[8] This study, which routinely used IV contrast at the initial CTC examination, underscores the utility of this diagnostic approach. In younger patients with less ominous symptoms, it is reasonable to avoid the use of IV contrast at the initial CTC examination because the majority will not ultimately have CRC or any other identifiable pathology.

Certain high-risk cohorts, such as patients with hereditary nonpolyposis colorectal cancer or longstanding inflammatory bowel disease, are generally better served by OC evaluation. However, in cases in which OC is incomplete or felt to be too risky, CTC can often provide a diagnostic evaluation and exclude CRC (Fig. 21-13) For patients with a history of prior CRC, the use of CTC

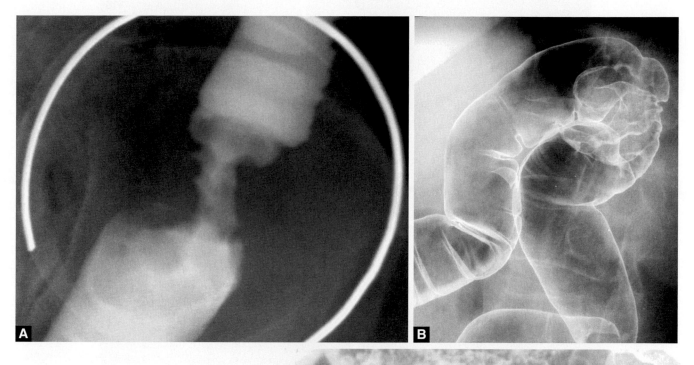

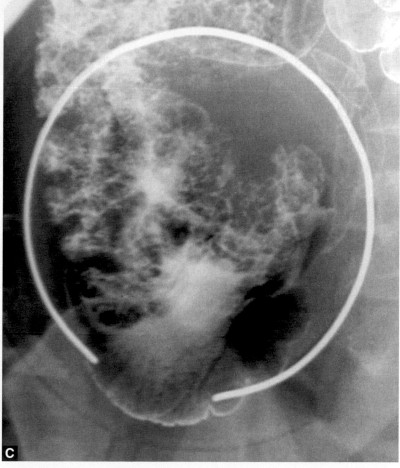

Figure 21-11   Symptomatic CRC at BE. Fluoroscopic images from barium enema in three different patients show typical "apple core" annular constricting masses in the first two (**A** and **B**) and a bulky villous tumor in the third patient (**C**).

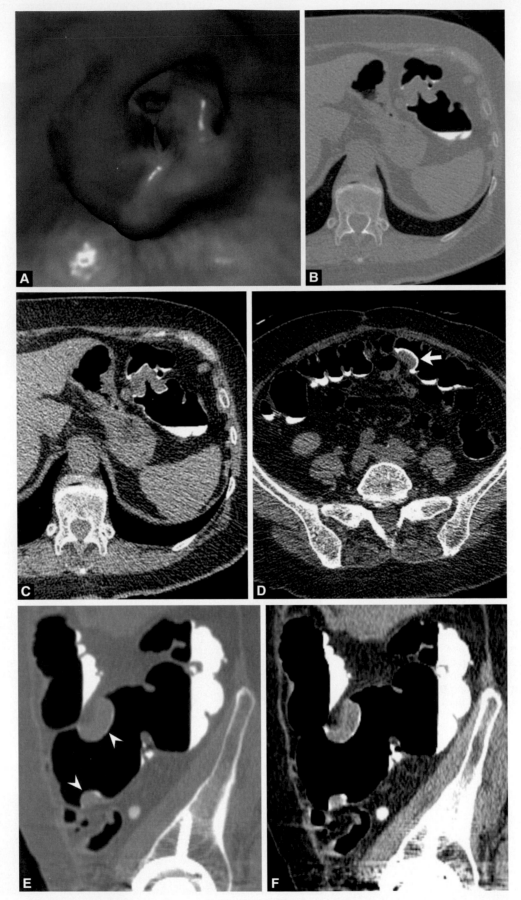

Figure 21-12 Synchronous CRC. 3D endoluminal CTC image **(A)** shows a nearly annular mass at the splenic flexure, which is easily confirmed on 2D images with polyp **(B)** and soft tissue **(C)** windowing. A second cancer was found in the midtransverse colon **(D,** *arrow).* The patient had undergone an incomplete screening OC 1 year earlier that was complicated by sigmoid perforation and failed to detect the cancers. 2D sagittal CTC images with polyp **(E)** and soft tissue **(F)** windows from a second patient show synchronous cecal cancers *(arrowheads). (*See associated video clip on DVD.)*

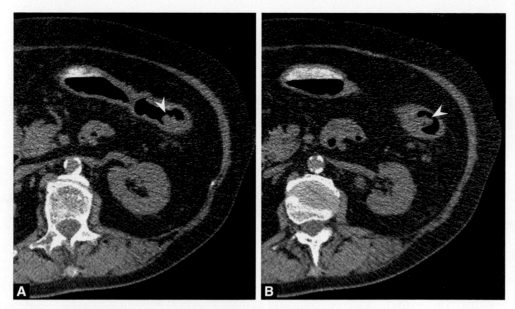

Figure 21-13 **Invasive CRC complicating longstanding Crohn's disease.** 2D transverse CTC images **(A** and **B)** show diffuse colonic wall thickening with associated luminal narrowing that is relatively uniform except a focal mass lesion *(arrowheads)*, representing CRC.

to evaluate for metachronous cancer may be reasonable (Fig. 21-14), although these patients have generally been followed with OC in the past.

EVALUATION FOLLOWING INCOMPLETE OC

CTC referral from incomplete OC because of either an occlusive cancer or other cause represented the first widely adopted clinical indication for CTC. Several early clinical studies documented the utility of CTC in this setting.[11-13] The primary goal of CTC evaluation for these patients is the evaluation for lesions proximal to where the endoscope reached and, if CRC is present, evaluation for metastatic disease (Figs. 21-15 and 21-16). In the case of occlusive CRC, because the diagnosis of cancer is known prior to CTC evaluation, a protocol using IV contrast is generally indicated if a prior staging CT for distant disease has not been performed (Fig. 21-15). When OC is incomplete because of a benign cause (e.g., excessive tortuosity, diverticular stricture, etc.), IV contrast is generally not used because the likelihood of CRC is considerably lower in most cases (Fig. 21-16). In general, the CTC examination is often performed on the same day as the incomplete OC to both expedite the workup and to avoid the need for additional bowel preparation. The lack of oral contrast tagging from the OC preparation can either be compensated by the presence of IV contrast or by the addition of a water-soluble iodinated oral contrast agent prior to CTC.

CRC DETECTION AT ASYMPTOMATIC SCREENING

As previously discussed, the primary goal of CRC screening in asymptomatic adults at average risk is cancer prevention through detection and removal of advanced adenomas. Of course, one would not want to miss an unsuspected CRC still at an early presymptomatic phase. Fortunately, because CTC technique and interpretation in this cohort are designed to optimize polyp detection, the occasional invasive CRC will generally be obvious. The rate of unsuspected CRC detection at asymptomatic screening is quite low. Based on our experience with more than 10,000 cases, the frequency has held steady at about 1 new case for every 500 adults screened (0.2%).[14] There are some interesting (and logical) morphologic differences in the CTC appearance of asymptomatic versus symptomatic CRC. It is not surprising that symptomatic cancers are more often annular with marked luminal narrowing, whereas asymptomatic tumors more often manifest as semiannular (Fig. 21-2), plaquelike (Fig. 21-17), or polypoid (Fig. 21-18) in morphology. However, a number of asymptomatic cancers will be annular at presentation but often without significant luminal compromise (Fig. 21-19). Malignant polyps are generally asymptomatic but are almost always greater than 1 cm and typically greater than 2 cm in size.[5] In our experience, primary CTC screening appears to be more sensitive than primary OC screening for detecting cases of unsuspected CRC in asymptomatic adults.[15] Other groups have also reported high miss rates for cancer at

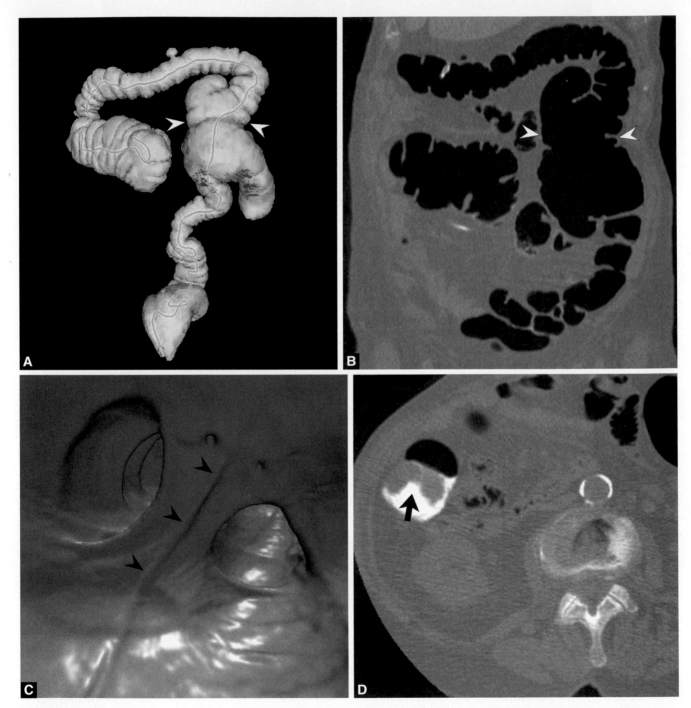

Figure 21-14 Metachronous CRC at CTC surveillance. 3D colon map **(A)**, 2D coronal **(B)**, and 3D endoluminal **(C)** CTC images from a patient with a history of CRC show postsurgical changes of segmental colonic resection with side-to-side anastomosis on the left *(arrowheads)*. Unfortunately, a new cancer was detected in the right colon **(D**, *arrow)*.

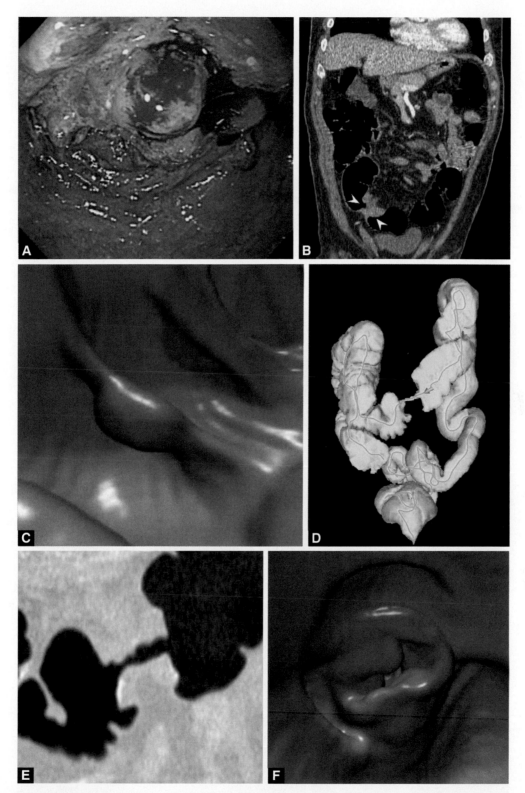

Figure 21-15 **Incomplete OC because of occlusive CRC.** Image from OC **(A)** shows an annular constricting sigmoid mass that precluded passage of the scope. 2D coronal CTC image **(B)** shows the occlusive mass. Note that IV contrast was administered to help assess for metastatic disease. 3D endoluminal CTC image **(C)** shows a large polyp proximal to the occlusive CRC. 3D colon map **(D),** 2D coronal **(E),** and 3D endoluminal **(F)** CTC images from a second patient show marked luminal narrowing of the midtransverse colon because of a large annular CRC. (Figs. B and C from Pickhardt PJ. Differential diagnosis of polypoid lesions seen at CT colonography (virtual colonoscopy). *Radiographics.* 2004;24:1535-1559.) *(*See associated video clip on DVD.)*

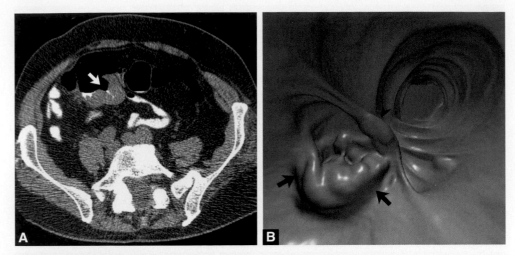

Figure 21-16 **Invasive CRC proximal to level of incomplete OC.** 2D transverse **(A)** and 3D endoluminal **(B)** CTC images from a patient who underwent incomplete OC to the level of the ascending colon earlier the same day show an irregular cecal mass *(arrows)* adjacent to the ileocecal valve *(arrowhead)*. Note how the mass is obscured from view in the ascending colon behind the ileocecal fold. *(*See associated video clip on DVD.)*

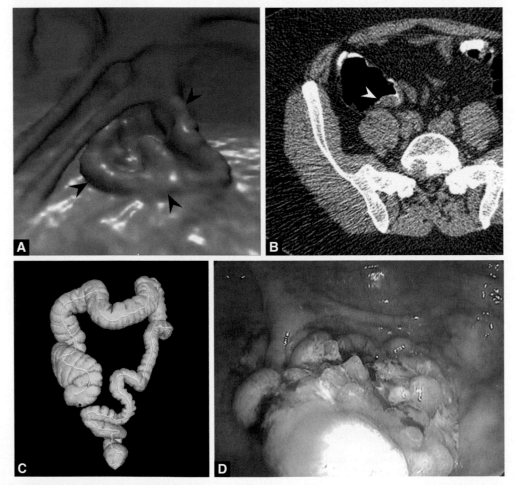

Figure 21-17 **Eccentric plaquelike CRC detected at asymptomatic screening.** 3D endoluminal **(A)** and 2D transverse **(B)** CTC images show an irregular plaquelike mass at the cecal base *(arrowheads)*. The 3D colon map **(C)** shows the location of the finding *(red dot)* and the relevant colorectal anatomy for the endoscopist. Image from same-day OC **(D)** confirms cecal carcinoma.

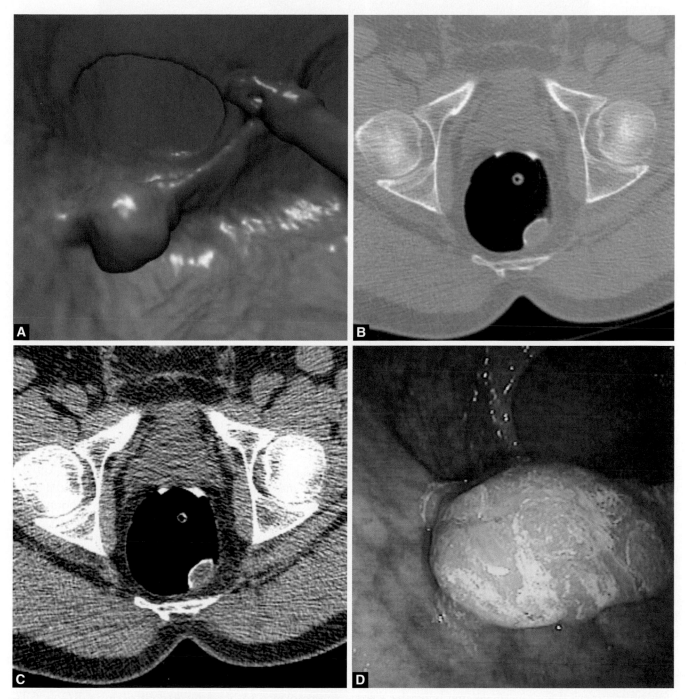

Figure 21-18 Polypoid CRC detected at asymptomatic screening. 3D endoluminal **(A)**, 2D polyp **(B)**, and 2D soft tissue **(C)** CTC images show a 2-cm polyp arising from a rectal valve. The thin etching of oral contrast on the polyp surface is very typical. The lesion was confirmed at same-day OC **(D)**. A well-differentiated adenocarcinoma arising within a tubulovillous adenoma was found at pathologic evaluation.

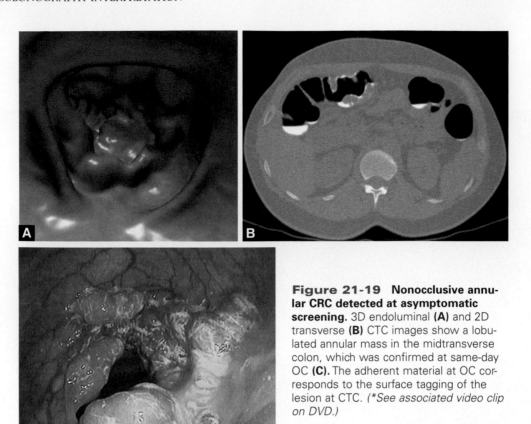

Figure 21-19 Nonocclusive annular CRC detected at asymptomatic screening. 3D endoluminal **(A)** and 2D transverse **(B)** CTC images show a lobulated annular mass in the midtransverse colon, which was confirmed at same-day OC **(C)**. The adherent material at OC corresponds to the surface tagging of the lesion at CTC. (*See associated video clip on DVD.)*

OC evaluation, which were prospectively detected at CTC and would have remained "occult" at OC if not for the CTC detection.[16]

For primary CTC screening in asymptomatic cohorts, IV contrast is generally not indicated. Therefore, patients with unsuspected CRC will generally require a subsequent diagnostic CT with IV contrast at some point during their workup.

IMAGING MIMICS OF CRC

A variety of neoplastic and non-neoplastic conditions can mimic the appearance of CRC at CTC and at other imaging tests such as OC and BE. Relatively common examples include serosal implants from endometriosis or extracolonic cancers, diverticular disease including both acute diverticulitis and chronic diverticular stricture, and transient colonic spasm. We have seen a number of cases of unsuspected endometriosis involving the colon in perimenopausal women that were detected at primary CTC examination. The specific findings vary considerably, ranging from a focal colorectal lesion to bulky peritoneal disease (Fig. 21-20). Malignant serosal invasion from peritoneal carcinomatosis or direct tumor invasion from an extracolonic malignancy can often be suggested from the combination of CT findings and clinical history (Fig. 21-21).

Diverticular disease, particularly involving the sigmoid colon, represents a common diagnostic challenge at CTC (see Chapter 20). Segmental spasm or stricture related to diverticular disease can mimic CRC, but tends to involve a relatively long segment, lacks a bulky or expansile soft tissue mass, and is clearly associated with advanced diverticulosis (Fig. 21-22). In cases where the abnormal segment cannot be confidently cleared by primary CTC, same-day flexible sigmoidoscopy without sedation can be an efficient means for completing the evaluation. In other cases, the indication for CTC will be incomplete OC from the diverticular stricture itself. When signs and symptoms suggesting acute diverticulitis are present, we would perform a standard diagnostic CT with IV contrast and avoid CTC technique in this acute setting. Appropriate followup can exclude the unlikely perforated cancer masquerading as diverticulitis (Fig. 21-9).

Focal colonic spasm will occasionally bear a superficial resemblance to an annular constricting CRC at CTC evaluation. However, in the case of focal spasm or collapse of an interhaustral fold, the very short segment of involvement, the smooth ringlike appearance, and the transient nature all help to easily exclude CRC (Fig. 21-23). Longer segments of spasm or collapse, often involving segments of advanced diverticular disease, can be more challenging if persistent on all views and positions. A third decubitus series will often help in excluding a

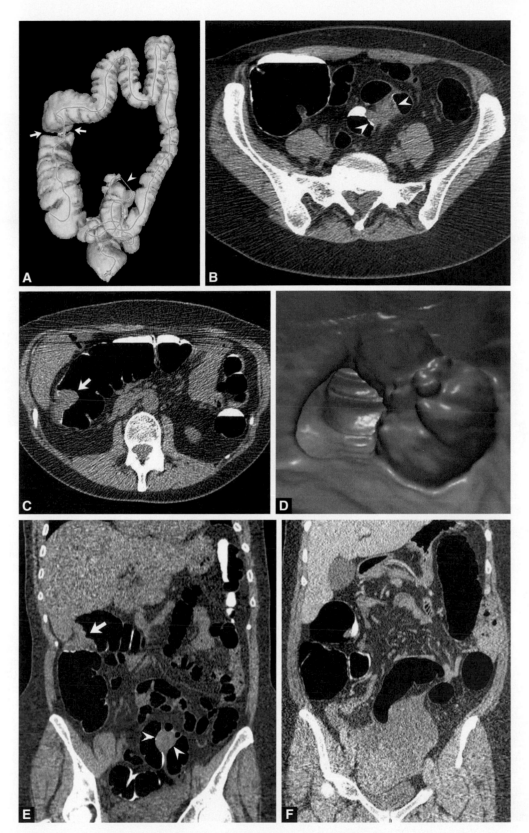

Figure 21-20   Unsuspected endometriosis with colonic involvement at CTC. 3D colon map **(A)** from an asymptomatic 50-year-old woman shows two regions of luminal compromise in the sigmoid *(arrowhead)* and ascending *(arrows)* colon. 2D transverse CTC image **(B)** shows a tight annular soft tissue lesion in the sigmoid *(arrowheads)*, which was occlusive at OC and proved to be endometriosis at surgery. 2D transverse **(C)** and 3D endoluminal **(D)** CTC images show a lobulated bulky mass *(arrow)* in the ascending colon, which could not be evaluated at OC but proved to be invasive CRC at surgery. 2D curved reformatted image **(E)** shows both the endometrial lesion *(arrowheads)* and the CRC *(arrow)*. 2D coronal CTC image from a second woman **(F)** shows a large peritoneal-based soft tissue mass that also proved to be endometriosis at surgery. (Figs. A-D from Pickhardt PJ, Kim DH. CT colonography: A primer for gastroenterologists. *Clin Gastroenterol Hepatol*. 2008;6:497-502.) (Fig. F from atlas.)

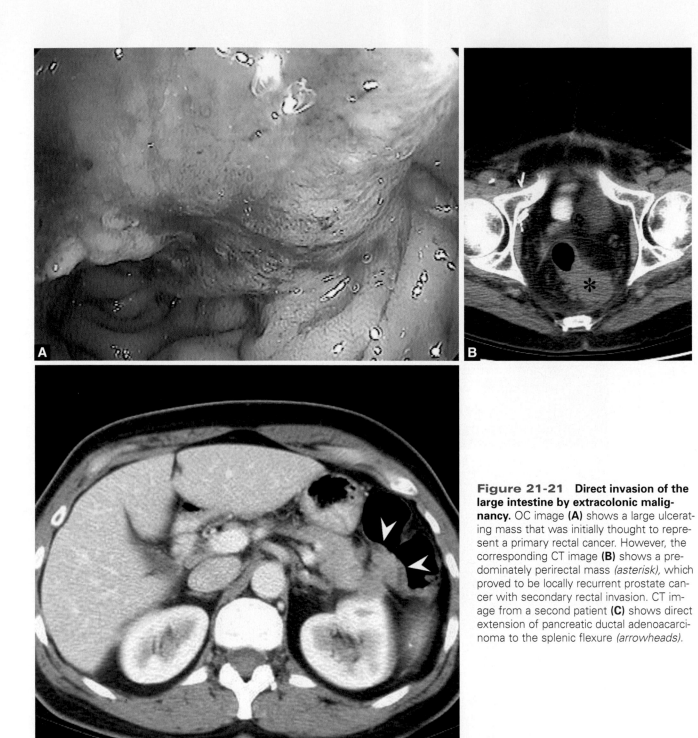

Figure 21-21   Direct invasion of the large intestine by extracolonic malignancy. OC image **(A)** shows a large ulcerating mass that was initially thought to represent a primary rectal cancer. However, the corresponding CT image **(B)** shows a predominately perirectal mass *(asterisk),* which proved to be locally recurrent prostate cancer with secondary rectal invasion. CT image from a second patient **(C)** shows direct extension of pancreatic ductal adenoacarcinoma to the splenic flexure *(arrowheads).*

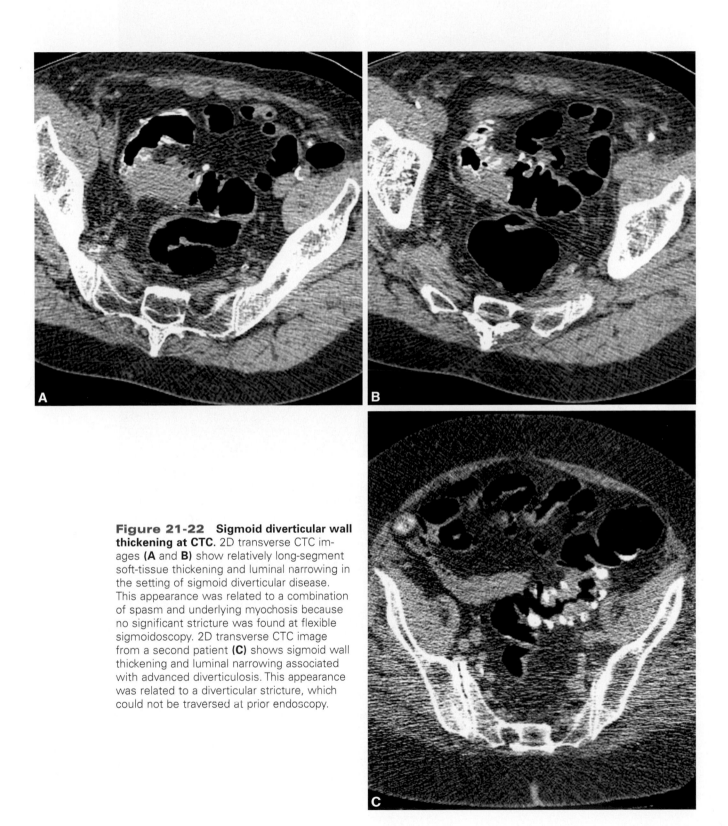

Figure 21-22   Sigmoid diverticular wall thickening at CTC. 2D transverse CTC images (**A** and **B**) show relatively long-segment soft-tissue thickening and luminal narrowing in the setting of sigmoid diverticular disease. This appearance was related to a combination of spasm and underlying myochosis because no significant stricture was found at flexible sigmoidoscopy. 2D transverse CTC image from a second patient (**C**) shows sigmoid wall thickening and luminal narrowing associated with advanced diverticulosis. This appearance was related to a diverticular stricture, which could not be traversed at prior endoscopy.

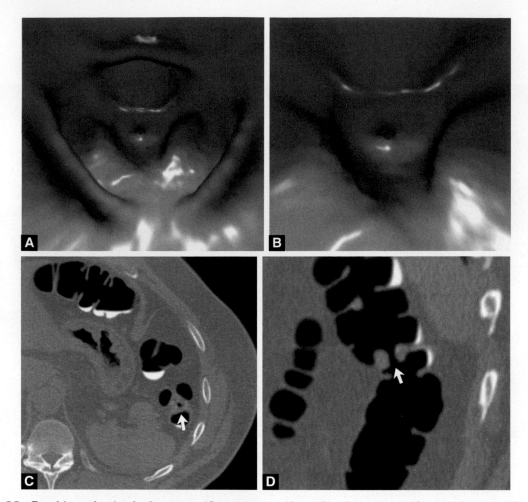

Figure 21-23 **Focal (transient) colonic spasm.** 3D endoluminal **(A and B)**, 2D transverse **(C)**, and 2D sagittal **(D)** CTC images show focal ringlike narrowing involving an interhaustral fold *(arrows)*, characteristic of focal spasm. Note the uniform nature, short segment, characteristic location, and lack of irregularity or shouldering. This should not be mistaken for an annular mass lesion.

true invasive mass lesion. In our experience, some cases with segmental areas of persistent collapse at CTC despite good technique will turn out to represent true pathology (e.g., benign stricture related to diverticular disease or radiation therapy).

Less common mimics of primary CRC include other malignant processes such as non-Hodgkin's lymphoma, hematogenous metastases, and rare nonepithelial colorectal malignancies (Fig. 21-24). The specific imaging features and pertinent clinical history will often point to a non-CRC process in these cases. Of special note are anal cancers, which may rarely be detected at CTC screening (Fig. 21-25). The majority of anal cancers will be squamous cell carcinoma, followed by adenocarcinoma. The anorectal region is a challenging area at CTC evaluation and is discussed in more detail in Chapter 20.

CONCLUSION

From its inception, CTC has been ideally suited for detection of invasive CRC. Based on data from the literature dating back to the early days of CTC, the sensitivity of this test for detecting CRC rivals or surpasses that of OC. The specific CTC protocol used will largely depend on the clinical scenario, which necessitates effective communication between the radiologist and referring clinician and correlation with the patient's clinical status. When CRC is known or highly suspected based on symptoms, CTC with IV contrast can effectively evaluate for primary colorectal lesions; for metastatic disease (if CRC is present); and for relevant extracolonic pathology, which may actually have given rise to the patient's symptoms.

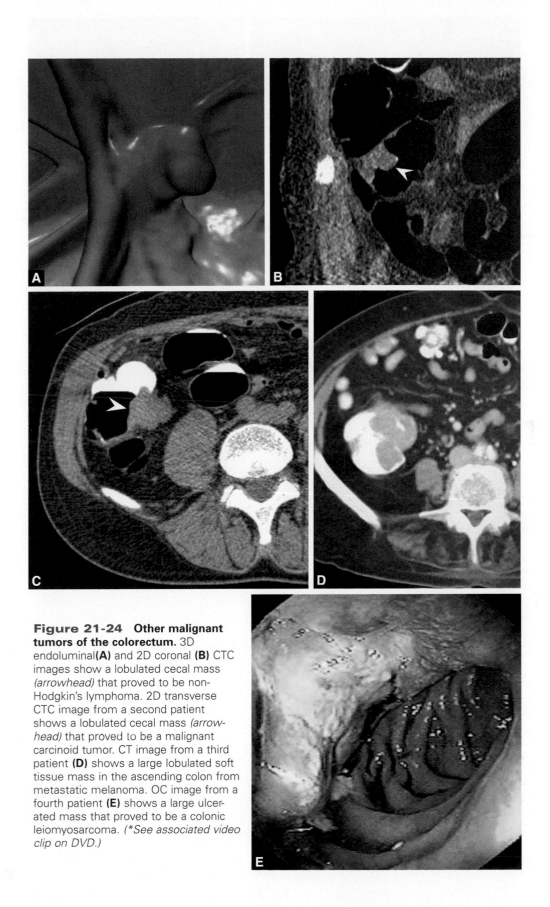

Figure 21-24   Other malignant tumors of the colorectum. 3D endoluminal **(A)** and 2D coronal **(B)** CTC images show a lobulated cecal mass *(arrowhead)* that proved to be non-Hodgkin's lymphoma. 2D transverse CTC image from a second patient shows a lobulated cecal mass *(arrowhead)* that proved to be a malignant carcinoid tumor. CT image from a third patient **(D)** shows a large lobulated soft tissue mass in the ascending colon from metastatic melanoma. OC image from a fourth patient **(E)** shows a large ulcerated mass that proved to be a colonic leiomyosarcoma. *(*See associated video clip on DVD.)*

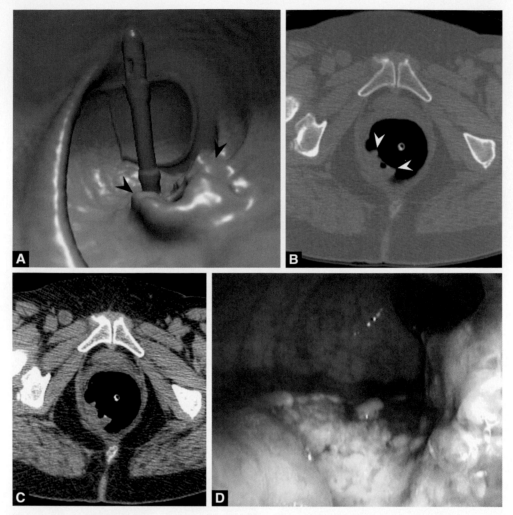

Figure 21-25   Anal cancer (squamous cell carcinoma) detected at CTC screening. 3D endoluminal **(A)** and 2D transverse **(B and C)** CTC images show a fixed, irregular mass *(arrowheads)* located eccentrically near the anorectal junction. Internal hemorrhoids are much more common, but the fixed masslike appearance and eccentric location triggered further evaluation in this case. A friable anorectal tumor was confirmed at OC **(D)**, which proved to be an invasive squamous cell carcinoma. *(*See associated video clip on DVD.)*

REFERENCES

1. Halligan S, Altman DG, Taylor SA, et al. CT colonography in the detection of colorectal polyps and cancer: Systematic review meta-analysis and proposed minimum data set for study level reporting. *Radiology.* 2006;238(3):893-904.

2. Balthazar EJ. CT of the gastrointestinal tract—Principles and interpretation. *Am J Roentgenol.* 1991;156(1):23-32.

3. Balthazar EJ, Megibow AJ, Hulnick D, Naidich DP. Carcinoma of the colon—Detection and preoperative staging by CT. *Am J Roentgenol.* 1988;150(2):301-306.

4. Ozel B, Pickhardt PJ, Kim DH, Bhargava N, Schumacher C, Pfau P. Detection of colorectal cancer on standard nontargeted CT evaluation. Chicago: Annual Meeting of the Society for Gastrointestinal Radiology; 2007.

5. Pickhardt PJ, Kim DH. Colorectal cancer screening with CT colonography: Key concepts regarding polyp prevalence, size, histology, morphology, and natural history. *AJR.* 2009 [in press].

6. Shinya H, Wolff WI. Morphology, anatomic distribution and cancer potential of colonic polyps. *Ann Surg.* 1979;190(6):679-683.

7. Muto T, Bussey HJR, Morson BC. Evolution of cancer of colon and rectum. *Cancer.* 1975;36(6):2251-2270.

8. Tolan DJM, Armstrong EM, Chapman AH. Replacing barium enema with CT colonography in patients older than 70 years: The importance of detecting extracolonic abnormalities. *Am J Roentgenol.* 2007;189(5):1104-1111.

9. Levin B, Lieberman DA, McFarland B, et al. Screening and surveillance for the early detection of colorectal cancer and adenomatous polyps, 2008: A joint guideline from the American Cancer Society, the US Multi-Society Task Force on Colorectal Cancer, and the American College of Radiology. CA *Cancer J Clin.* 2008;58(3):130-160.

10. Sahni VA, Burling D. The new NHS colorectal cancer screening programme and the potential role of radiology? *Br J Radiol.* 2007;80(958):778-781.

11. Fenlon HM, McAneny DB, Nunes DP, Clarke PD, Ferrucci JT. Occlusive colon carcinoma: Virtual colonoscopy in the preoperative evaluation of the proximal colon. *Radiology*. 1999;210(2): 423-428.

12. Macari M, Berman P, Dicker M, Milano A, Megibow AJ. Usefulness of CT colonography in patients with incomplete colonoscopy. *Am J Roentgenol*. 1999;173(3):561-564.

13. Morrin MM, Kruskal JB, Farrell RJ, Goldberg SN, McGee JB, Raptopoulos V. Endoluminal CT colonography after an incomplete endoscopic colonoscopy. *Am J Roentgenol*. 1999;172(4): 913-918.

14. Pickhardt PJ, Meiners RJ, Kim DH, Cash BD. Unsuspected cancers detected at CT colonography screening in over 10,000 asymtpomatic adults. Maui, HI: Annual meeting for the Society of Gastrointestinal Radiologists; 2009.

15. Kim DH, Pickhardt PJ, Taylor AJ, et al. CT colonography versus colonoscopy for the detection of advanced neoplasia. *N Engl J Med*. 2007;357(14):1403-1412.

16. Johnson CD, Fletcher JG, MacCarty RL, et al. Effect of slice thickness and primary 2D versus 3D virtual dissection on colorectal lesion detection at CT colonography in 452 asymptomatic adults. *Am J Roentgenol*. 2007;189(3):672-680.

Chapter 22

Submucosal Lesions at CTC

PERRY J. PICKHARDT, MD
DAVID H. KIM, MD

INTRODUCTION

The term "submucosal" can generically apply to any masslike protrusion into the lumen of the large intestine that originates deep in the overlying mucosa. On endoluminal examination, whether at virtual or optical colonoscopy (OC), submucosal lesions classically manifest as smooth, broad-based abnormalities.[1,2] These lesions may arise from the various layers of the intestinal wall itself (intramural) or from an extrinsic process (extramural). Some entities, such as extracolonic malignancy or endometriosis, may begin as an extramural process but secondarily invade the large intestine to become intramural as well. Although OC can accurately differentiate mucosal lesions from those of submucosal origin, the ability of this strictly luminal examination to fully characterize a submucosal abnormality is somewhat limited. Furthermore, the diagnostic yield of endoscopic biopsy for submucosal lesions is relatively low. Cross-sectional radiologic imaging modalities, however, can effectively evaluate the full thickness of the large intestinal wall and surrounding tissues and are therefore very useful in the workup of suspected submucosal abnormalities. In particular, computed tomography (CT), CT colonography (CTC), transrectal ultrasound (TRUS), and magnetic resonance (MR) imaging can all provide valuable information in this clinical setting. This chapter will focus on the utility of CT, with

or without colonography technique, in evaluating lesions of submucosal origin and will demonstrate the complementary nature of OC and CT for evaluation.

GENERAL PRINCIPLES OF EVALUATION

Detection of mucosal-based polyps and masses is the primary indication for CTC. However, because of the two-dimensional (2D) cross-sectional imaging ability of CTC, it can also be useful for evaluating lesions deep to the mucosal surface.[1,2] From a clinical standpoint, there are two distinct scenarios in which most submucosal lesions are encountered at CTC: (1) as a new finding at primary CTC evaluation, and (2) as a potential finding referred from OC for further evaluation. CTC and OC provide complementary assessment because some superficial submucosal lesions detected at CTC cannot be clearly differentiated from mucosal-based lesions and require further evaluation with OC, whereas other suspected submucosal lesions detected at OC can be more fully characterized at subsequent CTC. In fact, we have seen a number of referrals from OC for suspected intramural submucosal tumors that simply represent extrinsic impression from extracolonic structures at CTC.

We usually use our standard CTC protocol (see Chapter 29) for most suspected submucosal abnormalities referred from OC. However, intravenous contrast can be valuable for instances where the presence or absence of lesion enhancement may be a critical feature. When confronted with a focal polypoid lesion at CTC interpretation, characteristics that favor a submucosal over a mucosal location include a smooth, broad-based bulge that forms obtuse angles with the surrounding mucosal surface. The most commonly encountered intramural submucosal lesion—the colonic lipoma—is readily and definitively diagnosed at CTC as a result of its characteristic fat attenuation. However, some soft tissue lesions that reside within the superficial submucosal space (i.e.,

Table 22-1 ◻ Submucosal Lesions Involving the Colon and Rectum

NEOPLASTIC CAUSES	NONNEOPLASTIC CAUSES
Intramural Origin	Intramural Origin
Lipoma	Lymphoid polyps and hyperplasia
Carcinoid tumor	Vascular lesions
Lymphoma	Cystic lesions
Hemangioma	Hematoma
GI stromal tumor (GIST)	Pneumatosis cystoides
Other primary tumors	Extramural Origin
Hematogenous metastases	Endometriosis
Extramural Origin	Extrinsic impression
Invasion by extracolonic tumor	Presacral lesion
Peritoneal carcinomatosis	
Appendiceal tumors	

superficial to the muscularis propria) protrude into the lumen and cannot be easily differentiated from mucosal lesions at CTC. The remainder of this chapter will review the imaging findings of specific submucosal entities (Table 22-1), including examples at both OC and routine CT, in addition to CTC. For organizational purposes, submucosal lesions have been categorized according to both histology (neoplastic versus nonneoplastic) and site of origin (intramural versus extramural).

NEOPLASTIC CAUSES OF INTRAMURAL ORIGIN

A wide variety of primary submucosal neoplasms can arise from the large intestinal wall, most of which are benign in nature.[1] Most tumors, such as lipomas, carcinoid tumors, lymphomas, and hemangiomas, originate and remain superficial to the muscularis propria, whereas certain mesenchymal tumors such as gastrointestinal stromal tumors (GIST) arise from the deeper muscularis propria and most often demonstrate an exoenteric growth pattern. Among the various routes of spread to the colon by extracolonic malignancies, only the hematogenous route begins as an intramural process.

Lipoma

The colon is the most common gastrointestinal site for lipomas, which are more often right-sided.[3] At CTC, most lipomas appear as smooth, broad-based lesions (Fig. 22-1). At OC evaluation, lipomas typically have a pale-yellow appearance and are soft upon probing, which is termed the "pillow sign" (Fig. 22-2). However, despite their submucosal origin, they will occasionally evolve into pedunculated lesions (Fig. 22-3), which can serve as a lead point for intussusception (Fig. 22-4). Because some lipomas cannot be confidently diagnosed at OC, such indeterminate lesions may be referred to CTC for more definitive evaluation (Figs. 22-1 and 22-5). Although the 3D endoluminal appearance of lipomas at CTC remains nonspecific, the presence of fat attenua-

tion on 2D CT evaluation with soft tissue windowing is diagnostic. Of note, a lipomatous appearance to the ileocecal valve is extremely common and should not be confused for a colonic lipoma. Unless symptomatic, treatment for colonic lipomas is generally not indicated, even for large lesions (Fig. 22-2).

Carcinoid Tumor

Large intestinal carcinoid tumors are relatively uncommon but are more frequently encountered in the rectum, where they are typically small benign incidental lesions that often have a yellowish appearance at OC evaluation (Fig. 22-6).[4] At CTC and other radiologic imaging studies, smaller carcinoid tumors may be difficult to differentiate from mucosal-based lesions (Fig. 22-7). Lesions of significant size detected at CTC are generally referred to OC for further evaluation. Larger carcinoid tumors can ulcerate and present with lower gastrointestinal (GI) bleeding (Fig. 22-8). Proximal colonic carcinoid tumors tend to be bulkier and more aggressive in behavior than the smaller rectal lesions. Most proximal carcinoid tumors are located in the cecum or proximal ascending colon (Fig. 22-9). Appendiceal carcinoids are relatively common but are rarely symptomatic because most are subcentimeter and involve the distal appendix. Appendiceal carcinoids are rarely detectable at CTC.

Lymphoma

Primary lymphoma of the large intestine is relatively rare compared with gastric or small intestinal involvement. Nearly all cases represent non-Hodgkin's B-cell lymphoma.[5] The ileocecal region is most often involved (Fig. 22-10), followed by the rectosigmoid region. Appendiceal lymphoma is discussed later in this chapter. Patients who are immunocompromised, such as patients with AIDS or solid organ transplants, are at increased risk for extranodal lymphoproliferative disorders (Fig. 22-11). Clinical presentation is often nonspecific but may include

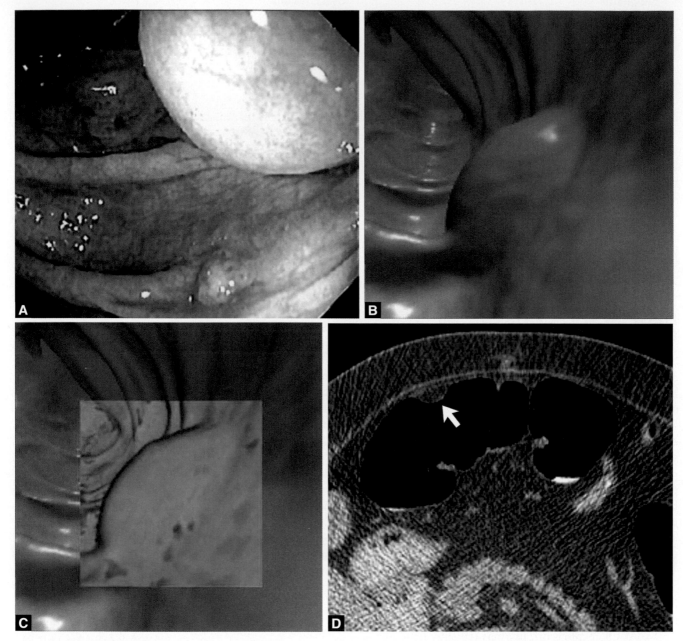

Figure 22-1 Colonic lipoma. OC image **(A)** shows a smooth, broad-based lesion, which was felt to be indeterminate in nature and was referred to CTC for further characterization. 3D endoluminal CTC image **(B)** shows the same submucosal lesion. With translucency rendering **(C)**, the internal green color signature indicates fat attenuation, which is confirmed on the 2D transverse CTC image **(D,** *arrow*).

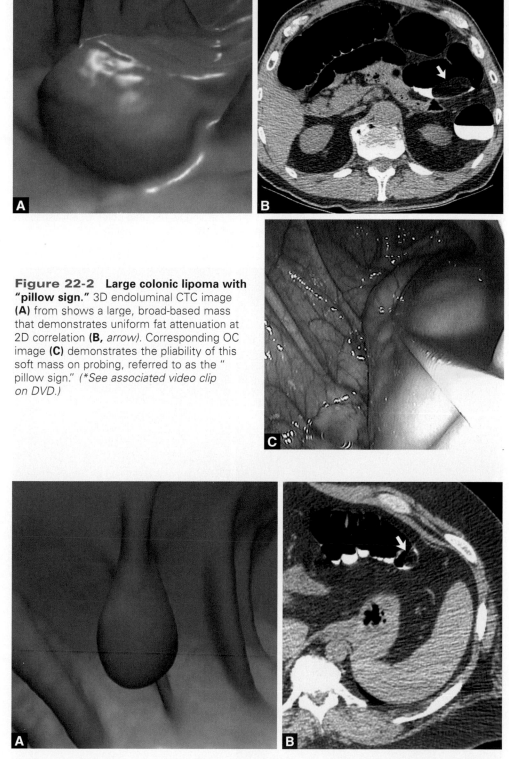

Figure 22-2   Large colonic lipoma with "pillow sign." 3D endoluminal CTC image **(A)** from shows a large, broad-based mass that demonstrates uniform fat attenuation at 2D correlation **(B,** *arrow). Corresponding OC image **(C)** demonstrates the pliability of this soft mass on probing, referred to as the " pillow sign." (*See associated video clip on DVD.)*

Figure 22-3   Pedunculated lipoma. 3D endoluminal CTC image **(A)** shows a smooth pedunculated polypoid lesion that is composed of uniform fat attenuation on the transverse 2D CTC image (**B,** *arrow*), which is diagnostic of a lipoma.

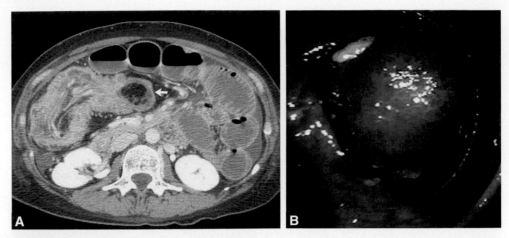

Figure 22-4 Colonic lipoma causing intussusception. Curved reformatted contrast-enhanced CT image **(A)** from a symptomatic patient shows a high-grade bowel obstruction from intussusception caused by a colonic lipoma *(arrow)* acting as a lead point. OC image **(B)** from a second patient shows another colonic lipoma acting as the lead point for intussusception. The usual pale-yellow appearance is absent as a result of mucosal edema and erythema.

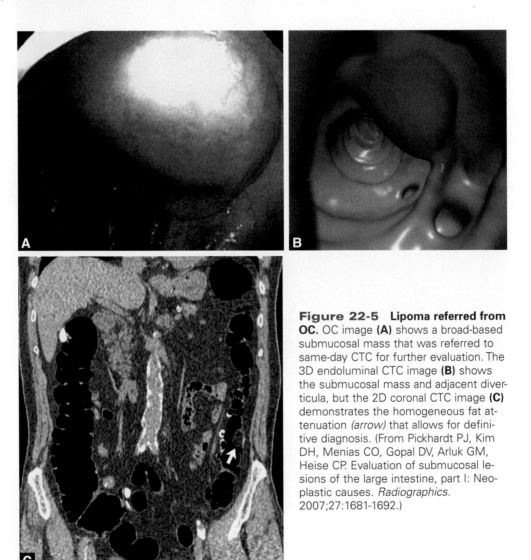

Figure 22-5 Lipoma referred from OC. OC image **(A)** shows a broad-based submucosal mass that was referred to same-day CTC for further evaluation. The 3D endoluminal CTC image **(B)** shows the submucosal mass and adjacent diverticula, but the 2D coronal CTC image **(C)** demonstrates the homogeneous fat attenuation *(arrow)* that allows for definitive diagnosis. (From Pickhardt PJ, Kim DH, Menias CO, Gopal DV, Arluk GM, Heise CP. Evaluation of submucosal lesions of the large intestine, part I: Neoplastic causes. *Radiographics.* 2007;27:1681-1692.)

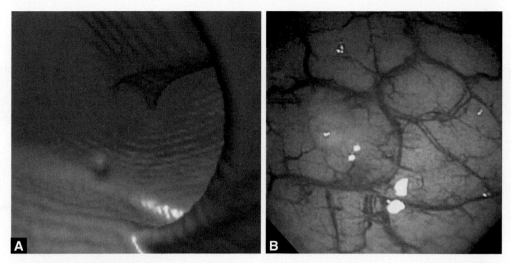

Figure 22-6 **Diminutive rectal carcinoid tumor.** 3D endoluminal CTC image **(A)** shows a nonspecific diminutive polyp in the rectum. Image from corresponding OC **(B),** performed as part of a clinical trial, shows a yellowish appearance to the lesion. The lesion proved to be a tiny carcinoid tumor.

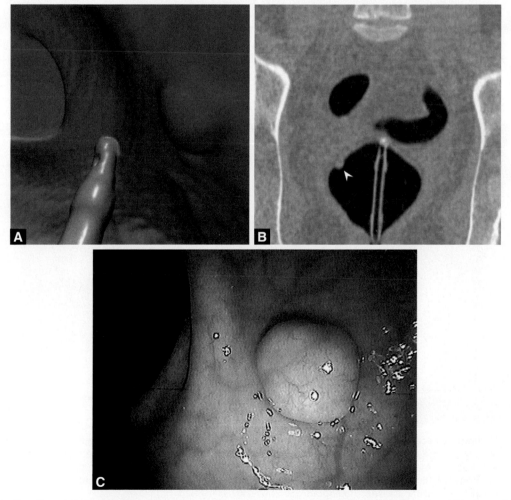

Figure 22-7 **Small rectal carcinoid tumor.** 3D endoluminal CTC image **(A)** shows a 9-mm polypoid lesion within the rectum, which is composed of soft tissue attenuation *(arrowhead)* on the 2D coronal CTC image **(B).** Note the adjacent rectal catheter on both images. This superficial submucosal lesion was resected at same-day OC **(C).** (From Pickhardt PJ, Kim DH, Menias CO, Gopal DV, Arluk GM, Heise CP. Evaluation of submucosal lesions of the large intestine, part I: Neoplastic causes. *Radiographics.* 2007;27:1681-1692.) *(*See associated video clip on DVD.)*

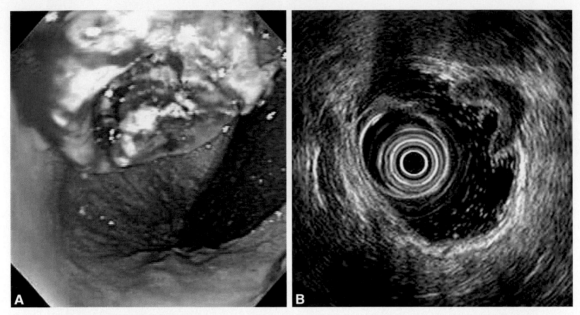

Figure 22-8 Large ulcerated carcinoid tumor. OC image **(A)** shows an ulcerated rectal mass. At TRUS **(B)**, the lesion appears hypoechoic and arises from the submucosal layer of the rectal wall. (From Pickhardt PJ, Kim DH, Menias CO, Gopal DV, Arluk GM, Heise CP. Evaluation of submucosal lesions of the large intestine, part I: Neoplastic causes. *Radiographics.* 2007;27: 1681-1692.)

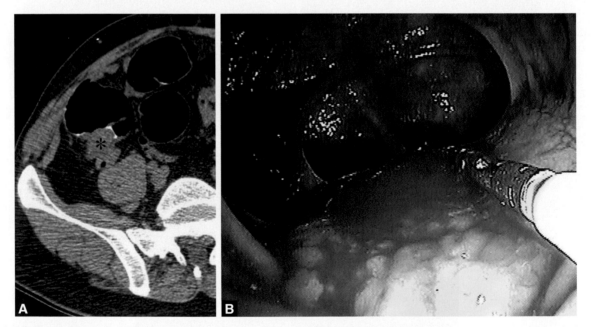

Figure 22-9 Malignant cecal carcinoid tumor. 2D transverse CTC image **(A)** shows an irregular submucosal soft tissue mass *(asterisk)* extending off the cecum. Image from same-day OC **(B)** shows broad-based mass effect on the cecum, which had a rigid appearance. At surgery, a malignant cecal carcinoid tumor was confirmed, with two of seven regional lymph nodes positive for spread of tumor. (From Pickhardt PJ, Kim DH, Menias CO, Gopal DV, Arluk GM, Heise CP. Evaluation of submucosal lesions of the large intestine, part I: Neoplastic causes. *Radiographics.* 2007;27:1681-1692.)

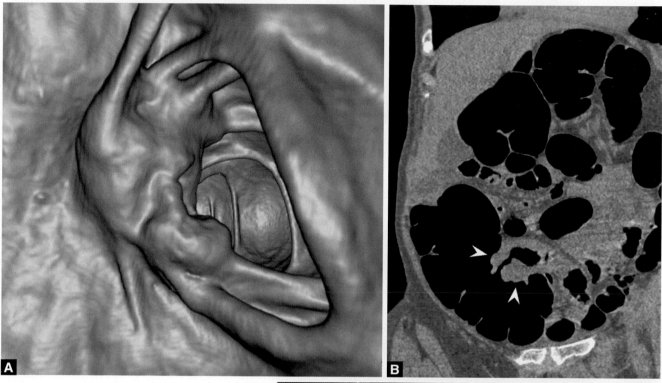

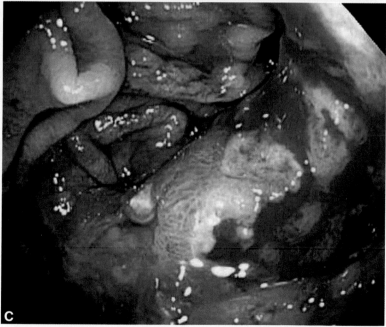

Figure 22-10 Ileocecal lymphoma. 3D endoluminal **(A)** and 2D coronal **(B)** CTC images show marked irregular fold thickening centered at the ileocecal valve *(arrowheads),* with extension into the terminal ileum. Irregular cecal fold thickening was also confirmed at OC **(C),** which provided the tissue diagnosis in this case. The patient responded well to chemotherapy. (From Pickhardt PJ, Kim DH, Menias CO, Gopal DV, Arluk GM, Heise CP. Evaluation of submucosal lesions of the large intestine, part I: Neoplastic causes. *Radiographics.* 2007;27:1681-1692.)

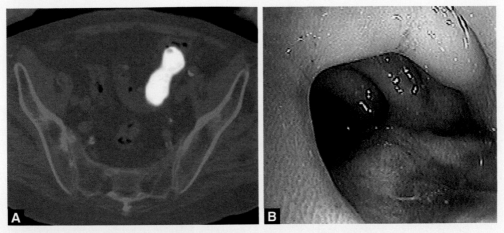

Figure 22-11   Colonic post-transplantation lymphoproliferative disorder (PTLD). Fused image from positron emission tomography (PET)-CT **(A)** in a heart transplant recipient shows intense segmental hypermetabolic activity conforming to the sigmoid colon. Subsequent OC **(B)** revealed a submucosal mass and biopsy suggested a lymphoproliferative process. PTLD was confirmed at laparoscopic sigmoid resection. (From Pickhardt PJ, Kim DH, Menias CO, Gopal DV, Arluk GM, Heise CP. Evaluation of submucosal lesions of the large intestine, part I: Neoplastic causes. *Radiographics.* 2007;27:1681-1692.)

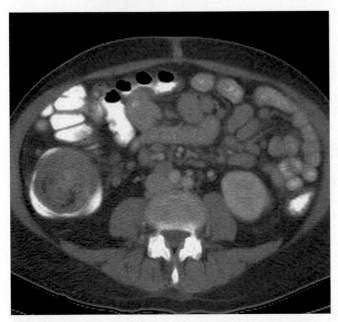

Figure 22-12   Ileocecal lymphoma causing intussusception. Contrast-enhanced CT image shows intussusception from ileocecal lymphoma, which is specifically suggested by the presence of extensive abdominal lymphadenopathy.

GI bleeding; obstruction is rare. Imaging manifestations of colonic lymphoma include solitary or multifocal polypoid or bulky masses, annular lesions, ulcerating masses, and long-segment nodular wall thickening. Polypoid lesions may predispose to intussusception (Fig. 22-12). Associated abdominal lymphadenopathy may be seen (see Fig. 22-12) but is often absent. Treatment usually consists of surgical resection, followed by adjuvant chemotherapy. For some cases of post-transplantation lymphoproliferative disorder (PTLD), reducing or withholding immunosuppression alone may be curative.[6,7]

Hemangioma

Colorectal cavernous hemangiomas are rare benign vascular neoplasms that most often involve the rectosigmoid region (Fig. 22-13). Hemangiomas may be seen as a solitary isolated finding or associated with an underlying condition, such as Klippel-Trénaunay-Weber syndrome, in which extensive disease may be present (i.e., hemangiomatosis). Rectal bleeding is the most common clinical manifestation.[8] At OC, cavernous hemangiomas manifest as a nonspecific submucosal mass or with a plum-red appearance from vascular congestion (Fig. 22-13). The presence of phleboliths at CT or other radiologic imaging test is highly suggestive or even diagnostic (Fig. 22-13).

Gastrointestinal Stromal Tumor

Gastrointestinal stromal tumors (GIST) represent the most common solid mesenchymal neoplasm of the GI tract and are distinct from smooth muscle and neural tumors. This unique tumor expresses the protein KIT (CD117) and is believed to derive from the interstitial cells of Cajal (gut pacemaker cells). GISTs typically arise in the muscularis propria layer and most commonly involve the stomach, followed by the small intestine, anorectum, colon, and esophagus, respectively. As with gastric and small intestinal lesions, colorectal GISTs tend to exhibit exoenteric growth and less commonly demonstrate a prominent intraluminal component.[9] Therefore, despite a relatively large size, these tumors may be subtle on luminal examinations such as OC, often demonstrating only a nonspecific broad-based impression that may be difficult to distinguish from an extrinsic structure (Figs. 22-14 and 22-15). These bulky tumors, however, are generally obvious at cross-sectional imaging studies such as CTC. Prominent enhancement of the tumor is usually apparent if intravenous (IV) contrast has been administered. Metastatic

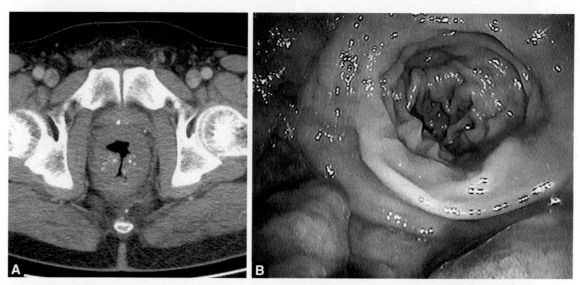

Figure 22-13 **Rectal hemangiomatosis in Klippel-Trénaunay-Weber syndrome.** Contrast-enhanced CT image **(A)** shows circumferential rectal wall thickening associated with multiple phleboliths, consistent with rectal hemangiomatosis. At OC **(B)** the purplish hue of the lesion seen peripherally stands out from the normal appearance of the more proximal rectosigmoid. MR angiography showed asymmetric involvement of the lower extremities by vascular malformations (not shown), which is typical for this syndrome. (From Pickhardt PJ, Kim DH, Menias CO, Gopal DV, Arluk GM, Heise CP. Evaluation of submucosal lesions of the large intestine, part I: Neoplastic causes. *Radiographics.* 2007;27:1681-1692.)

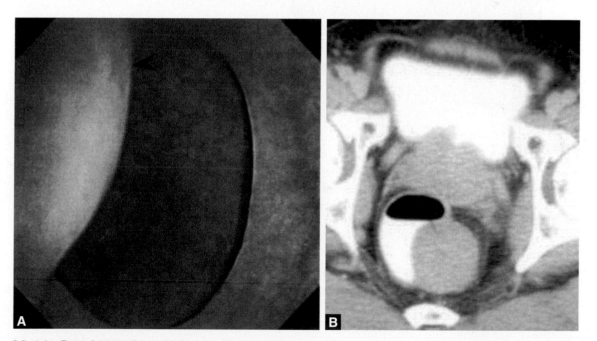

Figure 22-14 **Rectal gastrointestinal stromal tumor.** OC image **(A)** from a patient who presented with rectal bleeding shows a broad-based submucosal impression or mass within the rectum *(arrowheads)*. At CT **(B),** a solid rounded rectal mass demonstrating an exoenteric growth pattern is apparent. (From Pickhardt PJ, Kim DH, Menias CO, Gopal DV, Arluk GM, Heise CP. Evaluation of submucosal lesions of the large intestine, part I: Neoplastic causes. *Radiographics.* 2007;27:1681-1692.)

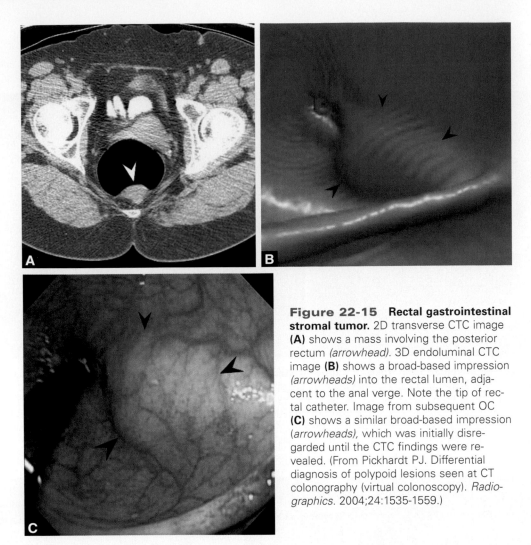

Figure 22-15 Rectal gastrointestinal stromal tumor. 2D transverse CTC image **(A)** shows a mass involving the posterior rectum *(arrowhead)*. 3D endoluminal CTC image **(B)** shows a broad-based impression *(arrowheads)* into the rectal lumen, adjacent to the anal verge. Note the tip of rectal catheter. Image from subsequent OC **(C)** shows a similar broad-based impression *(arrowheads)*, which was initially disregarded until the CTC findings were revealed. (From Pickhardt PJ. Differential diagnosis of polypoid lesions seen at CT colonography (virtual colonoscopy). *Radiographics.* 2004;24:1535-1559.)

spread to the liver and peritoneal cavity is typical of malignant GIST.

Other Primary Tumors

A variety of other submucosal primary colorectal neoplasms rarely can be seen at CTC.[1] Soft tissue mesenchymal tumors other than GIST include benign lesions such as leiomyoma and schwannoma, which may present as nonspecific polypoid lesions at imaging (Fig. 22-16). CTC may demonstrate an exoenteric component in some cases, which may be difficult to identify at OC (Fig. 22-16). Frankly malignant mesenchymal tumors arising from the colon such as leiomyosarcoma are extremely rare but are often large and ulcerative at presentation (Fig. 22-17). Other rare submucosal tumors include ganglioneuromas (Fig. 22-18) and granular cell tumors, which both tend to present as nonspecific polypoid lesions arising in the superficial submucosal space.

Hematogenous Metastases

Unlike secondary colonic involvement from peritoneal carcinomatosis or direct tumor invasion, hematogenous metastases begin as an intramural process, superficial to the muscularis propria. Melanoma is the most common primary tumor resulting in intestinal hematogenous spread, followed by lung cancer and breast cancer.[10] The lesions typically appear as well-defined submucosal nodules or masses, with or without central ulceration (Figs. 22-19 and 22-20). The colon and rectum are affected much less frequently than the small intestine.

NEOPLASTIC CAUSES OF EXTRAMURAL ORIGIN

Secondary involvement from an extracolonic tumor may be difficult to distinguish from normal extrinsic impression or a primary intramural lesion at OC, which is a purely luminal investigation. For extramural processes in particular, cross-sectional imaging studies such as CTC can be indispensable for evaluating the entire extent of disease. This section considers direct invasion by extracolonic malignancy; colonic involvement from peritoneal carcinomatosis; and appendiceal neoplasms, which represent a special subset of extramural neoplastic disease.

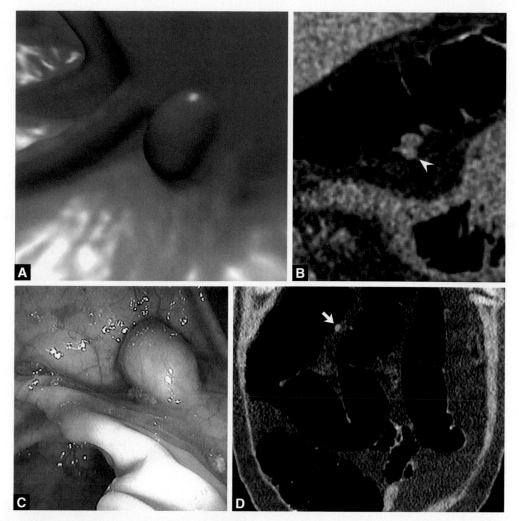

Figure 22-16   Colonic leiomyoma. 3D endoluminal CTC image **(A)** shows a 1.3-cm polypoid lesion in the transverse colon. The corresponding 2D coronal CTC image **(B)** not only confirms the soft tissue nature of the lesion, but also reveals a small lobule of exoenteric extension *(arrowhead)*, which would be highly atypical for a mucosal-based lesion. The intraluminal component was resected at subsequent OC **(C)** and proved to be a leiomyoma. The extraluminal component, which was not appreciated at OC, was still present at followup CTC evaluation two years later **(D,** *arrow). (*See associated video clip on DVD.)*

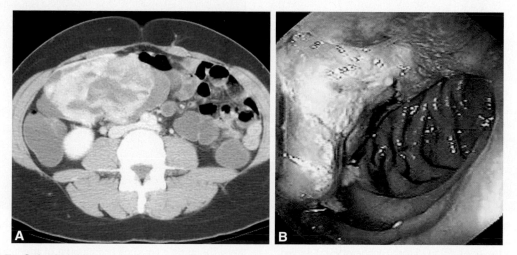

Figure 22-17   Colonic leiomyosarcoma. Contrast-enhanced CT **(A)** and OC **(B)** images from two different patients show large heterogeneous masses, which are predominantly exoenteric at CT and ulcerated at endoscopy. Both masses proved to be colonic leiomyosarcomas, which are rare.

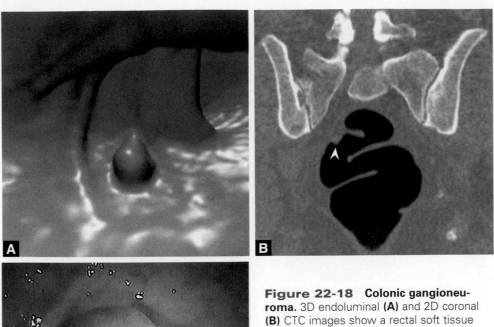

Figure 22-18 **Colonic gangioneuroma.** 3D endoluminal **(A)** and 2D coronal **(B)** CTC images show a rectal soft tissue polyp *(arrowhead)* that was confirmed at subsequent OC **(C)** and proved to be a submucosal ganglioneuroma at histologic evaluation. Determination of submucosal origin is not always possible based on imaging findings alone. (From Pickhardt PJ, Kim DH, Menias CO, Gopal DV, Arluk GM, Heise CP. Evaluation of submucosal lesions of the large intestine, part I: Neoplastic causes. Radiographics. 2007;27:1681-1692.)

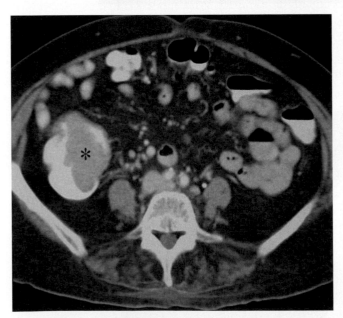

Figure 22-19 **Hematogenous metastasis (melanoma).** Contrast-enhanced CT image shows a large soft tissue metastasis *(asterisk)* in the right colon. (From Pickhardt PJ, Kim DH, Menias CO, Gopal DV, Arluk GM, Heise CP. Evaluation of submucosal lesions of the large intestine, part I: Neoplastic causes. Radiographics. 2007;27:1681-1692.)

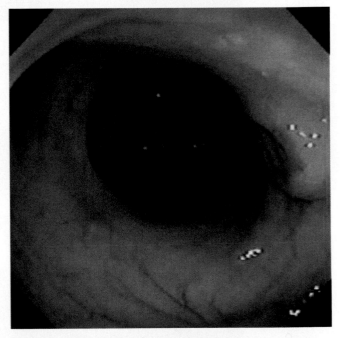

Figure 22-20 **Hematogenous metastasis (lung cancer).** OC image shows a small ulcerated submucosal lesion from metastatic small cell carcinoma of the lung.

Direct Invasion by Extracolonic Malignancy

Contiguous involvement of the colon or rectum by an extracolonic tumor can occur along connecting ligaments, which act as paths of least resistance, or simply as a result of direct spread from adjacent disease in close proximity. Clinical history often provides a clue to the diagnosis. The prototypical example of ligamentous spread is extension of gastric adenocarcinoma to the transverse colon via the gastrocolic ligament (Fig. 22-21). Similarly, adenocarcinoma of the transverse colon can spread to the greater curve of the stomach. At OC evaluation, extensive mural invasion from an extracolonic malignancy can manifest as luminal narrowing, irregular fold thickening, or ulceration (Figs. 22-21 and 22-22). Cross-sectional imaging, particularly CT, is effective for evaluating the entire extent of disease.

Peritoneal Carcinomatosis

Once malignant cells gain access to the peritoneal cavity, relatively unrestricted spread of tumor throughout this large potential space gives rise to peritoneal carcinomatosis. Nearly any malignancy has the potential to metastasize to the subperitoneal or peritoneal space, but GI and ovarian primaries are seen most frequently.[11] Serosal implants can involve and invade any portion of the large bowel that contacts the peritoneal space (Fig. 22-23). Because of anatomic considerations and peritoneal flow dynamics, the rectosigmoid and transverse colon are most frequently involved. The submucosal abnormalities seen at endoluminal

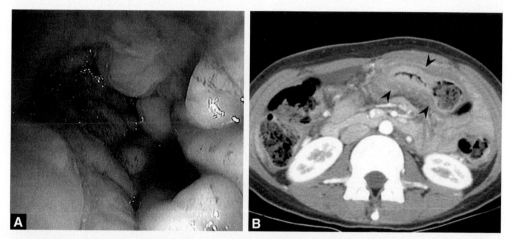

Figure 22-21 **Colonic extension of gastric adenocarcinoma via gastrocolic ligament.** OC image **(A)** shows fixed luminal narrowing and irregular fold thickening of the transverse colon. Contrast-enhanced CT image **(B)** show extensive soft tissue wall thickening of the transverse colon *(arrowheads),* which could be tracked up the gastrocolic ligament to the greater curvature of the stomach (not shown).

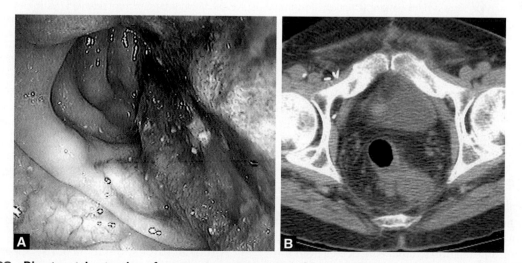

Figure 22-22 **Direct rectal extension of recurrent prostate cancer.** OC image **(A)** from a patient presenting with rectal bleeding shows a large ulcerated rectal mass. TRUS (not shown) demonstrated perirectal lymphadenopathy from this presumed primary rectal adenocarcinoma. Contrast-enhanced CT image **(B)** shows a predominately perirectal mass, atypical for primary rectal adenocarcinoma. Of note, this patient had been previously treated for prostate cancer. Final pathology after low anterior resection revealed metastatic adenocarcinoma of the prostate with rectal invasion. (From Pickhardt PJ, Kim DH, Menias CO, Gopal DV, Arluk GM, Heise CP. Evaluation of submucosal lesions of the large intestine, part I: Neoplastic causes. Radiographics. 2007;27:1681-1692.)

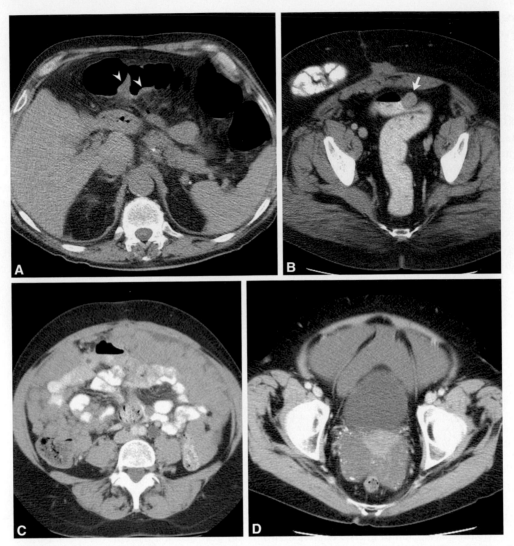

Figure 22-23   Peritoneal carcinomatosis. 2D transverse CTC image **(A)** in a patient with metastatic transitional cell carcinoma shows colonic wall thickening *(arrowheads)* and pericolonic stranding from peritoneal spread of tumor. CT image from a second patient **(B)** shows a rounded metastatic serosal implant *(arrow)* from ovarian cancer. A bowel-containing abdominal wall hernia is incidentally noted. CT image from a third patient **(C)** shows extensive peritoneal carcinomatosis from adenoid cystic carcinoma of the parotid gland, consisting of innumerable peritoneal-based soft tissue masses predominately involving the omentum. Mass effect on small and large bowel is present. CT image from a fourth patient **(D)** shows peritoneal fluid and calcification from an appendiceal mucinous cystadenocarcinoma (pseudomyxoma peritonei). (B and C from Pickhardt PJ, Kim DH, Menias CO, Gopal DV, Arluk GM, Heise CP. Evaluation of submucosal lesions of the large intestine, part I: Neoplastic causes. *Radiographics.* 2007;27:1681-1692.)

evaluation may result from soft tissue implants, loculated malignant ascites, or both (Fig. 22-23). Unlike strictly luminal examinations, CTC has the ability to detect peritoneal implants distant from the colon (Fig. 22-24).

Appendiceal Tumors

Appendiceal neoplasms represent a unique subset of submucosal tumors. Because of the constant anatomic relationship between the appendix and cecum, tumor location is an important diagnostic clue. Mucoceles from mucinous cystic neoplasms represent the most common appendiceal tumor, giving rise to a submucosal abnormality at imaging evaluation (Figs. 22-25 and 22-26). Occasionally, mucoceles will lead to symptomatic presentation

from intussusception, superinfection, or torsion (Fig. 22-27).[12-14] Because luminal-only evaluation visualizes only the "tip of the iceberg," cross-sectional imaging is critical for confirming the presence of an appendiceal neoplasm and providing comprehensive preoperative evaluation (Figs. 22-25 and 22-26). Complex mucoceles with an irregular soft tissue component are concerning for mucinous cystadenocarcinoma (Fig. 22-28A), which may give rise to pseudomyxoma peritonei if there is transgression of the appendiceal wall (Fig. 22-28B).

Although carcinoid tumors of the appendix are more common than mucinous cystic neoplasms, they are typically small and more often involve the distal appendix; therefore, these lesions only rarely give rise to an identifiable colonic submucosal abnormality. Other rare pri-

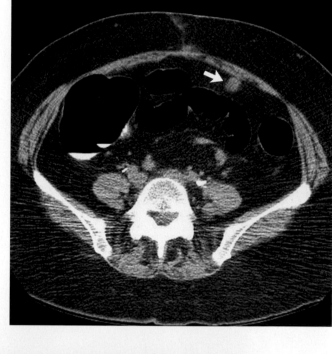

Figure 22-24 Peritoneal implant from unsuspected metastatic endometrial cancer. 2D transverse CTC image from a routine screening examination shows an omental soft tissue nodule *(arrow)*, which proved to be metastatic endometrial cancer. The patient had previously undergone hysterectomy for Stage I endometrial cancer that was presumed to be cured.

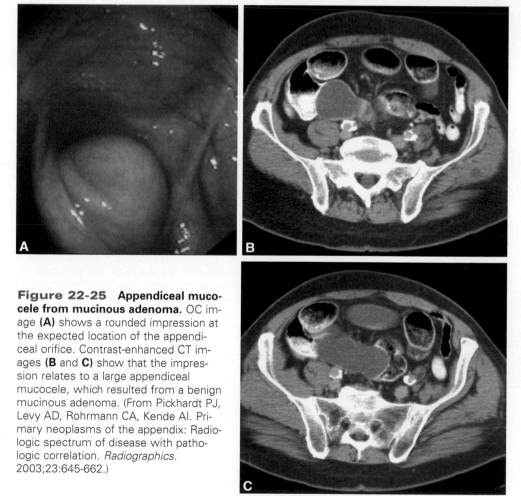

Figure 22-25 Appendiceal mucocele from mucinous adenoma. OC image **(A)** shows a rounded impression at the expected location of the appendiceal orifice. Contrast-enhanced CT images **(B** and **C)** show that the impression relates to a large appendiceal mucocele, which resulted from a benign mucinous adenoma. (From Pickhardt PJ, Levy AD, Rohrmann CA, Kende AI. Primary neoplasms of the appendix: Radiologic spectrum of disease with pathologic correlation. *Radiographics.* 2003;23:645-662.)

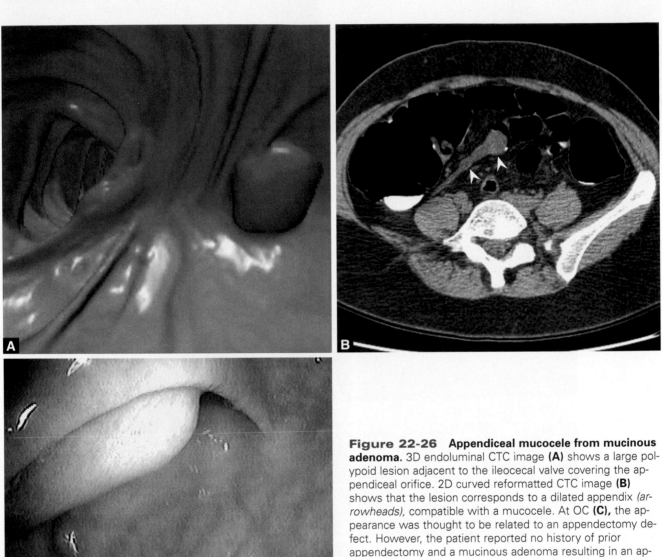

Figure 22-26 Appendiceal mucocele from mucinous adenoma. 3D endoluminal CTC image **(A)** shows a large polypoid lesion adjacent to the ileocecal valve covering the appendiceal orifice. 2D curved reformatted CTC image **(B)** shows that the lesion corresponds to a dilated appendix *(arrowheads)*, compatible with a mucocele. At OC **(C)**, the appearance was thought to be related to an appendectomy defect. However, the patient reported no history of prior appendectomy and a mucinous adenoma resulting in an appendiceal mucocele was confirmed at surgery. *(*See associated video clip on DVD.)*

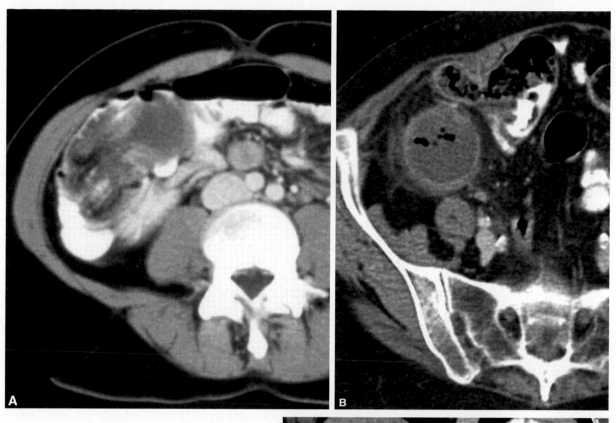

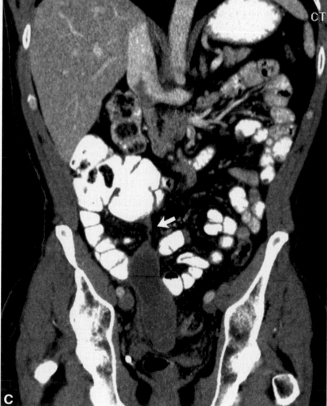

Figure 22-27 Symptomatic presentation of appendiceal mucoceles. CT image **(A)** shows an appendiceal mucocele causing intussusception. CT image from a second patient **(B)** shows an infected mucocele with internal gas bubbles and surrounding inflammatory changes. Curved reformatted CT image from a third patient **(C)** shows acute torsion of a mucocele about its base *(arrow)*. (C from Hebert JJ, Pickhardt PJ. MDCT diagnosis of an appendiceal mucocele with acute torsion. *Am J Roentgenol.* 2007;189:W4-6.)

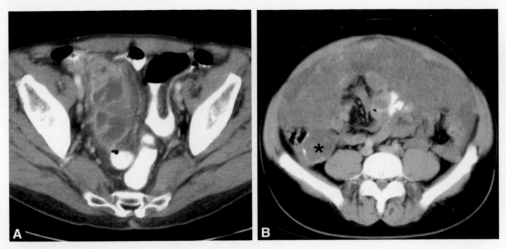

Figure 22-28 **Appendiceal mucinous adenocarcinoma.** Contrast-enhanced CT image **(A)** shows a complex cystic and solid mass in the right lower quadrant, which proved to be a malignant mucocele from mucinous adenocarcinoma. CT image from a second patient **(B)** shows a mucocele with rim calcification *(asterisk)*. The extensive peritoneal-based abnormalities represent metastatic disease (pseudomyxoma peritonei).

mary appendiceal neoplasms include colonic-type adenocarcinoma (Fig. 22-29), lymphoma (Fig. 22-30), and goblet cell carcinoid tumor, any of which may give rise to a luminal abnormality and/or obstructive symptoms if the base of the appendix is involved.[12,13,15]

NONNEOPLASTIC CAUSES OF INTRAMURAL ORIGIN

The nonneoplastic submucosal entities of intramural origin are a heterogeneous group of unrelated conditions that arise within the wall of the large intestine, deep to the mucosa, and may give rise to a focal submucosal abnormality at CTC or OC.[2]

Lymphoid Polyps and Hyperplasia

Benign lymphoid polyps are occasionally seen on endoluminal examination of the large intestine. Most lesions are diminutive in size and are sometimes categorized pathologically as mucosal tags with prominent lymphoid aggregates.[16] Some lymphoid polyps, however, can grow large enough to simulate significant mucosal pathology and rarely may even become pedunculated (Figs. 22-31 and 22-32).[2] The presence of small multifocal lymphoid polyps is referred to as nodular lymphoid hyperplasia and is more commonly seen in children (Fig. 22-33). Rarely, prominent cases may simulate lymphomatous polyposis.

Vascular Lesions

Nonneoplastic vascular lesions that may give rise to focal submucosal abnormalities include internal hemorrhoids, rectal varices, and venous malformations. At

OC, these vascular entities have characteristic appearances that preclude the need for biopsy, but not all lesions can be fully characterized at CTC. Internal hemorrhoids are a common incidental finding; complications include bleeding, thrombosis, and prolapse. At CTC, the specific anorectal location and often circumferential or hemi-circumferential appearance can usually distinguish internal hemorrhoids from a mucosal mass (Fig. 22-34), but correlation with physical examination is sometimes helpful (Fig. 22-35). Thrombosed hemorrhoids will generally demonstrate less effacement and less change between supine and prone positioning. Rectal varices are associated with portal hypertension, whereas hemorrhoids generally are not, and findings of cirrhosis and portal hypertension may be apparent at CT (Fig. 22-36). Distinguishing an isolated rectal varix from a rectal fold or normal funneling can be difficult on 2D evaluation (Fig. 22-37), but the tortuous and tubular morphology is generally apparent at 3D CTC (Fig. 22-38).

Small venous malformations or vascular "blebs" are associated with the rare blue rubber bleb nevus syndrome but are more commonly seen as an isolated finding at CTC and OC. Although the characteristic bluish hue is diagnostic at OC, these lesions demonstrate soft tissue attenuation at noncontrast CTC, thus mimicking mucosal-based polyps (Fig. 22-39).[17] In our experience, these lesions are often multiple, have a tendency to involve the transverse colon, and are almost always subcentimeter in size. Unnecessary OC related to subcentimeter vascular blebs detected at CTC represent yet another reason why a 10-mm referral threshold would be more a cost-effective, and clinically effective, CTC screening strategy.

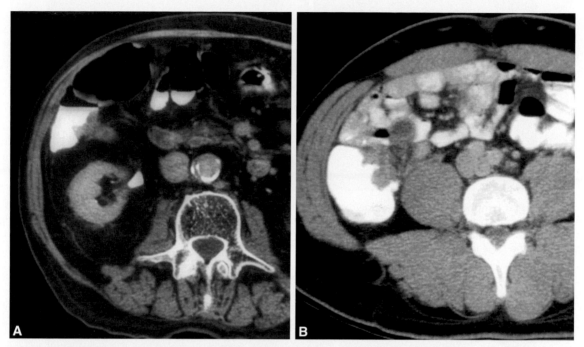

Figure 22-29 **Colonic-type adenocarcinoma of the appendix.** CT image **(A)** shows an appendiceal soft tissue mass with protrusion into the cecal lumen. CT image from a second patient **(B)** shows an appendiceal tumor with a similar appearance. Both proved to be colonic-type adenocarcinomas. (A from Pickhardt PJ, Levy AD, Rohrmann CA, Kende AI. Primary neoplasms of the appendix: Radiologic spectrum of disease with pathologic correlation. *Radiographics.* 2003;23:645-662.) (B from Pickhardt PJ, Levy AD, Rohrmann CA, Kende AI. Primary neoplasms of the appendix manifesting as acute appendicitis: CT findings with pathologic correlation. *Radiology.* 2002;224:775-781.)

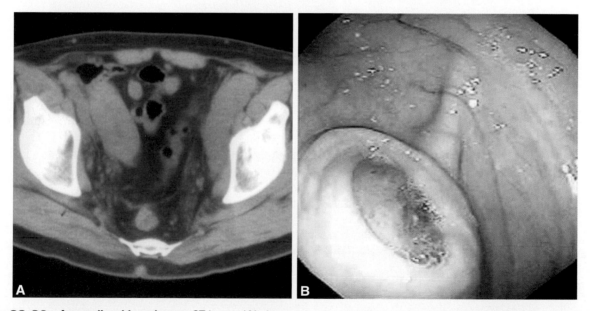

Figure 22-30 **Appendiceal lymphoma.** CT image **(A)** shows massive vermiform enlargement of the appendix with circumferential wall thickening but no mucocele formation. The appearance is typical of appendiceal lymphoma. OC image from a second patient **(B)** shows bulbous enlargement at the appendiceal base with abnormal mucosa protruding from the orifice. As with *A,* the entire appendix was enlarged by lymphoma. (A from Pickhardt PJ, Levy AD, Rohrmann CA, Abbondanzo SL, Kende AI. Non-Hodgkin lymphoma of the appendix: Clinical and CT findings with pathologic correlation. *Am J Roentgenol.* 2002;178:1123-1127.)

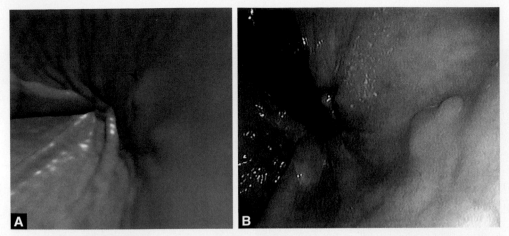

Figure 22-31 Flat lymphoid polyp. 3D endoluminal CTC image **(A)** shows a subtle, flat 8-mm lesion *(arrowheads)* located in the low rectum. Note the adjacent rectal catheter. Image from same-day OC **(B)** shows the lesion before snare cautery. Histologic evaluation revealed a lymphoid polyp. (From Pickhardt PJ, Kim DH, Menias CO, Gopal DV, Arluk GM, Heise CP. Evaluation of submucosal lesions of the large intestine, part II: Non-neoplastic causes. *Radiographics.* 2007;27:1693-1703.)

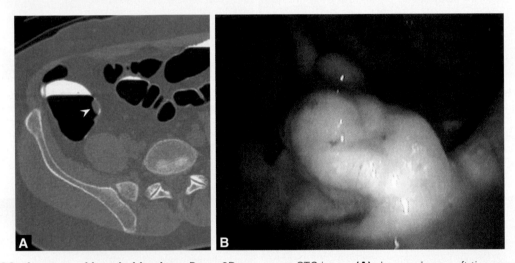

Figure 22-32 Large cecal lymphoid polyps. Prone 2D transverse CTC image **(A)** shows a large soft tissue polyp *(arrowhead)* within the cecum. Three lesions within close proximity measuring up to 1.5 cm were detected at CTC, all of which were confirmed at same-day OC **(B)** and proved to be lymphoid polyps. (From Pickhardt PJ, Kim DH, Menias CO, Gopal DV, Arluk GM, Heise CP. Evaluation of submucosal lesions of the large intestine, part II: Non-neoplastic causes. *Radiographics.* 2007;27:1693-1703.)

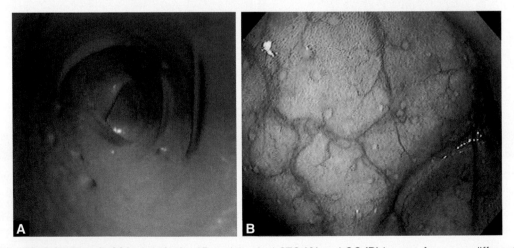

Figure 22-33 Nodular lymphoid hyperplasia. 3D endoluminal CTC **(A)** and OC **(B)** images from two different patients show multiple diminutive polypoid lesions representing nodular lymphoid hyperplasia. The nodules are particularly well seen at OC as a result of mild (pseudo)melanosis involving the background mucosa.

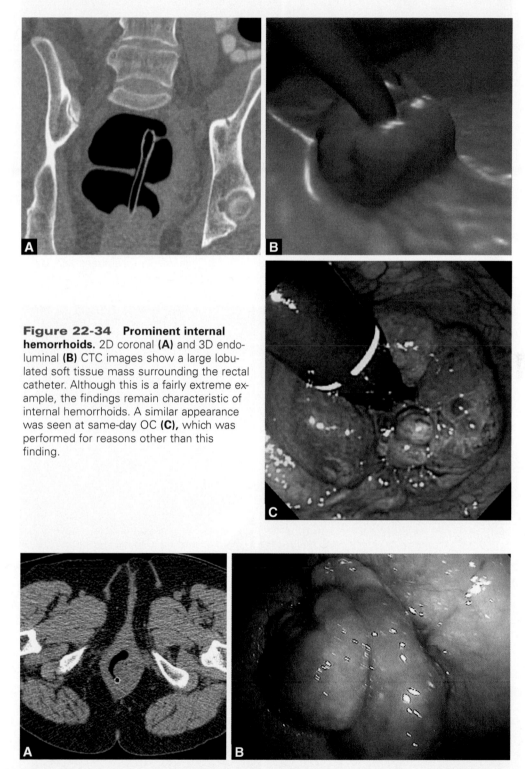

Figure 22-34   Prominent internal hemorrhoids. 2D coronal **(A)** and 3D endoluminal **(B)** CTC images show a large lobulated soft tissue mass surrounding the rectal catheter. Although this is a fairly extreme example, the findings remain characteristic of internal hemorrhoids. A similar appearance was seen at same-day OC **(C)**, which was performed for reasons other than this finding.

Figure 22-35   Hemorrhoids with prolapse at physical examination. 2D transverse CTC image **(A)** shows a large soft tissue lesion adjacent to and partially surrounding the rectal catheter. Image from subsequent OC **(B)** shows rectal prolapse of the hemorrhoids.

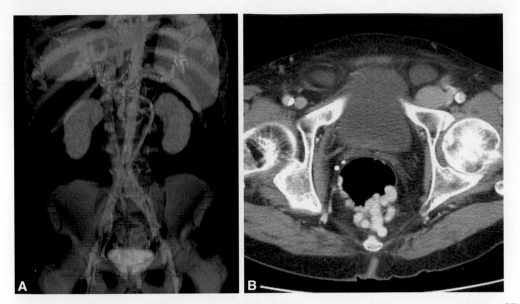

Figure 22-36 Rectal varices associated with portal hypertension. Coronal maximum intensity projection CT image **(A)** from a patient with cirrhosis and portal hypertension shows a nodular shrunken liver, splenomegaly, and dilated portomesenteric venous system. Prominent hemorrhoidal varices are associated with the large inferior mesenteric vein. Contrast-enhanced CT **(B)** from a different patient with portal hypertension shows multiple enhancing rectal varices.

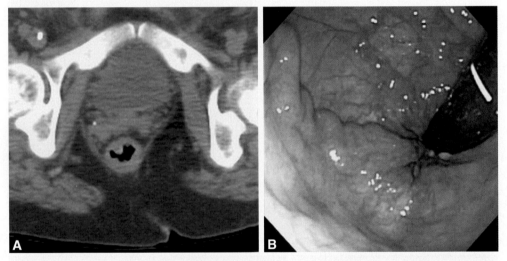

Figure 22-37 Rectal varix associated with portal hypertension. CT image **(A)** from a patient with portal hypertension from cirrhosis shows a prominent rectal varix which was also seen at OC **(B)**.

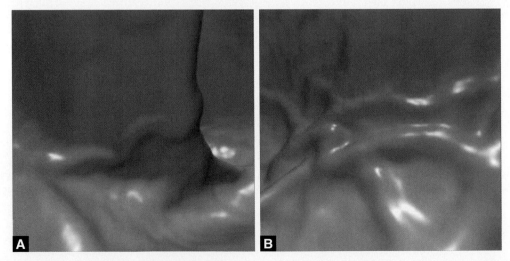

Figure 22-38 Rectal varices at 3D endoluminal CTC. 3D endoluminal CTC images **(A and B)** from two different patients show the typical appearance of a single prominent vein **(A)** and multiple submucosal veins **(B)**.

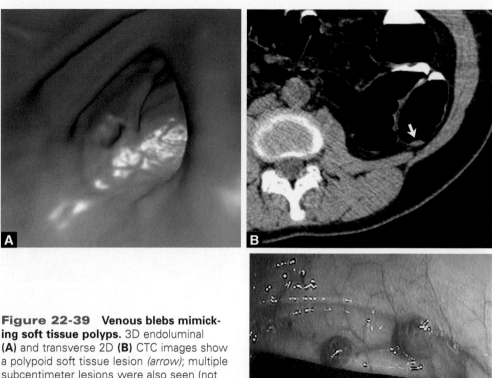

Figure 22-39 Venous blebs mimicking soft tissue polyps. 3D endoluminal **(A)** and transverse 2D **(B)** CTC images show a polypoid soft tissue lesion *(arrow)*; multiple subcentimeter lesions were also seen (not shown). At OC **(C),** all of the lesions corresponded to vascular blebs.

Cystic Lesions

Nonneoplastic cystic lesions arising from the colonic or rectal wall include duplication cysts, lymphangiomas, and colitis cystica profunda.[2] Cross-sectional imaging studies such as CTC, MR, and TRUS can demonstrate the cystic nature of these lesions. Enteric duplication cysts are uncommon congenital abnormalities that can occur anywhere along the GI tract. Large intestinal duplication cysts are rare but are most often seen in the rectum. Associated symptoms depend on the specific location but can include GI bleeding, pain, palpable mass, obstruction, and constipation. As with GISTs, these lesions tend to occupy a largely exoenteric location. Demonstration of mural layers to the cyst wall on US can be a highly suggestive feature. Cystic lymphangiomas of the colon are rare benign lesions that appear as well-defined cystic submucosal lesions, which are often pliable with compression at OC (Fig. 22-40). Internal septations may be apparent at cross-sectional imaging.[18] Colitis cystica profunda is a rare and poorly understood condition that shares some clinical features with the polypoid variant of solitary rectal ulcer syndrome, which is also poorly understood.[19] This chronic benign disorder is characterized by dilated mucin-filled submucosal rectal cysts (Fig. 22-41). Care must be taken to avoid misdiagnosis with other more common anorectal diseases.

Intramural Hematoma

Colonic intramural hematomas can be iatrogenic in nature (e.g., from colonoscopic polypectomy), related to other trauma, or represent a complication of an underlying condition such as a vasculitis or bleeding diathesis (Fig. 22-42).[20-22] A localized submucosal hematoma can act as a lead point for intussusception (Fig. 22-43). Surgical intervention may be required in some symptomatic cases of intramural hematoma.

Pneumatosis Cystoides

The presence of cystic or linear gas collections within the bowel wall is termed *pneumatosis* and can be submucosal or subscrosal in location. The two most important tasks in the evaluation of pneumatosis coli are (1) recognition of the entity and (2) differentiation of the benign form, for which no intervention is indicated, from the potentially life-threatening form.[23,24] Primary *pneumatosis cystoides coli* is a benign condition that favors the left colon. Unlike secondary pneumatosis, which tends to have a more linear appearance, the primary form typically manifests as a striking cluster of air-filled cysts involving the colon wall. At endoluminal evaluation such as OC or 3D CTC, the appearance can simulate

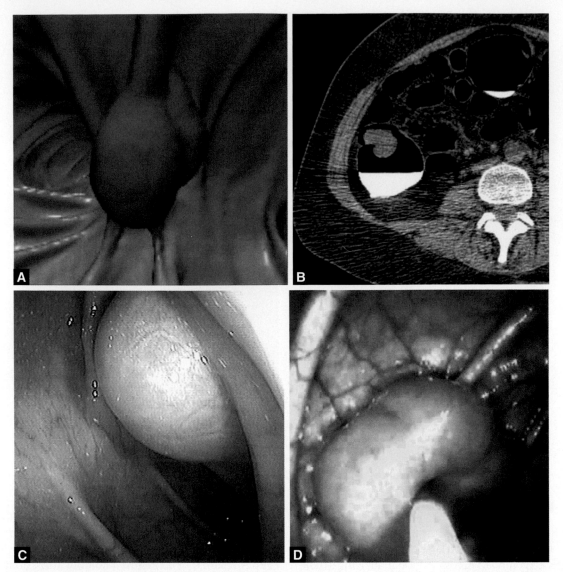

Figure 22-40 **Cystic lymphangiomas.** 3D endoluminal **(A)** and 2D transverse **(B)** CTC images show a lobulated cystic mass in the ascending colon. A tense-appearing bluish submucosal lesion was found at OC **(C)**. OC image from a second patient **(D)** shows the pliable nature of a cystic lymphangioma.

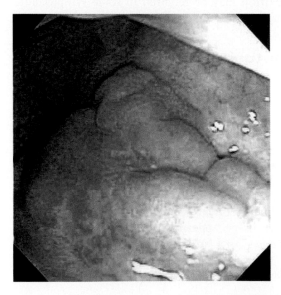

Figure 22-41 **Colitis cystica profunda.** OC image shows a smooth, lobulated submucosal abnormality within the rectum from colitis cystica profunda. (From Pickhardt PJ, Kim DH, Menias CO, Gopal DV, Arluk GM, Heise CP. Evaluation of submucosal lesions of the large intestine, part II: Nonneoplastic causes. *Radiographics.* 2007;27:1693-1703.)

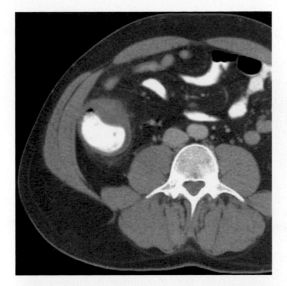

Figure 22-42 Postpolypectomy hematoma. Contrast-enhanced CT image from a patient admitted for a postpolypectomy syndrome following OC shows a submucosal hematoma at the biopsy site. (From Kim DH, Pickhardt PJ, Taylor AJ, Menias CO. Imaging evaluation of complications at optical colonoscopy. *Curr Probl Diagn Radiol.* 2008;37(4):165-177.)

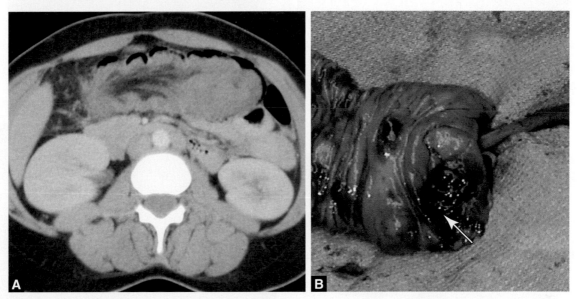

Figure 22-43 Cecal hematoma causing intussusception. CT image **(A)** shows colonic intussusception, which at surgery **(B)** proved to be from a cecal hematoma *(arrow)* related to cocaine use.

polyposis (Fig. 22-44). However, the diagnosis is clear from the internal air density at 2D CTC imaging (Fig. 22-45). The diagnosis can also be confirmed at OC by eliciting a release of gas with cyst puncture. Although the linear appearance of secondary pneumatosis is most concerning for ischemia (Fig. 22-46), this finding is nonspecific because it can also be seen as an innocuous imaging finding. Therefore, correlation with the presence of symptoms and the clinical setting is paramount in avoiding mismanagement of the patient.

In our experience, linear pneumatosis is a rare finding that can be encountered at CTC screening with carbon dioxide distention as an asymptomatic self-limited entity that has no apparent clinical significance (Fig. 22-47).[25] We have seen this finding at CTC with a frequency of about 1 case per 1000 screened. The right colon has been involved in all cases, and all patients remained asymptomatic. Because none of the patients required any treatment or intervention, this imaging finding should not be confused with frank colonic perforation. The precise etiology for asymptomatic pneumatosis at CTC is uncertain but likely multifactorial. Factors that could conceivably be involved to varying degrees include issues of mucosal permeability and defects, intraluminal pressure and colonic wall tension, cathartic preparation, and even bacterial flora. It is likely that asymptomatic pneumatosis at other colorectal examinations such as OC is under-recognized because there would be no clinical indication for pursuing CT imaging (see Chapter 15).

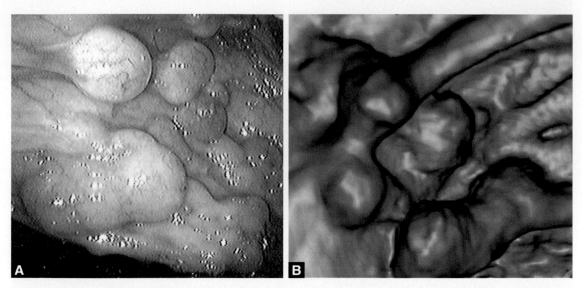

Figure 22-44 **Pneumatosis cystoides coli.** OC image **(A)** shows multiple polypoid lesions that were confirmed to represent pneumatosis at subsequent CT (not shown). 3D endoluminal CTC image from a second patient **(B)** shows a similar appearance from cystic pneumatosis. (From Pickhardt PJ, Kim DH, Menias CO, Gopal DV, Arluk GM, Heise CP. Evaluation of submucosal lesions of the large intestine, part II: non-neoplastic causes. *Radiographics*. 2007;27:1693-1703.)

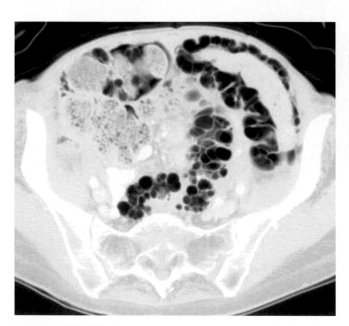

Figure 22-45 **Pneumatosis cystoides coli.** CT image with lung windows shows extensive pneumatosis cystoides involving the left colon, which is the typical distribution for this benign finding. (From Pickhardt PJ, Kim DH, Menias CO, Gopal DV, Arluk GM, Heise CP. Evaluation of submucosal lesions of the large intestine, part II: Non-neoplastic causes. *Radiographics*. 2007;27:1693-1703.)

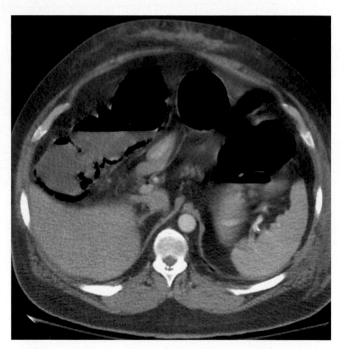

Figure 22-46 **Colonic pneumatosis related to necrosis.** Contrast-enhanced CT image shows linear gas tracking within the right colonic wall related to necrosis complicating sodium polystyrene sulfonate (Kayexalate) administration in a patient with renal disease. (From Pickhardt PJ, Kim DH, Menias CO, Gopal DV, Arluk GM, Heise CP. Evaluation of submucosal lesions of the large intestine, part II: Non-neoplastic causes. *Radiographics*. 2007;27:1693-1703.)

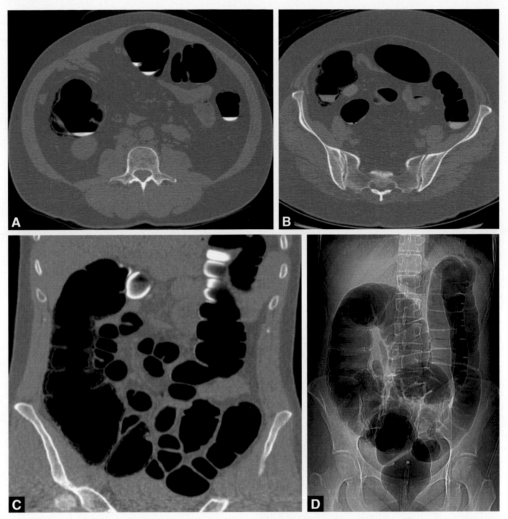

Figure 22-47 **Incidental asymptomatic pneumatosis related to luminal distention at CTC.** CTC images **(A-C)** from three healthy adults undergoing CTC screening show linear pneumatosis involving the right colon. Pneumatosis can also be seen on the scout view for the third case **(D).** All three remained asymptomatic throughout the procedure and afterward; no intervention or treatment was necessary. This finding at CTC should not be confused for perforation, which is exceedingly rare and has not occurred in our experience. Despite the similar imaging appearance with Fig. 22-46, the marked difference in clinical relevance underscores the need for clinical correlation. (From Pickhardt PJ, Kim DH, Taylor AJ. Asymptomatic pneumatosis at CT colonography: A benign self-limited imaging finding distinct from perforation. *Am J Roentgenol.* 2008;190:W112-117.)

NONNEOPLASTIC CAUSES OF EXTRAMURAL ORIGIN

Submucosal impression or invasion from an extracolonic process can be difficult to distinguish from an intramural submucosal entity at OC or other strictly luminal investigation. Simple extrinsic impression without mural invasion may be caused by normal adjacent structures or by an abnormal extracolonic lesion. Presacral lesions represent a subset of abnormal extrinsic lesions that will be discussed separately. Frank invasion of the colonic wall by endometriosis blurs the distinction between extramural and intramural submucosal processes.

Endometriosis

Symptomatic GI involvement by endometriosis is relatively uncommon but strongly favors the rectosigmoid region.[26] Intestinal involvement is characterized by serosal implantation with variable intramural extension. CTC is useful for defining the extent of disease when a submucosal lesion is identified at OC (Fig. 22-48). Deeply penetrating lesions often present with hematochezia and may mimic invasive malignancy on endoluminal examination and cross-sectional imaging (Fig. 22-49). Infiltrating peritoneal-based soft tissue masses from endometriosis can also mimic carcinomatosis on cross-sectional imaging (Fig. 22-50). Correlation with

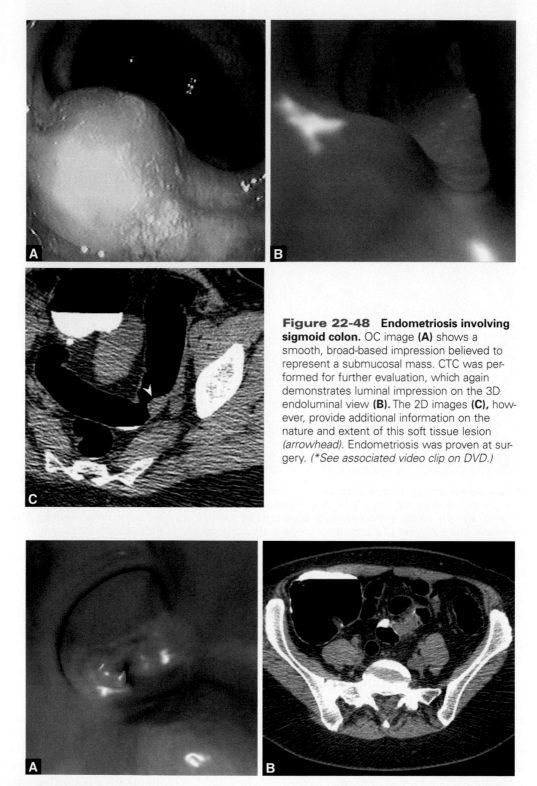

Figure 22-48 Endometriosis involving sigmoid colon. OC image **(A)** shows a smooth, broad-based impression believed to represent a submucosal mass. CTC was performed for further evaluation, which again demonstrates luminal impression on the 3D endoluminal view **(B).** The 2D images **(C),** however, provide additional information on the nature and extent of this soft tissue lesion *(arrowhead).* Endometriosis was proven at surgery. *(*See associated video clip on DVD.)*

Figure 22-49 Sigmoid stricture from endometriosis. 3D endoluminal CTC image **(A)** shows focal collapse of the sigmoid lumen, which can be seen with spasm or true mass lesion. The 2D transverse CTC image **(B)** shows a soft tissue mass, which could not be traversed at subsequent OC and proved to be endometriosis at surgery.

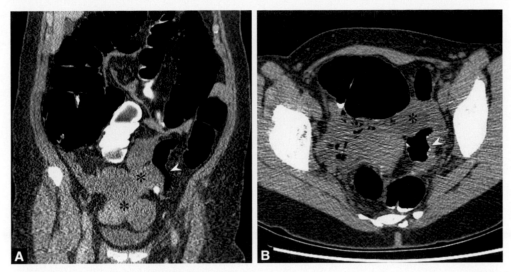

Figure 22-50 **Endometriosis mimicking peritoneal carcinomatosis.** 2D coronal **(A)** and transverse **(B)** CTC images from two different women undergoing screening show extensive peritoneal-based soft tissue masses *(asterisks)* that narrow the sigmoid colon *(arrowheads)*. Unsuspected endometriosis was proven in both cases.

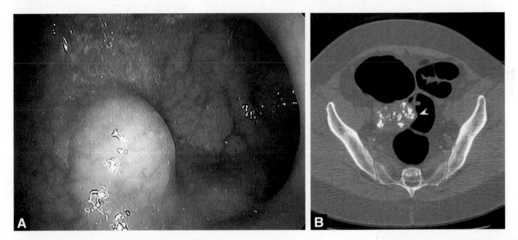

Figure 22-51 **Uterine fibroid mimicking colonic submucosal mass at OC.** OC image **(A)** shows a suspected submucosal mass, for which a biopsy was performed but was nondiagnostic, yielding only colonic mucosa. 2D transverse CTC image **(B)** shows that the colonic abnormality was simply caused by extrinsic impression of a degenerated uterine fibroid *(arrowhead)*. (From Pickhardt PJ, Kim DH, Menias CO, Gopal DV, Arluk GM, Heise CP. Evaluation of submucosal lesions of the large intestine, part II: Non-neoplastic causes. *Radiographics.* 2007;27:1693-1703.)

demographic and clinical history can be important for suggesting the diagnosis, but a history of endometriosis has often not been previously established. Surgery is often required both for diagnosis and therapy if hormonal manipulation is unsuccessful.

Extrinsic Impression

Any structure adjacent to the large intestine may impress upon the lumen. We have seen a number of referrals from OC for suspected intramural submucosal lesions that proved to result from both normal and abnormal extracolonic structures at CTC (Fig. 22-51). For this

reason, in addition to the low overall diagnostic success rate, attempted blind biopsy at OC should generally be avoided. The 2D MPR (multiplanar reformation) images at CTC allow for rapid correlation for any case of extrinsic compression seen on the 3D endoluminal view (Fig. 22-52). Common sources of extrinsic impression, whether normal or pathologic, include the uterus and adnexae in women, the aorta and common iliac arteries (Fig. 22-53), and the adjacent GI tract itself (Fig. 22-54). One finding at 3D endoluminal CTC that is characteristic of extrinsic impression from an extracolonic structure is inward displacement of an otherwise-preserved colonic fold, which we call the "continuous fold" sign (Fig. 22-55).

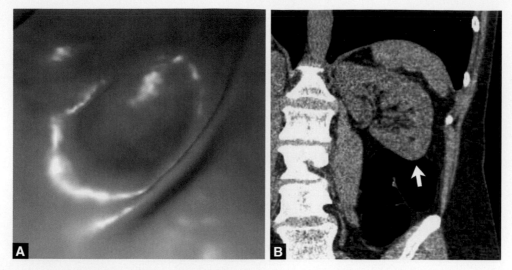

Figure 22-52 Extrinsic impression from normal kidney. 3D endoluminal CTC image **(A)** shows an apparent submucosal mass, which is found to simply represent extrinsic impression of the left lower pole kidney on the coronal 2D CTC image **(B,** *arrow*). *(*See associated video clip on DVD.)*

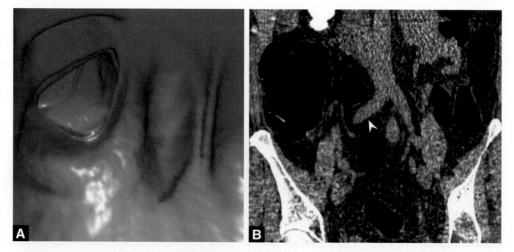

Figure 22-53 Extrinsic impression from iliac artery. 3D endoluminal CTC image **(A)** shows an elongated flat lesion, which is seen to represent extrinsic impression for the right common iliac artery on 2D coronal CTC image **(B,** *arrowhead*).

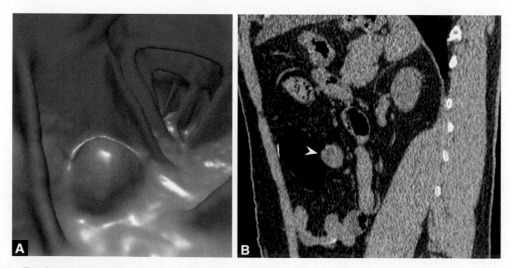

Figure 22-54 Extrinsic impression from small bowel loop. 3D endoluminal CTC image **(A)** shows an apparent submucosal mass, which is seen to represent an adjacent small bowel loop on the 2D sagittal CTC image **(B,** *arrowhead*).

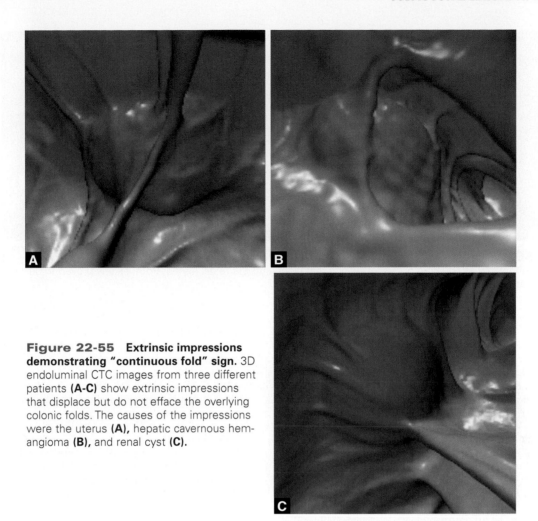

Figure 22-55 Extrinsic impressions demonstrating "continuous fold" sign. 3D endoluminal CTC images from three different patients **(A-C)** show extrinsic impressions that displace but do not efface the overlying colonic folds. The causes of the impressions were the uterus **(A)**, hepatic cavernous hemangioma **(B)**, and renal cyst **(C)**.

Presacral Lesions

Because of the relatively confined anatomic space of the presacral region, focal lesions often result in mass effect on the posterior rectum. Differential diagnostic possibilities include a heterogeneous array of entities, such as tailgut cysts (retrorectal cystic hamartoma), nerve sheath tumors, sarcomas, lymphoproliferative disorders, sacrococcygeal teratoma, anterior sacral meningocele, or any expansile sacral mass (e.g., giant cell tumor, chondrosarcoma, aneurysmal bone cyst, chordoma, etc). Benign tailgut cysts appear to represent the most frequent entity seen in asymptomatic adults (Fig. 22-56).[27]

SUMMARY

A wide variety of neoplastic and nonneoplastic entities of intramural and extramural origin may give rise to a submucosal abnormality at CTC or OC. The complementary nature of these two colorectal examinations provides for comprehensive evaluation of most submucosal lesions. Furthermore, both studies can generally be performed on the same day without the need for additional bowel preparation. In some cases, other imaging studies such as TRUS and MR may provide additional useful information. Regardless, close collaboration among radiologists, gastroenterologists, and colorectal surgeons is paramount for appropriate management of submucosal lesions.

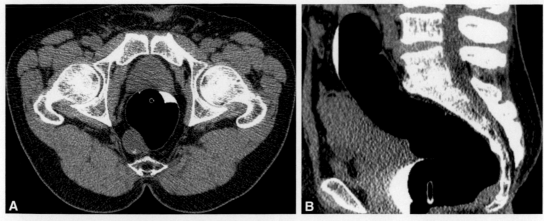

Figure 22-56 Retrorectal cystic hamartomas (tailgut cysts). 2D transverse **(A)** and sagittal **(B)** CTC images from two different patients show low attenuation presacral lesions that bulge into the rectal lumen. Both lesions proved to be retrorectal cystic hamartomas after resection. (*See associated video clip on DVD.)*

REFERENCES

1. Pickhardt PJ, Kim DH, Menias CO, Gopal DV, Arluk GM, Heise CP. Evaluation of submucosal lesions of the large intestine: Part 1. Neoplasms. *Radiographics*. 2007;27(6):1681-1692.
2. Pickhardt PJ, Kim DH, Menias CO, Gopal DV, Arluk GM, Heise CP. Evaluation of submucosal lesions of the large intestine: Part 2. Nonneoplastic causes. *Radiographics*. 2007;27(6):1693-1703.
3. Hancock BJ, Vajcner A. Lipomas of the colon—A clinicopathologic review. *Can J Surg*. 1988;31(3):178-181.
4. Levy AD, Sobin LH. From the archives of the AFIP—Gastrointestinal carcinoids: Imaging features with clinicopathologic comparison. *Radiographics*. 2007;27(1):237-U19.
5. Wong MTC, Eu KW. Primary colorectal lymphomas. *Colorectal Dis*. 2006;8(7):586-591.
6. Pickhardt PJ, Siegel MJ. Posttransplantation lymphoproliferative disorder of the abdomen: CT evaluation in 51 patients. *Radiology*. 1999;213(1):73-78.
7. Pickhardt PJ, Siegel MJ. Abdominal manifestations of posttransplantation lymphoproliferative disorder. *Am J Roentgenol*. 1998;171(4):1007-1013.
8. Dachman AH, Ros PR, Shekitka KM, Buck JL, Olmsted WW, Hinton CB. Colorectal hemangioma—Radiologic findings. *Radiology*. 1988;167(1):31-34.
9. Levy AD, Remotti HE, Thompson WM, Sobin LH, Miettinen M. Anorectal gastrointestinal stromal tumors: CT and MR imaging features with clinical and pathologic correlation. *Am J Roentgenol*. 2003;180(6):1607-1612.
10. Abrams HL, Spiro R, Goldstein N. Metastases in carcinoma; analysis of 1000 autopsied cases. *Cancer*. 1950;3(1):74-85.
11. Levitt RG, Koehler RE, Sagel SS, Lee JKT. Metastatic disease of the mesentery and omentum. *Radiol Clin North Am*. 1982;20(3):501-510.
12. Pickhardt PJ, Levy AD, Rohrmann CA, Kende AI. Primary neoplasms of the appendix manifesting as acute appendicitis: CT findings with pathologic comparison. *Radiology*. 2002;224(3):775-781.
13. Pickhardt PJ, Levy AD, Rohrmann CA, Kende AI. Primary neoplasms of the appendix: Radiologic spectrum of disease with pathologic correlation. *Radiographics*. 2003;23(3):645-662.
14. Hebert JJ, Pickhardt PJ. MDCT diagnosis of an appendiceal mucocele with acute torsion. *Am J Roentgenol*. 2007;189(1):W4-W6.
15. Pickhardt PJ, Levy AD, Rohrmann CA, Abbondanzo SL, Kende AI. Non-Hodgkin's lymphoma of the appendix: Clinical and CT findings with pathologic correlation. *Am J Roentgenol*. 2002;178(5):1123-1127.
16. Weston AP, Campbell DR. Diminutive colonic polyps: Histopathology, spatial distribution, concomitant significant lesions, and treatment complications. *Am J Gastroenterol*. 1995;90(1):24-28.
17. Lee AD, Pickhardt PJ, Gopal DV, Taylor AJ. Venous malformations mimicking multiple mucosal polyps on screening CT colonography. *Am J Roentgenol*. 2006;186(4):1113-1115.
18. Arluk GM, Drachenberg C, Darwin P. Colonic cystic lymphangioma. *Gastrointest Endosc*. 2004;60(1):98.
19. Sztarkier I, Benharroch D, Walfisch S, Delgado J. Colitis cystica profunda and solitary rectal ulcer syndrome-polypoid variant: Two confusing clinical conditions. *Eur J Intern Med*. 2006;17(8):578-579.
20. Calabuig R, Ortiz C, Sueiras A, Vallet J, Pi F. Intramural hematoma of the cecum - Report of two cases. *Dis Colon Rectum*. 2002;45(4):564-566.
21. Kim D, Pickhardt PJ, Taylor A, Menias CO. Imaging evaluation of complications at optical colonoscopy. *Curr Prob Diagn Radiol*. 2008;37(4):165-177.
22. Peterson CM, Menias CO, Balfe DM, Freeman BA. Adult intussusception due to cocaine-induced bowel wall hematoma: A case study. *Emerg Radiol*. 2006;12(4):177-179.
23. Heng Y, Schuffler MD, Haggitt RC, Rohrmann CA. Pneumatosis intestinalis—A review. *Am J Gastroenterol*. 1995;90(10):1747-1758.
24. Ho LM, Paulson EK, Thompson WM. Pneumatosis intestinalis in the adult: Benign to life-threatening causes. *Am J Roentgenol*. 2007;188(6):1604-1613.
25. Pickhardt PJ, Kim D, Taylor A. Asymptomatic pneumatosis at CT colonography: A benign self-limited imaging finding distinct from perforation. *Am J Roentgenol*. 2008;190(2): W112-W117.
26. Zwas FR, Lyon DT. Endometriosis—An important condition in clinical gastroenterology. *Digest Dis Sci*. 1991;36(3):353-364.
27. Lev-Chelouche D, Gutman M, Goldman G, et al. Presacral tumors: A practical classification and treatment of a unique and heterogenous group of diseases. *Surgery*. 2003;133(5):473-478.

3D Imaging Displays at CTC

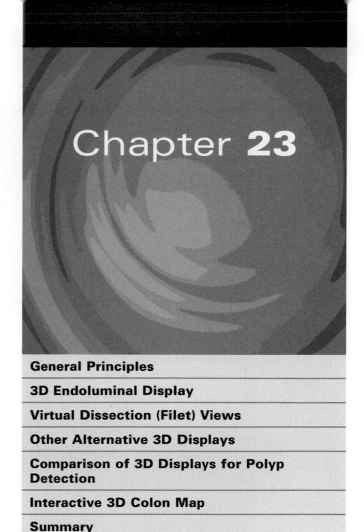

Chapter 23

PERRY J. PICKHARDT, MD
DAVID H. KIM, MD

GENERAL PRINCIPLES

A wide variety of three-dimensional (3D) displays have been developed to visualize the colonic lumen at CT colonography (CTC). This chapter is not intended to represent a detailed technical description of these advanced visualization techniques. Instead, this overview will present the various 3D imaging display techniques for CTC and discuss the relative advantages and disadvantages of each approach. One basic tenet that surfaces as a recurring theme is the tradeoff between mucosal visualization and geometric distortion. That is, certain 3D solutions that increase the amount of colonic surface visible at one time, which has the potential to reduce overall interpretation times, unfortunately also tend to result in greater spatial distortions that can negatively affect lesion detection. The key here is to find an optimal middle ground that combines efficient 3D surface visualization with effective polyp detection. The "standard" 3D endoluminal display will be considered first, with particular attention to the field-of-view (FOV) angle. The virtual dissection or filet view will be discussed next, including both static and dynamic formats. Beyond these two dominant approaches, a variety of other 3D views will be briefly discussed.

It is important to point out that only the standard 3D endoluminal projection has been clinically validated for screening. Therefore, these alternative 3D displays may be used to supplement standard 3D/2D CTC evaluation but should not be considered as a standalone technique for polyp detection at this time. One concern with the nonstandard 3D displays is that a more difficult learning curve could negate any gains related to decreased interpretation time. As emphasized throughout this textbook, the 2D display remains an essential companion for the ultimate characterization of findings, regardless of the 3D detection format that one uses.

3D ENDOLUMINAL DISPLAY

The standard 3D endoluminal view consists of a single camera vantage moving through the colonic lumen. The colonic wall is displayed using either a surface or volume rendering technique. The term "virtual colonoscopy" refers to this conventional endoluminal virtual reality projection because of the resemblance to conventional optical endoscopy (Fig. 23-1). In fact, it is probably incorrect to refer to primary 2D or alternative 3D visualization modes as "virtual colonoscopy" because they bear little or no resemblance to the appearance at optical colonoscopy (OC). Until recently, there were obvious differences in the image quality and navigational capabilities among the various CTC software systems.[1] Although clear differences persist in 3D performance, which results in widely disparate 3D interpretation times and variable polyp detection rates, the gap has closed considerably within the past few years. When choosing a CTC software system, it is critical to give it a thorough "test drive," which should include complete navigation in both automated and manual modes. Most CTC software systems provide for some sort of automated centerline that consists of a central axis path for facile navigation. The freedom and ease of manual, mouse-driven navigation, however, is variable among the

391

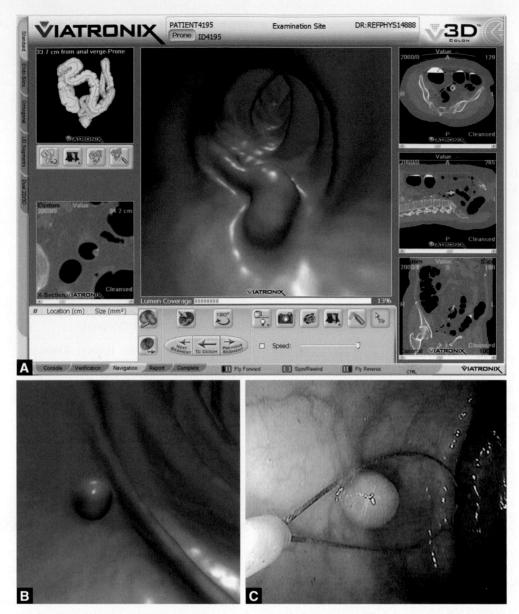

Figure 23-1 **The standard 3D endoluminal view.** Screen capture of the CTC system we use **(A)** shows the 3D endoluminal view in the center pane and the 2D MPR views and colon map to the side. The 3D endoluminal fly-through closely resembles the appearance at physical endoscopy, hence the term "virtual colonoscopy." The 3D endoluminal view allows for efficient and effective polyp detection, which can be rapidly confirmed on the 2D views. This large pedunculated polyp (tubular adenoma) was found in a patient several months after an incomplete screening OC was complicated by sigmoid perforation. 3D endoluminal CTC image **(B)** and corresponding OC image **(C)** from a second patient shows a 6-mm tubular adenoma. The 3D endoluminal CTC images can be made to closely match the OC findings. (*See associated video clip on DVD.)*

different systems. Furthermore, not all centerline navigations provide the same endoluminal coverage in the sense that some systems seem to "hug" the wall too closely, resulting in suboptimal evaluation. In addition, only some systems can keep track of which surfaces have been visualized, which increases diagnostic confidence and can greatly improve efficiency, particularly if one is interrupted during the interpretation.

The FOV angle is an important consideration for both virtual and optical colonoscopy. A 90-degree FOV is the typical default setting for a number of CTC systems. The main advantage of a 90-degree FOV is the lack of geometric distortion, allowing for a clear spatial depiction of findings. The main disadvantage is that luminal coverage from a single one-way fly-through is generally inadequate, requiring a second fly-through in the opposite direction. In our experience, approximately 75% of the lumen is visualized on average by unidirectional navigation, with more than 20% of the surface missed in more than 80% of cases (Fig. 23-2).[2] A second complete fly-through in the opposite direction increases coverage to 94% on average. To further increase diagnostic confidence for a

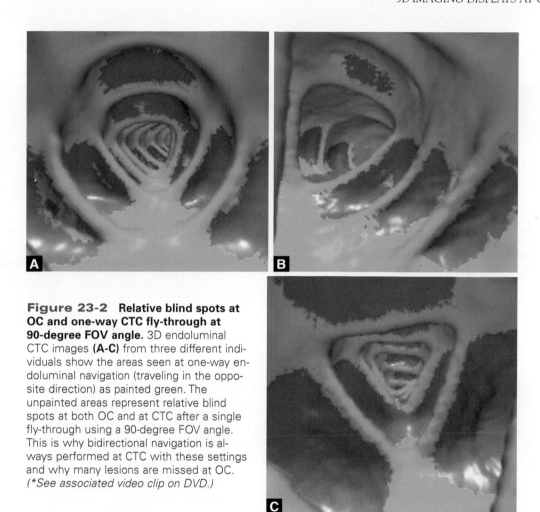

Figure 23-2   Relative blind spots at OC and one-way CTC fly-through at 90-degree FOV angle. 3D endoluminal CTC images **(A-C)** from three different individuals show the areas seen at one-way endoluminal navigation (traveling in the opposite direction) as painted green. The unpainted areas represent relative blind spots at both OC and at CTC after a single fly-through using a 90-degree FOV angle. This is why bidirectional navigation is always performed at CTC with these settings and why many lesions are missed at OC. (*See associated video clip on DVD.)

complete examination, a missed region tool allows the reader to quickly flip through unseen patches until coverage is essentially complete, adding only about 20 seconds to the interpretation time (Fig. 23-3). Although this approach has proven successful for accurate polyp detection,[3,4] it requires four complete endoluminal fly-throughs between the supine and prone views.

The need for four complete fly-through passes at a 90-degree FOV led us to investigate whether increasing the FOV angle could allow for a reduction in the total number of fly-throughs. However, any increase in luminal coverage should not be offset by unacceptable levels of geometric distortion that could negatively affect polyp detection. Our preliminary investigation (using the Viatronix V3D Colon Module) showed that a 150-degree FOV resulted in huge gains in mucosal coverage but at the expense of unacceptable distortion.[5] At a 120-degree FOV, however, the significant gains in coverage (approximately 90% coverage per flight) were balanced by an acceptable level of mild spatial distortion (Fig. 23-4)

The next phase of our investigation looked at actual polyp detection with a single pass at a 120-degree FOV compared with the clinically proven strategy of two-way fly-through at a 90-degree FOV.[6] Our 120-degree FOV

protocol consists of a retrograde pass toward the cecum on the supine view and an antegrade pass toward the rectum on the prone view. We found that the 120-degree setting allowed for a 50% reduction in fly-throughs (i.e., four to two) without any demonstrable dropoff in polyp detection. That is, all 104 polyps evaluated were seen on at least one of the two fly-throughs (and 83% were seen on both fly-throughs). In fact, we have noted some cases where polyps are clearly seen on one-way fly-through at 120 degrees but not clearly seen on two-way fly-through at 90 degrees (Fig. 23-5). In such a case, polyp detection at the 90-degree FOV setting would require visualization from a redundant backup such as the alternative supine/prone view, a primary 2D review, or the missed region tool. As a result of this study, the interpretive approach of single retrograde supine and antegrade prone fly-through (with the missed region tool to evaluate blind spots) has become a viable reading strategy in our practice, leading to large reductions in interpretation time. This paradigm is ideal for busy practices, avoiding the need for using any of the alternative 3D strategies discussed later in this chapter. When distention is suboptimal, however, we recommend bidirectional fly-through at 120 degrees on both supine and prone to maximize coverage.

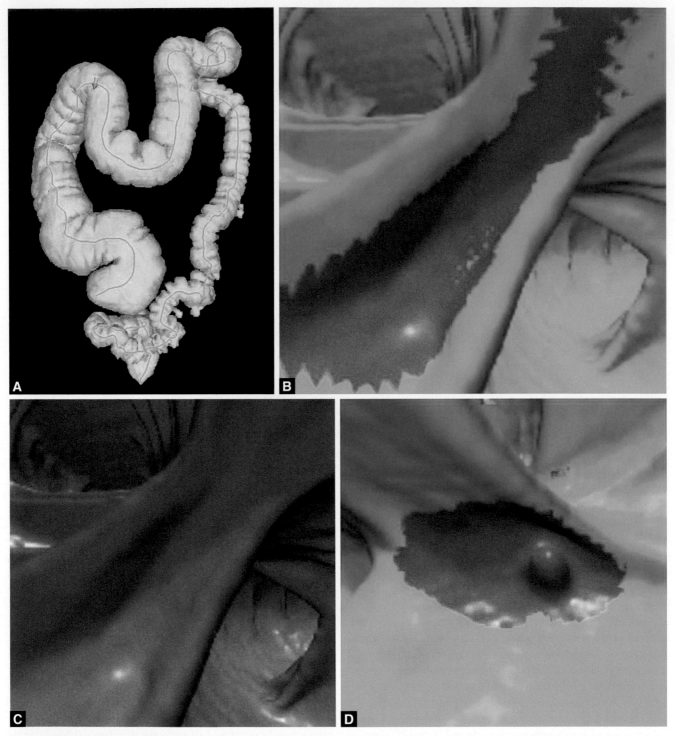

Figure 23-3 Missed region tool for 3D endoluminal evaluation. 3D colon map **(A)** shows the *blue arrow* directed toward the inner aspect of the hepatic flexure, which is a typical location for a missed patch of mucosa after endoluminal navigation along the centerline. 3D endoluminal CTC images with **(B)** and without **(C)** the paint function for visualized surfaces show the small missed patch. Clicking through the missed regions will uncover a polyp on only very rare occasions **(D),** but the process takes little time and increases reader confidence.

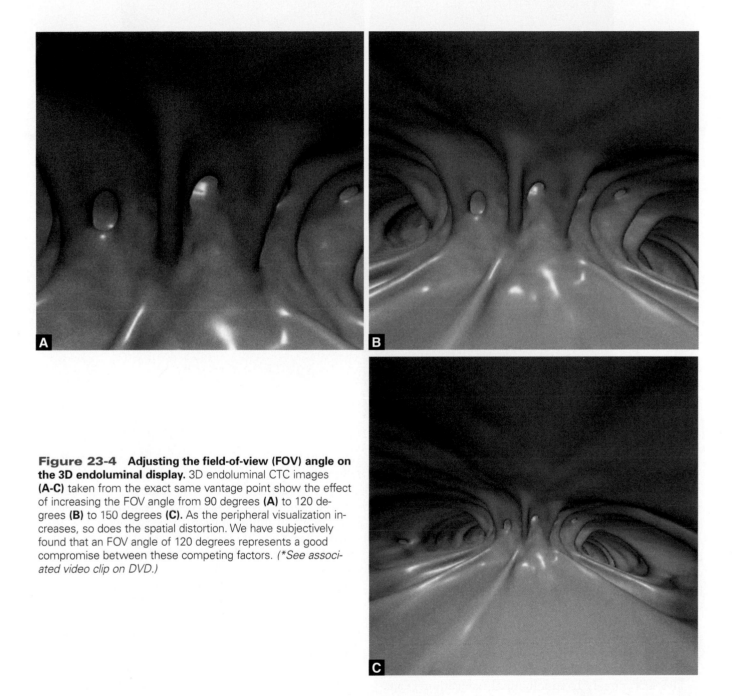

Figure 23-4 Adjusting the field-of-view (FOV) angle on the 3D endoluminal display. 3D endoluminal CTC images **(A-C)** taken from the exact same vantage point show the effect of increasing the FOV angle from 90 degrees **(A)** to 120 degrees **(B)** to 150 degrees **(C).** As the peripheral visualization increases, so does the spatial distortion. We have subjectively found that an FOV angle of 120 degrees represents a good compromise between these competing factors. *(*See associated video clip on DVD.)*

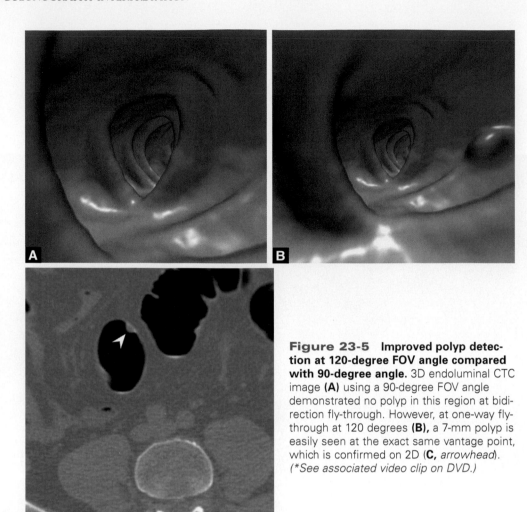

Figure 23-5 Improved polyp detection at 120-degree FOV angle compared with 90-degree angle. 3D endoluminal CTC image **(A)** using a 90-degree FOV angle demonstrated no polyp in this region at bidirection fly-through. However, at one-way fly-through at 120 degrees **(B),** a 7-mm polyp is easily seen at the exact same vantage point, which is confirmed on 2D **(C,** *arrowhead*). (*See associated video clip on DVD.*)

Interpretation times for 3D endoluminal CTC are highly dependent on the system used. Furthermore, because 2D correlation and secondary detection supplement the 3D evaluation, it can be misleading to report interpretation times as a pure 3D read. With the Viatronix V3D system, our typical interpretation times are generally in the 5- to 15-minute range, which includes a combined 3D/2D assessment and extracolonic evaluation. With certain other CTC systems, typical interpretation times may be as high as 25 to 40 minutes.[7-9]

VIRTUAL DISSECTION (FILET) VIEWS

The suboptimal 3D endoluminal navigational capabilities on some CTC systems and the need for four complete fly-throughs (at 90 degrees), resulting in long interpretation times, were likely the impetus for developing alternative 3D viewing strategies. Chief among these is the virtual dissection view, also referred to as the filet view or virtual pathology display.[8,10-13] In effect, the colon is (virtually) unravelled, dissected open, and flattened, which approximates the appearance of a pinned gross pathology specimen. In theory, this concept is appealing because the resulting strips or filets can be rapidly viewed, potentially resulting in dramatic reductions in interpretation time. However, the aforementioned tradeoff between increased surface visualization and geometric distortion has plagued this approach because even large polyps may be distorted beyond recognition. Distortion is particularly an issue at flexure points because not only may polyps be grossly distorted but folds may actually appear polypoid (Figs. 23-6 and 23-7). A more difficult learning curve is another concern when dealing with nonstandard 3D displays, which may further exacerbate polyp detection deficiencies. The initial clinical trials using the virtual dissection view have supported these considerations, reporting decreased interpretation times but at the expense of polyp detection rates that are generally much lower that what can be achieved with the more standard 3D endoluminal view.[8,12,13]

When comparing the various incarnations of the virtual dissection view at CTC, the two key features to

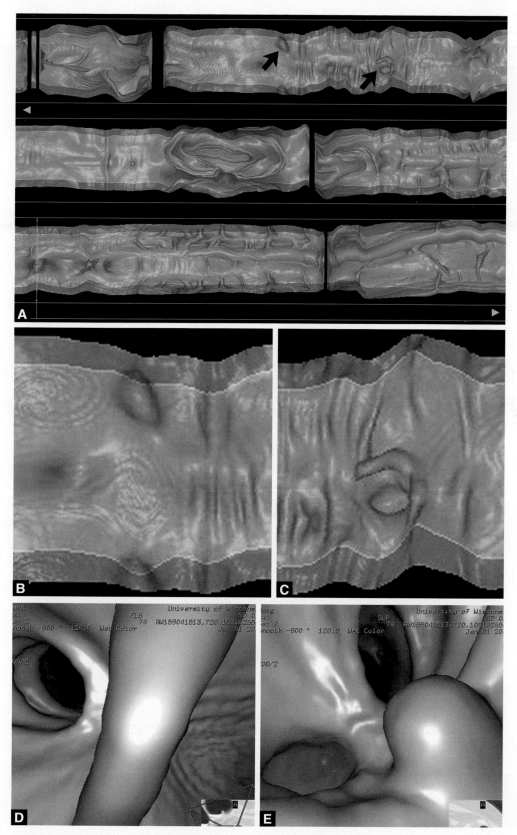

Figure 23-6 **Spatial distortion on the static 360-degree virtual dissection view.** Virtual dissection view **(A)** shows the entire colon in three strips (note rectal catheter in the upper left corner). Two other areas on the top strip *(arrows)* are magnified in *B* and *C.* The polypoid lesion **(B)** was seen to represent a colonic fold on the standard endoluminal view **(D).** The horizontal foldlike structure **(C)** corresponds to a 1.6-cm polyp on the endoluminal view **(E),** with an adjacent diverticulum. *(See associated video clip on DVD.)*

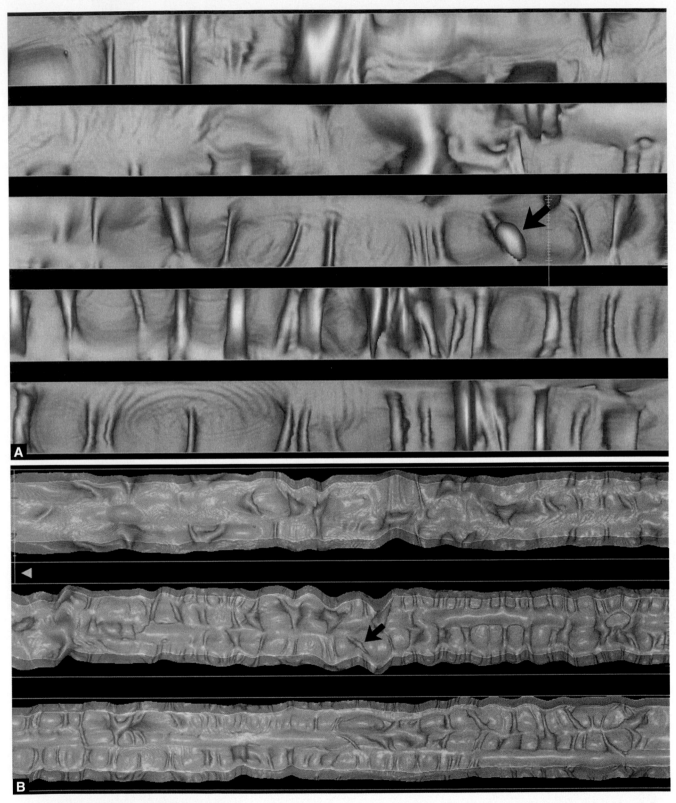

Figure 23-7 **Increasing spatial distortion on the virtual dissection going from 120-degree to 360-degree strips.** Virtual dissection view **(A)** with 120-degree strips shows an obvious polyp *(arrow)*. Not all 120-degree strips are included here. When the coverage per strip is increased beyond 360 degrees **(B)**, the lesion becomes more distorted and resembles a fold *(arrow)*.

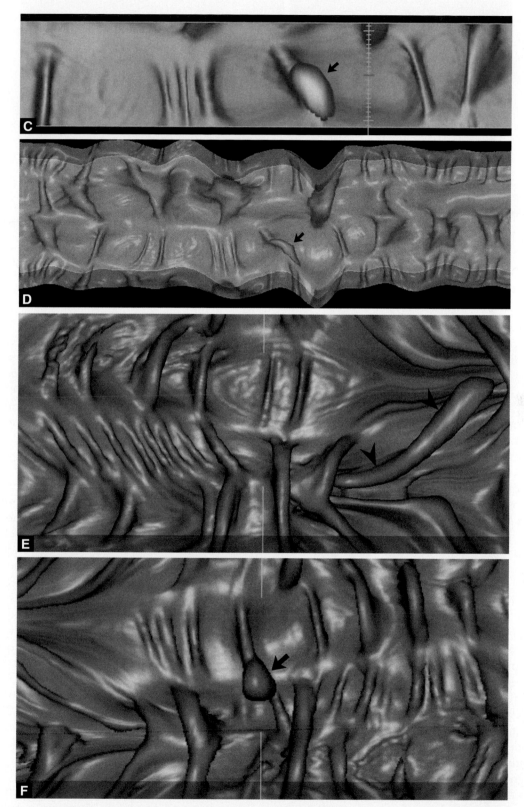

Figure 23-7 (Continued)   **Increasing spatial distortion on the virtual dissection going from 120-degree to 360-degree strips.** The areas of interest are magnified in **C** and **D**. Besides the distortion, which could preclude detection, note how the lesion also occupies less strip width. During "fly-over" with a dynamic 360-degree filet view, the same polyp appears foldlike during the early portion of its convolution (**E,** *arrowheads)* but then morphs into a polypoid structure as it rolls over the center pin (**F,** *arrow).*

Illustration continued on following page

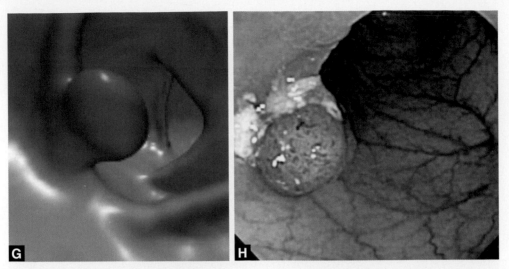

Figure 23-7 (Continued) **Increasing spatial distortion on the virtual dissection going from 120-degree to 360-degree strips.** This 1.2-cm pedunculated polyp is obvious on the 3D endoluminal fly-through **(G)** and proved to be a tubulovillous adenoma after poly-pectomy at OC **(H)**. *(*See associated video clip on DVD.)*

consider are the short-axis angle of coverage per strip and whether a static or dynamic viewing approach is used. Earlier versions of the static virtual dissection (e.g., from GE Medical Systems) provided thin strips in the range of 90 degrees to 120 degrees of short-axis coverage (Fig. 23-7 through 23-9).[13] One disadvantage of this approach was that multiple overlapping strips must be viewed to evaluate the entire luminal circumference. However, the relative advantages of the 120-degree strips compared with the subsequent 360-degree strips were that there was significantly less spatial distortion (Fig. 23-7) and that the lesions appeared larger relative to the strip size (Fig. 23-8). In fact, a spatial issue common to all flatten-ing views that produce a uniform strip width is that le-sions within a narrow portion of the colon such as the sigmoid will appear much larger relative to a cecal or rectal lesion, where the capacious lumen will markedly diminish the relative size of included lesions. Most current dissec-tion views, such as the GE AdvantageCTC, now consist of the full 360-degree coverage, with additional overlap included to avoid missing significant lesions at the edges. In our experience, the static 360-degree dissection view routinely causes a disturbing amount of distortion that can make even large polyps and masses difficult to discern, especially if relatively flat (Figs. 23-7 and 23-9). Further-more, readers must be cognizant of polyp size distortions and not assume a lesion is diminutive when located in a region of relatively large cross-sectional area (Fig. 23-8). Missing or ignoring important lesions would obviously negate any benefit related to a decreased interpretation time because sensitivity is the single most important crite-rion for clinical success.

One fairly elegant solution to the vexing spatial dis-tortion issue associated with full 360+-degree views is to dynamically change the projection. The "perspective filet view" on the Philips Extended Brilliance Work-space (Fig. 23-7) and the "band view" on the INFINITT

CTC system (Fig. 23-10) achieve this by rolling the unraveled strip over an imaginary center pin or con-veyer belt in the middle of the projected field.[11,14] As the reader scrolls through the 360-degree section (with an additional 20-degree overlap), the geometric distor-tion changes as it rolls over the central hump. As such, lesions that may be grossly distorted in a static dissec-tion view can often be detected during some phase of this dynamic convolution (Fig. 23-7). In addition, both sides of the colonic folds are visualized as the colon rolls over the tube (Fig. 23-11). It is not surprising that the "cost" of this improved detection capability is the in-creased time required to scroll through the entire colon, in effect resulting in a "fly-over" approach that resem-bles the task of the standard 3D endoluminal fly-through. Therefore, although this approach is attractive and certainly has merit, it may not offer a significant advantage in terms of interpretation time and lesion detection relative to a single-pass endoluminal ap-proach at 120 degrees. A number of diagnostic tools and techniques that were first applied to the standard 2D MPR (multiplanar reconstruction) or 3D endolumi-nal displays, such as translucency rendering, electronic cleansing, and computer-aided detection, are now be-ing applied to the dissection views (Fig. 23-12).

OTHER ALTERNATIVE 3D DISPLAYS

Beyond the various forms of the virtual dissection view discussed previously, there are a number of addi-tional advanced 3D displays that have been applied to CTC. The "unfolded cube" projection is an interest-ing approach that renders the six planar projections of a cube at 90-degree viewing angles, as seen from the center point.[15] The projections of the cube faces are then unfolded and flattened, resulting in a cross pattern

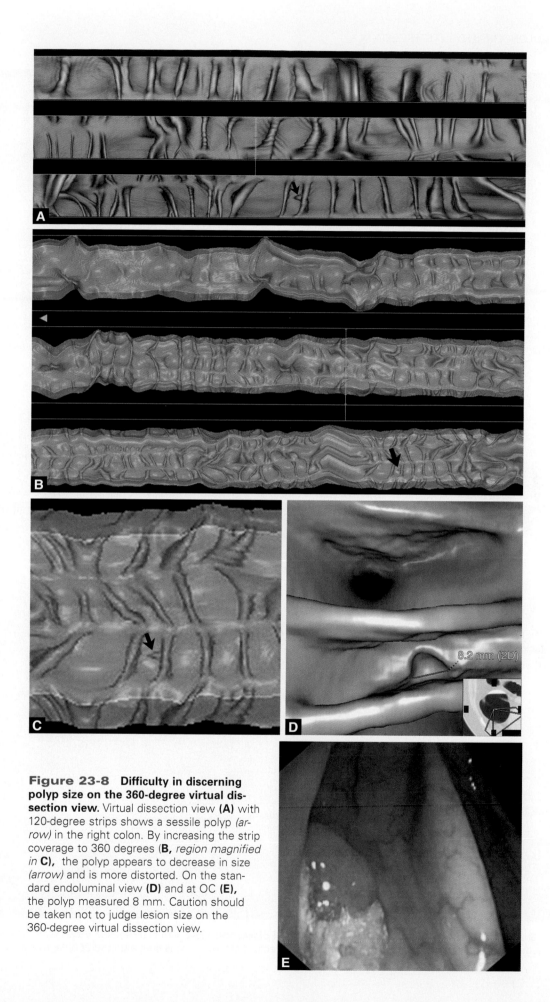

Figure 23-8 Difficulty in discerning polyp size on the 360-degree virtual dissection view. Virtual dissection view (**A**) with 120-degree strips shows a sessile polyp *(arrow)* in the right colon. By increasing the strip coverage to 360 degrees (**B**, *region magnified in* **C**), the polyp appears to decrease in size *(arrow)* and is more distorted. On the standard endoluminal view (**D**) and at OC (**E**), the polyp measured 8 mm. Caution should be taken not to judge lesion size on the 360-degree virtual dissection view.

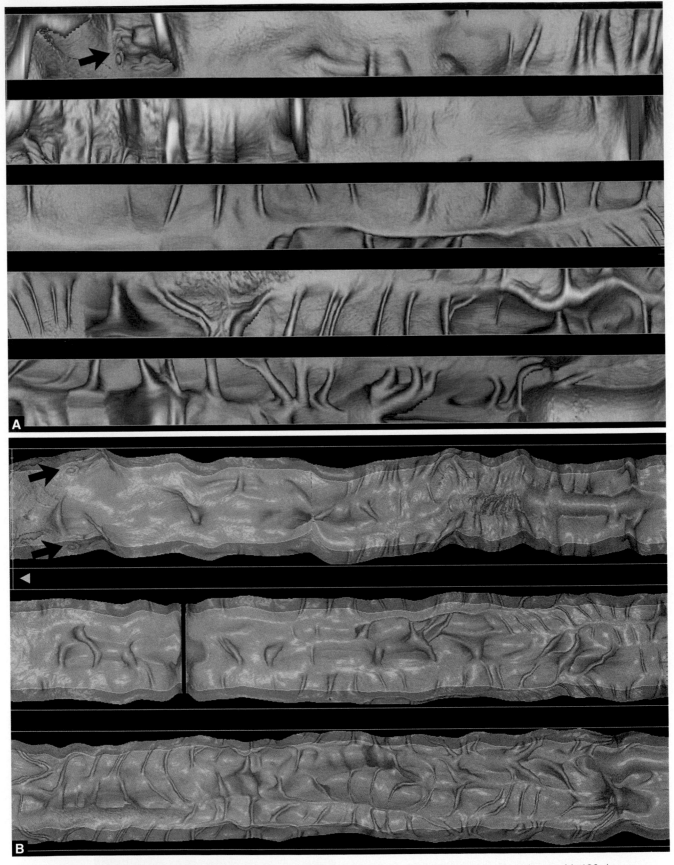

Figure 23-9 **Large flat mass (carpet lesion) on the virtual dissection view.** Virtual dissection views with 120-degree **(A)** and 360-degree **(B)** strips show an area of irregularity in the rectum *(arrows)* that is subtle on the 360-degree version.

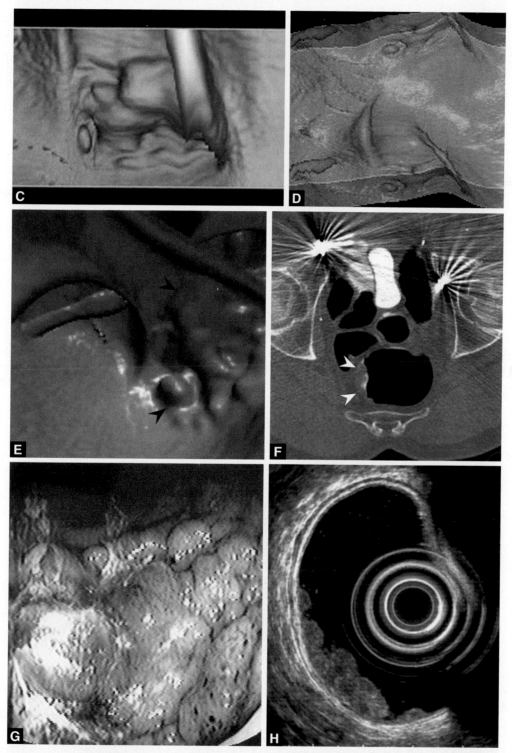

Figure 23-9 (Continued)   **Large flat mass (carpet lesion) on the virtual dissection view.** Magnified views of this region **(C** and **D)** are compared with 3D endoluminal **(E)** and 2D transverse **(F)** images, which show a large, relatively flat but lobulated mass *(arrowheads)* situated between rectal folds. A 5-cm villous adenoma with high-grade dysplasia was found at same-day OC **(G)** and TRUS **(H)**. *(*See associated video clip on DVD.)*

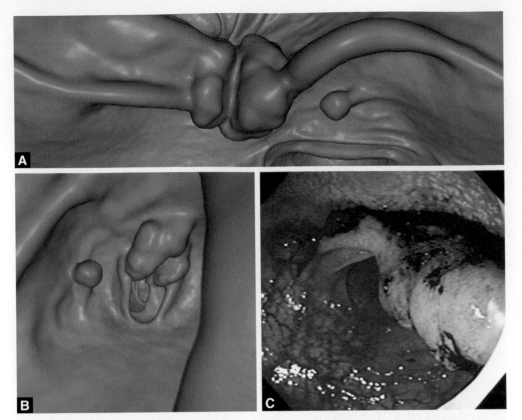

Figure 23-10 **Dynamic unfolded "band view."** Static images from the 3D panoramic band view **(A)** and standard 3D endo-luminal view **(B)** show an irregular 3-cm mass lesion and an adjacent 8-mm polyp. OC image **(C)** shows the mass, which proved to be invasive CRC, and the adjacent polyp, which was a tubular adenoma. (Case courtesy of Seong Ho Park, MD, Seoul, Korea.) (*See associated video clip on DVD.)

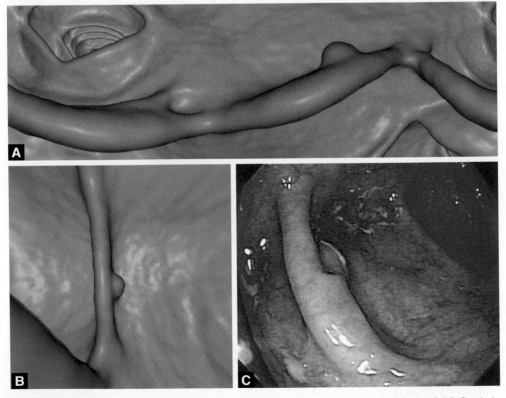

Figure 23-11 **Dynamic unfolded "band view" for detecting a small 6-mm polyp behind a fold.** Static images from the 3D panoramic band view **(A)** and standard 3D endoluminal view **(B)** show a small sessile polyp located on the backside of a fold. Because of the dynamic nature of the band view, polyps are generally visible on both sides of a fold, whereas two-way fly-through was needed for detection on the standard endoluminal view. The polyp proved to be a tubular adenoma after resection at OC **(C)**. (Case courtesy of Seong Ho Park, MD, Seoul, Korea.) (*See associated video clip on DVD.)

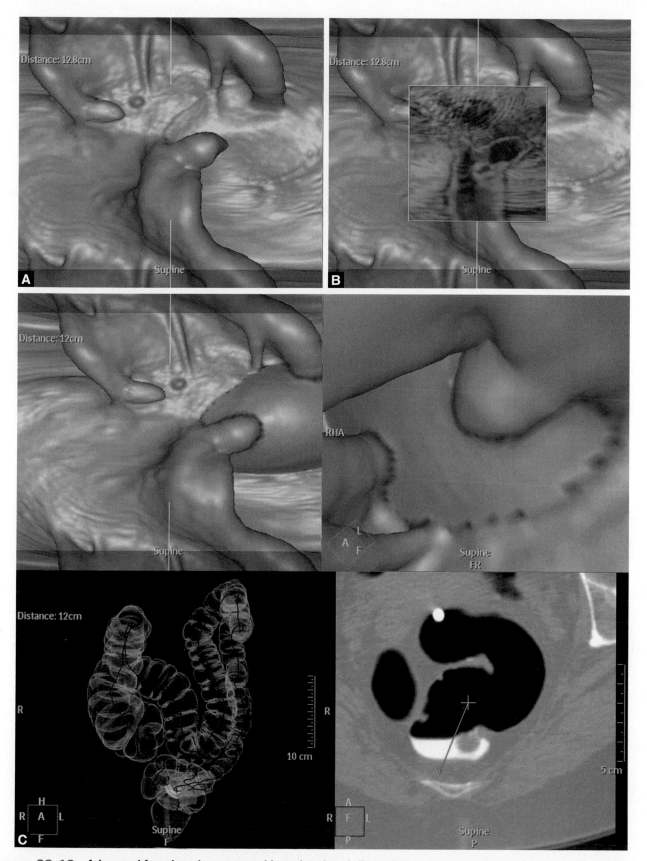

Figure 23-12   Advanced functions incorporated into the virtual dissection view. CTC software system with perspective filet view (Philips) has integrated functions such as attenuation color mapping **(A** and **B)**, electronic fluid cleansing (absent in **C)**

Illustration continued on following page

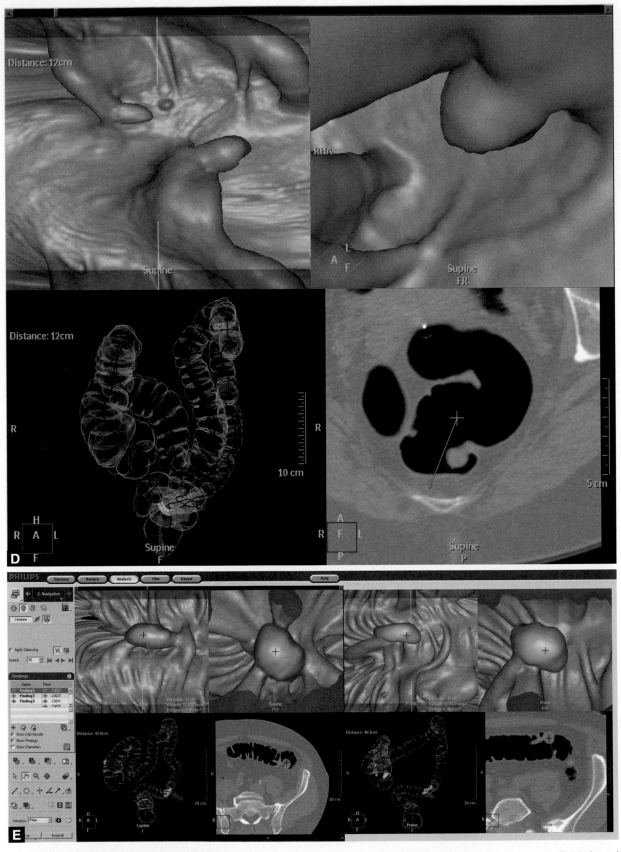

Figure 23-12 (Continued)   **Advanced functions incorporated into the virtual dissection view.** Electronic fluid cleansing (present in **D**), and computer-aided detection **(E)** into the dissection view.

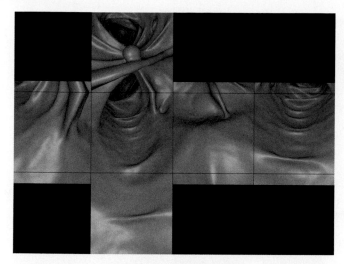

Figure 23-13 **Unfolded cube 3D view.** Static image shows the six sides of a cube flattened, which allows for simultaneous visualization of the incoming and outgoing lumen. A polyp is present that has just peeled off the incoming pathway and is starting to head away from the virtual camera. (*See associated video clip on DVD.*)

(Fig. 23-13). By navigating along the centerline, the reader simultaneously views both forward and reverse projections, with coverage of the entire colonic lumen in a single pass. Attention is focused primarily around the periphery of the central downstream pane where the folds appear to peel back, allowing for evaluation of both the front and back sides. As with the perspective filet view, the dynamic approach allows for improved polyp detection over the static dissection view. However, the compromise is once again the need to fly-through the entire colon.

Another interesting and potentially valuable approach is to virtually hinge open the colon like a clam shell (Fig. 23-14). One important benefit of this bisection approach is that the geometric distortion that limits the virtual dissection views is not introduced. One disadvantage is that the lack of straightening and need to evaluate both halves limit the amount of lumen that can be displayed at one time. Other approaches have included a volumetric slab that represents somewhat of a cross between 2D and 3D displays. A somewhat related view is a cube of volume, which can be cut away or grown in various planes. This rudimentary view has been used in the past for 3D correlation associated with primary 2D interpretation. Additional 3D displays such as the Mercator view have been investigated but do not appear to be clinically relevant solutions.[16] Given the difficulty cartographers have long faced in attempting to accurately depict the globe onto a flattened 2D map, it is not surprising that flattening an even more complex 3D structure such as the large intestine without introducing too much distortion has been such a challenge.

COMPARISON OF 3D DISPLAYS FOR POLYP DETECTION

To compare the detection capabilities of the various 3D displays, we performed two related retrospective multi-reader studies.[17,18] Specifically, we evaluated primary 3D polyp detection on the standard 3D endoluminal view (using Viatronix), the dynamic perspective filet view (using Philips/USA), and the "unfolded cube view" (using Philips/Netherlands). Three readers—an inexperienced radiology resident, an experienced body imaging fellow, and an expert CTC staff radiologist—each read a set of 30 endoscopically confirmed CTC cases on each system using primary 3D detection only (i.e., no secondary 2D detection was allowed). Each reader received hands-on applications training on each system. Because the purpose was only to compare 3D detection capabilities, the overall sensitivity for polyp detection by each system is underestimated. Cases were spaced with at least a 30-day washout period between each system to avoid recall bias, and the cases were arranged such that the 3D viewing order was different for each reader. For the standard 3D endoluminal interpretation, two-way fly-through at 90 degrees was performed.

The pooled sensitivity for 3D polyp detection at the 6-mm and 10-mm thresholds for the standard endoluminal, perspective filet, and unfolded cube views was 91% (63/69) and 98% (47/48), 72% (50/69) and 77% (37/48), and 81% (56/69) and 85% (41/48), respectively. Improvement in sensitivity at the 6-mm threshold for the expert staff compared with the experienced fellow and inexperienced resident averaged 13% for the standard endoluminal view and 28% for the both perspective filet and unfolded cube views. Therefore, the standard 3D endoluminal display showed improved polyp detection over the perspective filet and unfolded cube displays and had an easier learning curve for nonexpert readers. By combining all three systems for each reader, we found that increasing levels of experience correlated well with improved performance for 3D polyp detection. Sensitivity at the 6-mm and 10-mm threshold for the inexperienced (resident), experienced (fellow), and expert (staff) readers was 72% (50/69) and 77% (37/48), 75% (52/69) and 83% (40/48), and 97% (67/69) and 100% (48/48), respectively. The differences in sensitivity at both size thresholds were statistically significant between the inexperienced and expert reader ($p < 0.001$) and the experienced and expert reader ($p < 0.01$). By-patient specificity at 6-mm and 10-mm thresholds for the inexperienced, experienced, and expert readers was 86% and 95%, 90% and 98%, and 100% and 100%, respectively. The mean interpretation times for the inexperienced, experienced, and expert readers were similar at 9:39 ± 3:23, 10:00 ± 3:57, and 8:14 ± 2:50 minutes, respectively.

Our overall impressions were that (1) effective 3D polyp detection is attainable with minimal training; (2) although the nonexpert readers did well, perfor-

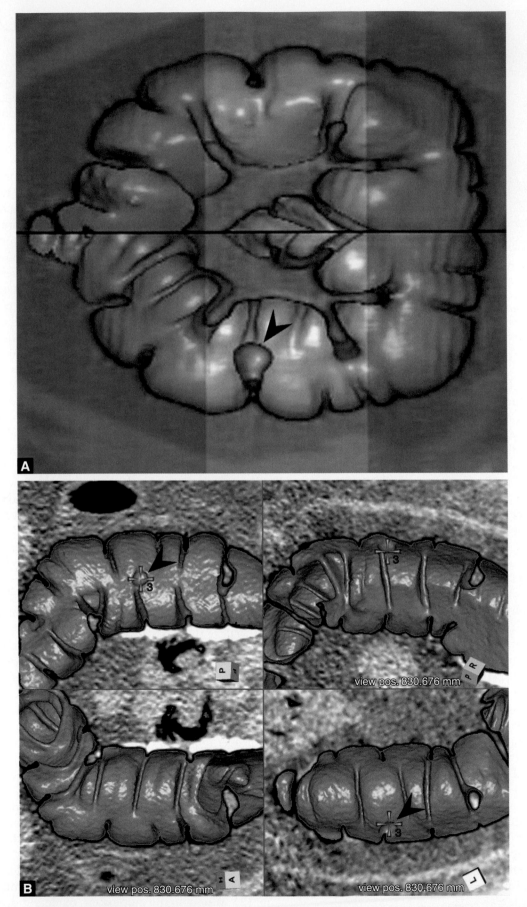

Figure 23-14 **Undistorted bisection segment view.** Images from two different vendors **(A** and **B)** demonstrate polyps *(arrowheads)* within segments that have been uncovered by this clamshell view. Note the lack of spatial distortion.

mance continues to improve up to the expert level; and (3) the learning curve for easiest for the standard endoluminal view.

INTERACTIVE 3D COLON MAP

An interactive 3D colon map is a vital CTC component for assessment of study quality, for CTC interpretation, and for effective communication of positive results (Fig. 23-15). Before CTC interpretation is performed, segmentation of the large intestine is required, including computation of an automated centerline. If a noncolonic gas-filled viscus (e.g., small bowel) is included in the model during the automated segmentation process, most systems allow the user to interact with the 3D map and extract only the relevant anatomy (Fig. 23-16). Prior to commencing CTC interpretation, the colon map allows for a rapid detailed assessment of luminal distention, including supine–prone correlation, to ensure diagnostic evaluation or to indicate areas of persistent underdistention.

For CTC interpretation, the 3D map and automated centerline are critical for effective and efficient 3D evaluation. The centerline allows for automated fly-through, largely reserving manual navigation for areas of potential concern. The 3D map also provides for precise localization in real time, allows for a display of bookmarks to indicate positive findings, and also allows for

efficient supine–prone correlation. In addition, the 3D map provides a way to rapidly and accurately reposition the desired vantage point. With regard to reporting of results, the 3D map effectively communicates location of positive findings (see Chapter 25) and depicts relevant anatomy, such as excessively tortuous cases (see Chapter 9).[19] Effective localization of positive results with the 3D map applies to both endoscopic and surgical referral and to CTC surveillance.

SUMMARY

In conclusion, 3D imaging displays complement 2D evaluation at CTC interpretation. The 3D endoluminal view gives rise to the term "virtual colonoscopy," but a host of alternative 3D displays that do not resemble OC have also been developed. In general, 3D volume rendered displays are intended to provide for effective and efficient polyp detection, leaving the 2D display primarily for confirmation of 3D-detected findings. However, among the advanced 3D projections, there is an important tradeoff between the degree of luminal surface visualized at one time and the amount of geometric distortion that is introduced. If spatial distortion is severe enough, or is not properly recognized, significant polyps may be missed. We believe that our modified interpretive approach that consists of single-pass evaluation through the 3D endoluminal display with a 120-degree FOV

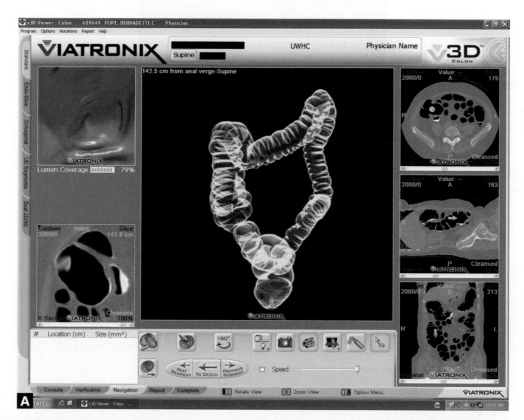

Figure 23-15   3D colon maps. Images from one vendor show examples of transparent **(A)**

Illustration continued on following page

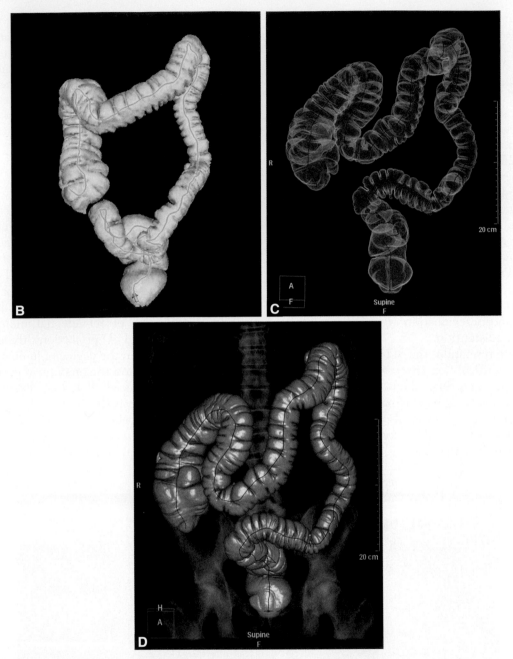

Figure 23-15 (Continued)   **3D colon maps.** and opaque **(B)** 3D maps. Images from another vendor also show examples of transparent **(C)** and opaque **(D)** versions of the colon map. We generally prefer opaque colon maps because bookmarks are better seen and the anatomy is easier to identify.

strikes an effective balance between efficiency and efficacy. However, continued interest and research in alternative views, in conjunction with expanded clinical implementation, should ultimately lead to an optimized hybrid interpretive approach that combines a variety of imaging displays (Fig. 23-17). Regardless of whether or not an alternative 3D view is used for polyp detection, displaying the positive results in such a format will likely cause confusion among referring physicians and endoscopists. Therefore, we would still recommend reporting, communicating, and archiving positive findings with standard nondistorting 2D and 3D displays.

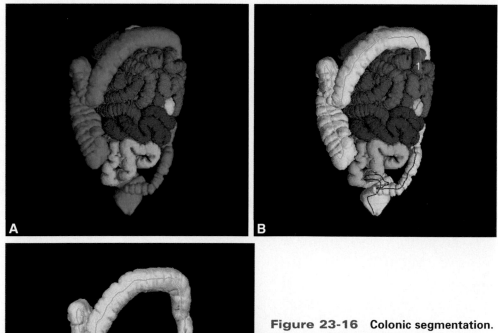

Figure 23-16 Colonic segmentation.
With most CTC software systems, the colon is automatically extracted and a centerline is determined. However, small bowel will often be included in the initial segmentation **(A),** which simply requires the user to select out the colon **(B),** which excludes any extracolonic structures **(C).**

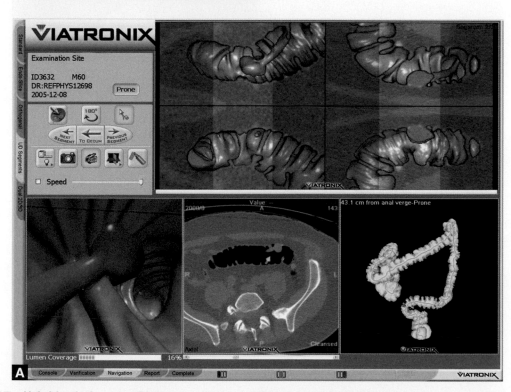

Figure 23-17   Hybrid solutions combining a number of different 2D and 3D display modes. Screen captures from three different vendors **(A-C)** show a variety of interpretive solutions that incorporate a number of different display modes. The individual user can generally choose a customized profile that he or she finds most suitable.   *Illustration continued on following page*

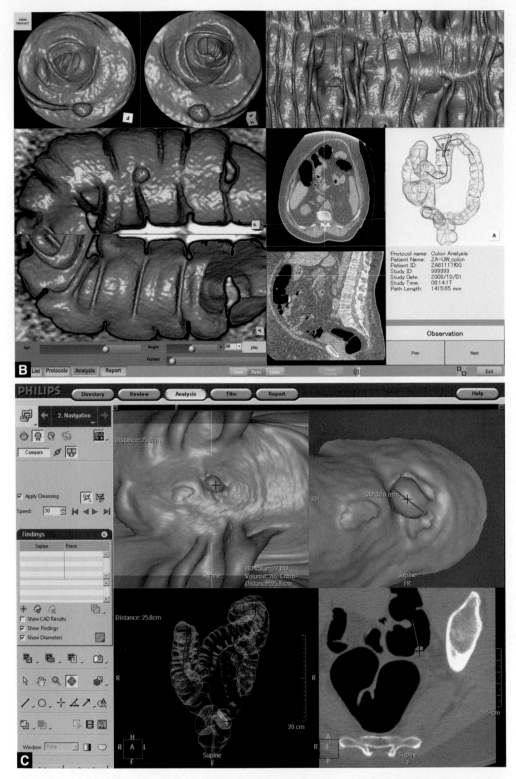

Figure 23-17 (Continued) **Hybrid solutions combining a number of different 2D and 3D display modes.**

REFERENCES

1. Pickhardt PJ. Three-dimensional endoluminal CT colonography (virtual colonoscopy): Comparison of three commercially available systems. *Am J Roentgenol.* 2003;181(6):1599-1606.

2. Pickhardt PJ, Taylor AJ, Gopal DV. Surface visualization at 3D endoluminal CT colonography: Degree of coverage and implications for polyp detection. *Gastroenterology.* 2006;130(6):1582-1587.

3. Pickhardt PJ, Choi JR, Hwang I, et al. Computed tomographic virtual colonoscopy to screen for colorectal neoplasia in asymptomatic adults. *N Engl J Med.* 2003;349(23):2191-2200.

4. Kim DH, Pickhardt PJ, Taylor AJ, et al. CT colonography versus colonoscopy for the detection of advanced neoplasia. *N Engl J Med.* 2007;357(14):1403-1412.

5. Schumacher C, Pickhardt PJ, Hinshaw JL, Kim DH. Effect of the field-of-view angle on 3D endoluminal surface coverage at CT colonography. Chicago: RSNA Scientific Assembly; 2007.

6. Pickhardt PJ, Schumacher C, Kim DH, Hinshaw JL. Increased field-of-view angle at 3D endoluminal CT colonography with one-way fly-through: Impact on polyp detection and interpretation time. Boston: 8th International VC Symposium; 2007.

7. Macari M, Milano A, Lavelle M, Berman P, Megibow AJ. Comparison of time-efficient CT colonography with two- and three-dimensional colonic evaluation for detecting colorectal polyps. *Am J Roentgenol.* 2000;174(6):1543-1549.

8. Juchems MS, Fleiter TR, Pauls S, Schmidt SA, Brambs HJ, Aschoff AJ. CT colonography: comparison of a colon dissection display versus 3D endoluminal view for the detection of polyps. *Eur Radiol.* 2006;16(1):68-72.

9. Johnson CD, Chen MH, Toledano AY, et al. Accuracy of CT colonography for detection of large adenomas and cancers. *N Engl J Med.* 2008;359(12):1207-1217.

10. Silva AC, Wellnitz CV, Hara AK. Three-dimensional virtual dissection at CT colonography: Unraveling the colon to search for lesions. *Radiographics.* 2006;26(6):1669-1686.

11. Kim SH, Lee JM, Eun HW, et al. Two-versus three-dimensional colon evaluation with recently developed virtual dissection software for CT colonography. *Radiology.* 2007;244(3):852-864.

12. Johnson CD, Fletcher JG, MacCarty RL, et al. Effect of slice thickness and primary 2D versus 3D virtual dissection on colorectal lesion detection at CT colonography in 452 asymptomatic adults. *Am J Roentgenol.* 2007;189(3):672-680.

13. Hoppe H, Quattropani C, Spreng A, Mattich J, Netzer P, Dinkel HP. Virtual colon dissection with CT colonography compared with axial interpretation and conventional colonoscopy: Preliminary results. *Am J Roentgenol.* 2004;182(5):1151-1158.

14. Carrascosa P, Capunay C, Lopez EM, Ulla M, Castiglioni R, Carrascosa J. Multidetector CT colonoscopy: Evaluation of the perspective-filet view virtual colon dissection technique for the detection of elevated lesions. *Abdom Imag.* 2007;32:582-588.

15. Vos FM, van Gelder RE, Serlie IWO, et al. Three-dimensional display modes for CT colonography: Conventional 3D virtual colonoscopy versus unfolded cube projection. *Radiology.* 2003;228(3):878-885.

16. Beaulieu CF, Jeffrey RB, Karadi C, Paik DS, Napel S. Display modes for CT colonography—Part II. Blinded comparison of axial CT and virtual endoscopic and panoramic endoscopic volume-rendered studies. *Radiology.* 1999;212(1):203-212.

17. Cubin E, Hinshaw JL, Meiners RJ, Pickhardt PJ. Polyp detection at 3D CT colonography according to reader experience level. Maui, HI: Annual Meeting of the Society for Gastrointestinal Radiology; 2009.

18. Cubin E, Hinshaw JL, Meiners RJ, Pickhardt PJ. Comparison of 3D polypdetection sensitivity on standard endoluminal, perspective filet, and unfolded cube displays at CT colonography. Boston: American Roentgen Ray Society Annual Meeting; 2009.

19. Hanson ME, Pickhardt PJ, Kim DH, Pfau PR. Anatomic factors predictive of incomplete colonoscopy based on findings at CT colonography. *Am J Roentgenol.* 2007;189(4):774-779.

Chapter 24

Computer-Aided Detection/ Diagnosis (CAD) in CT Colonography

DAVID H. KIM, MD
PERRY J. PICKHARDT, MD

INTRODUCTION

Computer-aided detection/diagnosis (CAD) is an area of considerable research and potential benefit to CT colonography (CTC). The task of detecting polyps within the long tubular structure of the colon lends itself to computerized algorithms to detect focal projections into the lumen. The true impact of CAD systems currently remains uncertain. Does CAD improve the interpretative performance at CTC, or does it simply increase sensitivity at the expense of specificity? This chapter will explore pertinent issues related to CAD devices including the major classes of devices, the common steps undertaken by CAD systems for device output, the various CAD reader paradigms, the polyp detection performance as documented in the current literature, and the factors that potentially optimize the CAD-reader interaction.

GENERAL PRINCIPLES

The overriding purpose of CAD is to improve the performance of the interpreting physician in regard to colorectal polyp detection and/or diagnosis. This is accomplished by reducing both perceptive and cognitive errors. Perceptive errors are errors in which the radiologist does not detect a polyp that in retrospect is visible on the examination, whereas cognitive errors are ones in which an abnormality is initially detected then discarded as normal. The hope for CAD is to increase a person's sensitivity for a given specificity or, in other words, to move the receiver operating characteristic (ROC) curve upward and toward the left. However, it is possible that the use of CAD may simply move a person along the curve, trading increased sensitivity for decreased specificity (Fig. 24-1). In a screening situation, this alone may be adequate if the increased sensitivity captures the important target lesions and the increase in false-positive results does not add significantly to risk or cost.

The excellent sensitivities at CT colonography by readers using a primary 3D approach unaided by CAD would initially suggest that there is little role for this device. However, the use of CAD adds redundancy to the examination in a positive fashion, assuming the additional time investment is minimal. There is an additional opportunity to detect polyps. Part of the success of CTC in polyp detection is related to the inherent redundancy in the interpretive scheme where multiple opportunities to detect polyps exist via multiple 3D fly-throughs, the missed region tool, and evaluation of multiple 2D series (e.g., supine and prone). Although the impact of CAD may be less for a primary 3D interpretive approach, this redundancy would likely be helpful to maintain high sensitivity. This is likely true particularly for the less experienced reader.[1,2] Perhaps the situation where CAD may hold the greatest benefit occurs for those radiologists (or nonradiologists) who use a primary 2D approach to CTC interpretation. Pure per-

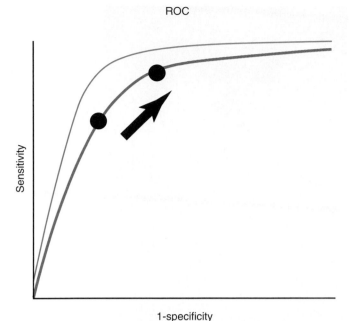

ROC

Sensitivity

1-specificity

Figure 24-1   Effect of CAD on reader performance.
ROC graph shows the potential effects of CAD on reader performance. The hope is that the ROC curve is shifted upward and to the left *(green line)*, consistent with a true improvement in interpretation accuracy, where there is an increase in both sensitivity and specificity. This is in distinction to a shift along the curve between two points *(red arrow)*. Here, increasing sensitivity is offset by decreasing specificity.

ceptual errors may occur with this reading paradigm where polyps are missed. These errors are prevalent, even for large lesions (Fig. 24-2). In one CTC series, 17 of the 30 false-negative results for polyps 10 mm or greater represented perceptual errors resulting from a primary 2D approach.[3] These perceptive errors would likely increase as screening volumes increase related to time constraints in case interpretation. Thus, CAD would be helpful for 2D readers to maintain adequate polyp sensitivities. In addition, it is important to realize that there are specific situations where a primary 2D CTC read is required. That is, although we would stress that a primary 3D evaluation should be the default manner for polyp detection in CTC interpretation, there are situations where it cannot be reasonably undertaken. One such instance is in the case of poor catharsis and large amounts of residual tagged stool in the colon (Fig. 24-3). A primary 3D approach would be difficult to use because of the numerous pseudopolyps related to stool that would require multiple 2D correlations. In such a case, a primary 2D approach is required. CAD would then be a useful adjunct to ensure that a large polyp is not overlooked given this approach. Along the same lines, CAD may be part of the solution for interpretation of tagged datasets of "prepless" (i.e., noncathartic) techniques.

Some pertinent issues currently concerning CAD involve both technical adaptations to the evolving CTC examination and the complex interaction between the device and the human reader. On the technical side, the tagging agents now in current use provide particular challenges to CAD related to the issues of pseudoenhancement and distortion of shape information.[4] Will CAD devices appropriately detect polyps on tagged datasets? In addition, questions related to CAD performance on ultra-low–dose CTC examinations are under investigation. On the device–individual interaction side, current issues include the appropriate reader paradigm for CAD (see later). What are the safeguards against the application of a first-reader paradigm for current applications? Will a first-reader paradigm ever be acceptable to the medical community or health care consumer? Other questions such as the effects of multiple false-positive CAD marks on the reader remain largely unknown (Fig. 24-4). Intuitively, multiple CAD false-positive marks or "hits" would presumably negatively affect reader performance, although there is some limited evidence to suggest that the effect may be neglible.[5] All of these issues are areas of continuing investigation and will ultimately have an impact on the overall usefulness and how CAD is used in CTC.

CADe AND CADx

CAD devices are broadly divided into detection devices (CADe) and diagnostic devices (CADx). CADe devices are those designed to influence detection tasks. The purpose is to reduce perceptual errors. The image is processed through the CADe algorithm, and an internal likelihood ratio is created for possible abnormal areas. If the number is higher than a set threshold, the "abnormality" is marked for reader review. Although the algorithm and purpose are detection, there is an element of diagnosis even at this step where the algorithm decides if an area meets the abnormal threshold (Fig. 24-5). Typically, CADe devices are set to mark a number of false positives to encompass the total population of true positives and minimize false negatives. The reader makes the final decision regarding the various potentially abnormal regions. With CADe devices, the reader is not provided with any information regarding the likelihood that a "hit" may be a true positive, such as a priority score or confidence level from the system. CADx devices add a layer of complexity where the identified abnormality is characterized. The algorithm generates a likelihood score for diagnosis (e.g., for a true polyp or for malignancy), which is presented to the reader (Fig. 24-5). The purpose of CAD in this situation is to decrease cognitive errors in addition to perceptive errors. Interfaces with CADx development for clinical CTC are only in their infancy at this time.

CAD devices use software algorithms to detect specific patterns within the presented radiologic images. This algorithm and the specific mathematic transforma-

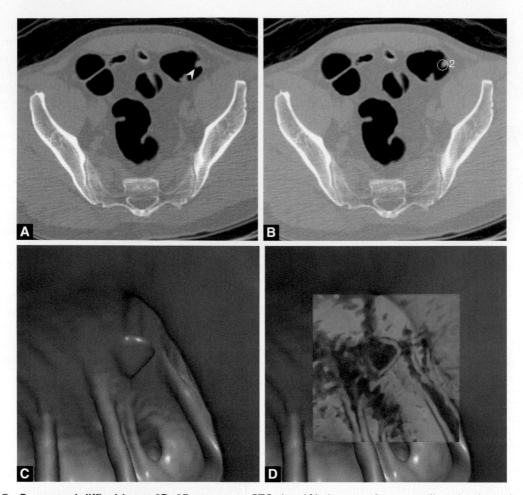

Figure 24-2 **Perceptual difficulties at 2D.** 2D transverse CTC view **(A)** shows a 10-mm sessile polyp *(arrowhead)* in the sigmoid colon. Despite its large size and the excellent prep and distention result, this lesion is somewhat difficult to distinguish from a fold and could be missed by a primary 2D approach. Thus, CAD may be helpful in this circumstance by successfully detecting this lesion (marked with an open circle, **B**). 3D endoluminal CTC image **(C)** clearly depicts the polyp morphology. Perceptual difficulties are less of an issue at primary 3D interpretation, in which polyps are easily distinguished from folds. The application of translucency **(D)** demonstrates the soft tissue nature of this lesion, which proved to be a tubular adenoma after resection at OC.

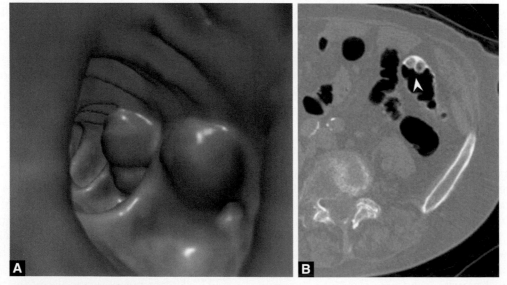

Figure 24-3 **Poorly prepped CTC and the need for a 2D approach.** 3D endoluminal view **(A)** shows multiple polypoid masses related to retained stool. In such poorly prepped cases, a primary 3D approach to polyp detection may be impossible, thus requiring a primary 2D approach **(B)** to interpretation. Here, the polypoid masses are noted to simply represent stool *(arrowhead)* in the sigmoid colon. CAD may be beneficial in enhancing performance in this situation, pointing out any potential true polyps amongst stool.

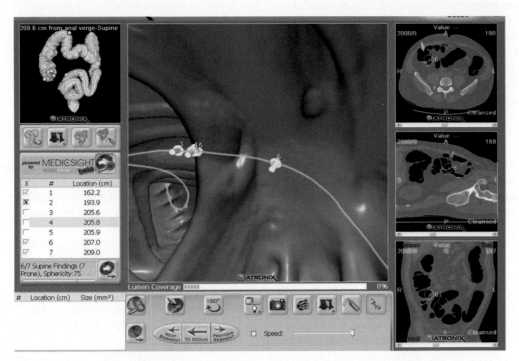

Figure 24-4   False-positive (FP) CAD marks. Screen capture of a CTC platform with active CAD demonstrates multiple false-positive marks *(arrows #3-5)*, which point out the ileocecal valve. Both the valve and the rectal catheter are the source of many FP marks, which are easily dismissed. Note the CAD mark pointing out a true polyp in the cecum *(arrow #6)*. The soft tissue nature is seen on the 2D MPR views *(right side of screen)*.

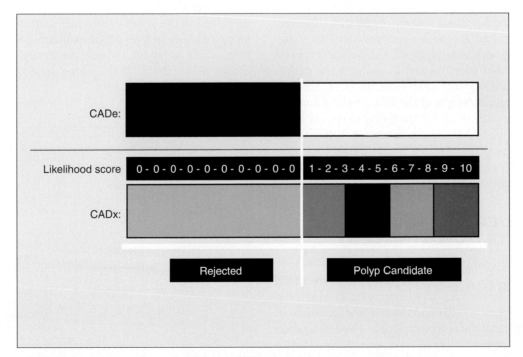

Figure 24-5   CADe versus CADx. Schematic diagram depicts the differences between detection and diagnosis devices. In actuality, they perform very similar functions. However, the output values of the CADx devices are reported to the user to give a confidence score for a real disease entity *(likelihood number or color-coded scale)*, whereas the CADe devices simply report whether a threshold for abnormality was met or not *(black versus white)* in a binary fashion.

tion and the manner in which this is accomplished typically are hidden away and unknown to the reader. These software algorithms are unique and the exact process for polyp detection is different from one CAD system to the next. However, there are some general common steps undertaken by all devices (Fig. 24-6).[6-9] The image to be assessed by CAD is postprocessed to facilitate reading, including such changes as alteration in image contrast or sharpening of structure edges within the image. The area of interest (here, the colon and rectum) is then segmented out for consideration, and a set of specific features are calculated within each pixel or voxel. Some examples of features that are considered include shape, size, and curvature, but many others may be used depending on the particular CAD system. The number and specific features are often different among CAD systems. The various features are then inserted into a learning algorithm or *classifier*. The learning algorithm may be a neural network, kernel machine, or decision tree. Typically, all of the features are transformed into a single numeric value resulting in a likelihood for disease. Thresholding is set and numbers higher than the set point are marked for reader consideration. If these values were to be presented to the reader, the CADe device would then be functioning as a CADx device.

Modifications to the features, learning algorithms, and thresholds are made during device optimization or training of the device. Akin to a radiologist gaining experience in evaluating CT examinations and learning to detect disease, the device is applied to a set of cases (the training set) and modifications are made to improve pattern recognition. Once the device is optimized, the device is applied to a new set of cases (the test set) to evaluate the performance of the CAD system. The cases must be different ones from the training set, and the test set should mimic the intended population of the device. It is important to remember that the CAD system detection is fixed after training and there is no adaptive learning over time with future cases. Further changes in device performance occur only with subsequent software revisions.

CAD READER PARADIGMS AND INTERPRETATION STRATEGY

Three reader paradigms for CAD exist. These include CAD as a *first reader*, *second reader*, and *concurrent reader* (Fig. 24-7). The first reader paradigm is one in which the CAD system interacts with the dataset and presents all potential polyp candidates to the reader. The reader then confirms or discards each mark as a true polyp. In this scenario, the entire examination is not reviewed by the reader. Instead, only the potentially abnormal areas pointed out CAD are examined. Such an approach leads to marked time savings. Currently, no CAD systems for CTC operate by this paradigm. The current CAD technology would likely lead to erroneous diagnoses and un-

acceptable results. One major reason involves the issue of colorectal masses. Most CAD systems are not optimized for large cancers but for simpler endoluminal projections/polyps. Certainly, cancer can be detected (typically recognized as multiple individual CAD "hits" on several discrete lobulations or focal projections; Fig. 24-8) but sensitivities can be unacceptably low (43% sensitivity for cancer by one CAD system).[2] In a situation in which the human reader evaluates the entire case, such deficiencies in CAD systems are not as much a problem because of the ease of human detection for large annular masses. However, in the first reader CAD paradigm, such deficiencies would hold significant negative consequences. In addition, such an adoption of a reader strategy would certainly represent a departure from the philosophy that the physician holds primary responsibility for the examination, where CAD is an adjunctive aid for the physician in interpretation.

The second reader paradigm is one in which the radiologist evaluates the examination as the first reader. Following a complete interpretation, the CAD results are then displayed. In other words, once the human interpretation is complete and all potential polyp candidates have been evaluated, the physician turns on the CAD system and evaluates any additional polyp candidates that are identified. The physician then determines if any of these additional polyp candidates are in fact true polyps. In this reader paradigm, the CAD device acts as a second reader to add redundancy in polyp detection. As described in the general principle section, this will likely be particularly helpful when evaluating the examination from a 2D approach, where perceptual errors may increase in number. Of the three strategies, the second

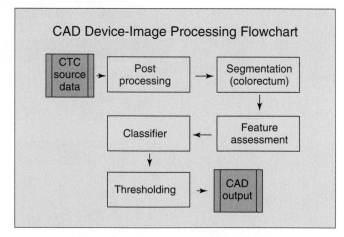

Figure 24-6 **CAD imaging processing flowchart.** Schematic shows the flowchart of steps that CAD devices undertake to the final output. Although the specific algorithms are unique to each CAD device, including how the image is postprocessed, the following generic steps are common to all: how the colon is segmented out, what polyps features are used, what classifier is applied, and what the threshold levels are.

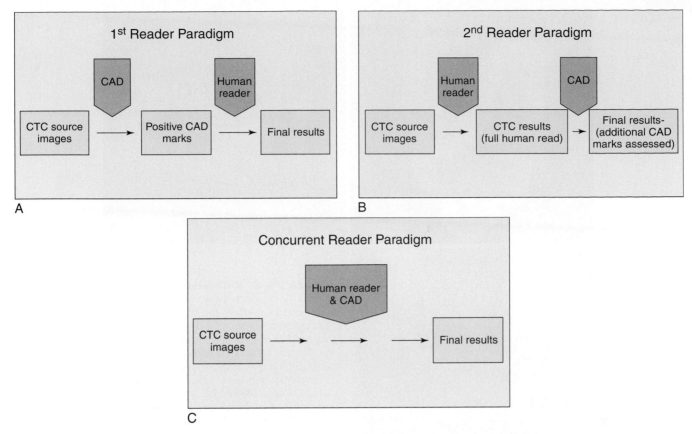

Figure 24-7 CAD reader paradigms. Various schematics demonstrate the possible reader strategies with CAD. The first reader paradigm **(A)** holds marked time savings where only the CAD marks, not the entire examination, are examined by the reader. In the second reader paradigm **(B)**, CAD is used as a double reader (or "spell checker") where it is applied only after the reader has completed full interpretation. In the concurrent reader paradigm **(C)**, CAD is operational as the reader initially evaluates the study.

reader approach for CAD is the one preferred by regulatory bodies such as the U.S. Food and Drug Administration. The main disadvantage of the second reader paradigm is one of increased time because it may add up to 4 minutes to the interpretation.[10]

The final potential strategy is the concurrent reader paradigm. Here, the CAD device is on while the physician undertakes initial evaluation of the entire case. The physician can assess both polyp candidates that he or she detects and the ones marked by CAD at the same time. Studies have demonstrated a time savings over the second read methodology.[10] However, the main concern with this paradigm is the possibility that the reader may migrate toward more of a first reader use. That is, it becomes tempting to relax vigilance for polyps and concentrate simply on the CAD marks with this method.

In our opinion, the interpretation strategy with CAD should revolve around the following: CAD should be used in the second reader paradigm. Polyp detection should be performed as in the unassisted case with a primary 3D approach with focused secondary 2D review, particularly for relatively collapsed areas and areas filled by opacified fluid (see Chapters 16 and 17). Following a complete, unassisted read, the CAD application should

be activated and the CAD polyp marks should be tabbed through on the 2D series, which can be done very quickly (Fig. 24-9). All polyp candidates that are potentially real should then be assessed on 3D to confirm polyp morphology and on the complementary 2D view to confirm soft tissue attenuation. Polyp candidates that meet these criteria should be seriously considered to represent true positives. The polyp list generated by both pre-CAD and post-CAD review can ultimately be combined.

CAD PERFORMANCE RESULTS

CAD devices are evaluated by two major study designs: standalone performance studies and reader performance studies. Both are important to determine the overall utility of CAD. Standalone performance determines the inherent sensitivity and specificity of the CAD system for the target lesion—in the case of CTC, the detection of polyps. By convention, the sensitivity and number of false positives per series (or study) are usually noted as the main output measures. CAD systems are typically set at a level to minimize the number of false negatives. In addition to overall polyp detection performance, the performance on specific substrata (subcatego-

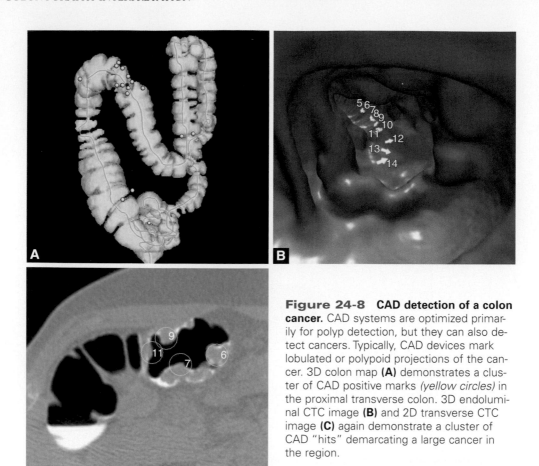

Figure 24-8 CAD detection of a colon cancer. CAD systems are optimized primarily for polyp detection, but they can also detect cancers. Typically, CAD devices mark lobulated or polypoid projections of the cancer. 3D colon map **(A)** demonstrates a cluster of CAD positive marks *(yellow circles)* in the proximal transverse colon. 3D endoluminal CTC image **(B)** and 2D transverse CTC image **(C)** again demonstrate a cluster of CAD "hits" demarcating a large cancer in the region.

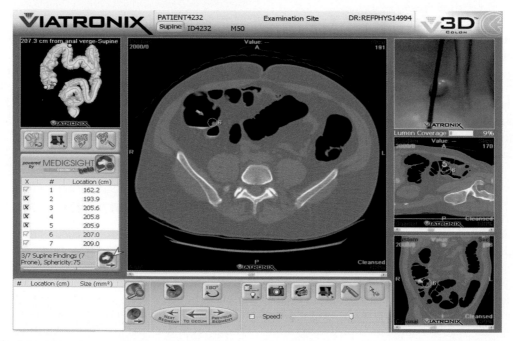

Figure 24-9 Second reader paradigm and workstation integration. Screen capture of the Viatronix platform with the Medicsight Colon-CAD module *(lower left on image)*. Our opinion is that CAD should be applied in the second reader paradigm. After full interpretation, the various CAD hits should be tabbed through on the 2D images by simply pressing a button *(arrowhead)*. The various CAD marks can be accepted *(green checkmarks)* or rejected *(red Xs)*.

ries) is important. For example, the detection performance for the CAD system can be assessed for sessile lesions, pedunculated lesions, and flat lesions. Thus, whether a CAD system maintains similar performance for flat lesions may be important because this is a subgroup recognized to be more difficult to detect compared to sessile lesions.[11-13] Other polyp subgroups such as those stratified by size or location can be assessed. The diagnostic performance in patient subgroups such as those with extensive diverticulosis can also be determined.

The second study type for CAD assessment involves reader performance studies. A CAD system may demonstrate intrinsic high performance for polyp detection on standalone studies yet only minimally improve overall detection during the human interaction. Reader performance studies are equally important for determining the overall utility of the CAD unit given the complex interaction between the CAD system and the reader using it. Such interaction may maintain or improve the standalone results or may woefully depress performance. For example, a CAD system may demonstrate adequate sensitivity yet produce too many CAD marks, leading the reader to discount even the true-positive CAD marks and thus decreasing performance. However, a CAD system may have low standalone sensitivity but tend to detect lesions that were missed by human readers, which may improve overall performance.[14] Accepted study de-

signs include multiple reader multicase (MRMC) studies to improve generalizability of results. ROC analysis is favored to assess true improvement as opposed to simply calculating sensitivity/false-positive rate measurements where an increase in sensitivity with a decrease in specificity may or may not represent true improvement.

Standalone performance studies of various CAD systems have demonstrated very good sensitivity results in the low 90% range for large ($\geq$10 mm) polyps and variable lower sensitivities ranging from 61% to 92% at the 6-mm threshold (Fig. 24-10). The number of false-positive marks per patient ranged from 2 to 14 per case in these studies.[6,15-18] Unfortunately, the majority of the standalone performance studies have involved fairly small test samples. In addition, the actual performance could ultimately differ depending on the specific substrata. For example, the sensitivity for flat lesions by the CAD system may not be as robust as the reported overall sensitivity. In one study of flat T1 cancers, sensitivities ranged from 83% (20/24) to 54% (13/24) dependent on various CAD settings.[19] Of the standalone studies, one study that was conducted on a large subset of asymptomatic screening individuals from the Department of Defense (DoD) CTC trial is of particular merit.[16] The test evaluation set for this study comprised 792 cases randomly selected from the total patient population of the original DoD trial, thus closely approximating an

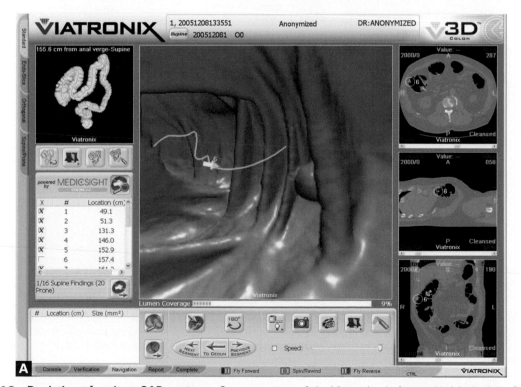

Figure 24-10 Depiction of various CAD systems. Screen capture of the Viatronix platform with Medicsight Colon-CAD module **(A)** demonstrates a static image from a concurrent read paradigm. Here, the CAD is operational and the CAD marks are seen on the 3D endoluminal display as arrows pointing to the abnormality off the automated centerline. These are visible during the dynamic endoluminal fly-through.

Illustration continued on following page

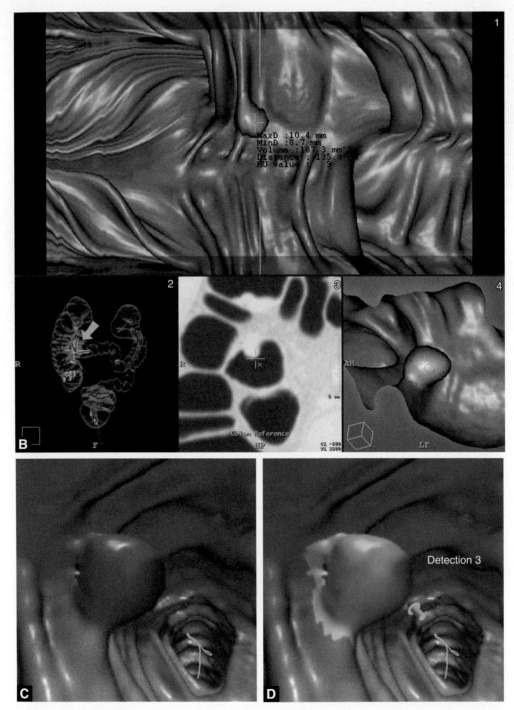

Figure 24-10 (Continued) **Depiction of various CAD systems.** Screen capture of the Philips EBW platform with perspective filet and Philips CAD **(B)** shows a CAD-detected polyp in blue. The maximum linear size and volume are calculated automatically. 3D endoluminal CTC image without **(C)** and with CAD **(D)** from a National Institutes of Health CAD module using the Viatronix platform depicts a large polyp painted in blue by CAD.

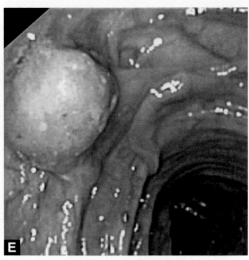

Figure 24-10 (Continued) **Depiction of various CAD systems.** The polyp was confirmed at OC **(E).** (C-E from Summers RM, Yao JH, Pickhardt PJ, et al. Computed tomographic virtual colonoscopy computer-aided polyp detection in a screening population. *Gastroenterology.* 2005;129(6):1832-1844.)

asymptomatic average-risk screening population. The CAD sensitivity was 89% on a per-polyp analysis for adenomatous polyps 10 mm or greater in size. There were 2.1 false positives marked per case. Given the large population size and the application of the CAD in a test case scenario that closely parallels a screening population, there is increased confidence in the generalizability of this study's CAD results.

Reader performance CAD studies have demonstrated an interesting and consistent observation. CAD may be more helpful for inexperienced readers and less so for experienced readers.[1,2,10,20] For the experienced readers, there may not be a substantial increase in sensitivity as seen with inexperienced readers; instead, simply an increased false-positive rate may occur with the use of CAD.[10] For both groups, there is some evidence that CAD may function to shift a person along the ROC curve as opposed to shifting the curve upward and toward the left (and thus representing improved accuracy). In a well-conceived study, Petrick et al.[21] demonstrated that reader performance with CAD increased sensitivity by approximately 15% for polyps 6 mm or greater over unassisted reads but at the expense of specificity, which decreased by 14%. No significant differences were seen in the area under the curve (AUC) for the ROC curve for the different polyp size thresholds. Although this would argue against true improvement in interpretation with CAD, one could argue that in the screening situation, increased sensitivity at the expense of specificity may be worthwhile if the increase in false positives does not significantly increase costs and complications. In general, CAD in the second reader paradigm adds about 3 minutes to the interpretation time, as seen in the Petrick study[21] and in several other studies.[1,5,10]

FACTORS OPTIMIZING CAD PERFORMANCE

The primary purpose of CAD applications is to improve reader performance in polyp detection. This involves many factors, including the intrinsic capability of the CAD and the complex interaction between the system and the reader. From a reader perspective, several factors should be optimized to maximize the capabilities of the CAD system. The end user should be aware of the intended use of the CAD system and its appropriate application (e.g., the specific reader paradigm) to apply CAD in the correct situation. Although the reader does not need to know the intricacies of the underlying diagnostic algorithm, knowledge of the general processes of the system would be helpful. For example, knowledge that the system analyzes the surface characteristics of an abnormal area such as curvature or sphericity can be helpful. In this case, for those lesions that are minimally raised or flat, CAD may have difficulty and the reader would understand why a true lesion may not be marked by the system. It is also important that the reader is aware of the performance characteristics for specific substrata. Knowledge that the sensitivity is 90% for sessile polyps greater than or equal to 10 mm but only 60% for similar-sized flat lesions is helpful. Likewise, poor performance in segments with advanced diverticular disease would be important to recognize if a potential polyp in such an area that looks real is not called by the CAD.

Training in the use of the CAD system is paramount to appropriately use the device. It also is important that the end user obtain feedback through pathologic correlation and longitudinal followup regarding the called (and uncalled) CAD marks and outcomes to gain experience in how CAD affects his or her individual performance in a specific patient population. Without such feedback and learning, polyp detection with CAD will suffer. Halligan et al.[20] demonstrated this in a group of abdominal radiologists equipped with CAD but without formal CTC or CAD training. In this study, CAD positive marks were ignored presumably because of this lack of training. The standalone performance for the CAD system was 90% for greater than or equal to 10 mm polyps, yet the final CAD-assisted sensitivity for the readers was only 51% where true CAD-marked polyps were erroneously discarded.

SUMMARY

CAD holds promise in improving the overall performance in CTC interpretation. At the very least, it holds a role in added redundancy to prevent large important lesions from being missed. In a few specific situations, such as the poorly cleansed colon, it may represent a very useful tool related to the need for a primary 2D read. As screening volumes increase, requiring physicians to more rapidly interpret the CTC dataset, the utility of CAD may increase correspondingly. It remains important that the reader–CAD interface is optimized by education and training specific to the use of CAD. Longitudinal followup with appropriate feedback is a key element for each reader to improve performance with CAD.

REFERENCES

1. Baker ME, Bogoni L, Obuchowski NA, et al. Computer-aided detection of colorectal polyps: Can it improve sensitivity of less-experienced readers? Preliminary findings. *Radiology.* 2007; 245(1):140-149.
2. Mang T, Peloschek P, Plank C, et al. Effect of computer-aided detection as a second reader in multidetector-row CT colonography. *Eur Radiol.* 2007;17(10):2598-2607.
3. Fletcher JG, Johnson CD, Welch TJ, et al. Optimization of CT colonography technique: Prospective trial in 180 patients. *Radiology.* 2000;216(3):704-711.
4. Nappi J, Yoshida H. Fully automated three-dimensional detection of polyps in fecal-tagging CT colonography. *Acad Radiol.* 2007;14(3):287-300.
5. Taylor SA, Greenhalgh R, Ilangovan R, et al. CT colonography and computer-aided detection: Effect of false-positive results on reader specificity and reading efficiency in a low-prevalence screening population. *Radiology.* 2008;247(1):133-140.
6. Yoshida H, Nappi J, MacEneaney P, Rubin DT, Dachman AH. Computer-aided diagnosis scheme for detection of polyps at CT colonography. *Radiographics.* 2002;22(4):963-979.
7. Summers RM, Johnson CD, Pusanik LM, Malley JD, Youssef AM, Reed JE. Automated polyp detection at CT colonography: Feasibility assessment in a human population. *Radiology.* 2001;219(1): 51-59.
8. Summers RM, Franaszek M, Miller MT, Pickhardt PJ, Choi JR, Schindler WR. Computer-aided detection of polyps on oral contrast-enhanced CT colonography. *Am J Roentgenol.* 2005;184 (1):105-108.
9. Jerebko AK, Summers RM, Malley JD, Franaszek M, Johnson CD. Computer-assisted detection of colonic polyps with CT colonography using neural networks and binary classification trees. *Med Phys.* 2003;30(1):52-60.
10. Taylor SA, Charman SC, Lefere P, et al. CT colonography: Investigation of the optimum reader paradigm by using computer-aided detection software. *Radiology.* 2008;246(2):463-471.
11. Pickhardt PJ, Nugent PA, Choi JR, Schindler WR. Flat colorectal lesions in asymptomatic adults: Implications for screening with CT virtual colonoscopy. *Am J Roentgenol.* 2004;183(5):1343-1347.
12. Park SH, Ha HK, Kim AY, et al. Flat polyps of the colon: Detection with 16-MDCT colonography—Preliminary results. *Am J Roentgenol.* 2006;186(6):1611-1617.
13. Park SH, Lee SS, Choi EK, et al. Flat colorectal neoplasms: Definition, importance, and visualization on CT colonography. *Am J Roentgenol.* 2007;188(4):953-959.
14. Summers RM, Jerebko AK, Franaszek M, Malley JD, Johnson CD. Colonic polyps: Complementary role of computer-aided detection in CT colonography. *Radiology.* 2002;225(2):391-399.
15. Taylor SA, Halligan S, Burling D, et al. Computer-assisted reader software versus expert reviewers for polyp detection on CT colonography. *Am J Roentgenol.* 2006;186(3):696-702.
16. Summers RM, Yao JH, Pickhardt PJ, et al. Computed tomographic virtual colonoscopy computer-aided polyp detection in a screening population. *Gastroenterology.* 2005;129(6):1832-1844.
17. Kim SH, Lee JM, Lee JG, et al. Computer-aided detection of colonic polyps at CT colonography using a Hessian matrix-based algorithm: Preliminary study. *Am J Roentgenol.* 2007;189(1):41-51.
18. Nappi J, Okamura A, Frimmel H, Dachman A, Yoshida H. Region-based supine-prone correspondence for the reduction of false-positive CAD polyp candidates in CT colonography. *Acad Radiol.* 2005;12(6):695-707.
19. Taylor SA, Iinuma G, Saito Y, Zhang J, Halligan S. CT colonography: computer-aided detection of morphologically flat T1 colonic carcinoma. *Eur Radiol.* 2008;18(8):1666-1673.
20. Halligan S, Altman DG, Mallett S, et al. Computed tomographic colonography: Assessment of radiologist performance with and without computer-aided detection. *Gastroenterology.* 2006;131 (6):1690-1699.
21. Petrick N, Haider M, Summers RM, et al. CT colonography with computer-aided detection as a second reader: Observer performance study. *Radiology.* 2008;246(1):148-156.

Endoscopic and Surgical Referral from CTC

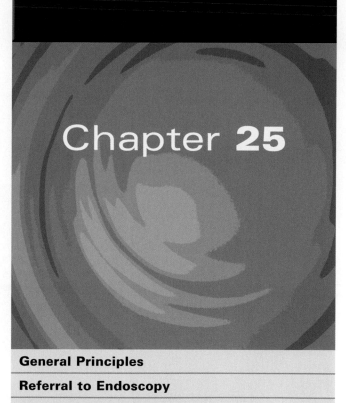

Chapter 25

PERRY J. PICKHARDT, MD
DAVID H. KIM, MD

General Principles

Referral to Endoscopy

Preoperative Assessment with CTC

GENERAL PRINCIPLES

CT colonography (CTC) is a minimally invasive yet accurate test for colorectal evaluation. As such, CTC can avoid the need for more invasive investigations such as optical colonoscopy (OC) or surgery in the majority of cases by excluding relevant pathology. For those patients in whom CTC detects a significant lesion, referral to endoscopy is generally indicated. For more complex or likely malignant lesions, surgical resection may be necessary. As discussed later in this chapter, CTC can provide detailed information that is valuable to both the endoscopist and the surgeon. CTC is currently underused by colorectal surgeons for preoperative assessment, but its role will undoubtedly increase once its utility is better appreciated.

REFERRAL TO ENDOSCOPY

There are a number of indications for referral to OC following CTC examination. The most common indication by far is for significant polyps detected at CTC. In our practice, this is primarily for large polyps (≥10 mm), corresponding to C-RADS (CT Colonography Reporting and Data System) category C3, where polypectomy is clearly indicated. However, a significant fraction of OC referrals are for small polyps (6-9 mm), including individuals with one or two small polyps (C-RADS category C2) who opt for immediate polypectomy instead of CTC surveillance and a small minority with three or more small polyps (C-RADS category C3) where OC is generally recommended (Fig. 25-1).[1] In symptomatic and asymptomatic patients, an invasive mass (C-RADS category C4) detected at CTC will generally undergo preoperative OC for tissue diagnosis, although the added benefit of this additional invasive test for obvious cancers could be questioned in some cases. Beyond detection of significant pol-

yps and masses, nondiagnostic segmental evaluation as a result of persistent collapse, spasm, or stricture (C-RADS category C0) is another potential indication for endoscopic referral. Because such nondiagnostic evaluation almost always involves the left colon related to diverticular disease (sigmoid > descending), same-day flexible sigmoidoscopy (FS) without sedation may be performed to avoid the need for additional preparation (Fig. 25-2). Rare indications for OC referral from CTC may include newly diagnosed terminal ileitis (Fig. 25-3), atypical colitis (in the appropriate clinical setting), or innumerable lesions of diminutive size, for which OC may be used to confirm and sample a representative lesion or two.

For the typical referral of a positive CTC study to OC for polypectomy, some standard information is supplied to the endoscopist. Via the PACS system, we routinely network images of the 3D colon map and pertinent 2D and endoluminal 3D images (Fig. 25-4). The 3D map not only indicates the specific location of detected polyps, it also provides an excellent overview of the colonic anatomy and length. This anatomic information can be valuable to the gastroenterologist, particularly in cases with extreme tortuosity, elongation, or diverticular disease (Fig. 25-5). In some of these cases, the patient may have had an incomplete prior OC examination that led to CTC in the first place. In this setting, a case-by-case determination must be made as to whether repeat OC or surgical referral is indicated. Factors that influence this decision include the potential importance of the CTC-detected lesion, the reason for the initial incomplete OC, the specific colorectal anatomy and lesion location, and the skill of the endoscopist involved.

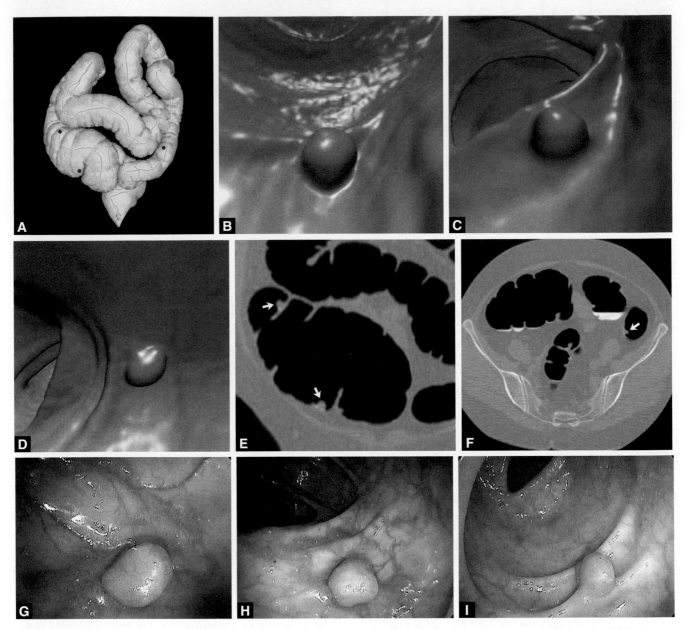

Figure 25-1 **OC referral for C-RADS category C3 finding.** 3D map **(A)** and 3D endoluminal images **(B-D)** from CTC screening study show three small sessile lesions, including a 9-mm cecal polyp **(B)**, 6-mm ascending polyp **(C)**, and 8-mm descending polyp **(D)**. Coronal **(E)** and transverse **(F)** 2D images confirm the soft tissue nature of the three lesions *(arrows)*. Endoscopy was recommended given the C-RADS C3 findings, and all three polyps were subsequently removed at same-day OC **(G-I)** and proved to be tubular adenomas at histologic examination. *(*See associated video clip on DVD.)*

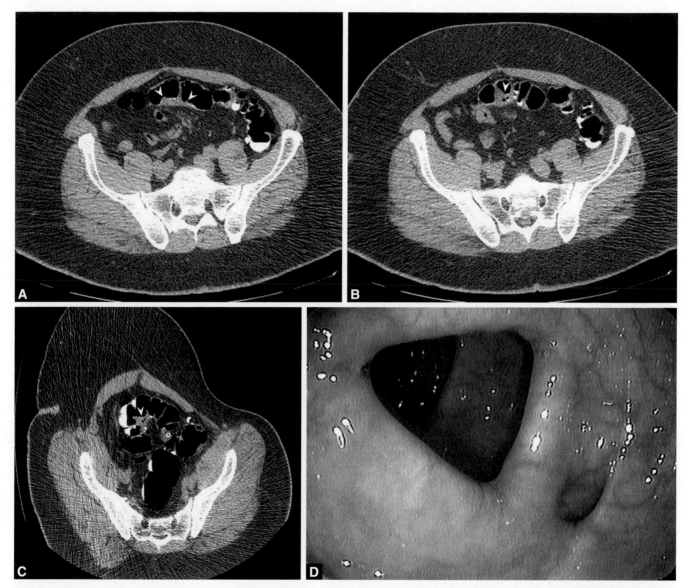

Figure 25-2 **Same-day unsedated flexible sigmoidoscopy (FS) for nondiagnostic CTC evaluation (C-RADS C0).** Supine **(A** and **B)** and right-lateral decubitus **(C)** 2D transverse images show eccentric wall thickening and diverticular changes involving the sigmoid colon *(arrowheads)* that persisted on all views (prone images not shown). Although an atypical appearance of diverticular disease was strongly favored as the underlying cause, same-day flexible sigmoidoscopy without sedation was performed to exclude an unlikely neoplasm given the eccentric wall thickening. Sigmoid diverticular disease without focal mass was confirmed at sigmoidoscopy **(D).**

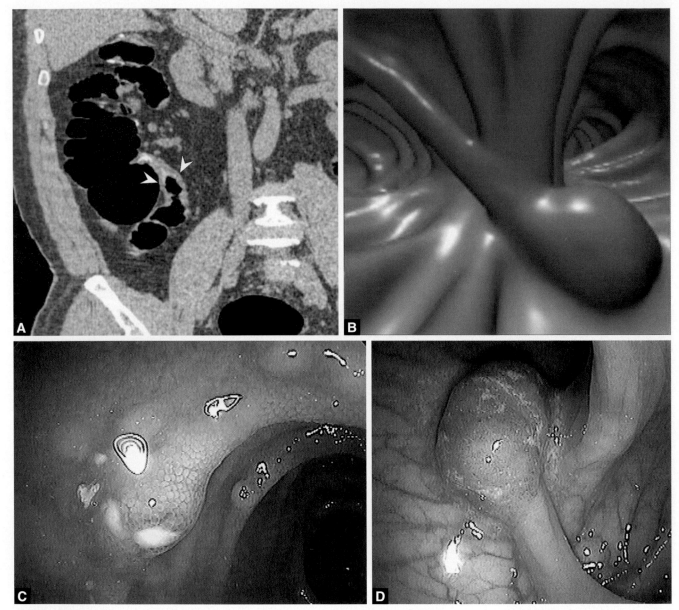

Figure 25-3 OC referral for large sigmoid polyp and suspected terminal ileitis detected at CTC screening. 2D coronal image from CTC screening **(A)** shows irregular wall thickening involving the terminal ileum *(arrowheads)*. The patient also had a 1.2-cm pedunculated polyp in the sigmoid colon **(B)**. At OC, ulceronodular inflammatory changes were seen in the terminal ileum **(C)**. The pedunculated sigmoid polyp **(D)** proved to be a large tubular adenoma.

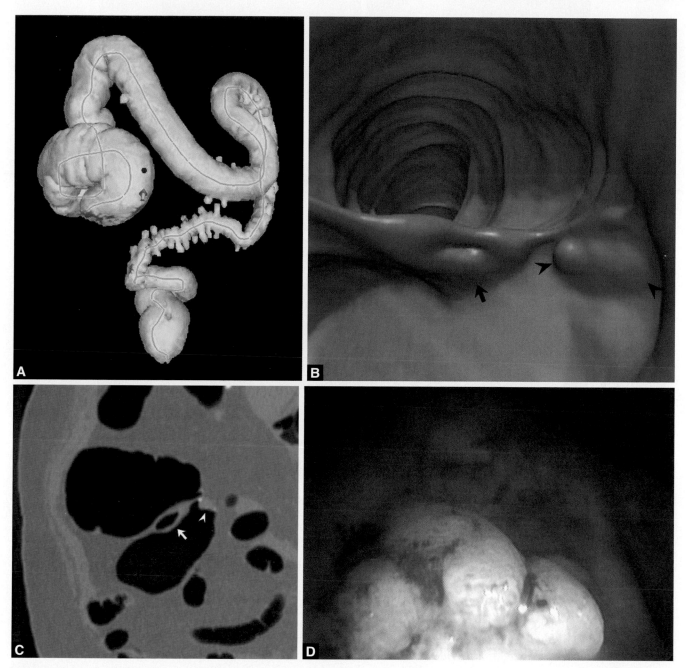

Figure 25-4   **Difficult polyp location for detection and polypectomy at OC.** The standard CTC information provided to endoscopists for positive referral includes a 3D colon map **(A)**, 3D endoluminal images **(B)**, and 2D MPR (multiplanar reconstruction) images **(C)**. The colon map in this case **(A)** shows the precise anatomic location of a CTC-detected cecal polyp *(red dot)*. The map demonstrates the colon anatomy for the endoscopist, including extensive sigmoid diverticulosis in this case. The 3D endoluminal image **(B)** was obtained from the perspective of the cecal tip and shows a relatively subtle 1.5-cm sessile polyp *(arrowheads)* located behind a fold and adjacent to the ileocecal valve *(arrow)*. The 2D coronal image **(C)** confirms a soft tissue lesion *(arrowhead)* next to the ileocecal valve *(arrow)*. The polyp was found and removed at OC and proved to be a tubulovillous adenoma with high-grade dysplasia. However, because of its difficult location, the gastroenterologist noted that he would have missed this lesion without the detailed advanced knowledge of its existence provided by CTC. Furthermore, the polyp was only partially removed at the initial examination, demonstrating progression at followup OC **(D)**. The darker area in the background is an India ink tattoo placed at the prior OC study. (From Pickhardt PJ. Screening CT colonography: How I do it. *Am J Roentgenol.* 2007;189:290-298.) *(*See associated video clip on DVD.)*

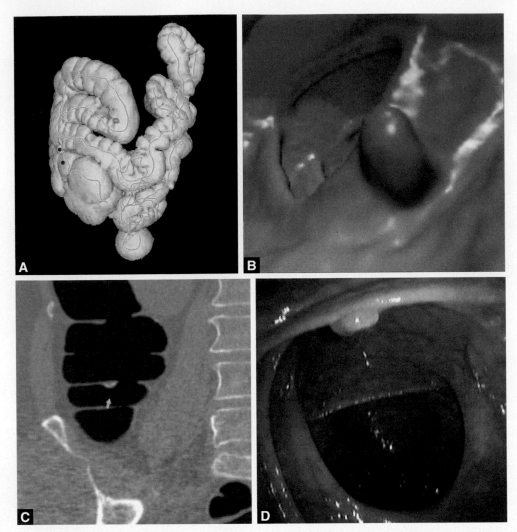

Figure 25-5 **Markedly tortuous colon referred to OC for large right-sided lesions detected at CTC.** The patient had previously undergone several attempted OC and barium enema examinations elsewhere prior to CTC, all of which were incomplete. The 3D map **(A)** shows extensive colonic redundancy and tortuousity, with a total length of more than 260 cm and 16 acute-angle flexure points. The location of two large right-sided polyps is denoted by the red-dot bookmarks. 3D endoluminal **(B)** and 2D coronal **(C)** CTC images show one of these sessile polyps *(arrow)* located on the backside of a fold in the ascending colon. With this CTC knowledge, an experienced endoscopist successfully negotiated the entire colon, confirming and removing large adenomas **(D)** in the process.

For each lesion detected at CTC, representative 2D multiplanar and 3D endoluminal images are provided (Fig. 25-4). In some cases, we also provide a short movie clip that shows the polyp at 3D endoluminal fly-through to simulate the endoscopic view. Basic polyp information that is communicated includes lesion size, morphology, and segmental location. Of note, one should refrain from reporting CTC polyp distances from the anorectal junction. Although these measurements are precise, the endoscopic distance will be considerably less as a result of telescoping and straightening, which could cause unnecessary confusion. Special communication is made for lesions in potentially challenging locations at OC, such as behind a fold or near an inner turn of a flexure (Fig. 25-4). We also score the diagnostic confidence for a given CTC finding on a 3-point scale (3 = most confi-

dent, 1 = least confident). For subtle abnormalities ("soft calls") that have a lesser chance of representing true pathology, communicating this lower confidence to the gastroenterologist may prevent excess evaluation time for false-positive calls (Fig. 25-6).[2]

Depending on the specific situation and the clinical practice pattern, the OC examination stemming from CTC referral can be performed on the same day as CTC, on the following day, or at a later date. In our CTC screening program at the University of Wisconsin, the overwhelming majority of cases referred to OC will be performed on the same day the lesion is found. This avoids the need for additional or repeat bowel preparation—a program feature that is highly valued by our patients. In the American Gastroenterological Association's comments submitted for the CMS National

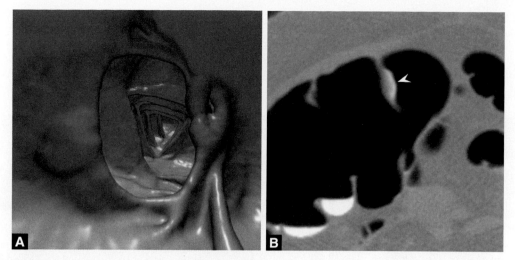

Figure 25-6 **Presumed false-positive CTC finding assigned a lower diagnostic confidence.** 3D endoluminal CTC image **(A)** shows a subtle flat 12-mm lesion behind a cecal fold opposite the ileocecal valve. On 2D correlation **(B)**, this focal abnormality was primarily related to oral contrast *(arrowhead)*, but an underlying soft tissue lesion that slightly thickens the fold was suggested. No corresponding lesion could be identified at subsequent OC. Despite the potentially difficult endoscopic location behind a fold in the right colon, this discordant result was felt to most likely represent a CTC false positive and not an OC false negative on retrospective review.

Coverage Analysis for CTC screening, it identified the "appropriate episode of care" with same-day studies as the optimal model for CTC screening. For same-day studies to occur, patients must be appropriate candidates for OC and will need to arrange for a driver following the invasive procedure because of the use of sedation. Some programs considering this "one-stop shop" approach to integrated CTC–OC screening have raised the concern that providing this same-day OC option will be too onerous. However, one must keep in mind that our OC referral rate from CTC screening is less than 10%,[3] which means that a screening volume greater than 10 CTC cases per morning is needed to average just a single OC referral each day. Even if all patients with CTC-detected polyps ≥6 mm were referred to OC, our referral rate would still be just 13%. It would take very large CTC screening volumes to generate enough OC referrals to substantially affect a capable clinical endoscopy service. Nonetheless, for practices where same-day OC is not feasible, another viable option that avoids the need to repeat catharsis is to perform OC on the following day, keeping the patient on a clear-liquid diet. The oral contrast agents used in our CTC bowel preparation (i.e., 2% barium and diatrizoate) have never caused a problem such as obscuration of colonic mucosa or clogging of colonoscopic channels or ports at same-day OC. This represents a combined experience of nearly 2000 positive referred cases dating back to the multicenter trial. For patients receiving anticoagulation therapy with warfarin, we generally do not recommend stopping this medication prior to CTC, weighing the relatively low risk of a positive finding that may require invasive OC against the potential risks of reversing the anticoagulation. In fact, a higher threshold for OC referral is prudent for

many of these patients. Also, because relatively few patients screened by CTC will require OC, we do not require that chauffeur arrangements be made prior to CTC; instead we address this issue only when it becomes necessary.

PREOPERATIVE ASSESSMENT WITH CTC

Preoperative assessment at CTC may be unanticipated, related to an unsuspected new surgical finding, or expected, as in the case of an occlusive cancer referred because of incomplete OC. The primary difference between these scenarios is that one can plan ahead for an intravenous (IV) contrast protocol in the latter situation to evaluate for metastatic disease. When an obvious colonic mass diagnostic of invasive cancer is identified at a primary noncontrast CTC evaluation, an astute CT technologist should notify the responsible radiologist between the supine and prone series acquisitions to inquire whether IV contrast is indicated. Using an IV contrast protocol in this setting can provide for complete preoperative evaluation. Our specific protocol for diagnostic CTC with IV contrast is covered in Chapter 14. As mentioned previously, preoperative OC is typically performed to obtain a tissue diagnosis for new cancers detected at CTC, but this may not be absolutely necessary in all cases. In fact, we have had cases where the preoperative OC examination was incomplete and could not reach a CTC-detected cancer to obtain a biopsy (Figs. 25-7 and 25-8). Perhaps in the future OC evaluation will not automatically be considered a necessary preoperative procedure for obvious surgical lesions detected at CTC; instead perhaps it will be reserved for cases where there is some diagnostic uncertainty.

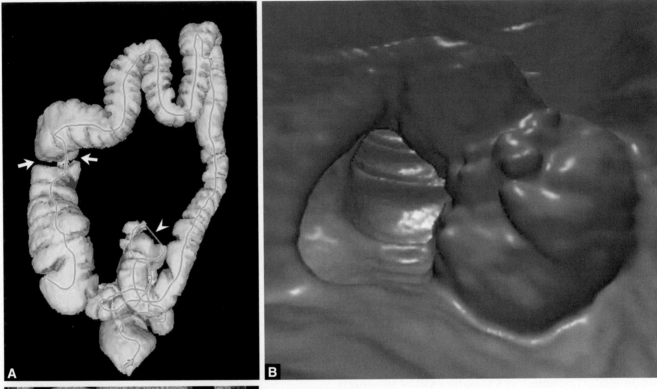

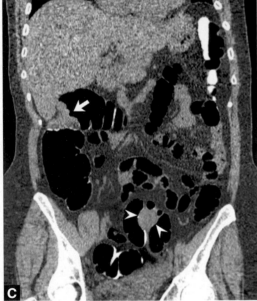

Figure 25-7 Surgical referral for right-sided cancer and sigmoid endometriosis detected at screening CTC examination in an asymptomatic average-risk 50-year-old woman. The 3D colon map **(A)** marks the location of two colonic abnormalities identified at CTC, one in the ascending colon near the hepatic flexure *(arrows)* and the other in the mid-sigmoid colon *(arrowhead)*. 3D endoluminal CTC image **(B)** shows a large, lobulated mass in the distal ascending colon, which measured 5 cm and was highly concerning for invasive cancer. Curved reformatted 2D coronal CTC image **(C)** simultaneously shows the ascending colon mass *(arrow)* and a mid-sigmoid annular lesion *(arrowheads)*, which precluded passage of the endoscope at same-day OC. At surgery, the sigmoid lesion proved to be endometriosis and the ascending mass proved to be Stage I adenocarcinoma. (From Pickhardt PJ, Kim DH. CT colonography: A primer for gastroenterologists. *Clin Gastroenterol Hepatol.* 2008;6:497-502.)

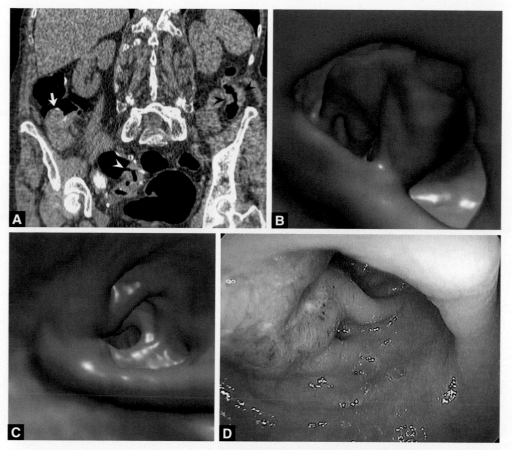

Figure 25-8 **Multiple synchronous cancers detected at CTC with subsequent incomplete OC in a symptomatic 82-year-old woman.** Curved reformatted 2D coronal CTC image **(A)** shows three masses located in the sigmoid *(white arrowhead)*, descending *(black arrowheads)*, and ascending *(arrow)* colon, all of which were concerning for invasive cancer. 3D endoluminal images **(B** and **C)** show the ascending **(B)** and sigmoid **(C)** masses. At subsequent OC, the scope could not extend past the occlusive sigmoid mass **(D)**, but all lesions ultimately proved to be cancer at surgery.

CTC evaluation associated with incomplete OC examination resulting from an occlusive colon cancer (or other cause) can provide important preoperative information for the surgeon, regardless of whether the OC or CTC was performed first. Several published series have demonstrated the ability of CTC to detect significant colorectal lesions proximal to a lesion that is occlusive to OC (Figs. 25-7 through 25-9).[4-7] The term "occlusive" generally applies only to OC because diagnostic CTC evaluation proximal to these stenotic lesions is almost always achievable (Figs. 25-7 through 25-11). The use of IV contrast at CT, whether as part of the CTC study itself or a separate diagnostic examination, allows for assessment of distant metastatic disease (Fig. 25-10). In addition, important information regarding the primary tumor can also be obtained, including T staging and improved anatomic localization.[7] As discussed in Chapter 26, CTC allows for precise and reproducible localization of colorectal abnormalities, whereas OC does not.

Incorrect localization of cancer at OC is not uncommon and may have important implications for the surgeon (Fig. 25-11).[7] The accuracy and utility of CTC for preoperative TNM staging of CRC has not been well established, but a number of reports suggest a promising role.[7,8] In addition, an integrated positron emission tomography (PET)–CTC approach has shown significant potential for preoperative staging of CRC.[9-11]

Beyond obvious cancers, a number of large and advanced but still benign CTC-detected lesions will not be completely resectable at subsequent OC. Repeat OC will be performed in some cases (Fig. 25-4), whereas others will go straight to surgical resection (Figs. 25-12 and 25-13). For these cases, CTC provides superior localization for the surgeon. In fact, given the utility of this additional information, colorectal surgeons should consider sending more OC-detected surgical lesions for preoperative CTC assessment, regardless of whether the OC evaluation was "complete."

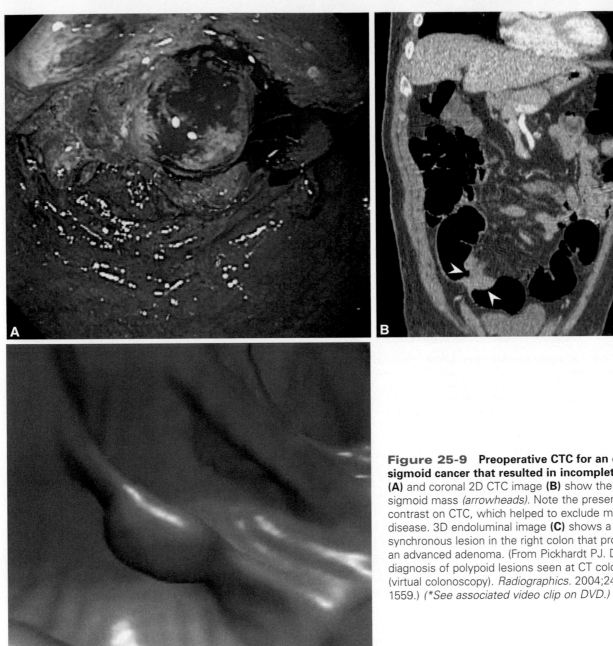

Figure 25-9 Preoperative CTC for an occlusive sigmoid cancer that resulted in incomplete OC. OC **(A)** and coronal 2D CTC image **(B)** show the annular sigmoid mass *(arrowheads)*. Note the presence of IV contrast on CTC, which helped to exclude metastatic disease. 3D endoluminal image **(C)** shows a 1.5-cm synchronous lesion in the right colon that proved to be an advanced adenoma. (From Pickhardt PJ. Differential diagnosis of polypoid lesions seen at CT colonography (virtual colonoscopy). *Radiographics.* 2004;24:1535-1559.) *(*See associated video clip on DVD.)*

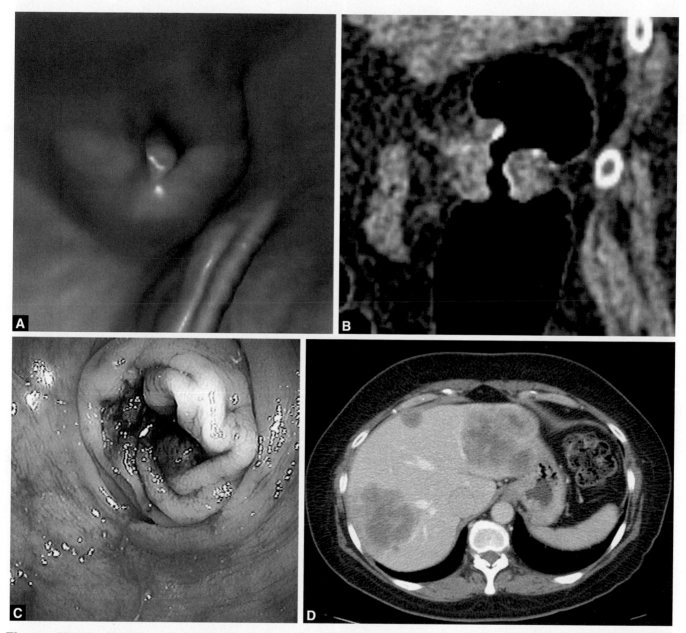

Figure 25-10 **Unsuspected metastatic colon cancer in an otherwise-healthy asymptomatic 55-year-old woman.** 3D endoluminal **(A)** and 2D coronal **(B)** images from screening CTC show an annular cancer in the descending colon, which was occlusive an attempted OC evaluation **(C).** Preoperative CT with IV contrast **(D)** confirmed advanced hepatic metastatic disease that was suggested on the noncontrast CTC examination.

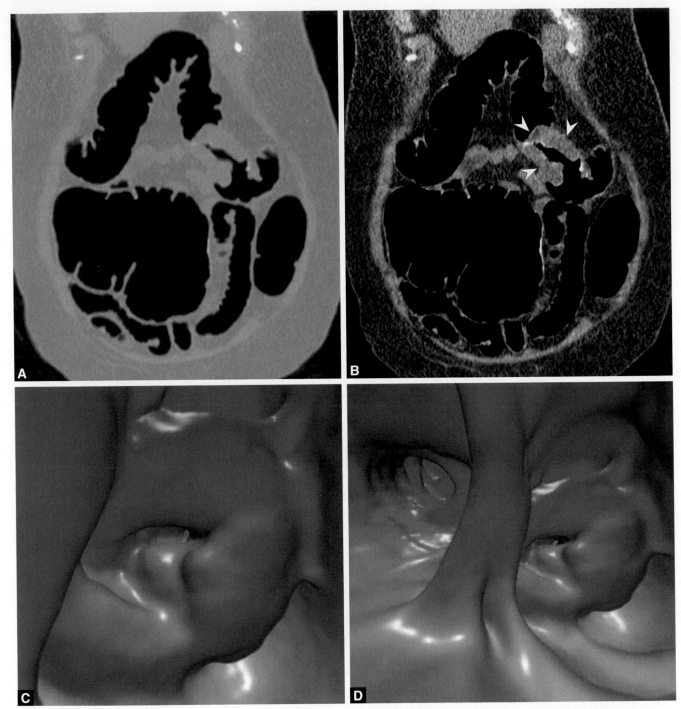

Figure 25-11   Cancer near splenic flexure incorrectly localized to cecum at OC. The patient was initially evaluated by OC, where the endoscopist encountered a cancer that he believed involved the cecal base. The colorectal surgeon referred the patient for preoperative CTC to confirm OC localization. 2D coronal CTC images **(A** and **B)** with polyp **(A)** and soft tissue **(B)** window settings show an annular mass *(arrowheads)* in the distal transverse colon. Close-up **(C)** and pulled-back **(D)** 3D endoluminal views of the mass show its morphology and relationship to the splenic flexure. Without preoperative CTC, the entire right colon would not have been evaluated and could have lead to an incorrect surgical approach. *(*See associated video clip on DVD.)*

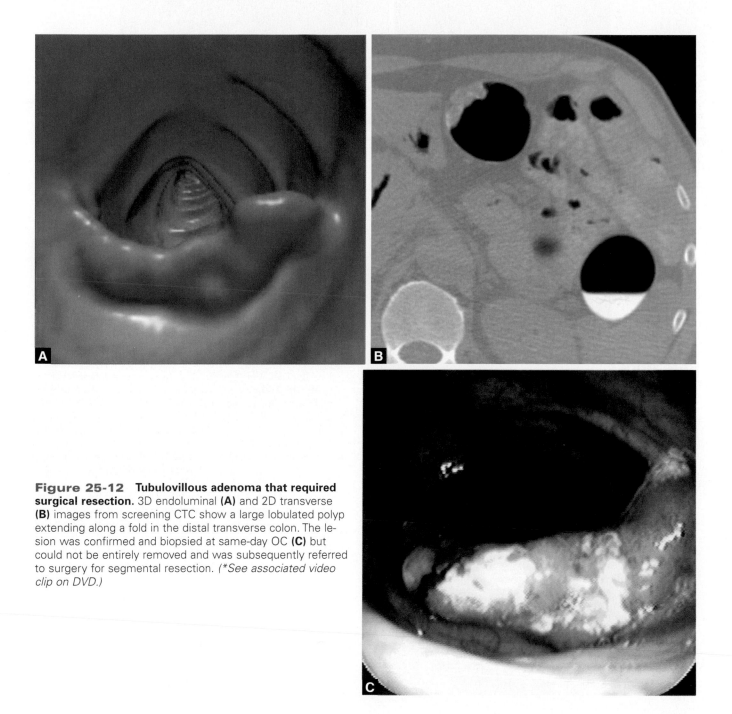

Figure 25-12 **Tubulovillous adenoma that required surgical resection.** 3D endoluminal **(A)** and 2D transverse **(B)** images from screening CTC show a large lobulated polyp extending along a fold in the distal transverse colon. The lesion was confirmed and biopsied at same-day OC **(C)** but could not be entirely removed and was subsequently referred to surgery for segmental resection. *(*See associated video clip on DVD.)*

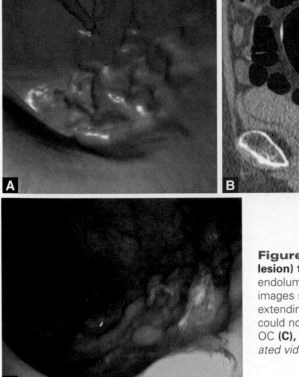

Figure 25-13 **Villous adenoma (carpet lesion) that required surgical resection.** 3D endoluminal **(A)** and 2D sagittal **(B)** CTC images show an extensive flat carpet lesion extending to the anorectal junction, which could not be entirely removed at subsequent OC **(C),** necessitating surgery. *(*See associated video clip on DVD.)*

References

1. Zalis ME, Barish MA, Choi JR, et al. CT colonography reporting and data system: A consensus proposal. *Radiology.* 2005;236(1):3-9.
2. Pickhardt PJ, Choi JR, Nugent PA, Schindler WR. The effect of diagnostic confidence on the probability of optical colonoscopic confirmation of potential polyps detected on CT colonography: Prospective assessment in 1,339 asymptomatic adults. *Am J Roentgenol.* 2004;183(6):1661-1665.
3. Kim DH, Pickhardt PJ, Taylor AJ, et al. CT colonography versus colonoscopy for the detection of advanced neoplasia. *N Engl J Med.* 2007;357(14):1403-1412.
4. Fenlon HM, McAneny DB, Nunes DP, Clarke PD, Ferrucci JT. Occlusive colon carcinoma: Virtual colonoscopy in the preoperative evaluation of the proximal colon. *Radiology.* 1999;210(2):423-8.
5. Morrin MM, Kruskal JB, Farrell RJ, Goldberg SN, McGee JB, Raptopoulos V. Endoluminal CT colonography after an incomplete endoscopic colonoscopy. *Am J Roentgenol.* 1999;172(4):913-918.
6. Neri E, Giusti P, Battolla L, et al. Colorectal cancer: Role of CT colonography in preoperative evaluation after incomplete colonoscopy. *Radiology.* 2002;223(3):615-619.
7. Kim JH, Kim WH, Kim TI, et al. Incomplete colonoscopy in patients with occlusive colorectal cancer: Usefulness of CT colonography according to tumor location. *Yonsei Med J.* 2007;48:934-941.
8. Utano K, Endo K, Togashi K, et al. Preoperative T staging of colorectal cancer by CT colonography. *Dis Colon Rectum.* 2008;51(6):875-881.
9. Veit-Haibach P, Kuehle CA, Beyer T, et al. Diagnostic accuracy of colorectal cancer staging with whole-body PET/CT colonography. *JAMA* .2006;296(21):2590-2600.
10. Nagata K, Ota Y, Okawa T, Endo S, Kudo SE. PET/CT colonography for the preoperative evaluation of the colon proximal to the obstructive colorectal cancer. *Dis Colon Rectum.* 2008;51(6):882-890.
11. Kinner S, Antoch G, Bockisch A, Veit-Haibach P. Whole-body PET/CT-colonography: A possible new concept for colorectal cancer staging. *Abdom Imag.* 2007;32:606-612.

Discordant Findings at CTC—Endoscopic Evaluation

PERRY J. PICKHARDT, MD
DAVID H. KIM, MD

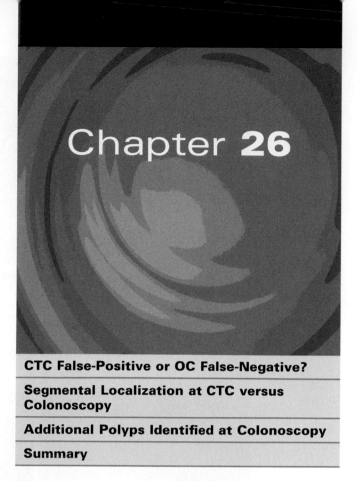

Chapter 26

CTC False-Positive or OC False-Negative?

Segmental Localization at CTC versus Colonoscopy

Additional Polyps Identified at Colonoscopy

Summary

INTRODUCTION

CT colonography (CTC) and optical colonoscopy (OC) are complementary imaging tests for colorectal evaluation. Colorectal lesions that tend to be missed by one examination are often detected by the other.[1] Because no infallible gold standard exists, it can be difficult to know which test result is correct when there is a discrepancy in the findings. When a discordant result occurs between the CTC and OC findings, the first step is to determine whether the disagreement is of potential clinical significance. The most important clinical scenario to be considered involves a positive finding at CTC that cannot be confirmed at OC because there is the potential for leaving an important lesion behind. If a case is discordant by segmental localization only, it is likely that the OC localization was incorrect. Of secondary importance is the situation in which additional polyps are found at OC that were not reported at CTC. This chapter explores the issues related to discordant findings between CTC and OC.

CTC FALSE-POSITIVE OR OC FALSE-NEGATIVE?

For patients referred to OC for significant polyps or masses detected at CTC, it is imperative to supply the endoscopist with the relevant polyp features and anatomic location (see Chapter 25). In particular, care must be taken for lesions situated behind a fold, at the inner turn of a flexure, within the right colon, within the distal rectum, or with a flat (nonpolypoid) morphology. All of these situations can contribute to missed lesions at conventional endoscopy (Figs. 26-1 through 26-6).[1] After completion of

the OC examination, it is important to confirm that all the relevant colorectal findings identified at CTC were also found at OC. For significant CTC-detected lesions not seen at OC (especially large lesions), we generally review the case as a group and make a consensus determination as to whether the discordant finding most likely represents a CTC false-positive call or a missed lesion at OC. As past experiences with barium enema and our own clinical experiences with CTC have shown,[1,2] one should not automatically assume that the OC results are correct.

For presumed CTC false-positive results, no further action is needed with regard to patient care (Figs. 26-7 and 26-8). Formal review of the case, however, still provides beneficial feedback for education and quality improvement. For cases where there is a realistic chance that a significant lesion was missed at OC, we will generally try to arrange for a short-interval CTC follow-up (Figs. 26-1 through 26-4). The time interval for CTC followup will depend on the specific circumstances (e.g., the size and nature of the lesion and the age and health of the patient). The rationale behind repeating the CTC study prior to repeating OC is that if the lesion is not seen again on CTC, it can be assumed to represent a false positive on the original CTC (or perhaps a lesion that regressed in the interval). However, if the same polyp is identified at follow-up CTC, a decision regarding the need for immediate OC can be made based on the lesion size, the presence of any interval change, and the clinical status of the patient. For cases where an obvious lesion at CTC was

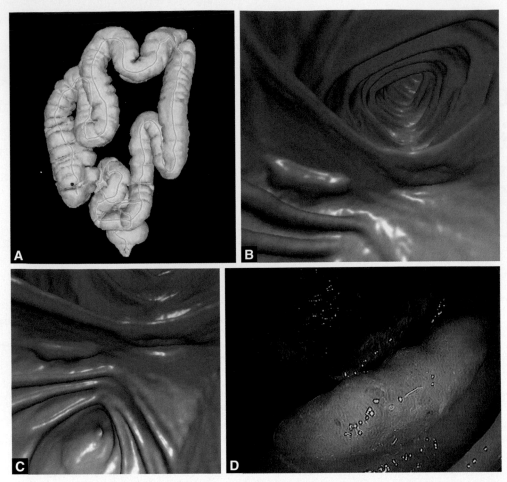

Figure 26-1 **OC false-negative result (2-cm adenoma) related to polyp location.** 3D map **(A)** from CTC screening shows a moderately tortuous colon and a bookmark *(red dot)* for a polyp identified in the cecum. 3D endoluminal CTC image **(B)** as viewed from the cecal tip shows an elongated 2-cm sessile polyp located on the backside of a fold adjacent to the ileocecal valve. At same-day OC, the lesion could not be found, despite multiple attempts and retroflexion of the scope within the cecum. Because the CTC confidence level was high, a repeat CTC examination was performed 9 months later, which again showed the same cecal polyp **(C).** The lesion had grown slightly in the interval. Note adjacent ileocecal valve and appendiceal orifice. Same-day OC was again performed, this time by a more experienced endoscopist, and the large lesion was confirmed **(D)** and removed. *(*See associated video clip on DVD.)*

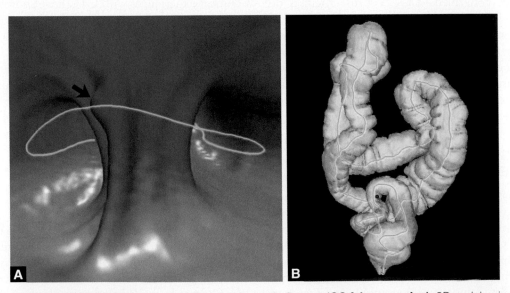

Figure 26-2 **Polyp situated at the inner turn of an acute-angle flexure (OC false negative).** 3D endoluminal CTC image **(A)** shows a 6-mm polyp *(arrow)* located behind a fold and at the inner turn of a sharp rectosigmoid bend. The green line represents the automated centerline. The 3D colon map **(B)** viewed from behind shows the polyp location *(red dot)*. A followup CTC (not shown) performed 3 years later confirmed the presence of this polyp, which had grown to 8 mm in the interval. *(*See associated video clip on DVD.)*

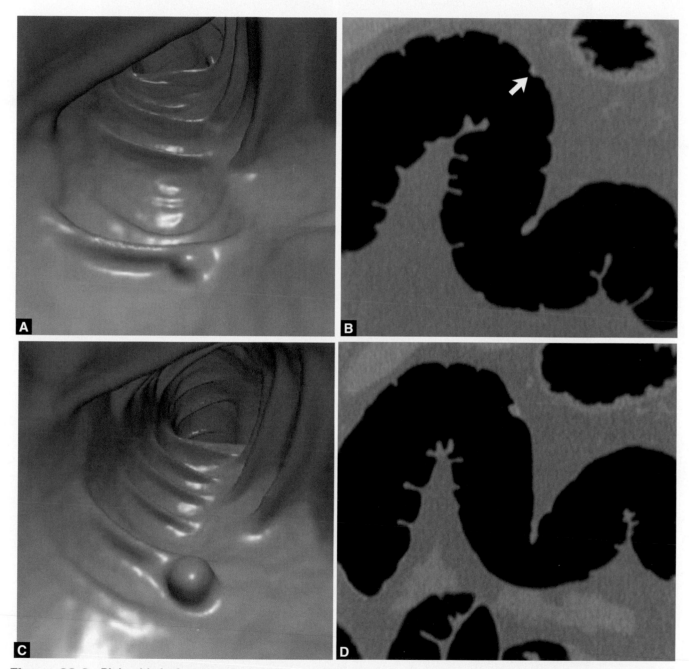

Figure 26-3 **Right-sided adenoma missed at OC but detected at repeat examination after CTC showed interval growth.** 3D endoluminal **(A)** and 2D coronal **(B)** images from CTC screening show a 6-mm polyp *(arrow)* located on a fold near the hepatic flexure. The lesion was not seen at the initial OC examination, but two other small CTC-detected polyps were identified. Repeat CTC **(C** and **D)** performed 1.5 years later shows interval growth of the polyp to 8 mm. The lesion was confirmed and removed at subsequent OC.

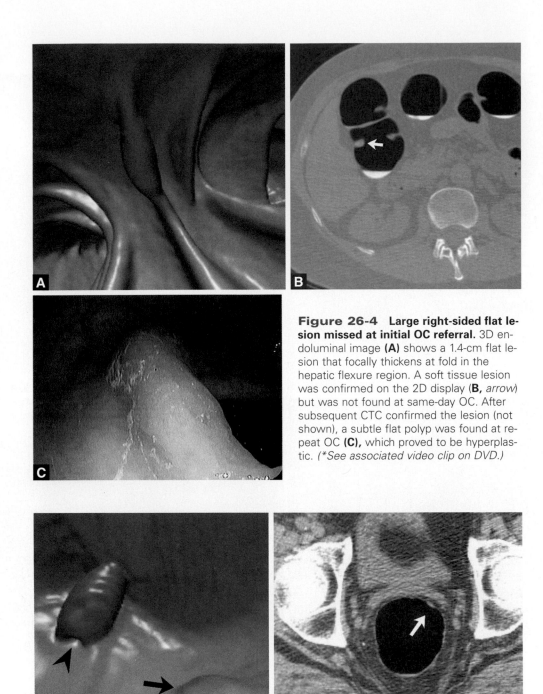

Figure 26-4 Large right-sided flat lesion missed at initial OC referral. 3D endoluminal image **(A)** shows a 1.4-cm flat lesion that focally thickens at fold in the hepatic flexure region. A soft tissue lesion was confirmed on the 2D display **(B,** *arrow*) but was not found at same-day OC. After subsequent CTC confirmed the lesion (not shown), a subtle flat polyp was found at repeat OC **(C),** which proved to be hyperplastic. (*See associated video clip on DVD.*)

Figure 26-5 Flat 7-mm adenoma near the anorectal junction missed at prospective OC evaluation in the DoD trial. 3D endoluminal CTC image **(A)** simulating a retroflexed OC view of the rectum shows a subtle flat lesion *(arrow)* in the distal rectum (note adjacent rectal catheter tip; *arrowhead*). 2D transverse image **(B)** with soft tissue window settings confirms the lesion *(arrow)*, which was missed at prospective OC evaluation prior to unblinding of CTC results. (From Pickhardt PJ, Nugent PA, Mysliwiec PA, Choi JR, Schindler WR. Location of adenomas missed at optical colonoscopy. *Ann Intern Med.* 2004;141:352-359.)

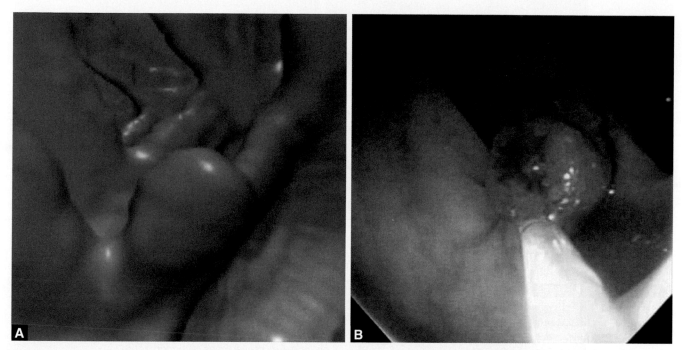

Figure 26-6 Right-sided cancer missed at prospective OC evaluation in the DoD trial. 3D endoluminal CTC image **(A)** shows a large polypoid lesion, which was located near the hepatic flexure. The lesion was missed at initial OC evaluation and at several attempts after unblinding of CTC results as a result of repeated slippage of the endoscope. The lesion, however, was eventually identified at OC **(B)** and proved to be an invasive adenocarcinoma. (From Pickhardt PJ, Nugent PA, Mysliwiec PA, Choi JR, Schindler WR. Location of adenomas missed at optical colonoscopy. *Ann Intern Med.* 2004;141:352-359.)

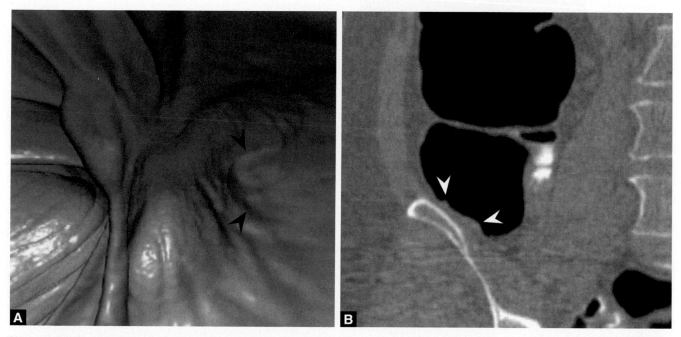

Figure 26-7 CTC-detected flat lesion presumed to represent a false positive. 3D endoluminal **(A)** and 2D coronal **(B)** CTC images show a subtle 2-cm flat lesion *(arrowheads)* in the cecum (note ileocecal valve on 3D). The lesion could not be confirmed at OC and presumably represents a CTC false positive.

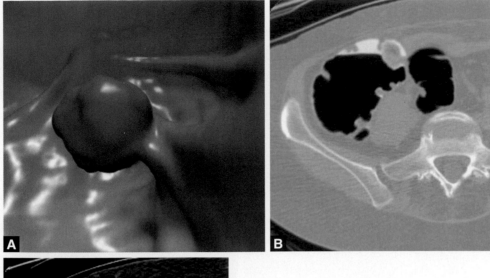

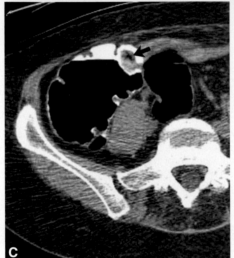

Figure 26-8 **CTC false positive from large, adherent untagged collection of solid stool.** 3D endoluminal CTC image **(A)** shows a large, pedunculated 3-cm mass at the base of the cecum. On 2D imaging with polyp windowing **(B)**, this pedunculated lesion could be mistaken for a soft tissue mass, although some internal heterogeneity is present. However, on 2D imaging with soft tissue windowing **(C)**, the internal low attenuation *(arrow)* consistent with untagged stool is much more apparent. This case is very unusual in that most untagged stool balls of this size are neither adherent nor pedunculated in appearance and are generally recognized as such.

clearly missed at the initial OC, repeat CTC may not be necessary. However, for more difficult or questionable cases, performing the OC as the initial followup step may lead to uncertainty if the finding is not confirmed at this modality. Thus, for this reason we prefer to proceed with the study that saw the lesion in the first place. Therefore, the appropriate followup management of these discordant cases is largely determined on a logical case-by-case basis.

A number of factors contribute to the retrospective assessment of a discordant finding. One important CTC criterion is the diagnostic confidence level from the prospective interpretation. For every positive call at CTC, we prospectively assign a diagnostic confidence level (level 3 = highest, level 2 = intermediate, level 1 = lowest), which strongly correlates with the likelihood of finding the lesion at OC (Fig. 26-9).[3] This subjective but valuable measure simultaneously combines a number of features, including quality of the bowel preparation and distention, and characteristics of the polyp itself. Other important anatomic factors that increase the likelihood of missing a CTC-detected lesion at OC include a polyp location on the backside of a fold, at the inner turn of a flexure point, in the right

colon, or near the anorectal junction (Figs. 26-1 through 26-6).[1] Combinations of these anatomic factors likely have a negative synergistic effect on OC detection. In our experience, relatively large right-sided lesions may be missed at OC. A flat (nonpolypoid) polyp morphology also increases the likelihood that a CTC-detected lesion will not be found at OC. In this situation it can be difficult to determine whether the finding represents a CTC false-positive (Fig. 26-7) or OC false-negative (Figs. 26-4 and 26-5) result. For a large pedunculated soft tissue polyp in a well-prepared, well-distended colon detected at CTC, there can be nearly 100% certainty that the finding is real. This is not the case, however, for a subtle flat lesion in a poorly prepared or untagged colon. Lack of a correlate at subsequent OC for a high-confidence finding will likely be viewed as an endoscopic miss but is more easily accepted as a CTC false positive for a lower-confidence CTC finding. As discussed later in this chapter, anatomic localization is precise at CTC but can be fraught with error at OC.[4] This factor must be considered if the discrepancy is simply one of localization and the lesion is found because there is no clinical dilemma in such a case (Fig. 26-10).

Figure 26-9 Correlation between diagnostic confidence level at CTC and a matching lesion at OC in the DoD trial. As diagnostic confidence increased from low (= 1) to high (= 3), the likelihood of finding a corresponding polyp at OC significantly increased. With current CTC and OC techniques, our concordance rate is now much higher than it was in this trial. (From Pickhardt PJ, Choi JR, Nugent PA, Schindler WR. The effect of diagnostic confidence on the probability of optical colonoscopic confirmation for potential polyps detected at CT colonography: Prospective assessment in 1339 asymptomatic adults. *Am J Roentgenol.* 2004;183:1661-1665.)

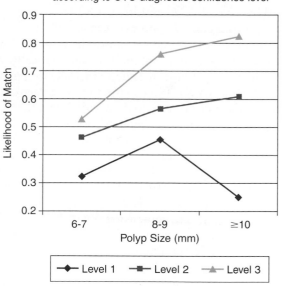

Likelihood of finding a matched polyp at OC according to CTC diagnostic confidence level

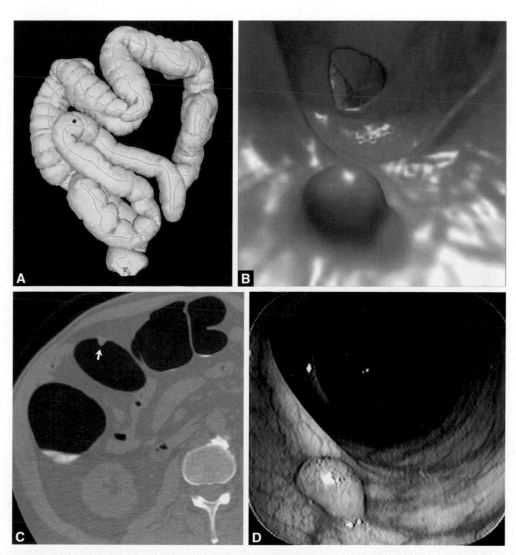

Figure 26-10 Incorrect segmental localization of a polyp at OC. 3D colon map **(A)** shows the location of a CTC-detected 7-mm adenoma *(red dot)* within a redundant sigmoid colon. 3D endoluminal **(B)** and 2D transverse **(C)** CTC images show the polyp *(arrow),* which was felt to be located near the splenic flexure at OC **(D)** related to the redundant sigmoid. (From Pickhardt PJ, Taylor AJ, Kim DH, Reichelderfer M, Gopal DV, Pfau PR. Screening for colorectal neoplasia with CT colonography: Initial experience from the first year of coverage by third-party payers. *Radiology.* 2006;241:417-425.) *(*See associated video clip on DVD.)*

Unblinding of CTC results at OC in a prospective validation trial can be done in a segmental fashion after initial blinding of the endoscopist.[5] In routine clinical practice, however, such "unblinding" automatically takes place when the patients are referred to OC for polypectomy by a positive CTC examination. Segmental unblinding from our clinical trial provided important data on OC performance for polyp detection[1] but still underestimated the OC miss rate because some lesions may be missed even after repeated unblinded OC evaluation. This notion is supported by our experience with discordant cases in the University of Wisconsin (UW) screening program, where CTC-detected polyps not seen on initial colonoscopy are detected at repeat CTC and then found by repeat OC. Nonetheless, by using segmental unblinding of CTC results, we showed a 12% miss rate for large adenomas at OC evaluation.[1] This miss rate has been confirmed in subsequent OC studies.[6] In clinical practice, we do not blind the endoscopist from the CTC findings but rather provide as much helpful information as possible. Occasionally, our gastroenterologists will freely admit that they would have likely missed a significant lesion referred from CTC had they not had the advance knowledge of its existence. Furthermore, we have seen a number of discordant cases in which only by virtue of CTC followup (or by unblinding of results if part of a trial) can we prove that the CTC-detected abnormality is real (Figs. 26-1 through 26-6). Because of this phenomenon, the OC performance results obtained with segmental unblinding only represent a lower limit of the actual endoscopic miss rate.

There is also evidence from several CTC studies that suggests that in addition to an increased miss rate for polyps, the OC miss rate for colorectal *cancers* may be considerably higher than the 5% rate that has been previous reported in the gastrointestinal literature.[7,8] In the Department of Defense (DoD) screening trial, one of the two cancers was missed at OC prior to segmental unblinding (Fig. 26-6).[5] In a recent Mayo Clinic study, four of five CTC-detected cancers (80%) were missed at the index OC evaluation but were subsequently found after repeat OC evaluation.[9] Finally, in large, well-matched screening populations with more than 3000 adults in each cohort, primary CTC found more than three times as many cancers as did primary OC evaluation.[10] In comparison, the cancer detection rate at CTC has been more than 96%, even when older CTC trials are included.[11]

From the previous discussion, it becomes clear that the true positive predictive value (PPV) of CTC is underestimated somewhat as a result of OC false negatives and the lack of a true gold standard for reference. However, PPV remains an acceptable term to describe the concordance rate between CTC and OC. Because of advances in bowel preparation, bowel distention, and interpretive software, we have seen a marked increase in the PPV (or concordance) for positive CTC results, which may be further enhanced by increased reader experience. From the initial DoD screening trial, the PPV for all polyps 6 mm and greater was about 60%.[5,12] For our CTC screening program at the UW, the PPV has remained steady at more than 90%.[13,14] Sources of false-positive interpretation and other pitfalls are covered in detail in Chapter 20. Residual untagged stool is a very rare cause of false positives with our CTC methodology, which combines a cathartic agent with dilute barium and diatrizoate tagging agents (see Chapter 12). Without the use of an effective oral contrast tagging regimen, however, the rate of false-positive interpretations related to residual solid stool can quickly escalate. When there is a clear correlate at OC, whether a true soft tissue polyp or pitfall such as a vascular bleb or appendiceal stump, there is generally no need for further action (Figs. 26-11 and 26-12).

SEGMENTAL LOCALIZATION AT CTC VERSUS COLONOSCOPY

CTC allows for precise and reproducible anatomic localization of colorectal abnormalities, which can provide valuable preoperative information for surgeons (see Chapter 25). At OC, however, precise localization is not possible unless the lesion is near the ileocecal valve, appendiceal orifice, or anorectal junction. This uncertainty in localization at OC has implications for correlation with CTC and for potential surgery. Beyond the obvious problems with CTC–OC polyp localization for validation trials, the issue of segmental matching in actual clinical practice is of less importance, as long as the lesion is found at OC (26-10). However, if the lesion is surgical in nature, it is important for the colorectal surgeon to understand that the CTC localization is much more accurate than OC. Incorrect localization of cancer at OC is not uncommon and can have important implications for the surgical approach (see Chapter 25).[4] If a cancer is occlusive at OC or there is any uncertainty in localization, a preoperative CTC can provide vital information to the surgeon.

Of note, although CTC systems provide precise unperturbed centerline distances of polyp location from the anorectal junction, we purposefully refrain from reporting this distance to the endoscopist. The reason for this is that the telescoping and foreshortening of the measured distances at OC may lead to confusion. Although a correction factor normalized to total colonic length can be applied, we instead prefer to report the segmental location of polyps, in addition to polyp size, morphology, confidence level, and any other relevant information (e.g., located behind a fold).

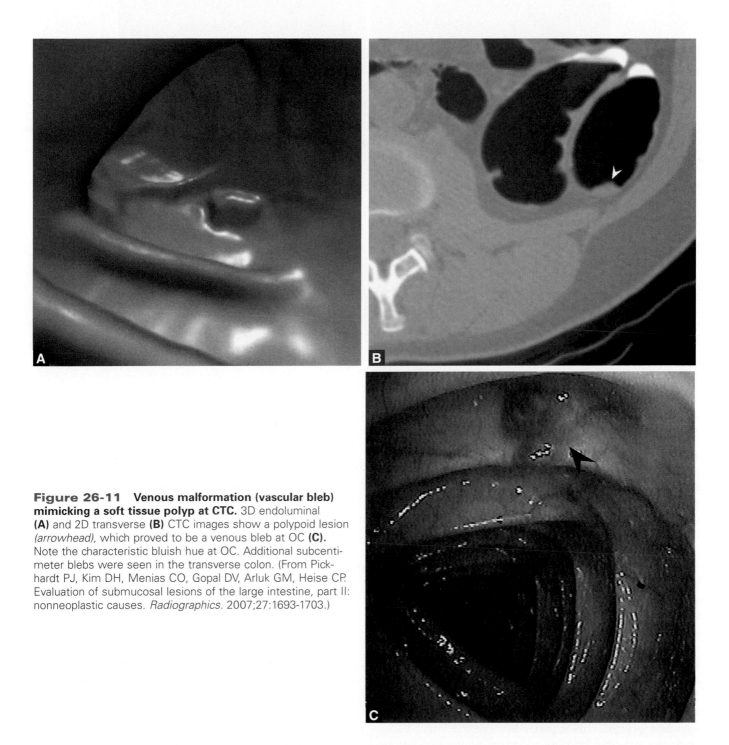

Figure 26-11 Venous malformation (vascular bleb) mimicking a soft tissue polyp at CTC. 3D endoluminal **(A)** and 2D transverse **(B)** CTC images show a polypoid lesion *(arrowhead),* which proved to be a venous bleb at OC **(C).** Note the characteristic bluish hue at OC. Additional subcentimeter blebs were seen in the transverse colon. (From Pickhardt PJ, Kim DH, Menias CO, Gopal DV, Arluk GM, Heise CP. Evaluation of submucosal lesions of the large intestine, part II: nonneoplastic causes. *Radiographics.* 2007;27:1693-1703.)

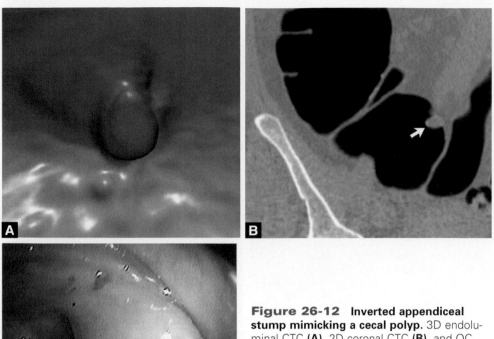

Figure 26-12 **Inverted appendiceal stump mimicking a cecal polyp.** 3D endoluminal CTC **(A)**, 2D coronal CTC **(B)**, and OC **(C)** images show a prominent inverted appendiceal stump *(arrow)*, which can mimic a true polyp at both examinations.

ADDITIONAL POLYPS IDENTIFIED AT COLONOSCOPY

The situation in which lesions are identified at OC in addition to those prospectively called at CTC is less problematic than the issue of determining CTC false positive versus OC false negative, as outlined earlier. In fact, the great majority of additional polyps found at OC are of little or no clinical significance and largely relate to nonreporting of diminutive lesions at CTC. In our experience, more than 70% of additional polyps seen at OC are diminutive, more than 90% are subcentimeter, and more than 80% are hyperplastic.[14] In addition to a predominately diminutive size, even nondiminutive hyperplastic polyps are generally more difficult to detect at CTC, often related to an atypical morphology and the tendency to flatten out with colonic distention (Fig. 26-13).[15]

Although we intentionally refrain from reporting isolated diminutive lesions at CTC (see Chapter 28), we will make an exception for cases that are positive for nondiminutive polyps. This is partly because the larger polyps erase the potential harm of reporting diminutive lesions, but also because of the way the subsequent OC findings may be communicated to the patient. For example, suppose that one or two large polyps identified at CTC are subsequently confirmed at OC but that several diminutive lesions are also seen at OC. If these results are not properly communicated to the patient, he or she may be left with the impression that CTC missed the majority of the polyps, without any explanation regarding polyp size or the reasoning behind nonreporting of diminutive lesions at CTC. Depending on the specific situation, this has led us on occasion to note that additional diminutive lesions may be present, even though we clearly state in every dictation that "CTC is not intended for the detection of diminutive colonic polyps, the presence or absence of which will not change management of the patient." It is important to note that we have seen a number of significant complications arise from the resection of meaningless isolated diminutive lesions at OC (Fig. 26-14). These unfortunate complications are avoided with primary CTC screening.

On occasion, a small (6-9 mm) or large (≥10 mm) adenoma may be identified at OC that was not prospectively called at CTC. However, in nearly every case, the additional lesion is less important (e.g., smaller or nonadvanced) than the CTC-detected lesion(s) and almost never upstages the C-RADS category from the prospective CTC assessment. In fact, for patients in whom CTC finds only left-sided polyps, the yield of full OC compared with flexible sigmoidoscopy is so low that the additional costs, risks, and time associated with the more

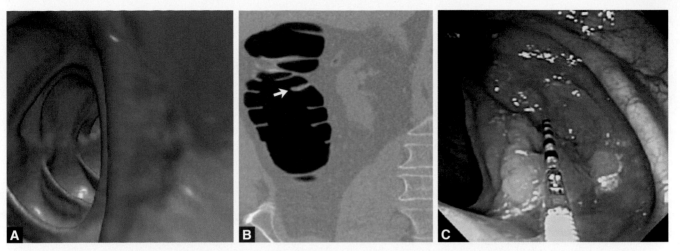

Figure 26-13   Large hyperplastic polyp missed at prospective CTC evaluation in the DoD trial. 3D endoluminal **(A)** and 2D coronal **(B)** CTC images show a flat lesion that causes subtle irregular thickening of a colonic fold *(arrow)*. This lesion was missed at prospective CTC but found at subsequent OC **(C)**. In our experience, most subtle flat lesions with this appearance at CTC that prove to be real are hyperplastic in nature (as was the case in this example).

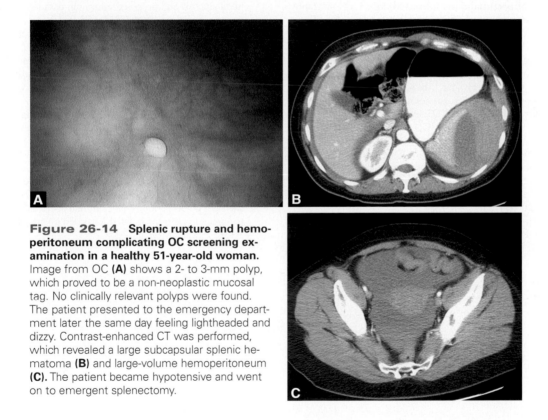

Figure 26-14   Splenic rupture and hemoperitoneum complicating OC screening examination in a healthy 51-year-old woman. Image from OC **(A)** shows a 2- to 3-mm polyp, which proved to be a non-neoplastic mucosal tag. No clinically relevant polyps were found. The patient presented to the emergency department later the same day feeling lightheaded and dizzy. Contrast-enhanced CT was performed, which revealed a large subcapsular splenic hematoma **(B)** and large-volume hemoperitoneum **(C)**. The patient became hypotensive and went on to emergent splenectomy.

invasive procedure are not justified. In our experience with 139 adults with isolated left-sided polyps at CTC screening that went on to complete OC, no large polyps or advanced adenomas were found proximal to the splenic flexure.[16] In a number of cases involving patients who were debilitated or frail and thus at higher risk for OC complications, our gastroenterologists wisely have chosen to limit endoscopic examination to a flexible sigmoidoscopy if no right-sided polyps were identified at

CTC. Nonetheless, for the majority of healthy adults, a complete OC examination is still being performed by most gastroenterologists on referral from CTC.

SUMMARY

Neither CTC nor OC are infallible tests, and each will miss relevant colorectal lesions on occasion. Fortunately, these tests are complementary in nature, likely resulting in few if any important findings that will be missed on both examinations. This suggests the possibility for an alternating CTC–OC hybrid screening strategy in the future to maximize detection. Multidisciplinary conferences involving both radiologists and colonoscopists are the optimal approach for discussing cases with discordant findings between CTC and OC. At the very least, for all positive CTC cases referred to OC, the final results should be compared and any significant discrepancies should be addressed. This exercise establishes important CTC performance data such as positive predictive values and false positive rates, although it should be recognized that some discordant cases are the result of OC false negatives and not CTC error. When a discrepancy is felt to be more likely the result of a missed lesion at OC, an appropriate followup plan must be devised. This will usually consist of a CTC followup examination to confirm whether the earlier CTC finding was real prior to repeating the more invasive examination that failed to demonstrate the finding in the first place.

REFERENCES

1. Pickhardt PJ, Nugent PA, Mysliwiec PA, Choi JR, Schindler WR. Location of adenomas missed by optical colonoscopy. *Ann Intern Med.* 2004;141(5):352-359.
2. Glick SN, Teplick SK, Balfe DM, et al. Large colonic neoplasms missed by endoscopy. *Am J Roentgenol.* 1989;152(3):513-517.
3. Pickhardt PJ, Choi JR, Nugent PA, Schindler WR. The effect of diagnostic confidence on the probability of optical colonoscopic confirmation of potential polyps detected on CT colonography: Prospective assessment in 1,339 asymptomatic adults. *Am J Roentgenol.* 2004;183(6):1661-1665.
4. Kim JH, Kim WH, Kim TI, et al. Incomplete colonoscopy in patients with occlusive colorectal cancer: Usefulness of CT colonography according to tumor location. *Yonsei Med J.* 2007;48:934-941.
5. Pickhardt PJ, Choi JR, Hwang I, et al. Computed tomographic virtual colonoscopy to screen for colorectal neoplasia in asymptomatic adults. *N Engl J Med.* 2003;349(23):2191-2200.
6. Heresbach D, Barrioz T, Lapalus MG, et al. Miss rate for colorectal neoplastic polyps: A prospective multicenter study of back-to-back video colonoscopies. *Endoscopy.* 2008;40(4):284-290.
7. Rex DK, Rahmani EY, Haseman JH, Lemmel GT, Kaster S, Buckley JS. Relative sensitivity of colonoscopy and barium enema for detection of colorectal cancer in clinical practice. *Gastroenterology.* 1997;112(1):17-23.
8. Bressler B, Paszat LF, Vinden C, Li C, He JS, Rabeneck L. Colonoscopic miss rates for right-sided colon cancer: A population-based analysis. *Gastroenterology.* 2004;127(2):452-456.
9. Johnson CD, Fletcher JG, MacCarty RL, et al. Effect of slice thickness and primary 2D versus 3D virtual dissection on colorectal lesion detection at CT colonography in 452 asymptomatic adults. *Am J Roentgenol.* 2007;189(3):672-680.
10. Kim DH, Pickhardt PJ, Taylor AJ, et al. CT colonography versus colonoscopy for the detection of advanced neoplasia. *N Engl J Med.* 2007;357(14):1403-1412.
11. Halligan S, Altman DG, Taylor SA, et al. CT colonography in the detection of colorectal polyps and cancer: Systematic review meta-analysis and proposed minimum data set for study level reporting. *Radiology.* 2006;238(3):893-904.
12. Pickhardt PJ. Limitations of virtual colonoscopy—In response. *Ann Intern Med.* 2005;142(2):155.
13. Pickhardt PJ, Taylor AJ, Kim DH, Reichelderfer M, Gopal DV, Pfau PR. Screening for colorectal neoplasia with CT colonography: Initial experience from the 1st year of coverage by third-party payers. *Radiology.* 2006;241(2):417-425.
14. Cornett D, Barancin C, Roeder B, et al. Findings on optical colonoscopy after positive CT colonography exam. *Am J Gastroenterol.* 2008;103(8):2068-2074.
15. Pickhardt PJ, Choi JR, Hwang I, Schindler WR. Nonadenomatous polyps at CT colonography: Prevalence, size distribution, and detection rates. *Radiology.* 2004;232(3):784-790.
16. Durick NA, Pickhardt PJ, Kim DH. Negative CT colonography of the right colon permits change in management from colonoscopy to sigmoidoscopy for isolated left-sided polyps. Washington, DC: ARRS Annual Meeting; 2008.

Extracolonic Findings at CTC

PERRY J. PICKHARDT, MD
DAVID H. KIM, MD

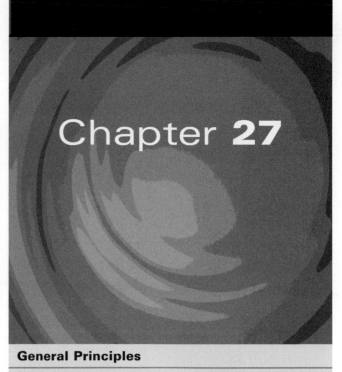

Chapter 27

General Principles

Technique, Classification, and Reporting

Extracolonic Findings of Potential Significance

Cost Implications

Summary

GENERAL PRINCIPLES

The primary indication for performing CT colonography (CTC) is the detection of colorectal polyps and masses. CTC is a clinically validated and cost-effective colorectal screening test of proven value, which justifies its existence. By comparison, there are currently insufficient scientific data to support the routine use of self-referred whole-body CT screening. The reality for CTC, however, is that the extracolonic abdomen and pelvis are unavoidably "screened" in a limited fashion with low-dose, noncontrast CT. In effect, the extracolonic portion of the CTC examination amounts to "half-body CT screening." Therefore, it is important for radiologists involved in CTC screening to appreciate the unique aspects that surround CT evaluation of healthy adults, in which the likelihood of harboring a clinically significant extracolonic finding is relatively low—but not zero. If not handled appropriately, the potential for CTC screening to open a floodgate of downstream workups for incidental extracolonic findings is a legitimate concern for referring physicians. Radiologists who tend to "overcall" findings in a defensive manner will only exacerbate this issue. However, findings on CT that are incidental to the clinical indication for the examination are encountered every day in radiology practice. The only real difference in the case of CTC screening is that the "patient" is generally an otherwise healthy individual.

Extracolonic evaluation at CTC should be viewed as a double-edged sword.[1] The potential benefits include personal reassurance for the vast majority of adults for whom nothing ominous is found and, in a small minority, discovery of an unsuspected but clinically significant process, whether malignant (Fig. 27-1) or nonmalignant (Fig. 27-2) in nature. The potential limitations include the undue anxiety and added costs stemming from additional workup for findings that eventually prove to be of no consequence. When considering extracolonic findings at CTC, one must keep in mind that many *poten-* *tially* significant findings will prove to be of no real concern after more definitive evaluation has been completed. Furthermore, it is important to specify the patient population under consideration because the frequency of relevant extracolonic findings, and their implications, can be quite different. For example, substantial differences in the rate of important extracolonic findings will be seen between an asymptomatic screening cohort[1,2] and a symptomatic elderly cohort.[3] This chapter will explore this intriguing issue of extracolonic findings at CTC. Specific topics will include the techniques for CT acquisition and interpretation, classification and reporting, and extracolonic findings of potential clinical significance. Emphasis will be placed on the evaluation of asymptomatic screening populations.

TECHNIQUE, CLASSIFICATION, AND REPORTING

Technique

At our institution, multidetector CT (MDCT) scanning for CTC examination entails thin collimation with a low-dose, noncontrast technique (see Chapter 14). However, for evaluation of extracolonic structures, we perform an automatic retrospective reconstruction of the supine series in all cases, consisting of 5-mm sections at 3-mm intervals. The advantages of this approach include fewer images to review, decreased image noise, and easier

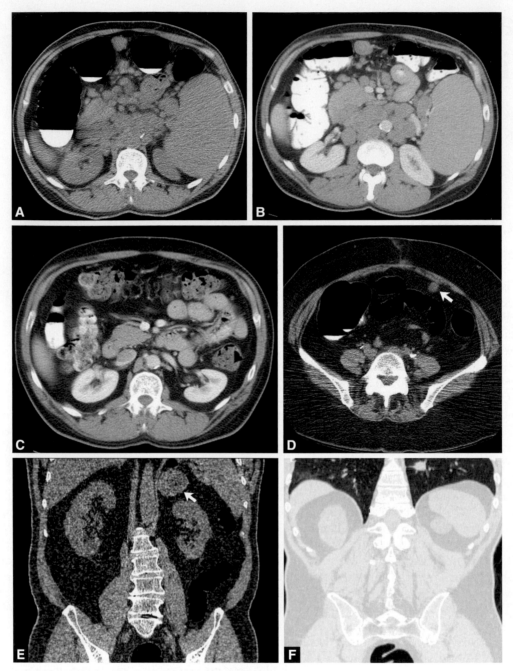

Figure 27-1 **Unsuspected extracolonic malignancies identified at CTC screening (C-RADS category E4).** Two-dimensional (2D) extracolonic CTC image (i.e., reconstruction of noncontrast low-dose supine dataset with 5-mm slice thickness; **A**) shows spleno-megaly and extensive abdominal lymphadenopathy, which is better depicted on the subsequent diagnostic CT examination with IV contrast **(B)**. Mantle cell non-Hodgkin's lymphoma was confirmed on image-guided core needle biopsy. Followup diagnostic CT **(C)** fol-lowing chemotherapy shows resolution of the abnormalities. 2D extracolonic CTC image **(D)** from a second individual shows a small omental implant *(arrow)* that proved to represent unsuspected metastatic disease from a previous Stage I endometrial cancer. 2D cor-onal CTC image **(E)** from a third individual shows a large left adrenal mass *(arrow),* which proved to be Stage I adrenocortical carci-noma. 2D coronal image with lung window settings **(F)** from a fourth individual shows a spiculated left lower lobe nodule, which proved to be Stage I bronchogenic adenocarcinoma. (Figs. A-C from Pickhardt PJ, Hanson ME, Vanness DJ, Lo J, Kim DH, Taylor AJ, et al. Unsuspected extracolonic findings at screening CT colonography: Clinical and economic impact. *Radiology.* 2008;249:151-159.)

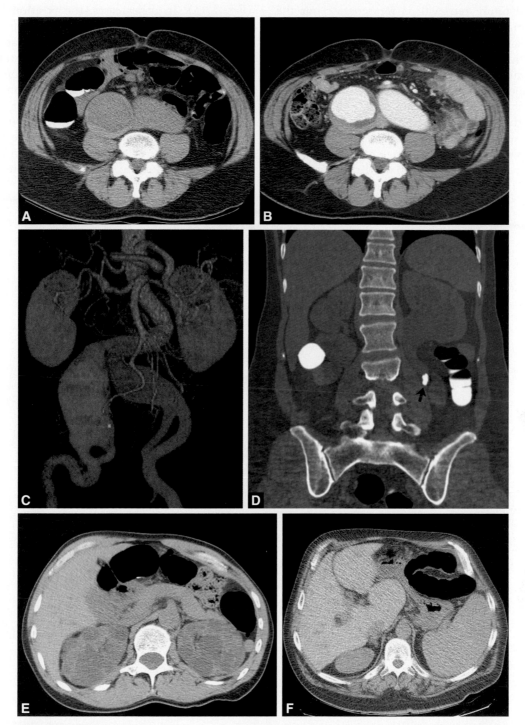

Figure 27-2 **Important non-neoplastic extracolonic findings at CTC screening (C-RADS category E4).** 2D extracolonic CTC image **(A)** shows massive bilateral iliac artery aneurysms, right greater than left. Intramural high attenuation wall thickening involving the right common iliac artery aneurysm suggests hemorrhage and impending rupture. 2D transverse **(B)** and 3D volume-rendered **(C)** images from subsequent preoperative CT angiography better demonstrate the vascular pathology. The patient, who was not yet symptomatic, underwent successful bypass surgery shortly after the incidental detection at CTC. 2D curved reformatted coronal CTC image **(D)** from a second individual shows an unsuspected large, obstructing left ureteral calculus *(arrow)* resulting in prominent hydronephrosis. The stone was successfully treated with extracorporeal shock-wave lithotripsy. 2D extracolonic CTC image **(E)** from a third individual shows innumerable bilateral renal cysts from previously undiagnosed autosomal dominant polycystic disease. 2D extracolonic CTC image from a fourth individual **(F)** shows a hyperdense liver (75-80 HU) with a cirrhotic morphology and splenomegaly from portal hypertension. Unsuspected cirrhosis from hereditary hemochromatosis was subsequently diagnosed. (Figs. A-E from Pickhardt PJ, Hanson ME, Vanness DJ, Lo J, Kim DH, Taylor AJ, et al. Unsuspected extracolonic findings at screening CT colonography: clinical and economic impact. *Radiology.* 2008;249:151-159.)

archiving and future retrieval as we separate out the image-rich, thin-section CTC source data. In effect, this creates a series that superficially resembles a noncontrast CT examination performed for urolithiasis evaluation. For extracolonic evaluation at CTC, however, it is important to remember that the thin-section source images are still available if needed. In particular, one must keep in mind that the prone series often extends more cephalad than the supine series. We have seen a number of clinically important thoracic findings, including several lung cancers, which were only seen on the prone display (Fig. 27-3). In other cases, the positional change between supine and prone may provide useful information with regard to the mobile or stationary nature of certain findings (Fig. 27-4). Occasionally, an astute CT technologist may identify a potentially important extracolonic finding before the examination is completed, which may allow for more definitive evaluation with intravenous (IV) contrast during the initial encounter. Alternatively, some programs may require online image review by the radiologist before the examination is concluded. In general, we prefer to interpret the entire CTC exami-

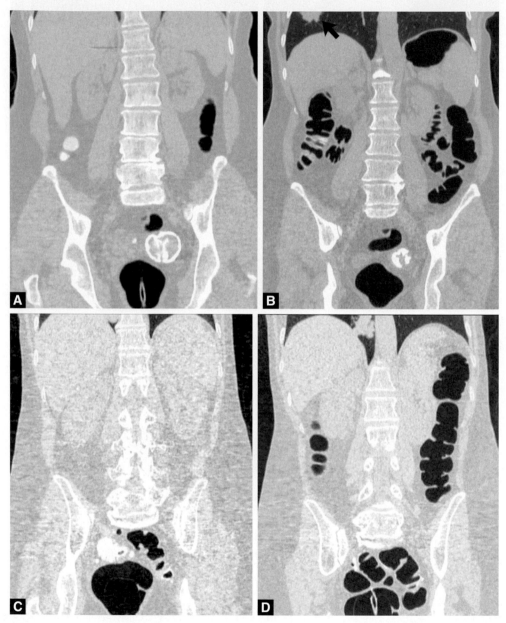

Figure 27-3 **Lung cancers imaged only on the prone acquisition.** Supine **(A)** and prone **(B)** 2D coronal CTC images show a large, spiculated lung mass in the right lower lobe *(arrow),* which is only seen on the prone view as a result of greater cephalad coverage and would have been missed on supine-only extracolonic review. Supine **(C)** and prone **(D)** images from a second individual show a similar situation with a right lower lobe mass. Primary bronchogenic adenocarcinoma was subsequently proven in both cases. Although we routinely reconstruct the supine series for extracolonic evaluation, it is advisable to check the lung bases on the prone series as well because of the greater coverage.

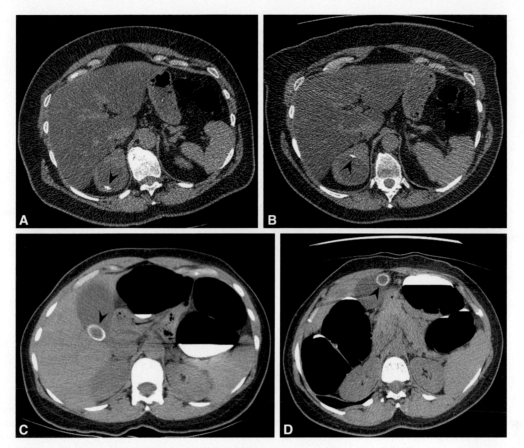

Figure 27-4 **Utility of positional change between supine and prone series.** Supine **(A)** and prone **(B)** 2D CTC images show a large complex renal cyst involving the upper pole of the right kidney. The peripheral high attenuation *(arrowheads)* could have been mistaken for mural calcification on one view, but its dependent shift within the cyst indicates dense luminal debris, which is of less clinical concern. Hepatic steatosis is incidentally noted. The positional change at CTC can provide information in other areas as well, such as demonstrating mobility of gallstones **(C** and **D,** *arrowheads)*, thus excluding impaction.

nation for all relevant colonic and extracolonic findings before performing or recommending any further tests.

In an attempt to circumvent the issue of extracolonic findings altogether, some have advocated for exclusion of all "extraneous" extracolonic regions via a postprocessing step. However, withholding or not reviewing irradiated and imaged regions raises obvious clinical and ethical concerns, especially given the finite potential for harboring a clinically relevant finding. As such, the medicolegal implications of ignoring scanned areas are probably more severe than responsibly managing them. We believe that judicious handling of extracolonic findings at CTC is the best course of action, taking care not to practice "defensive medicine," in which further workup is recommended for findings that are overwhelmingly benign (e.g., uncomplicated hepatic or renal cysts). It is important to realize that extracolonic evaluation is rather limited to begin with as a result of the low-dose, noncontrast nature of CTC (Fig. 27-5). As technical advances such as tube current modulation allow for further dose reduction at CTC, this may further decrease the ability to detect extracolonic abnormalities. This limited evaluation is probably not such a negative consequence because, in practice, the

hope is that most extracolonic findings with a legitimate chance to be truly clinically relevant will still be identifiable but that the many incidental lesions of little no significance become more obscured.

Classification

It is important to approach extracolonic findings detected at CTC in a systematic fashion. One important distinction is to separate those findings that require further attention (e.g., more definitive imaging, future surveillance, clinical correlation, or treatment) from those that do not. Beyond this binary distinction, the CT Colonography Reporting and Data System (C-RADS)[4] provides a useful framework for handling extracolonic findings, including verification of appropriate follow-up for concerning findings. We have used the C-RADS classification system from the very start of our clinical program but have slightly modified the meaning of the various "E" categories from the original description. For example, we have never used the C-RADS E0 classification ("limited examination—compromised by artifact") in any case because we feel that extracolonic evaluation

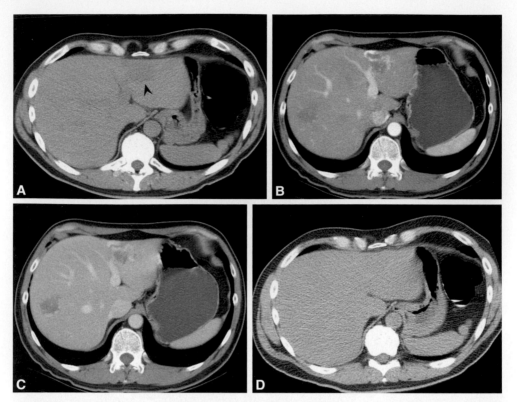

Figure 27-5 **Limitations of extracolonic evaluation at low-dose, noncontrast CTC.** 2D extracolonic CTC image **(A)** obtained at 175 mAs shows a subtle indeterminate lesion *(arrowhead)* in the left hepatic lobe, which proved to simply represent a cavernous hemangioma at diagnostic IV contrast-enhanced CT **(B** and **C).** The second hemangioma in the right lobe is not well seen at the initial CTC study. However, a subsequent CTC (performed for surveillance of a small polyp) that was obtained at 80 mAs fails to show either hepatic lesion. As CTC protocols continue toward lower doses, extracolonic evaluation becomes even more limited (which may be desirable for asymptomatic screening).

at CTC is limited by definition (again, perhaps a good thing). We simply do not have a definable threshold for what constitutes an evaluation that is "too limited," and we do not want to imply to clinicians that further evaluation might be indicated. The subsequent categories of C-RADS E1, E2, E3, and E4 roughly correspond to extracolonic findings of no, low, moderate, and high clinical importance, respectively. It is important to keep in mind, however, that many E3 and E4 findings should be considered to be only of *potential* importance, pending further evaluation. Many will ultimately prove to be of little or no actual significance, especially in healthy asymptomatic adults. In our opinion, the boundary between E1/2 and E3/4 is critical because this separates findings into the relevant binary categories noted earlier, in which further evaluation is generally indicated for findings above this threshold.

We treat the C-RADS E1 category ("normal exam") as a completely unremarkable extracolonic examination in which not even incidental findings are noted, regardless of how insignificant. However, as any practicing radiologist knows, nearly all adults undergoing CT evaluation have some "finding" that could conceivably be reported. Of course, the vast majority of these relate to normal variations or simply evidence of normal aging

(e.g., mild degenerative changes of the lumbar spine). We generally refrain from commenting on such normal variants or typical senescent changes. If a "finding" is felt to be clinically unimportant yet worth noting in the report, we classify this as E2, which deviates slightly from the original C-RADS description.

The C-RADS E2 category ("clinically unimportant finding") constitutes a broad spectrum of incidental lesions. Once an insignificant extracolonic finding is noted in the CTC report, we categorize this as E2 rather than try to distinguish it from an unimportant E1 finding/variant. In practice, however, we generally lump E1 and E2 together for both clinical and accounting purposes ("E1/2") because the more relevant dividing line is really between E2 and E3. Common incidental E2 findings encountered on a daily basis include uncomplicated renal or hepatic cysts, arterial vascular calcifications, calcified granulomata, uncomplicated hernias (particularly hiatal and inguinal), various benign skeletal findings, and incidental adrenal adenomas (Fig. 27-6). Except for unusual or extreme cases, these findings do not require further evaluation (if so, they are more appropriately classified as E3). In particular, we feel that benign-appearing low-attenuation renal and hepatic lesions do not require further workup (such

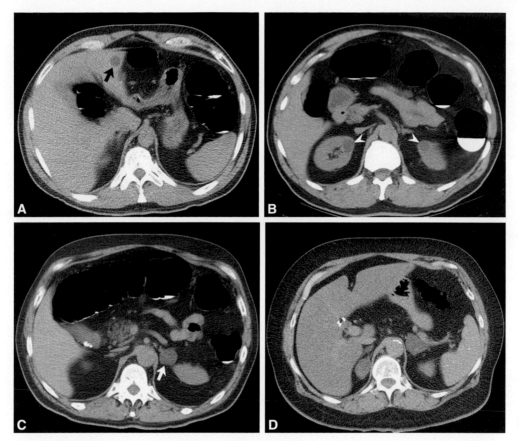

Figure 27-6 **Typical C-RADS category E2 extracolonic findings of no clinical significance.** 2D extracolonic CTC images from two different individuals show benign-appearing liver (**A,** *arrow*) and kidney (**B,** *arrowheads*) cysts, both of which are extremely common findings that should not trigger further workup. 2D extracolonic CTC image (**C**) from a third individual shows an incidental lipid-rich left adrenal adenoma *(arrow),* which measured less than 10 HU and requires no further imaging evaluation. Uncomplicated calcified gallstones are present, which are also an E2 level finding. 2D extracolonic image (**D**) from a fourth individual shows multiple incidental E2 findings, including bilateral adrenal adenomas, aortic calcification, punctate splenic calcifications from old healed benign granulomatous disease, hepatic steatosis, and prior cholecystectomy.

as ultrasound) unless unequivocal complexity is present.[1,2] Care must be taken in how these findings are described or relayed because some referring physicians will instinctively work up lesions that are clearly benign if there is any hint of doubt or uncertainty in the report. Many radiologists may reasonably choose not to mention many of these findings in their report. In particular, we refrain from mentioning small sliding hiatal hernias because we surmise that this often represents simply a physiologic response to colonic distention and is seen in more than 40% of cases (Fig. 27-7).

A second tier of E2 findings exist that, although not of immediate importance in an asymptomatic person undergoing CTC screening, could conceivably become relevant at some point in the future. Prime examples include incidental nephrolithiasis (Fig. 27-8) and cholelithiasis (Fig. 27-9), which are both seen at CTC in 5% to 10% of asymptomatic adults.[1,5] Another interesting example is fatty liver, which we commonly see at routine CTC screening—6% to 46% of asymptomatic adults, depending on the specific Hounsfield unit criterion used

for defining steatosis (Fig. 27-10).[6] These borderline findings are largely distinguished from E3 findings by the fact that, in isolation and without associated symptoms, they generally do not require additional imaging evaluation for further characterization. Nonetheless, knowledge of these incidental findings may prove useful if the patient were to develop symptoms in the future.

C-RADS E3 categorization ("likely unimportant—incompletely characterized") represents an important dividing point from E1/2-level findings, primarily because further workup may be indicated. Prime examples include moderately complicated renal cysts, prominent cystic adnexal lesions in women, indeterminate pulmonary nodules, and indeterminate liver lesions (Fig. 27-11). In nearly all cases in which such findings are identified at routine CTC screening in otherwise-healthy adults, these lesions prove to be benign. However, many of these findings undergo further workup, such as renal ultrasound or CT for complex renal cysts, pelvic ultrasound and sometimes even laparoscopy for adnexal cystic lesions, chest CT surveillance for indeterminate lung nodules, and contrast-enhanced CT or

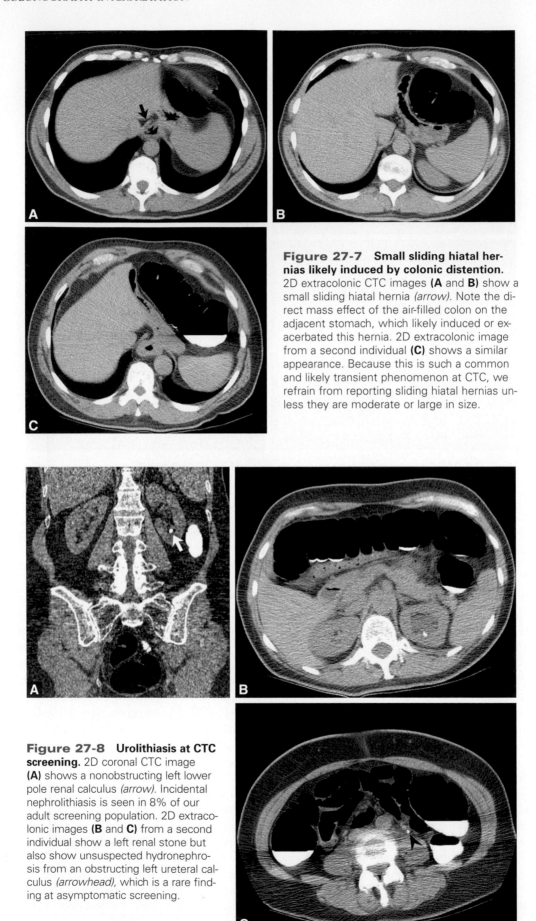

Figure 27-7 Small sliding hiatal hernias likely induced by colonic distention. 2D extracolonic CTC images (**A** and **B**) show a small sliding hiatal hernia *(arrow)*. Note the direct mass effect of the air-filled colon on the adjacent stomach, which likely induced or exacerbated this hernia. 2D extracolonic image from a second individual (**C**) shows a similar appearance. Because this is such a common and likely transient phenomenon at CTC, we refrain from reporting sliding hiatal hernias unless they are moderate or large in size.

Figure 27-8 Urolithiasis at CTC screening. 2D coronal CTC image (**A**) shows a nonobstructing left lower pole renal calculus *(arrow)*. Incidental nephrolithiasis is seen in 8% of our adult screening population. 2D extracolonic images (**B** and **C**) from a second individual show a left renal stone but also show unsuspected hydronephrosis from an obstructing left ureteral calculus *(arrowhead),* which is a rare finding at asymptomatic screening.

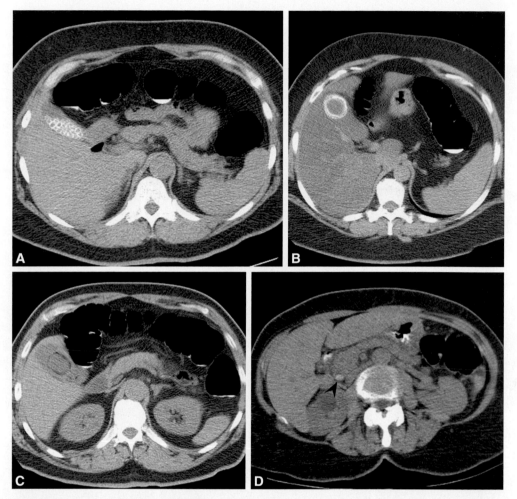

Figure 27-9   Cholelithiasis and choledocholithiasis at CTC screening. 2D extracolonic CTC images from three different adults **(A-C)** show gallstones with attenuation components varying from calcification to less than water density. 2D CTC image from a fourth individual **(D)** shows unsuspected nonobstructing choledocholithiasis with a slightly dense stone in the distal common bile duct *(arrowhead)*. Incidental choledocholithiasis is a rare finding at CTC screening. Note the cyst (C-RADS E2) in the right kidney.

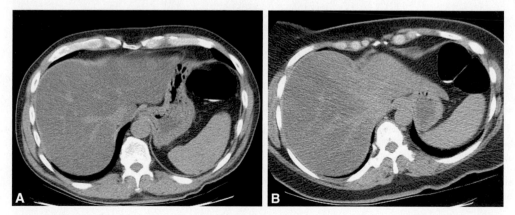

Figure 27-10   Incidental hepatic steatosis at CTC screening. 2D extracolonic CTC images from two different individuals show diffuse **(A)** and right lobar **(B)** distribution patterns of fatty liver. Steatosis is a common incidental finding at CTC screening, which is of uncertain but doubtful significance and does not require further imaging evaluation.

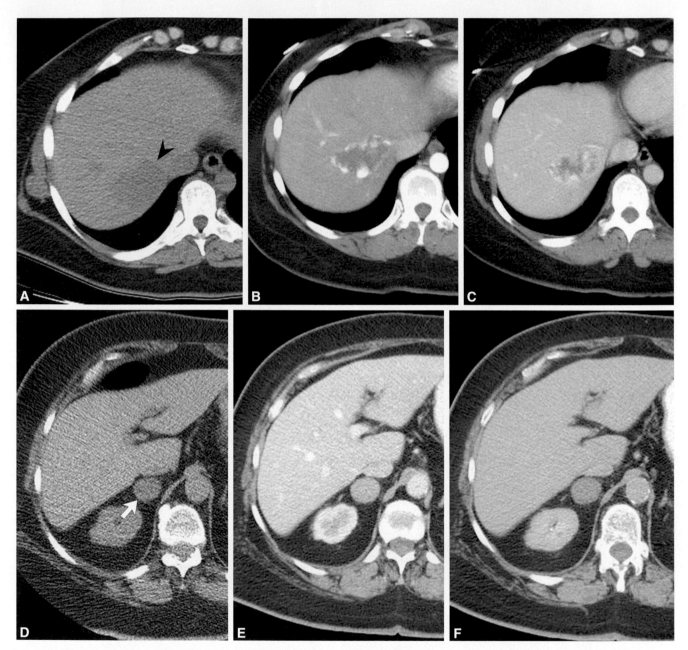

Figure 27-11 **Typical C-RADS category E3 extracolonic findings, which are probably not clinically important but are incompletely characterized.** 2D extracolonic CTC image **(A)** shows a subtle indeterminate liver lesion *(arrowhead)*, which proved to be a cavernous hemangioma at biphasic contrast-enhanced CT **(B** and **C)**. 2D extracolonic CTC image from a second individual **(D)** shows a 2.7-cm right adrenal lesion *(arrow)* that measured 27 HU in attenuation, which is indeterminate but likely a lipid-poor adenoma in a low-risk screening individual. Adrenal CT demonstrates enhancement on portal venous phase **(E,** 86 HU) with greater than 50% washout on delayed phase **(F,** 40 HU), diagnostic of a benign lipid-poor adenoma.

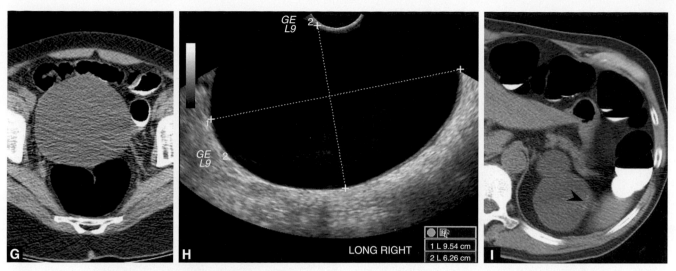

Figure 27-11 (Continued)   **Typical C-RADS category E3 extracolonic findings, which are probably not clinically important but are incompletely characterized.** 2D CTC image from a third individual **(G)** shows a large, benign-appearing adnexal cyst, which had a simple appearance at pelvic ultrasound **(H)**. This ovarian lesion was removed at laparoscopy and proved to be a serous cystadenoma. 2D extracolonic CTC image from a fourth individual **(I)** shows left upper pole renal cysts and cholelithiasis. The larger renal cyst demonstrates subtle wall calcification *(arrowhead),* which may also be slightly thickened. Comparison with an outside CT performed 7 years earlier, however, showed no interval change.

MR imaging for indeterminate liver lesions (which invariably seem to be benign cavernous hemangiomas). Excessive E3 categorization with subsequent diagnostic workup will drive up programmatic costs and yield relatively little benefit. Therefore, it behooves the interpreting radiologist to limit the number of these workups whenever possible because very few will ultimately prove to be clinically important.

C-RADS E4 classification ("potentially important finding") should be reserved for findings that are either of clear clinical significance (e.g., large abdominal aortic aneurysm) or should be assumed to be of high potential clinical significance until proven otherwise (e.g., worrisome masses or lymphadenopathy; Figs. 27-1 and 27-2). Some form of workup and/or treatment is usually indicated for E4 findings, such as more definitive imaging, needle biopsy, or surgery. Direct communication of unsuspected E4 results to the referring physician is generally indicated to ensure appropriate further management. Of course, not all concerning E4 findings will ultimately prove to be malignant, or even important, after definitive investigation (Fig. 27-12). Furthermore, because the dividing line between E3 and E4 is not always clearcut (Fig. 27-13), it can be useful to simply dichotomize extracolonic findings into E1/2 and E3/4 to emphasize the threshold for additional workup. The use of C-RADS classification in our clinical CTC database allows for easy tracking of these cases to ensure proper followup (Fig. 27-14).

Use of the C-RADS classification system as part of a clinical CTC database allows for continual quality assessment of the program, ensures appropriate patient care, and provides for direct comparison with other programs. From the initial 2500 adults screened at the University of Wisconsin CTC program, the frequency of

C-RADS E0, E1/2, E3, and E4 classification was 0%, 90.0%, 7.8%, and 2.2%, respectively.[7] These preliminary findings provide an initial benchmark against which future CTC screening programs can be compared.

Reporting

Beyond detection alone, how one actually reports the extracolonic findings seen at CTC is very important. Responsible reporting implies that there are no ambiguities with regard to the potential importance of a particular finding or with the need for further evaluation. Confusion may arise from the reporting of the overall frequency of extracolonic "findings" (not otherwise specified), which has ranged as high as 70%.[8-11] Because of the difficulty in defining what truly represents a finding versus normal variant or expected age-related change, it may be best to avoid reporting this poorly defined variable altogether. Because of the relative limitations of extracolonic evaluation related to CTC technique, we include the following statement in our standard report template: *"extracolonic evaluation is limited by the lack of IV contrast and low-dose CT technique."* Although this statement may not confer any substantial medicolegal coverage, it at least provides referring physicians and their patients with more reasonable expectations. Although we extensively use the C-RADS classification system for internal tracking, for quality assurance, and as a guide for clinical management, we do not explicitly include C-RADS verbiage in our dictated report. We feel this complicates the report and may unnecessarily confuse referring physicians and patients. Rather, we describe any notable findings in the body of the report and clearly state in the impression whether any findings are deemed

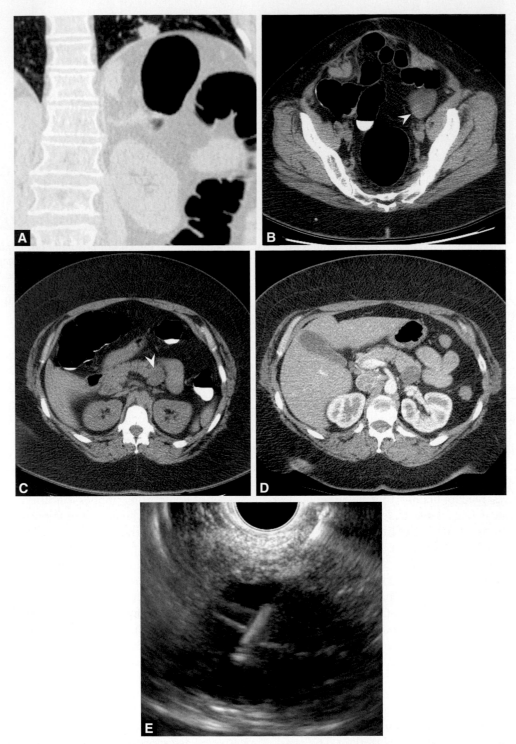

Figure 27-12 C-RADS category E4 extracolonic findings that ultimately proved to be benign at subsequent evaluation.
2D coronal CTC image **(A)** shows a spiculated nodule at the left lung base, which was metabolically active at subsequent PET study. Final pathology after surgical resection was a necrotizing granuloma. 2D extracolonic CTC image from a second individual **(B)** shows a suspicious left adnexal cystic lesion with an apparent mural soft tissue nodule *(arrowhead)*. The lesion proved to be a non-neoplastic paraovarian inclusion cyst after laparoscopic resection. 2D extracolonic CTC image from a third individual **(C)** shows a cystic pancreatic lesion *(arrowhead)*. Septations were demonstrated at contrast-enhanced CT **(D)** and endoscopic ultrasound **(E).** The lesion proved to be a benign mucinous cystic neoplasm.

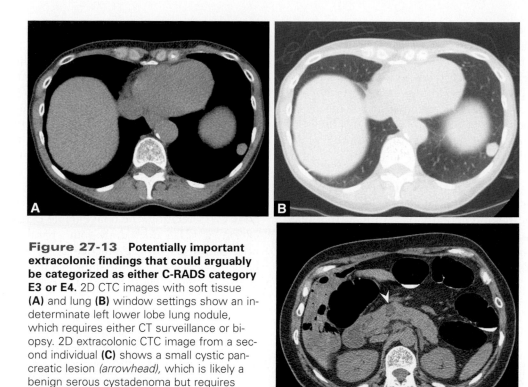

Figure 27-13 Potentially important extracolonic findings that could arguably be categorized as either C-RADS category E3 or E4. 2D CTC images with soft tissue **(A)** and lung **(B)** window settings show an indeterminate left lower lobe lung nodule, which requires either CT surveillance or biopsy. 2D extracolonic CTC image from a second individual **(C)** shows a small cystic pancreatic lesion *(arrowhead)*, which is likely a benign serous cystadenoma but requires more definitive imaging evaluation.

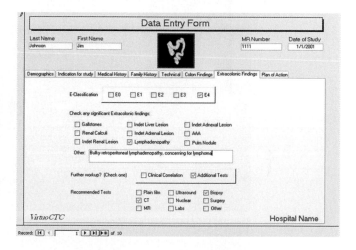

Figure 27-14 Tracking of extracolonic findings through use of a clinical database. Our CTC database allows for efficient followup of patients with potentially important extracolonic findings. We use the C-RADS categorization for our database (but not in our dictated report to clinicians). In addition, we track our frequency for recommending additional testing. (Note, the demographic information for this database entry is fictitious.)

to be of potential significance and whether further evaluation is required or should be considered. In some cases, the need for further workup depends on the specific clinical context, which may require correlation on behalf of the referring physician.

For most unsuspected extracolonic findings of potentially high significance (corresponding to C-RADS E4 classification), we directly communicate both the finding itself and recommended course of action to the referring physician. Although we immediately notify patients as to whether significant polyps were identified (to facilitate same-day colonoscopy, if needed), we generally do not relay extracolonic findings directly to patients. This allows the referring physician, who has presumably built a rapport

with the patient and is ultimately responsible for arranging further workup, the ability to maintain appropriate control of communication of such findings. We do, however, keep a careful log of potentially important extracolonic findings (through our patient database), which we periodically check to confirm clinical resolution or outcome.

EXTRACOLONIC FINDINGS OF POTENTIAL SIGNIFICANCE

Although most prior studies on extracolonic findings at CTC have involved symptomatic or high-risk cohorts, the findings from our asymptomatic screening experience are similar to a number of these studies in many respects.

The rate of extracolonic findings of at least moderate potential significance has been within a rather narrow range of 7.4% to 11.4% in a number of published studies involving largely nonscreening cohorts.[9-12] Similarly, the rate of unsuspected findings of moderate or greater potential significance from our screening experience is 8% to 9%, corresponding to new E3 and E4 level findings.[2] However, a study from the United Kingdom involving symptomatic elderly patients with an average age of 80 years old reported a 29% frequency of significant extracolonic findings, which emphasizes the need for considering the specific population under consideration.[3]

Recommending and actually obtaining further diagnostic workup are additional important parameters that can be compared between programs. In our screening experience, we have recommended or suggested further evaluation in 7% of cases, which is similar to that reported by Yee et al.[12] Additional diagnostic workup was performed in 6% of our total screening population. The actual workup rate is slightly less than the "recommended" rate, in part because further evaluation was only suggested in some E3-level cases, which ultimately depends on the clinical judgment of the referring physician, after appropriate correlation. The workup rate is slightly inflated, however, by inappropriate evaluation performed for incidentally noted E2 findings, which ac-

counted for 14% of additional workups in our series.[2] Examples of studies ordered by referring physicians following a negative CTC examination include ultrasound or contrast-enhanced CT examination for benign-appearing renal or hepatic cysts (Fig. 27-15). This underscores the importance of clearly placing all extracolonic findings in their proper context within the dictated report. Language that clearly indicates that further imaging workup is not needed for incidentally noted E2 findings may be necessary for some practice settings. Although CTC is a targeted screening study distinct from the controversial realm of self-referred whole-body CT screening, the unavoidable extracolonic evaluation at CTC does draw some parallels. Relatively little data exist on the practice of nontargeted whole-body CT screening. In one study of 1192 adults undergoing nontargeted whole-body CT screening in a private-practice setting, the frequency for recommending further testing was an alarming 37%—more than five times the rate seen in our CTC screening program.[13] This shows the potential for abuse from irresponsible or overly defensive interpretation of noncontrast CT scans, which could lead to excessive program costs and poor clinical practice.

As previously noted, although many unsuspected extracolonic findings of at least moderate potential signifi-

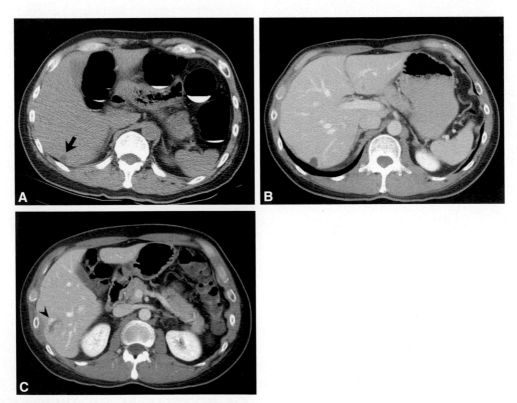

Figure 27-15 **Inappropriate workup of C-RADS category E2 extracolonic findings.** 2D CTC image **(A)** shows a well-defined subcentimeter low-attenuation lesion involving the peripheral aspect of the right hepatic lobe *(arrow)*. This was prospectively categorized as E2, no further evaluation was recommended, and the dictation stated "in the screening setting, this is almost certainly a benign finding." Nonetheless, the referring physician ordered a diagnostic CT with IV contrast for further evaluation **(B),** which confirmed a benign cystic lesion. A cavernous hemangioma *(arrowhead)* was also identified on the contrast-enhanced study **(C),** which was not appreciated on the low-dose, noncontrast CTC study.

cance will ultimately prove to be of little or no clinical significance, a substantial minority will remain clinically important. In our experience, nearly 30% of all potentially important findings (or 2.6% of the total screening population) proved to be relevant after further workup. The great majority of these will be prospectively categorized as E4 findings, but some will be labeled as E3. This underscores the importance of responsible reporting and handling of incidental imaging findings because the likelihood of harboring a clinically significant disease is relatively low—but is not zero. The probability of finding a clinically relevant alternative diagnoses is typically higher in other symptomatic groups undergoing CT evaluation for other indications. For instance, 10% to 30% of symptomatic patients being evaluated by noncontrast CT for suspected ureteral calculi will have a clinically relevant alternative diagnosis.[14]

Certain specific examples of extracolonic findings deserve further consideration. Detection of extracolonic malignancy is perhaps most noteworthy. On average, we identify one unsuspected extracolonic cancer for every 300 asymptomatic adults undergoing CTC screening, compared with a colorectal cancer detection rate of approximately of 1 in 500.[15] This may seem paradoxical at first, but it serves as an important reminder that colorectal screening of asymptomatic adults is primarily intended for cancer prevention through detection and removal of advanced but benign adenomas, with cancer detection itself an important but secondary concern. The most commonly identified extracolonic cancers are renal cell carcinoma, bronchogenic carcinoma, and lymphoma, but we have seen a number of other malignancies as well (Figs. 27-1 and 27-16). Early detection of these cancers in a presymptomatic phase appears to have resulted in a more favorable outcome.[15] Detection of asymptomatic vascular aneurysms represents another side benefit of CTC screening. Most aneurysms involve the abdominal aorta but significant iliac, mesenteric, and splenic artery

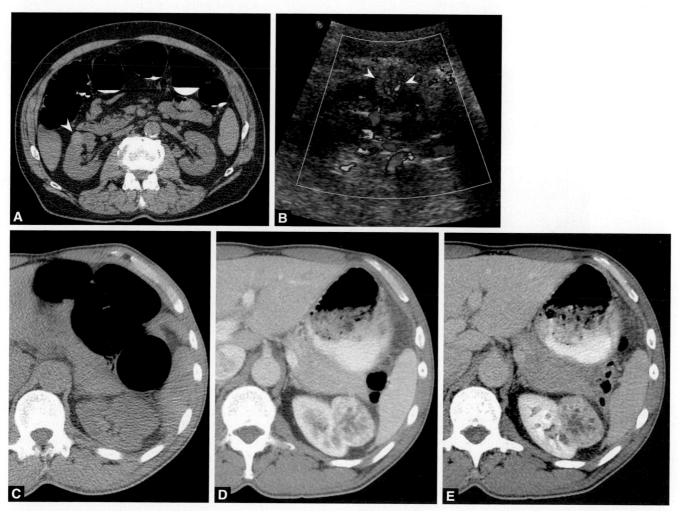

Figure 27-16 **Unsuspected extracolonic cancers detected at CTC screening.** 2D extracolonic CTC image **(A)** shows a small right renal lesion demonstrating high attenuation *(arrowhead)*. Subsequent renal ultrasound **(B)** to differentiate a hyperdense cyst from a solid lesion shows a hyperechoic mass *(arrowheads)* with internal blood flow on Doppler interrogation. This proved to be a small renal cell carcinoma. 2D extracolonic CTC image from a second individual **(C)** shows a large exophytic isodense left renal lesion, which demonstrated obvious enhancement on dedicated renal CT **(D** and **E)** and also proved to be a renal cell carcinoma.

Illustration continued on following page

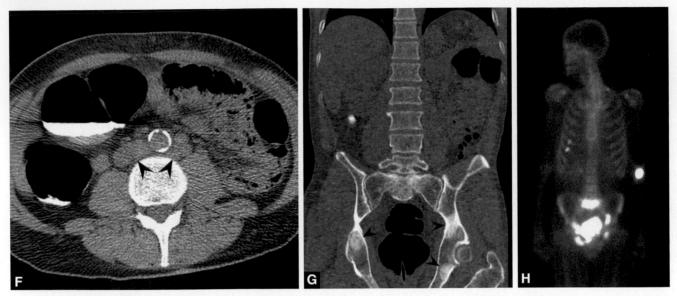

Figure 27-16 (Continued) **Unsuspected extracolonic cancers detected at CTC screening.** 2D extracolonic CTC image from a third individual **(F)** shows para-aortic retroperitoneal lymphadenopathy *(arrowheads).* 2D coronal reformatted image **(G)** with bone windows shows multiple blastic bone lesions *(arrowheads).* The prostate gland was not grossly enlarged, but a prostate specific antigen (PSA) level was drawn and found to be more than 7000 ng/mL. Metastatic prostate cancer was subsequently diagnosed and treated. Note the blastic osseous metastatic disease on skeletal scintigraphy **(H).**

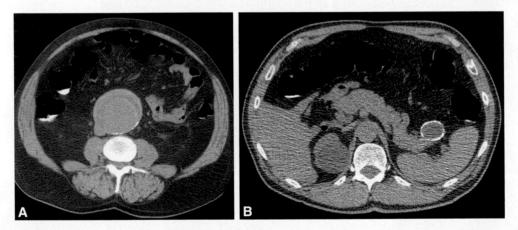

Figure 27-17 **Asymptomatic abdominal aneurysms detected at CTC screening.** 2D extracolonic CTC image **(A)** shows a large 8-cm abdominal aortic aneurysm, which was subsequently repaired. 2D extracolonic CTC image from a second patient **(B)** shows a 3-cm rim-calcified splenic artery aneurysm.

aneurysms are also seen on occasion (Figs. 27-2 and 27-17). As discussed later, detection of unsuspected but clinically significant aneurysms positively contributes to the overall cost effectiveness of CTC screening.

In contradistinction to extracolonic cancers and arterial aneurysms, further workup of indeterminate adnexal and hepatic lesions has proved to be of very low yield in terms of important pathology in our experience. Because most women undergoing CTC are either perimenopausal or postmenopausal, prominent cystic adnexal lesions often necessitate ultrasound followup. Findings range from simple-appearing unilocular ovarian or paraovarian cysts that are almost certainly benign to more complex solid and cystic masses that require surgical evaluation (Fig.

27-18). Most uniform solid adnexal lesions, however, are likely to represent pedunculated fibroids extending into the broad ligament. Indeterminate hepatic soft tissue lesions identified at asymptomatic screening CTC almost always are shown to represent cavernous hemangiomas of essentially no clinical importance on IV contrast–enhanced studies (Fig. 27-19). In some straightforward cases, ultrasound may represent a more efficient means for confirming cavernous hemangiomas.

A variety of incidental extracolonic gastrointestinal lesions may be identified in the distal esophagus, stomach, small bowel, and appendix.[16] Examples that we have seen include gastrointestinal lipomas, ileal carcinoid tumors, small bowel hamartomas, lymphangiomas, and

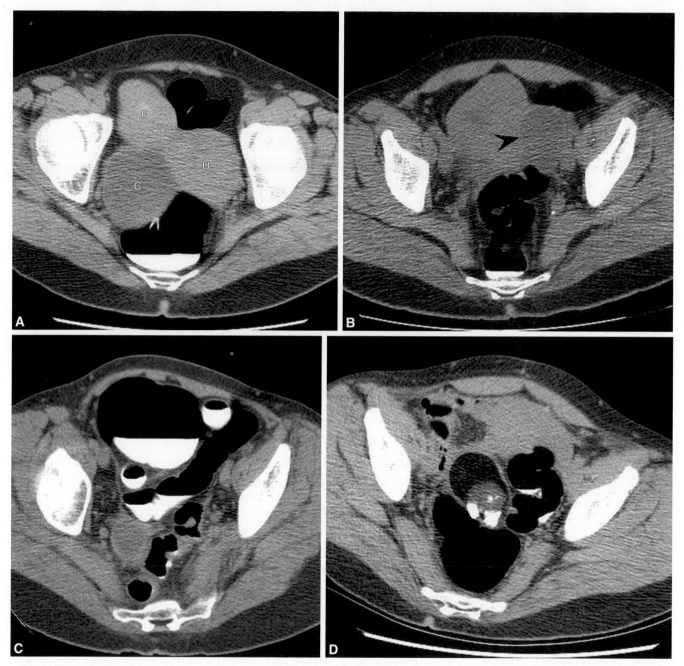

Figure 27-18   Adnexal findings in women undergoing CTC screening. 2D extracolonic CTC image **(A)** shows both solid- and cystic-appearing right adnexal lesions displacing the uterus (U). The solid lesion represents an exophytic fibroid **(F)** and the cystic lesion **(C)** is simply a functional ovarian cyst. 2D extracolonic CTC image from a second woman **(B)** shows a cystic left adnexal lesion *(arrowhead)* that proved to be an endometrioma. 2D extracolonic CTC image from a third woman **(C)** shows a thick-walled left adnexal cystic lesion that proved to be an ovarian cystadenofibroma. 2D extracolonic CTC image from a fourth woman **(D)** shows a fat-containing ovarian mass, consistent with a mature teratoma. Soft tissue and calcific components are also present. (Part A from Pickhardt PJ, Taylor AJ. Extracolonic findings identified in asymptomatic adults at screening CT colonography. *Am J Roentgenol.* 2006;186:718-728.)

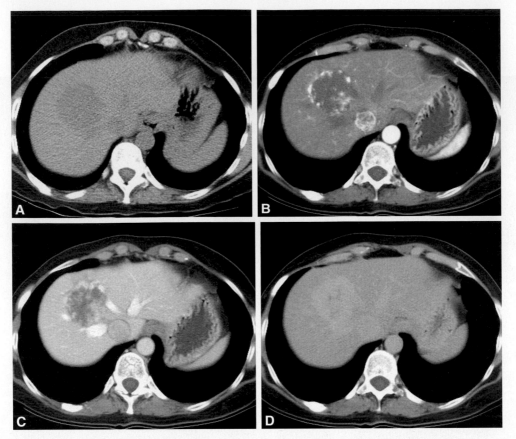

Figure 27-19 **Cavernous hemangioma manifesting as an indeterminate hepatic lesion at CTC.** 2D extracolonic CTC image **(A)** shows a subtle but large liver lesion centrally that is higher in attenuation than a simple cyst. Images from subsequent postcontrast diagnostic CT **(B-D)** show the pathognomonic enhancement pattern of a cavernous hemangioma.

appendiceal mucinous adenomas forming mucoceles (Fig. 27-20). Unsuspected incidental malrotation and other congenital abnormalities will also be encountered on occasion, which may be clinically relevant in some cases (Fig. 27-21).[17] Lipomas are of low clinical significance and can be confidently diagnosed at noncontrast CTC evaluation, as can other fat-containing lesions in the abdomen and pelvis (Fig. 27-22). Benign adrenal adenomas and incidental urolithiasis are other conditions in which imaging-specific diagnosis is possible and no further workup is generally needed (Figs. 27-6 and 27-8). Urolithiasis is seen in about 8% of our screening population and typically consists of nonobstructing renal calculi, although asymptomatic ureteral stones with or without evidence of obstruction are rarely seen (Fig. 27-2 and 27-8).

In some cases, the existence of an important extracolonic condition will already be known (Fig. 27-23). Although this is not a dilemma for the patient in any way, it does create some difficulty in terms of proper C-RADS categorization and program quality metrics. If important but previously established extracolonic findings are categorized as E3 or E4, it will artificially inflate the workup rate, which should be restricted to unsuspected findings.

However, E2 classification may be also inappropriate if these findings are of clinical importance. A special subcategory should perhaps be considered to account for known conditions.

COST IMPLICATIONS

It is important to consider the economic implications of detecting extracolonic findings at CTC. Our cost estimates for additional diagnostic imaging workup of $31 per patient[2] agrees with prior studies that have clustered within a remarkably narrow range of $24 to $34 per patient.[9,11,12,18] Although this represents only a small fraction of overall CTC costs, these cost considerations do not include the cost of surgical procedures and inpatient hospitalization required as a part of the diagnostic workup, which averaged $67.54 per patient screened in our study.[2] Of course, these additional costs must be balanced against the potential benefits derived from early detection of a wide variety of relevant extracolonic pathology. This would require a detailed longitudinal analysis of the ultimate clinical outcomes, which is not yet possible. Mathematic modeling, however, has been helpful in this regard. We have modeled the cost-effectiveness of CTC when

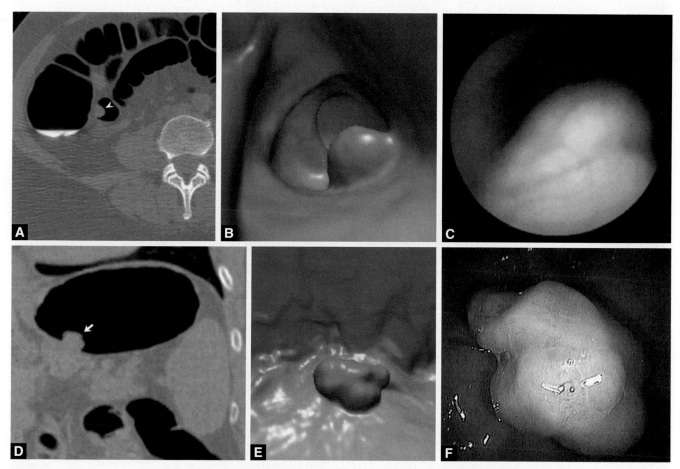

Figure 27-20   **Noncolonic gastrointestinal lesions detected at CTC screening.** 2D transverse **(A)** and 3D endoluminal **(B)** CTC images show a polypoid soft tissue lesion *(arrowhead)* within the ileum, which was confirmed on capsule endoscopy **(C)** and proved to be a benign lymphangioma after surgical resection. 2D coronal **(D)** and 3D endoluminal **(E)** CTC images from a second individual show a polypoid soft tissue lesion *(arrow)* within the proximal stomach, which proved to be a fundic gland polyp after endoscopic resection **(F)**. (From Pickhardt PJ, Kim DH, Taylor AJ, Gopal DV, Weber SM, Heise CP. Extracolonic tumors of the gastrointestinal tract detected incidentally at screening CT colonography. *Dis Colon Rectum.* 2006;50:1-8.) *(*See associated video clips on DVD.)*

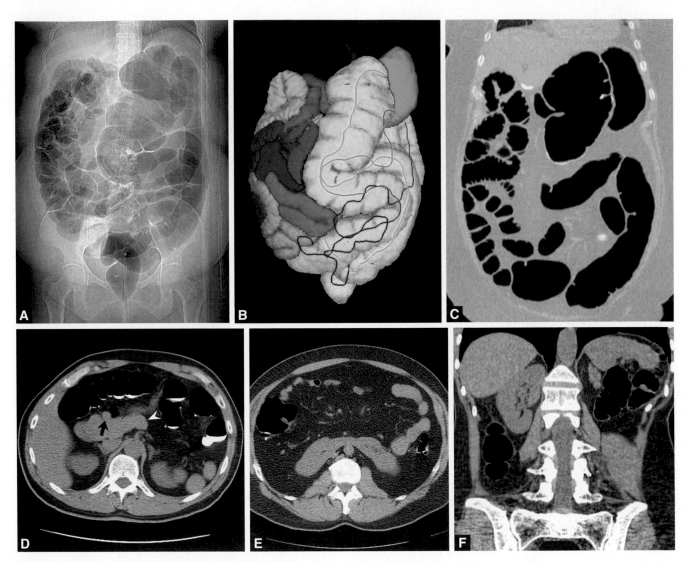

Figure 27-21 Unsuspected congenital anomalies and variants identified at CTC screening. Scout radiograph for CTC **(A)** suggests that the gas-filled colon is predominately left-sided and the gas-filled small bowel is predominately right-sided. 3D colon map **(B)** and 2D coronal CTC image **(C)** confirm the abnormal bowel position, consistent with malrotation (nonrotation). 2D extracolonic CTC image from a second individual **(D)** shows multiple spleens, abrupt cutoff of the pancreatic body *(arrowhead)*, and a preduodenal portal vein *(arrow)*, consistent with polypsplenia. 2D extracolonic CTC image from a third individual **(E)** shows a horseshoe kidney without complication. 2D coronal CTC image **(F)** from a final individual shows congenital agenesis of the left kidney.

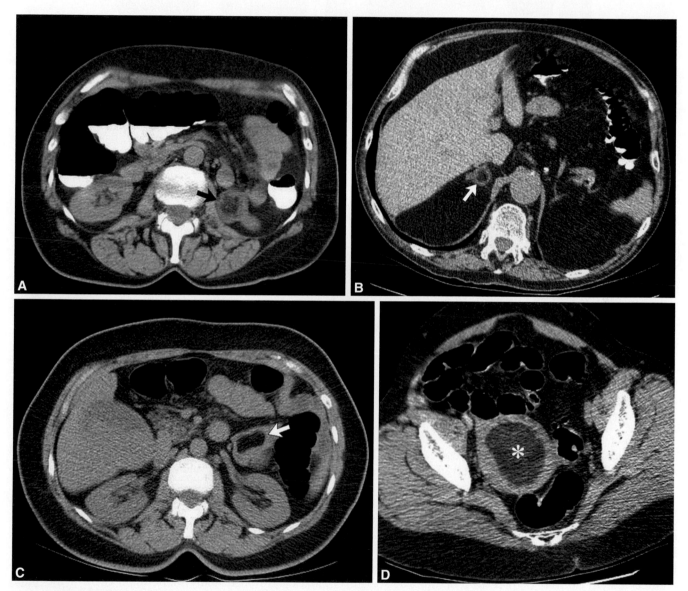

Figure 27-22   Fat-containing extracolonic lesions. 2D CTC images from four different individuals show an exophytic renal angiomyolipoma (**A,** *arrow*), adrenal myelolipoma (**B,** *arrow*), jejunal lipoma (**C,** *arrow*), and uterine lipoleiomyoma (**D,** *asterisk*). The presence of detectable fat allows for the diagnosis in each case. (Part A from Pickhardt PJ, Taylor AJ. Extracolonic findings identified in asymptomatic adults at screening CT colonography. *Am J Roentgenol.* 2006;186:718-728.)

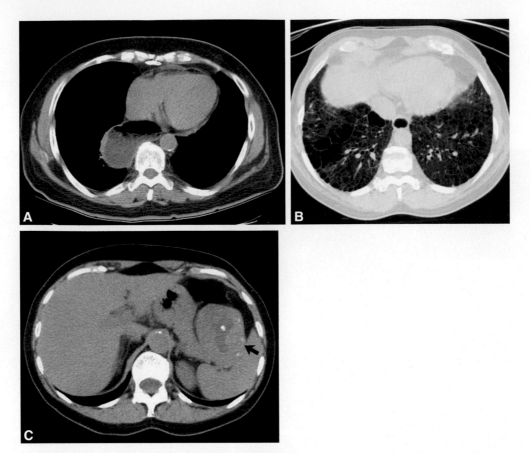

Figure 27-23 **Important but already-established extracolonic findings at CTC screening.** 2D extracolonic CTC image **(A)** shows a massively dilated, debris-filled esophagus in a patient with longstanding achalasia. 2D extracolonic CTC image from a second patient **(B)** shows chronic interstitial lung disease related to a known connective tissue disorder (note also the air-filled esophagus). 2D extracolonic CTC image from a third patient **(C)** shows a heterogeneous left upper quadrant soft tissue mass *(arrow)* with areas of cystic change and calcification, which was presumed to represent a mesenchymal tumor and had been stable for many years (the patient refused surgery for this finding).

detection of extracolonic cancers and aortic aneurysms are also considered.[19] This simulation showed that CTC dominated optical colonoscopy screening, being both more cost effective and clinically effective in terms of life-years gained. Furthermore, when considering the relative cost effectiveness of CTC screening versus optical colonoscopy screening, the additive costs related to extracolonic evaluation are dwarfed by the disparity in costs related to the two screening tests. In fact, the charge for CTC at our institution is three to four times less than colonoscopy charges, a situation that is not reflected in published cost-effectiveness analyses.[19,20]

SUMMARY

Extracolonic evaluation at CTC screening is an unavoidable yet diagnostically limited examination. This aspect of CTC constitutes a double-edged sword because there is the potential for both significant benefit and possible harm. As such, this subplot of CTC screening should not be underestimated because it represents a major concern for some referring clinicians. It is important to make referring physicians and their patients aware of this evaluation, including the possibility that additional workup may be necessary in some cases. Some welcome this added dimension of CTC evaluation, whereas others do not. Regardless, defensive-minded overcalling by the interpreting radiologist could lead to excessive diagnostic workups and associated costs.

Regardless of whether extracolonic evaluation is viewed as a net benefit or liability, it is a responsibility that must be handled with care by the interpreting radiologist. Although many "abnormalities" will inevitably be uncovered, the pretest probability of clinically relevant disease is considerably low among average-risk asymptomatic adults. In terms of receiver operating characteristic (ROC) curve analysis considerations, one needs to "slide down" the ROC curve somewhat to decrease the false-positive fraction and avoid overcalling extracolonic findings in screening cohorts, which could have a negative impact on both cost effectiveness and overall patient care. Although the vast majority of extracolonic "findings" do not require further workup, a finite number of important disease processes will nonetheless be found. Judicious use of further diagnostic evaluation will help to keep the additive costs in check.

REFERENCES

1. Pickhardt PJ, Taylor AJ. Extracolonic findings identified in asymptomatic adults at screening CT colonography. *Am J Roentgenol.* 2006;186(3):718-728.
2. Pickhardt PJ, Hanson ME, Vanness DJ, et al. Unsuspected extracolonic findings at screening CT colonography: Clinical and economic impact. *Radiology.* 2008;249(1):151-159.
3. Tolan DJM, Armstrong EM, Chapman AH. Replacing barium enema with CT Colonography in patients older than 70 years: The importance of detecting extracolonic abnormalities. *Am J Roentgenol.* 2007;189(5):1104-1111.
4. Zalis ME, Barish MA, Choi JR, et al. CT colonography reporting and data system: A consensus proposal. *Radiology.* 2005;236(1):3-9.
5. Pickhardt PJ, Choi JR, Hwang I, et al. Computed tomographic virtual colonoscopy to screen for colorectal neoplasia in asymptomatic adults. *N Engl J Med.* 2003;349(23):2191-2200.
6. Boyce CJ, Pickhardt PJ, Hinshaw JL et al. Noncontrast CT for detection of fatty liver: Evaluation in 3,357 consecutive asymptomatic adults. Presented at the 2008 ARRS meeting.
7. Pickhardt PJ, Kim DH, Taylor AJ, Burnside ES. CT colonography reporting and data system (C-RADS): Prospective categorization for screening in 2,501 patients. Chicago: RSNA Scientific Assembly; 2006.
8. Hellstrom M, Svensson MH, Lasson A. Extracolonic and incidental findings on CT colonography (virtual colonoscopy). *Am J Roentgenol.* 2004;182(3):631-638.
9. Gluecker TM, Johnson CD, Wilson LA, et al. Extracolonic findings at CT colonography: Evaluation of prevalence and cost in a screening population. *Gastroenterology.* 2003;124(4):911-916.
10. Edwards JT, Wood CJ, Mendelson RM, Forbes GM. Extracolonic findings at virtual colonoscopy: Implications for screening programs. *Am J Gastroenterol.* 2001;96(10):3009-3012.
11. Hara AK, Johnson CD, MacCarty RL, Welch TJ. Incidental extracolonic findings at CT colonography. *Radiology.* 2000;215(2):353-357.
12. Yee J, Kumar NN, Godara S, et al. Extracolonic abnormalities discovered incidentally at CT colonography in a male population. *Radiology.* 2005;236(2):519-526.
13. Furtado CD, Aguirre DA, Sirlin CB, et al. Whole-body CT screening: Spectrum of findings and recommendations in 1192 patients. *Radiology.* 2005;237(2):385-394.
14. Rucker CM, Menias CO, Bhalla S. Mimics of renal colic: Alternative diagnoses at unenhanced helical CT. *Radiographics.* 2004;24:S11-S28.
15. Pickhardt PJ, Meiners RJ, Kim DH, Cash BD. Unsuspected cancers detected at CT colonography screening in over 10,000 asymptomatic adults. Presented at the 2009 SGR scientific session.
16. Pickhardt PJ, Kim DH, Taylor AJ, Gopal DV, Weber SM, Heise CP. Extracolonic tumors of the gastrointestinal tract detected incidentally at screening CT colonography. *Dis Colon Rectum.* 2007;50(1):56-63.
17. Pickhardt PJ, Bhalla S. Intestinal malrotation in adolescents and adults: spectrum of clinical and imaging features. *Am J Roentgenol.* 2002;179(6):1429-1435.
18. Chin M, Mendelson R, Edwards J, Foster N, Forbes G. Computed tomographic colonography: Prevalence, nature, and clinical significance of extracolonic findings in a community screening program. *Am J Gastroenterol.* 2005;100(12):2771-2776.
19. Hassan C, Pickhardt P, Laghi A, et al. Computed tomographic colonography to screen for colorectal cancer, extracolonic cancer, and aortic aneurysm. *Arch Intern Med.* 2008;168(7):696-705.
20. Pickhardt PJ, Hassan C, Laghi A, Zullo A, Kim DH, Morini S. Cost-effectiveness of colorectal cancer screening with computed tomography colonography—The impact of not reporting diminutive lesions. *Cancer.* 2007;109(11):2213-2221.

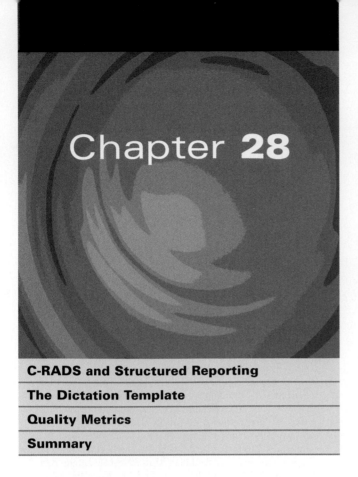

Chapter 28

Reporting of Results and Quality Metrics in CTC

DAVID H. KIM, MD
PERRY J. PICKHARDT, MD

INTRODUCTION

Effective and efficient reporting of results is a central component to a successful CT colonography (CTC) program. Consistency between institutions will be vital given the large numbers involved in a national screening effort. The benefits of structured reporting are well documented from the mammography experience and translate well into the colorectal cancer (CRC) screening realm. This chapter explores structured reporting at CTC in the context of CT Colonography Reporting and Data System (C-RADS), the components for a complete CTC report, and the various important quality metric measures that all CTC programs should undertake.

C-RADS AND STRUCTURED REPORTING

The reporting of results in the context of population screening is a very different circumstance from the usual reporting of diagnostic examinations for a specific symptomatic indication or patient complaint. Whereas individualized reports are useful to provide the necessary nuances for a specific clinical situation, it significantly hampers the utility of the examination in the screening setting. Consistency of reports between individuals and institutions is paramount to allow valid comparisons of screened individuals in both the clinical and research realms. A common lexicon with set categories based on

examination results allows for valid outcome measurements and defined management options.

C-RADS represents the structured reporting vehicle for colorectal cancer screening by CT colonography.[1] It is a consensus statement on reporting written by the Working Group on Virtual Colonoscopy, which was an international group of radiologists active in the early development of CTC. C-RADS comprises three main components: a lexicon, a classification schema for polyps, and a parallel schema for extracolonic findings.

Lexicon and Polyp Descriptors

The importance of a standardized lexicon cannot be overstated. It creates a common language for the examination. In addition to the standardization of various terms, it attempts to specify how these various descriptors should be applied to increase uniformity. For example, by C-RADS convention, the long axis of the polyp head (with exclusion of the polyp stalk) constitutes the reported size measurement of the polyp (see later).

In the lexicon, a *polyp* is defined as a focal protrusion of soft tissue attenuation into the colonic lumen. The distinction between a polyp and a colonic *mass* is arbitrarily set at 3 cm. When a polyp or mass is identified, four standard descriptors should be applied to characterize the lesion in a CT colonography report. These descriptors include *size, morphology, location,* and *attenuation*.

Size is perhaps the most important polyp descriptor because it represents the main determinant for the various C categories of the polyp classification schema (see later). Polyp size is a linear measurement of the long axis of the polyp (Fig. 28-1). For pedunculated polyps, only the long axis of the polyp head is measured and the polyp

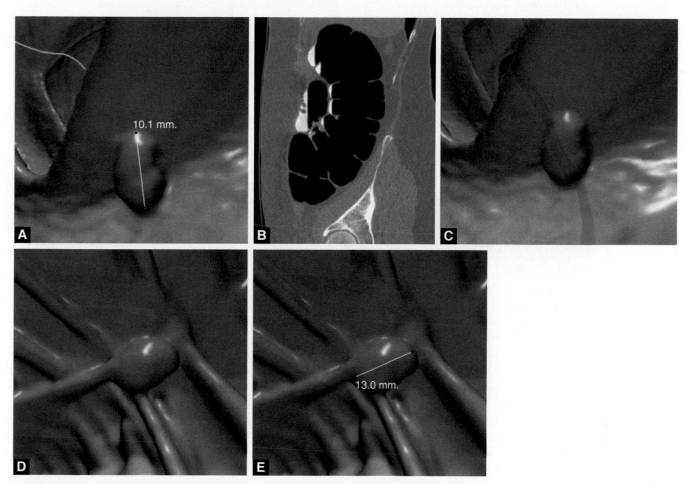

Figure 28-1   Determination of polyp size. Polyp size is determined by the length of the long axis of the polyp. Both 3D and 2D views are used where one may be favored over the other depending on the specific case. 3D endoluminal view **(A)** shows linear measurement of a polyp at 3D. In this case, the "optimized" sagittal 2D CTC image **(B),** where the polyp *(blue arrow)* is the largest among the three orthogonal planes, would underestimate the true size of the polyp because the sagittal plane is obliqued **(C,** *green line*) in relation to the true long axis of the polyp. Thus, the reported measurement in this case should reflect the 3D measurement. 3D endoluminal CTC image **(D)** in another patient demonstrates the accepted convention for measurement of a pedunculated polyp where the polyp head is measured **(E)** with exclusion of the polyp stalk. This polyp was a villous adenoma at pathology.

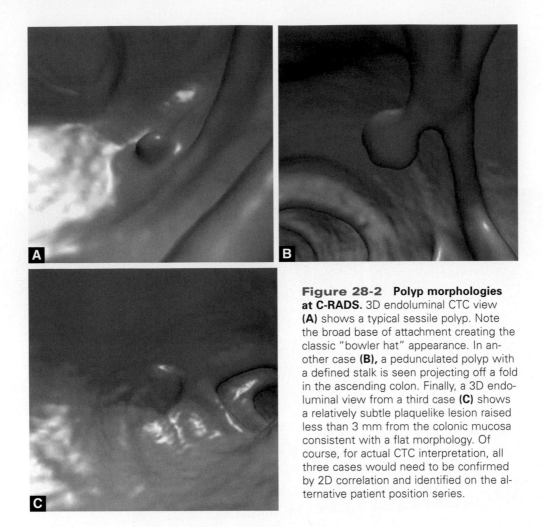

Figure 28-2   Polyp morphologies at C-RADS. 3D endoluminal CTC view **(A)** shows a typical sessile polyp. Note the broad base of attachment creating the classic "bowler hat" appearance. In another case **(B),** a pedunculated polyp with a defined stalk is seen projecting off a fold in the ascending colon. Finally, a 3D endoluminal view from a third case **(C)** shows a relatively subtle plaquelike lesion raised less than 3 mm from the colonic mucosa consistent with a flat morphology. Of course, for actual CTC interpretation, all three cases would need to be confirmed by 2D correlation and identified on the alternative patient position series.

stalk is excluded. Both two-dimensional (2D) and 3D series should be used in the determination of maximum linear size.[2] Specific window settings to optimize visualization of the polyp should be used for measurement determination on the 2D images (window width/level settings of 2000/0 are the optimal values in our opinion). There are three main size categories for polyps. Large polyps are ≥10 mm in size. Small polyps are 6 to 9 mm in size. Diminutive polyps measure ≤5 mm. Size allows for stratification of polyps related to inherent risk for cancer and for future development of cancer. Large size correlates well with an increased risk because the 10-mm threshold captures the vast majority of advanced adenomas (see Chapter 2).[3]

Morphology is defined by three main descriptors: sessile, pedunculated, and flat (Fig. 28-2). Sessile morphology is applied to polyps with a broad base of attachment to the colonic mucosa. Pedunculated polyps are characterized by the presence of a defined stalk that attaches to the colonic mucosa. Consequently, there is typically a more bulbous region representing the polyp head. Flat polyps are a subset of sessile lesions having a plaquelike appearance with a broad base of attachment. Flat polyps

are defined as lesions raised less than 3 mm from the colonic surface (with the exception of carpet lesions, which are flat masses 3 cm or larger that may exceed 3 mm in height). It is important to realize that there are differing definitions of flat morphology in both the optical colonoscopy (OC) and CT colonography literature. For example, some define flat lesions as those that have a height less than half the width of the base. At C-RADS, however, a more restrictive definition has been adopted with a 3-mm maximal raised distance. In addition to the three classic morphologic descriptors, we have found additional terms helpful for the morphologic characterization of larger masses (e.g., 3 cm in size or greater). These include carpet, saddle, hemi-circumferential, and annular. Carpet lesions are laterally spreading lesions that are characterized by a large area of involvement of several centimeters. Overall, the lesion is relatively flat, although there may be projections that measure up to 1 cm in height. These lesions are typically located in the rectum or cecum.[4] They often create a bizarre pattern of ridges and projections that are generally detectable but can be somewhat subtle at CTC (Fig. 28-3). They are important to detect because many contain advanced

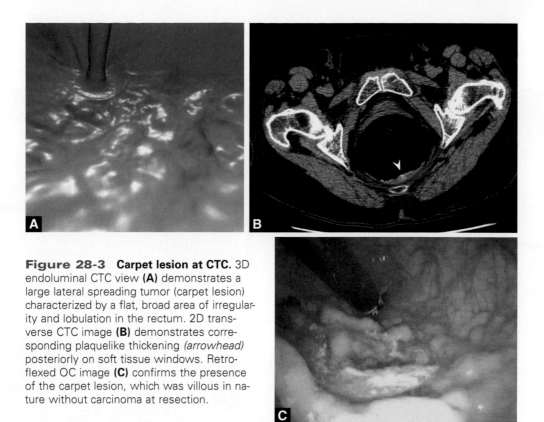

Figure 28-3 Carpet lesion at CTC. 3D endoluminal CTC view **(A)** demonstrates a large lateral spreading tumor (carpet lesion) characterized by a flat, broad area of irregularity and lobulation in the rectum. 2D transverse CTC image **(B)** demonstrates corresponding plaquelike thickening *(arrowhead)* posteriorly on soft tissue windows. Retroflexed OC image **(C)** confirms the presence of the carpet lesion, which was villous in nature without carcinoma at resection.

histology. The morphologic terms of saddle, hemicircumferential, and annular are helpful in the description of large masses involving the circumference of the colon (Fig. 28-4). These are typically malignant in nature (see Chapter 21).

Polyp location is described in terms of colonic segmental anatomy. For location, the colon is divided into six segments including the cecum, ascending colon, transverse colon, descending colon, sigmoid colon, and rectum (Fig. 28-5). The hepatic and splenic flexures can be applied as optional modifiers but should not be used as a specific location for polyp position because it is difficult to correlate such a location at optical colonoscopy. There are several important borders to keep in mind to properly locate a polyp. The dividing line between cecum and the ascending colon is the ileocecal valve where polyps at or inferior to the valve are in the cecum and those superior reside in the ascending colon (Fig. 28-5). The hepatic flexure denotes the dividing line between the ascending colon and transverse colon. The transverse colon spans from the hepatic flexure to the splenic flexure. It is important to note that the flexure positions may vary somewhat from person to person (and indeed within a person between prone and supine positions). The descending colon spans from the splenic flexure to a characteristic anterior bend in the left lower quadrant where the colon transitions from a retroperitoneal structure to an intraperitoneal structure on a mesentery. The dividing border between the sigmoid colon and rectum is

the third/proximal rectal fold and is easily identified at both 2D and 3D CTC (Fig. 28-5). In many CTC software programs, a centerline distance measurement from the anorectal junction to a given polyp is calculated. It is important to realize that this distance is accurate for its purpose but correlates poorly with distances obtained at optical colonoscopy. Because of telescoping of the bowel by the endoscope and lack of constant distention, the OC distances are often half that of the centerline measurements at CTC in our experience, even for distal right-sided lesions. Reporting out the CTC centerline distances for polyp location as opposed to segmental location descriptors would thus likely cause confusion for the colonoscopist.

Attenuation is the final classic descriptor. True polyps are of homogenous soft tissue gray appearance at CTC. It is often helpful to qualitatively assess attenuation by comparing the appearance of the polyp against muscle such as the psoas (see Chapter 18). Lipomas may present morphologically as well-defined polyps but will demonstrate much lower fatty attenuation with negative HU values. The main importance regarding attenuation concerns the distinction of pseudopolyps related to stool from true soft tissue polyps (see Chapter 20). Untagged stool can usually be differentiated by attenuation characteristics where these "polyps" are typically more heterogeneous in appearance as a result of the presence of air density. However, they can be indistinguishable from true soft tissue polyps with a relatively homogenous gray

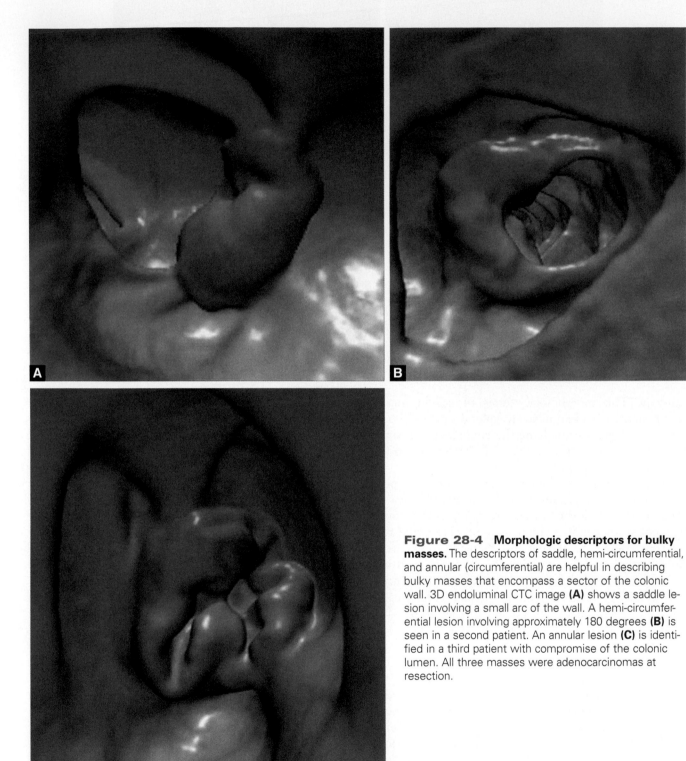

Figure 28-4 Morphologic descriptors for bulky masses. The descriptors of saddle, hemi-circumferential, and annular (circumferential) are helpful in describing bulky masses that encompass a sector of the colonic wall. 3D endoluminal CTC image **(A)** shows a saddle lesion involving a small arc of the wall. A hemi-circumferential lesion involving approximately 180 degrees **(B)** is seen in a second patient. An annular lesion **(C)** is identified in a third patient with compromise of the colonic lumen. All three masses were adenocarcinomas at resection.

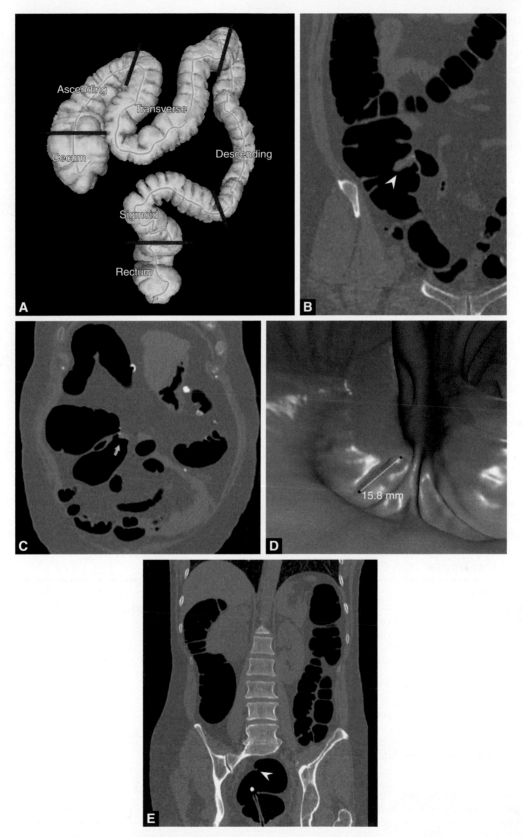

Figure 28-5 Segmental anatomy of the large intestine. Polyp locations are best described by segmental anatomy. 3D co-lon map **(A)** demonstrates the six named segments. 2D coronal image **(B)** shows the ileocecal valve *(arrowhead)* along the medial wall of the right colon. This landmark allows accurate delineation between the ascending colon and the cecum. Another case dem-onstrates a cecal polyp on 2D **(C,** *blue arrow)* and 3D **(D,** *calipers)*, which is located on the proximal side of the ileocecal fold, adja-cent to the valve. 2D coronal CTC image **(E)** in another patient shows the three rectal valves (of Houston), which allow accurate delineation between the sigmoid and rectum. The third/proximal valve (counting up from the distal rectum) is the dividing line *(ar-rowhead)*. Note the rectal catheter contacting the middle valve. Indentation from the balloon near the anorectal junction simulates a more distal fold.

appearance, requiring movement between supine and prone series for confirmation. In addition, true soft tissue polyps can appear somewhat mottled when low-dose techniques are applied, making the distinction even more difficult. When tagged, stool is easily distinguished from a polyp with marked increased attenuation values and a white appearance. As seen with measurement, appropriate window/level settings are important for the accurate assessment of attenuation. Polyp windows set at 2000/0 appear to be optimal. This allows high contrast between the air-filled colonic lumen and the soft tissue nature of the protruding polyp. However, this high contrast does not obscure the more subtle differences in attenuation between the soft tissue of the colonic wall and the adjacent pericolonic fat, as seen with some other window level settings (e.g., 1500/-200).

Finally, *diagnostic confidence* assignment for a polyp is not yet formally incorporated into the C-RADS lexicon but has been a helpful descriptor in our experience.[5] C-RADS suggests that it be used by clinical investigators for research, but it has also been very helpful for us in routine clinical practice. We use a three-point scale where a score of 1 indicates lowest confidence for a true polyp, 2 indicates moderate/intermediate confidence, and 3 indicates highest confidence (a score of zero—not used in practice—would indicate that the lesion is felt to be a pseudopolyp—below the threshold of diagnosis). In practical terms, we generally score a polyp with a diagnostic confidence of 3 when a focal fixed soft tissue lesion is seen on both the supine and prone series. If it is clearly seen on only one of the two series, the confidence score would drop to 1 or 2. In general, a score of 1 is given when a polyp represent a "soft call" where we would not be surprised if there was no OC correlate. A typical example is a possible subtle flat lesion covered by a thick coat of contrast. The clinical scenario in which the diagnostic score has been most useful concerns the situation where a CTC-reported polyp is not seen at therapeutic OC. In our experience, the positive predictive value according to diagnostic confidence score is 95% (554/585) for highest confidence (score = 3), 83% (106/127) for intermediate confidence (score = 2), and 63% (17/27) for least confidence (score = 1). A level 2 or 3 confidence more often yielded a matching lesion at OC than level-1 confidence (93% [660/712] versus 63% [17/27]; *p* <0.0001).[6] Therefore, if a diagnostic confidence is low (score = 1), the gastroenterologist is more reassured that they are not missing a true lesion and that the reported polyp more likely represented a CTC false-positive result. However, if a score of 3 was given by the interpreting radiologist, the colonoscopist will often examine the area more extensively because it is more likely that this polyp represents an initial OC false-negative result. This scoring system is also important in evaluating discordant cases to determine whether additional examinations are required (please see later in program metrics and Chapter 26).

Colonic and Extracolonic Classification Schemas

The two final and most visible components of C-RADS are the two classification schemas for examination results. Colorectal polyp findings are grouped into specific C *categories* where each category represents a homogenous population of results. Tied to each category is an inferred level of future risk and suggested management options.

Table 28-1 ◘ Colorectal "C" Categories of C-RADS

C0: Inadequate study
- Inadequate prep: cannot exclude lesions ≥10 mm owing to presence of fluid/feces
- Inadequate insufflation: one or more colonic segments collapsed on both views
- Awaiting prior colon studies for comparison

C1: Normal colon or benign lesions*
- No visible abnormalities of the colon
- No polyp ≥6 mm
- Lipoma or inverted diverticulum
- Nonneoplastic findings (e.g., colonic diverticula)

C2: Intermediate (small) polyp or indeterminate finding†
- Intermediate (small) polyp 6-9 mm, <3 in number
- Indeterminate finding, cannot exclude polyp ≥6 mm in technically adequate examination

C3: Polyp, possibly advanced adenoma‡
- Polyp ≥10 mm
- ≥3 polyps, each 6-9 mm

C4: Colonic mass, likely malignant§
- Lesion compromises bowel lumen, demonstrates extracolonic invasion

*Routine screening every 5-10 years.
†Surveillance or colonoscopy recommended. Evidence suggests surveillance can be delayed at least 3 years, subject to individual patient circumstance.
‡Followup colonoscopy recommended.
§Surgical consultation recommended. Communicate to referring physician as per accepted guidelines for communication, such as the ACR Practice Guideline for Communication: Diagnostic Radiology. Subject to local practice, endoscopic biopsy may be indicated.
Adapted from Zalis ME, Barish MA, Choi JR, et al. CT colonography reporting and data system: A consensus proposal. *Radiology.* 2005;236(1):3-9

The extracolonic findings detected on the CTC examination are handled similarly where they are grouped into specific *E categories*. As on the colonic side, each category conveys a level of future risk and provides acceptable management options.

For colorectal findings, there are 5 categories ranging from C0 to C4 (Table 28-1). C0 refers to examinations that are <u>nondiagnostic</u> as result of one of three reasons. First, the bowel preparation is inadequate where residual stool precludes exclusion of large polyps (≥10 mm). Second, there is a segment of colon that remains collapsed on all performed series and thus cannot be evaluated. Third, the comparison examinations for a person in CTC surveillance for a small polyp are not available and thus the assessment for interval change cannot be made. At the University of Wisconsin (UW), we have used our C0 category as a quality metric to assess the rate of technically inadequate examinations. If the rare third reason (waiting for comparison examinations) were a large component of C0s, obviously these cases would need to be separated out if the C0 rate is to be used in this manner.

The *C1* category represents a *negative* examination where no nondiminutive polyps (≥6 mm) are identified or only innocuous lesions such as a colonic lipoma are seen. As a rule, diminutive lesions (≤5 mm) are not reported if identified in isolation without relevant polyps. The specificity for diminutive lesions decreases for CTC, and they are difficult to match at OC even when real. Most important, diminutive lesions are highly unlikely to represent an advanced adenoma or a malignant polyp (see Chapter 2). Patients in the C1 category are relegated to routine screening. The interval is currently set at 5 years, although a range up to 10 years may not be unreasonable.

The C2 category is applied to patients with one or two small polyps (6-9 mm) detected on their CTC examination (Fig. 28-6). Acceptable management recommendations include colonoscopy with polypectomy or imaging surveillance in up to 3 years. The exceedingly low likelihood that a polyp of this size harbors carcinoma or would progress to carcinoma over this timeframe makes imaging surveillance a very reasonable option. The C2 polyp is somewhat analogous to a BI-RADS (Breast Imaging Reporting and Data System) 3 lesion (i.e., a likely benign lesion with a management option of imaging followup). The C2 category lesion fulfills the precedent set at mammography for imaging followup where (1) there is clearly less than 2% chance that the lesion represents carcinoma (for subcentimeter polyps, this risk is more on the order of 0.2% or less)[7-9] and (2) cancers seen at surveillance would likely present as early Stage I cancers. In the Hofstad

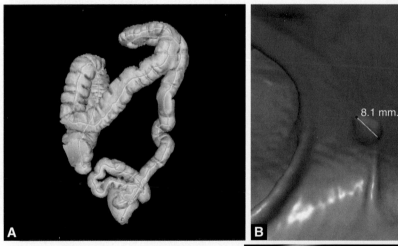

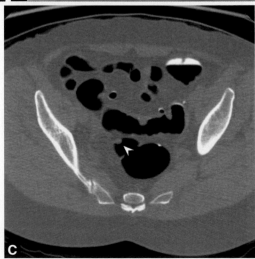

Figure 28-6 C-RADS category C2 designation. 3D colon map **(A)** bookmarks a polyp in the sigmoid colon *(red dot)*. 3D endoluminal CTC image **(B)** shows an 8-mm sessile polyp just proximal to the proximal rectal valve (dividing line between sigmoid and rectum). On the corresponding 2D transverse CTC image **(C),** the soft tissue nature of the polyp *(arrowhead)* is confirmed. One or two small polyps (6-9 mm) place the patient in the C2 category. Although imaging surveillance is an option, this patient elected for immediate polypectomy, which demonstrated a tubular adenoma without high-grade dysplasia.

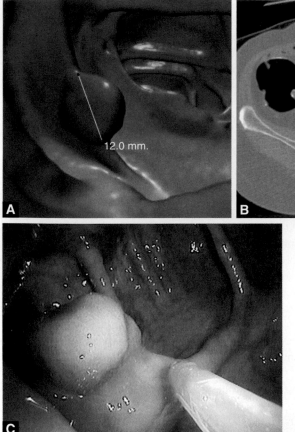

Figure 28-7 **C-RADS category C3 designation.** 3D endoluminal CTC view **(A)** shows a large, smooth polyp in the cecum that measures 12 mm. 2D transverse CTC view **(B)** confirms a homogeneous soft tissue core with a minimal surrounding coat of contrast. A polyp ≥10 mm places the patient in the C3 category. A tubulovillous adenoma was removed at OC **(C).** A designation of C3 is also given for cases where three or more small polyps measuring 6 to 9 mm in size are present.

colonoscopic surveillance series, the one incident cancer presented as an early cancer.[10] To date, we have not seen any cancers develop related to CTC surveillance of small polyps. The C2 category can also be applied to examinations that are technically adequate but somehow indeterminate for relevant lesions. We apply this second criterion to potential lesions of lowest diagnostic confidence (score = 1), such as a subtle flat lesion, in which the likelihood of a positive match at OC is low. This can include low-likelihood flat lesions that measure large (≥10 mm). In this case, a C2 designation can be assigned and the recommended followup interval can be decreased from the standard 5-year interval for a negative result to a shorter time interval (e.g., 2-3 years).

The C3 category is applied for the true target lesions of CTC screening. A C3 category designation is given for an examination with a polyp that measures 10 mm in size or greater or for an examination with three or more small 6- to 9-mm polyps (Fig. 28-7). The second criterion based on multiplicity of small polyps is a loose surrogate for the observation that multiple adenomas confer increased risk for future advanced neoplasia.[11] The polyps in the C3 category have a much higher likelihood to represent advanced neoplasia, either advanced adenomas (more likely) or carcinoma. For polyps 1 to 2 cm in size, recent series suggest a 1% rate of cancer (see Chapter 2). In our series, 95% of advanced adenomas are captured with a 10-mm polyp size threshold.[3] The clinical management for a C3

examination is referral to optical colonoscopy for polypectomy. Imaging surveillance generally would not be an appropriate option in this setting.

The C4 category is applied when an obvious mass is seen narrowing the lumen (Fig. 28-8). The majority of C4 lesions will represent cancers. Although direct surgical referral would be reasonable for many of the straightforward C4 malignancies, preoperative OC is currently used for histologic confirmation in most cases. Large polypoid masses measuring 3 cm or more are usually classified as C4, although most will not yet be malignant but still at the advanced adenoma stage. A small fraction of C4 lesions will be nonneoplastic, most often from mass-forming sigmoid diverticular strictures. Such strictures can usually be distinguished from cancer at CTC, and many will have already come from incomplete OC. However, as with suspected cancers, surgical consultation is the recommended course of action for most benign but high-grade strictures.

For the extracolonic lesions, a parallel classification schema is present ranging from E0 to E4 (Table 28-2). Similar to the colorectal findings, this allows the creation of relatively homogenous categories regarding extracolonic findings to stratify risk for significant findings. Appropriate management options are associated with each category. The issue of extracolonic findings and the overall approach should be handled carefully (see Chapter 27). Certainly, there are significant lesions outside of the large bowel that can be detected incidentally during

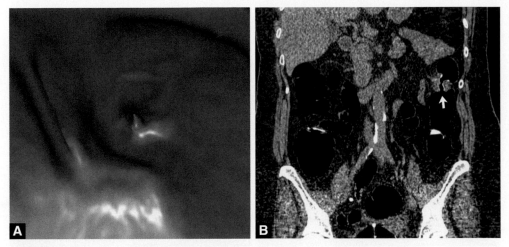

Figure 28-8   C-RADS category C4 designation. 3D endoluminal CTC view **(A)** shows an annular mass narrowing the descending colon consistent with a C4 lesion. 2D coronal CTC image **(B)** with soft tissue window/level settings confirms the focal soft tissue mass *(arrow)* circumferentially involving the colon in this area.

Table 28-2 ▣ Extracolonic "E" Categories of C-RADS

E0: Limited examination.
• Compromised by artifact; evaluation of extracolonic soft tissues is severely limited
E1: Normal examination or anatomic variant.
• No extracolonic abnormalities visible.
  • Example: retroaortic left renal vein
E2: Clinically unimportant finding.
• No workup indicated.
  • Examples: benign-appearing renal and hepatic cysts; uncomplicated cholelithiasis
E3: Likely unimportant finding, incompletely characterized.
• Subject to local practice and patient preference, workup may be indicated.
  • Examples: complex renal or ovarian cyst
E4: Potentially important finding.
• Communicate to referring physician as per accepted practice guidelines.
  • Examples: lymphadenopathy, solid organ-based mass, aortic aneurysm

From Zalis ME, Barish MA, Choi JR, et al. CT colonography reporting and data system: A consensus proposal. *Radiology*. 2005; 236(1):3-9.

screening where subsequent evaluation can make a marked positive impact. However, many of these extracolonic findings will likely be determined to be of no clinical significance, sometimes only after an extensive evaluation. This leads to increased medical costs, increased risks of complications related to procedures, and increased undue anxiety for the patient and referring physician. A judicious approach to this issue is warranted to decrease unnecessary examinations.[12]

The E0 category is intended for examinations where extracolonic evaluation is decreased and findings may be missed (e.g., marked streak artifact from spinal hardware decreasing evaluation of the pelvis). In our opinion, the E0 category is not relevant for CTC screening. The CTC examination is designed as a low-dose, noncontrast examination with inherent limitations. If positive findings are seen, they should be categorized. However, categorizing an examination as additionally limited over its limited baseline is not particularly helpful. Therefore, as a rule, we do not use the E0 category.

The E1 category is applied to examinations where normal anatomy or normal variants are seen (Fig. 28-9). Thus, there are no findings of any clinical significance and no other evaluation is suggested. The E2 category is applied to extracolonic findings that hold no acute significance or require additional evaluation to determine its likely benign nature (Fig. 28-9). Some examples would include benign-appearing hepatic and renal cysts. Incidental cholelithiasis and urolithiasis would also generally result in an E2 designation, unless the person was symptomatic or had obvious complications that would require attention.

E3 extracolonic findings are still most likely unimportant but are incompletely characterized. Thus, they remain possibly of some clinical significance (Fig. 28-10). One example is a potentially complicated renal cyst. Another example would be a cystic adnexal mass in a premenopausal woman. In both cases, although likely benign, additional evaluation is often required. Thus, indeterminate E3 lesions are best defined by the need for further studies for evaluation yet fall short of the E4 threshold. Management of E3 lesions usually involves further investigation with an additional imaging test to confirm the finding's presumed benign status.

E4 lesions are those that are potentially significant and of greater clinical concern, such as a solid-appearing parenchymal mass (liver, renal, pancreas, etc.) or vascular aneurysm (Fig. 28-10). In our experience, E4 findings are identified in about 2% of examinations. The unsuspected extracolonic cancer rate for our screening program has held steady at about 1 for every 300 patients screened.

The distinction between E2 and E3 is the crucial dividing line in the extracolonic classification of C-RADS.

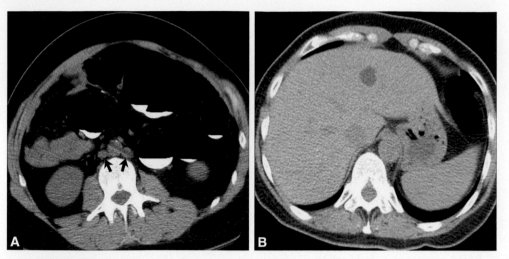

Figure 28-9 C-RADS category E1 and E2 designations. 2D transverse CTC image **(A)** shows a duplicated inferior vena cava *(arrows).* This anatomic vascular variant would still keep the patient in the E1 category. Individuals with no extracolonic findings to comment on would also maintain E1 status. 2D transverse CTC image **(B)** in another patient demonstrates a well-circumscribed low-attenuation lesion consistent with a benign hepatic cyst and an E2 status. Radiologists must be able to comfortably diagnose benign hepatic and renal cysts on this low-dose, noncontrast examination. Otherwise, an excessively high rate of additional imaging studies will be undertaken unnecessarily.

For E2 findings, no additional evaluation is required. In distinction, although likely benign, E3 findings may require additional evaluation for confirmation. The percentage of E1/E2 versus E3/E4 category lesions for a given screening population is a key statistic that may indicate a given program's approach to extracolonic evaluation (i.e., "overcalling" versus "undercalling" tendencies) and ultimately help determine the overall cost effectiveness of CTC screening.

THE DICTATION TEMPLATE

Each CTC report should contain several standard elements (Fig. 28-11). The indication for the examination (whether screening, diagnostic, or polyp followup) should be included. The technique should be outlined including the type of bowel preparation and method of distention. The results sections should hold a statement reflecting the quality of examination regarding the fidelity of the bowel preparation and colonic distention. Each identified polyp should have appropriate applied C-RADS descriptors, as discussed earlier, including size measurement, morphologic type, and segmental location. It is also helpful to provide a diagnostic score with each polyp, as discussed earlier. A statement regarding pertinent extracolonic findings should be in the report. The summary/conclusion/impression statements should reflect the various C and E categories of C-RADS. Although it is not necessary to explicitly state the specific C-RADS category in the report (which would likely not be understood by the referring physician), the summary statements should reflect the underpinnings of the C-RADS categories (both colonic and extracolonic) and a defined management recommendation should be present. For example, we would report out a C1/E2 case as a

"Negative CTC examination. Recommend routine colorectal screening in approximately five years. No significant extracolonic findings."

We have found it helpful to place disclaimer statements in the report template. For diminutive lesions, we add to each report that "*CT colonography is not intended for the detection of diminutive colonic polyps (i.e., tiny polyps ≤5 mm), the presence or absence of which will not change management of the patient.*" For extracolonic findings, we add that "*Extracolonic evaluation is limited by the low dose CT technique and lack of IV contrast.*"

QUALITY METRICS

In addition to allowing valid comparisons of examination results among institutions, structured reporting through C-RADS also allows for the generation of various quality metrics. In the context of colorectal cancer screening with CTC, quality metrics are measures that reflect a program's effectiveness in various key defined areas. Auditing a program through quality metrics is necessary to quantitatively gauge quality and helps determine deficiencies in a particular area. In addition, these measures are also helpful for comparison between different programs. An acceptable range for a given quality metric can be determined, and evaluation for outlier programs can then be made. Quality metrics will be a necessary key to maintaining quality as CTC implementation expands nationally. Without such measures, polyp detection rates may suffer or extracolonic workup rates may increase to unacceptably high levels related to overcalling. CTC screening programs should institute appropriate quality metrics to monitor and maintain acceptable standards. It is hoped that such measures will feed back into OC screening programs in which there currently are no national quality metrics in

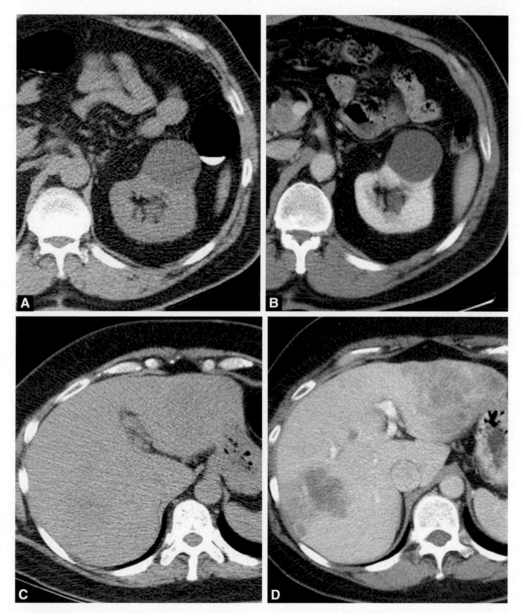

Figure 28-10 **C-RADS category E3 and E4 designations.** 2D transverse CTC image **(A)** demonstrates a potentially complicated cystic lesion in the left kidney. The possibility of a mural soft tissue component could not be confidently excluded. A status of E3 was given and a contrast-enhanced CT was recommended, which ultimately confirmed the benign nature of this lesion **(B).** 2D transverse CTC image **(C)** in another patient shows subtle but large low-attenuation masses in the liver. These potentially significant E4 lesions were seen in the context of an unsuspected annular mass in the descending colon at CTC screening (see Fig. 28-8) and therefore were concerning for metastatic disease. Subsequent contrast-enhanced CT **(D)** confirms the extensive metastatic disease from the previously unrecognized, asymptomatic adenocarcinoma of the colon.

UW Screening CT Colonography Dictation Template

INDICATION: Routine colorectal cancer screening. [Revise if other indication]

TECHNIQUE: The patient underwent UW virtual colonoscopy bowel preparation the day before the exam, consisting of oral [magnesium citrate/PEG], 2% barium, and diatrizoate. Following automated carbon dioxide insufflation per rectum, low-dose supine and prone CT images were obtained without IV contrast. Images were sent to the Viatronix V3D workstation for combined 2D-3D evaluation of the colorectum for polyps.

FINDINGS:

COLON: [Comment on quality of prep and distention. Describe size, morphology, and location of any large (≥10 mm) or small (6-9 mm) polyps]

Note: CT colonography is not intended for the detection of diminutive colonic polyps (i.e., tiny polyps ≤5 mm), the presence or absence of which will not change management of the patient.

EXTRACOLONIC: [Note any relevant findings and specify in the impression whether additional work-up should be considered]

Note: Extracolonic evaluation is limited by the low-dose CT technique and the lack of IV contrast.

IMPRESSION: [Include relevant findings and follow-up recommendations]

Figure 28-11 Dictation template. Reprint of the dictation template in use for the UW CTC screening program. Note the disclaimer statements regarding diminutive polyps and extracolonic findings.

place. Cecal withdrawal time is but one potential measure of interest for OC. Barclay et al. demonstrated a marked decrease in advanced neoplasia yield for colonoscopists with cecal withdrawal times less than 6 minutes compared with those with greater than 6 minutes within a large community group.[13]

The specific metrics for CTC are in evolution. The following are some that we have found very helpful to track for the University of Wisconsin screening program (Table 28-3). However, it is important to realize that the ultimate set of accepted quality metrics (defined perhaps by groups such as the American College of Radiology) may differ somewhat from this list.

One quality metric we use is the *program C0 rate*. The C0 rate is helpful to assess the frequency of nondiagnostic examinations (number of C0 examinations divided by total number of examinations). For an asymptomatic young screening population, it is our opinion that this rate for a well-established CTC screening program should be 1% to 2% or less (the UW rate has been well under 1% for more than 5000 patients). Higher percentages should institute investigations into potential reasons. A high rate may be related either to technical causes or to interpretation (any C0 examinations coded for those awaiting comparison examinations should be subtracted from this number, but this occurrence is exceedingly rare). In the

technical realm, there may be problems with the specific bowel preparation protocol leading to increased stool or problems in the distention protocol leading to colonic collapse. Once the cause is identified, a solution can then be implemented with subsequent protocol alterations. On the other hand, it may be related to an interpreter's comfort level with less-than-optimal examinations. Here, the solution involves increased training and exposure to both positive and negative cases in this situation to allow increased confidence in accepting these segments as adequately evaluated. For example, one common issue is relative underdistention of the sigmoid colon associated with diverticular disease. Early in interpretative experience, there may be a tendency to categorize examinations as C0 when the sigmoid is not completely distended on both series, which can occur not infrequently with diverticular-diseased segments. However, if at least one series is partially open (with smooth diffuse wall thickening without asymmetry), it is highly unlikely to hide pathology and should be cleared as diagnostic (Fig. 28-12). Complete distention in these cases is rare as a result of the deposition of fibroelastic material in the colonic wall from this disease process (i.e., myochosis).

The *OC concordance rate* is a measure that represents the rate at which there is a structural correlate at optical colonoscopy for a lesion called at CTC. Structural OC correlates include adenomas, hyperplastic and other non-neoplastic polyps, venous blebs, submucosal masses, and so on. Pseudopolyps related to stool would not count as a structural correlate. For those polyps with an assigned diagnostic confidence of 3, this rate should generally be more than 90%.[6] The percentage may be considerably lower for scores of 2 or 1. This rate should be taken in the

Table 28-3 ◻ CTC Quality Metrics

Metric	Calculation	Range from UW Experience
C0 nondiagnostic rate	No. of C0 exams/total no. of exams	≤1%
OC concordance rate	No. of matched CTC-OC findings/No. of CTC positive findings	≥90%
OC referral rate	No. of OC exams/no. of total CTC exams	5-13%*
Advanced neoplasia rate	No. of exams with advanced neoplasia/total no. of exams	3-4% prevalence
C and E category breakdown	No. of each C/E category/total no. of exams	See Chapter 30

*The lower range represents the referral rate if all C2 category patients elected imaging followup, whereas the higher number represents the rate if all patients in the C2 category are sent to OC.

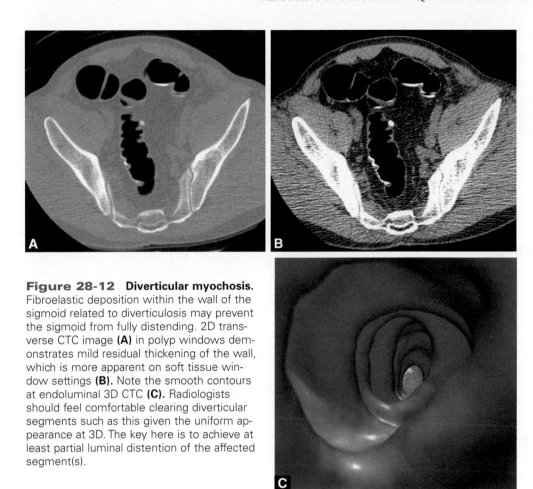

Figure 28-12   Diverticular myochosis. Fibroelastic deposition within the wall of the sigmoid related to diverticulosis may prevent the sigmoid from fully distending. 2D transverse CTC image **(A)** in polyp windows demonstrates mild residual thickening of the wall, which is more apparent on soft tissue window settings **(B).** Note the smooth contours at endoluminal 3D CTC **(C).** Radiologists should feel comfortable clearing diverticular segments such as this given the uniform appearance at 3D. The key here is to achieve at least partial luminal distention of the affected segment(s).

context of the OC referral rate. If a program had a very low OC referral rate (well below the accepted range), it could artificially inflate the OC correlation rate where only the truly obvious lesions are sent. Presumably, however, there would be an associated unacceptably low advanced neoplasia programmatic yield in this situation. The situation is somewhat analogous to the negative appendectomy rate for surgeons. A complementary metric is the *discordant case rate* (see Chapter 30), which is a reflection of the disagreement between a CTC positive examination result and the OC therapeutic examination result. In addition, the discordant case rate is a per-patient measurement as opposed to the OC concordance rate, which is a per-polyp measure.

The OC *referral rate* measures the number of patients that are sent to endoscopy from a positive CTC examination result. This represents the percentage of patients that undertake both examinations (number of OC examinations divided by total number of CTC examinations). In our experience this number should be less than 10% but may be as high as 13% to 15% if all C2 lesions are sent on to colonoscopy. A very low rate (e.g., less than 5%) should suggest that polyp detection sensitivity is suboptimal and lesions are being

missed. In these circumstances, the yield/prevalence of advanced neoplasia should be assessed for lower-than-expected numbers.

The *program advanced adenoma or neoplasia rate* is a quality measure that reflects the program's sensitivity for detecting truly significant lesions, which is also reflected by the C3/C4 rate. Both the absolute number and prevalence of advanced neoplasia should be calculated for a given CTC screening program. It should be taken in the context of the demographics of the screening population because these factors will affect this measure. For example, a high fraction of female or younger patients would tend to decrease the number of advanced neoplasms. For a generally healthy, truly asymptomatic, average-risk screening population, this rate should be around 3% to 4% in our experience.[14] Lower rates should prompt review of potential reasons for decreased sensitivity. Calculation of individual reader percentages may be helpful to detect outliers in performance.

The *program complication rate* is important to consider. In addition to perforations (which should be nearly nonexistent for screening), it is important to include significant complications related to the bowel preparation.

Capture of the perforations related to therapeutic OC for positive CTC cases also should be done.

Finally, we have found it helpful to track the percentages of the various C and E categories of C-RADS. We have found these categories to be remarkably stable over our program's existence (see Chapter 30). Drift of these category percentages should prompt a review. Of these categories, we pay particular attention to the breakdown of C1 versus C2 to C4 rates, and E1/E2 versus E3/E4 rates. For our screening program, the C2 to C4 and E3/E4 rates have remained steady at about 13% and 10%, respectively.

SUMMARY

C-RADS with structured reporting represents one of the foundation keys to effective screening by CTC. It consists of a lexicon with defined descriptors, a classification schema for colorectal polyps, and a parallel schema for extra-colonic findings. C-RADS allows for communication via a common language where valid comparisons can be made between examinations and between programs. In addition, it allows the generation of various quality metrics to assess and maintain program effectiveness.

REFERENCES

1. Zalis ME, Barish MA, Choi JR, et al. CT colonography reporting and data system: A consensus proposal. *Radiology.* 2005;236(1):3-9.
2. Pickhardt PJ, Lee AD, McFarland E.G., Taylor AJ. Linear polyp measurement at CT colonography: In vitro and in vivo comparison of two-dimensional and three-dimensional displays. *Radiology.* 2005;236(3):872-878.
3. Kim DH, Pickhardt PJ, Taylor AJ. Characteristics of advanced adenomas detected at CT colonographic screening: Implications for appropriate polyp size thresholds for polypectomy versus surveillance. *Am J Roentgenol.* 2007;188(4):940-944.
4. Rubesin SE, Saul SH, Laufer I, Levine MS. Carpet lesions of the colon. *Radiographics.* 1985;5(4):537-552.
5. Pickhardt PJ, Choi JR, Nugent PA, Schindler WR. The effect of diagnostic confidence on the probability of optical colonoscopic confirmation of potential polyps detected on CT colonography: Prospective assessment in 1,339 asymptomatic adults. *Am J Roentgenol.* 2004;183(6):1661-1665.
6. Wise SM, Pickhardt PJ, Kim DH. Positive predictive value for polyps detected at screening CT Colonography. Maui, HI: Annual meeting for the Society of Gastrointestinal Radiologists; 2009.
7. Lieberman D, Moravec M, Holub J, Michaels L, Eisen G. Polyp size and advanced histology in patients undergoing colonoscopy screening: Implications for CT colonography. *Gastroenterology.* 2008;135(4):1100-1105.
8. Church JM. Clinical significance of small colorectal polyps. *Dic Colon Rectum.* 2004;47(4):481-485.
9. Odom SR, Duffy SD, Barone JE, Ghevariya V, McClane SJ. The rate of adenocarcinoma in endoscopically removed colorectal polyps. *Am Surg.* 2005;71(12):1024-1026.
10. Hofstad B, Vatn MH, Andersen SN, et al. Growth of colorectal polyps: Redetection and evaluation of unresected polyps for a period of three years. *Gut.* 1996;39(3):449-456.
11. Obrien MJ, Winawer SJ, Zauber AG, et al. The National Polyp Study—Patient and polyp characteristics associated with high-grade dysplasia in colorectal adenomas. *Gastroenterology.* 1990;98 (2):371-379.
12. Pickhardt PJ, Hanson ME, Vanness DJ, et al. Unsuspected extra-colonic findings at screening CT colonography: Clinical and economic impact. *Radiology.* 2008;249(1):151-159.
13. Barclay RL, Vicari JJ, Doughty AS, Johanson JF, Greenlaw RL. Colonoscopic withdrawal times and adenoma detection during screening colonoscopy. *N Engl J Med.* 2006;355(24):2533-2541.
14. Kim DH, Pickhardt PJ, Taylor AJ, et al. CT colonography versus colonoscopy for the detection of advanced neoplasia. *N Engl J Med.* 2007;357(14):1403-1412.

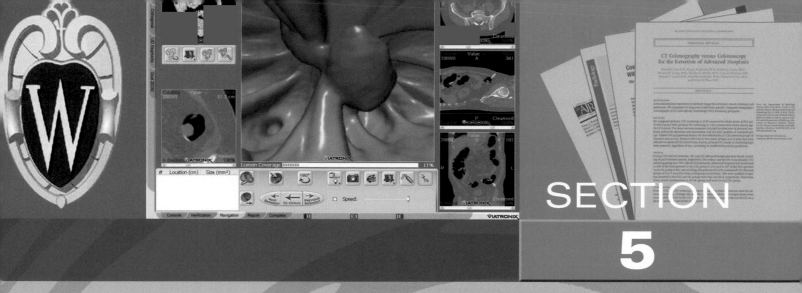

CT Colonography at the University of Wisconsin

CT Colonography at the University of Wisconsin: How We Do It

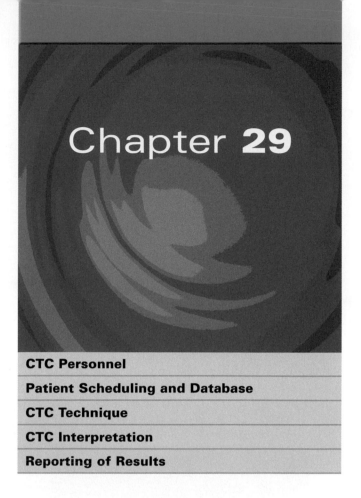

Chapter 29

PERRY J. PICKHARDT, MD
DAVID H. KIM, MD

CTC Personnel

Patient Scheduling and Database

CTC Technique

CTC Interpretation

Reporting of Results

INTRODUCTION

This chapter provides an overview of the organization and execution of the CT colonography (CTC) program at the University of Wisconsin (UW). The program has evolved from its origins tracing back to the National Naval Medical Center in Bethesda, MD. Because screening CTC examinations at UW has been covered by local third-party payers since April 2004, long before any other program in the United States, we have unique insight into the various challenges involved in setting up a high-volume practice. We have learned many lessons along the way and now hope to educate other groups that are just getting started so that they may avoid or at least minimize the hurdles that will be encountered. Time is of the essence because it appears that expanded coverage for CTC screening is on the horizon.

Although many of the topics discussed herein have been covered in previous chapters throughout this book, this chapters represents a more specific and encapsulated synthesis of "how we do it." This practical overview will summarize our current programmatic and interpretive approaches, which have continued to simplify and improve on our earlier methods that were validated in the Department of Defense (DoD) CTC screening trial.[1,2] It is not our intention to provide an exhaustive review or to compare and contrast the various CTC techniques currently in use elsewhere. We do not mean to imply that other approaches are not worthy or valid, but it is important to keep in mind that our methods have been extensively tested and have proved effective in both clinical trial and real-world settings.[2,3] It is our hope that this chapter can serve as a template for groups interested in offering high-quality colorectal screening. This gratifying clinical service can provide a valuable complement to an existing practice and could ultimately represent a major workload component given the millions of American adults in need of effective screening.

CTC PERSONNEL

In setting up a clinical CTC program, there is a tendency to place the initial focus on the capital and equipment needs and not on the critical personnel needs. However, for a typical radiology practice, the most expensive component (the multidetector CT [MDCT] scanner) will already be in place and the remaining equipment needs are minimal, consisting of a CO_2 insufflator and dedicated CTC software. For nonradiology groups looking to break into CTC, securing a CT scanner could represent a major new investment and direction. Beyond the MDCT scanner, of paramount importance is the need to assemble a motivated CTC team, consisting of a program coordinator, CT technologists, and interpreting physicians. At UW, we have been fortunate to have a stellar crew, consisting of a nurse program coordinator, assistant program coordinator, office assistant, motivated CT technologists, and specialized abdominal radiologists, all of whom are dedicated and take great pride in their contribution to the CTC program. Additional help provided by numerous students, radiology residents, and abdominal imaging fellows bolster both the clinical and research enterprises. The program coordinators and CT technologists truly represent the "face" of the program through their daily interactions with our patients. The coordinators handle all patient queries before and after the actual examination, and the CTC technologists (i.e., CT technologists with expertise in CTC) perform the entire procedure, including the appropriate quality assurance and need for additional views.

The CTC program coordinator, who is preferably a registered nurse, is invaluable for both the startup and maintenance of a successful clinical program (Fig. 29-1). With the likelihood that multiple CT technologists and radiologists will contribute to a typical CTC program, the coordinator provides a constant for the program and can ensure quality and uniformity. Many of the questions and concerns that patients have will require the medical acumen of a health professional, such as a registered nurse. Otherwise, many of these queries would need to be fielded by a radiologist, who is often already busy with

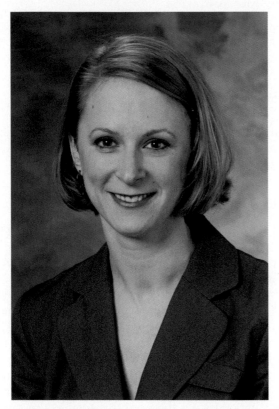

Figure 29-1 CTC clinical program coordinator. The clinical coordinator serves as the linchpin for any CTC program, including both the startup and operational phases. For a larger program, a registered nurse is preferable, but a CT technologist may suffice for smaller operations. Our program coordinator for the UW CTC program, Holly Casson, RN, BSN, has been an indispensable member of our clinical team. A constant and knowledgeable presence is critical for the daily functioning of a CTC program. We are greatly indebted to Holly and her staff for the success of our clinical service.

the clinical workload. Our nurse coordinator is the unifying force behind maintaining the CTC schedule, communicating study results, coordinating referral to optical colonoscopy (OC), overseeing the maintenance of the clinical database, ensuring appropriate patient followup, handling insurance coverage issues, developing community outreach activities, assisting in research activities, and so on. It should be easy to see how this person represents the true linchpin of a successful CTC program.

The second key personnel component to a successful CTC program is the CTC technologist. When first starting out, it is helpful to identify at least one capable CT technologist who is motivated and willing to nurture a nascent program. This specialized CTC technologist will serve as the go-to person for technical issues related to colonic distention and scanning and for training of additional technologists. Rapid diffusion of CTC training across the CT technology staff is desirable (and feasible) so that any available tech can properly handle a case. Once properly trained, these individuals are primarily responsible for obtaining a diagnostic examination, with active input from the radiologist generally restricted only to unusual circumstances. It remains critical, however, that the interpreting radiologist provides continual feedback on examination quality and decisions regarding an additional decubitus series. By cleanly dividing between image acquisition and study interpretation, the radiologist can maximize reading efficiency. In our experience, even the technologists who were initially reluctant to perform CTC generally come to enjoy this procedure, which is now favored by many of our technologists. Compared with most other body CT scans, screening CTC does not entail a temporally demanding intravenous (IV) contrast protocol and most "patients" are healthy adults and not sick inpatients. Because the CTC technologist interacts closely with the individual undergoing the examination, it is critical from a public relations standpoint that he or she exude a positive attitude with regard to the program and screening in general.

The final core member of the CTC program is the interpreting physician, presumably a board-certified radiologist. With ultimate responsibility for the entire program and its clinical results, the physician must first build a strong clinical team. Accurate image interpretation is of obvious importance and is covered in detail later in this chapter. Although we have entrusted communication of the same-day polyp findings largely to our program coordinators, many physicians will choose to relay these results to patients directly themselves until study volume precludes it. Effective communication of potentially important extracolonic findings is also an integral component to study interpretation and patient care. Where it is felt to be warranted, we communicate important extracolonic findings directly to the referring physician, along with offering a recommended course of action for further workup. The interpreting physician is also ultimately responsible for ensuring an accurate clinical database and for monitoring program quality metrics. When a discordant case arises as a result of a CTC-detected abnormality not being found at subsequent OC, we perform a joint review of the case by all available CTC radiologists to determine whether further action is needed (see Chapter 26). A close collaborative spirit among the radiologists and gastroenterologists involved in colorectal screening is helpful. In particular, information regarding CTC-detected polyps that are considered to be in a potentially difficult location for endoscopy should be effectively communicated, including pertinent two-dimensional (2D) and 3D images (see Chapter 25).

PATIENT SCHEDULING AND DATABASE

Given the elective nature of colorectal screening, examination scheduling has a forgiving nature that allows flexibility for both patients and the program itself. For asymptomatic adults, the examination can be planned and scheduled many months in advance—a luxury not common to most imaging procedures. We schedule our screening CTC examinations in a 7:00 am to 10:00 am block, which not only allows fasting adults to return to their regular activities sooner, but also allows time to secure a same-day OC slot for polypectomy, if needed. From the radiologist's perspective, the schedule can be conveniently blocked off during times when staffing is particularly light. With studies restricted to the morning, the radiologist in the "VC am" slot is free to staff other services or perform other tasks in the afternoon. Unlike mammography screening, we currently require a physician referral for CTC screening. Although this has decreased our initial volume somewhat, the rationale behind this decision is that we do not want to exclude the primary care provider (PCP) from the process. Not only might this alienate an important referral base (NB: The PCP, not the gastroenterologist, is the gatekeeper for screening referral), but you may also encounter an important extracolonic finding. Without a referring physician on the CTC order, the radiologist must then assume responsibility for this finding, which is uncharted and unwanted territory to most radiologists. A final reason for requiring physician referral is that it provides a mechanism for someone familiar with the patient to choose the most appropriate bowel preparation, if different options are available.

As a part of the routine scheduling process, we gather pertinent information on our intake form regarding specific study indication, patient demographics, medical history, and insurance coverage. Specific medical history obtained includes personal history of any cancer, history of abdominal surgery, and family history of colorectal cancer. If the insurance provider is outside the group of carriers that cover screening CTC at UW, then preau-

thorization is sought. Although our nurse coordinator was originally given the task of filling out the history portion of the intake form, we soon realized that it was too time consuming and would be much more efficient to train the radiology schedulers for these duties. These intake data are entered into the CTC clinical database along with the technique and findings from the examination itself. See Figures 29-2 and 29-3, which illustrate the workflow process for preappointment (Fig. 29-2) and appointment (Fig. 29-3) of CTC.

A viable CTC program needs to create and maintain an active clinical database that records all enrolled patients and examination results. It is much more efficient and practical to set up or otherwise obtain a database on the front end than attempt to gather the information after the fact. Data inputs should include demographic information, patient historical information, technical parameters of the examination, polyp findings, extracolonic findings, findings at subsequent OC and pathology, and the clinical followup plan. With regard to colorectal and extracolonic findings, we would strongly encourage use of the CT Colonography Reporting and Data System (C-RADS).[4] This database information is needed to generate program quality metrics, maintain appropriate followup lists, and keep track of discordant cases. This will allow for both internal comparison among readers and external comparison against other CTC programs. With a dedicated database, many of these functions can be automated, allowing for easy and customized generation of reports. Our clinical database was constructed using Microsoft Access, which allows for rapid queries involving any data points. Much of the patient demographic data can be entered by the program coordinator or other personnel (we employ student help as well). However, the primary responsibility for the integrity of important clinical results, and reconciliation with OC and pathology findings, rests with the physician.

CTC TECHNIQUE

The basic concept behind successful CTC is straightforward: by imaging a properly prepared and distended colon with MDCT, clinically relevant polyps and masses should be readily detectable with dedicated CTC software. If all facets of the CTC examination (i.e., bowel preparation, colonic distention, MDCT scanning, and image interpretation) are adequately addressed, effective evaluation is much easier than many realize. Although each technical component will be discussed separately in this chapter, it is crucial to recognize the interdependence of these factors because any weak link can damage the outcome. Even the best CTC software system will fail in the setting of inadequate colonic preparation or distention. Similarly, optimal preparation and distention cannot compensate for an inadequate CTC software system or an ineffective interpretive approach.

Virtual Colonoscopy Preappointment Process

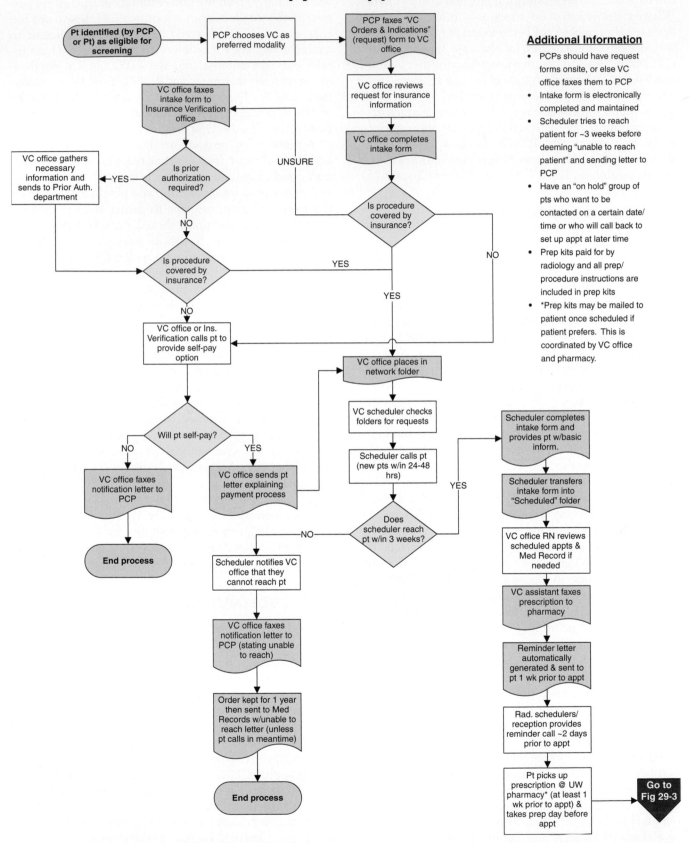

Figure 29-2 Preappointment process for CTC screening at UW. This flow chart demonstrates the process of ordering and scheduling a screening CTC examination. The preappointment process includes insurance coverage considerations and obtaining the bowel prep kit.

Virtual Colonoscopy Appointment Process

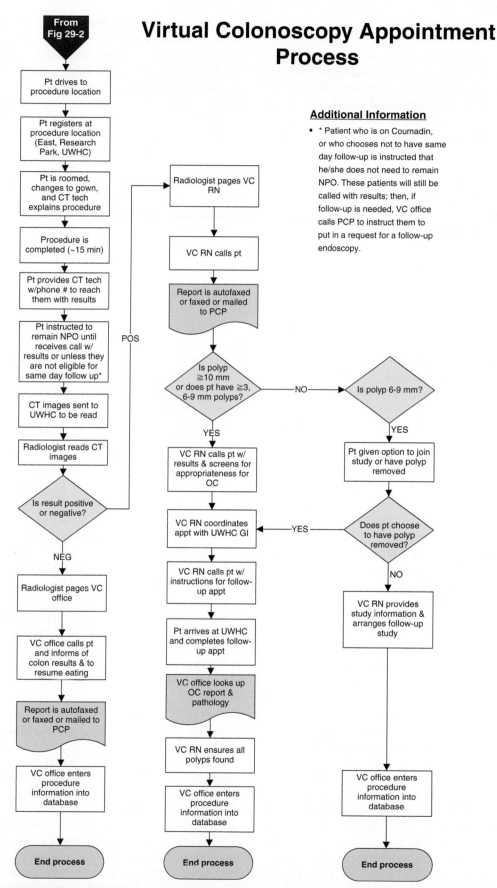

Additional Information

• * Patient who is on Coumadin, or who chooses not to have same day follow-up is instructed that he/she does not need to remain NPO. These patients will still be called with results; then, if follow-up is needed, VC office calls PCP to instruct them to put in a request for a follow-up endoscopy.

Figure 29-3   Appointment process for CTC screening at UW. This flow chart describes the course of action for a patient on the day of the CTC screening examination. Beyond the procedure itself, the reporting of results and subsequent course of action are explicitly outlined.

Bowel Preparation

Robust colonic preparation for screening CTC is critical for accurate polyp detection and involves both cleansing and tagging (alternative approaches for certain diagnostic indications are considered later). We have been satisfied with our current low-volume CTC preparation that combines three basic components: a laxative for catharsis, dilute 2% barium for tagging of any solid residual stool, and iodinated water-soluble contrast (diatrizoate) for opacification of luminal fluid (see www.virtuoctc.com for specific bowel regimens). This 1-day preparation has been greatly simplified from the one used previously in the multicenter DoD trial, with clinical validation of the modifications, including a decrease in residual luminal fluid.[5-7] We have received surprisingly few complaints from patients about our low-volume preparation. The streamlined nature of this preparation is designed with working adults in mind because it does not require taking a day off to complete. Perhaps more important, we have not yet encountered any significant prep-related complications in more than 6000 patients dating back to the screening trial. In addition to the main prep components, which are taken the evening before the examination, the patient also maintains a clear-liquid diet throughout the day and takes bisacodyl tablets around noon. Bisacodyl (dulcolax) will generally not cause diarrhea but serves to "prime the pump" for later on. Because the prep includes both over-the-counter laxatives and prescription oral contrast agents, we currently have our central pharmacy combine the constituents into one convenient kit, which can then be mailed directly to patients or dispensed at a number of local satellite pharmacies.[8] In addition to the prep instructions, we provide a pamphlet containing general information about colorectal screening and CTC within the kit. The issue of getting the prep kit to your patients requires one to survey the local situation to derive a customized solution. We are hopeful that a commercialized version of the bowel preparation kit will become available, which would obviate the need for a special solution to delivery.

The specific choice of laxative depends on the health status of the individual. Although our nurse coordinator initially screened all patients for pertinent health concerns to determine the most appropriate preparation,[1,8] we found it much more efficient and logical to provide the referring physicians with our guidelines and have them choose the best preparation for their patients as part of the CTC order form. For the initial 4 years of our CTC screening program at UW, the laxative for our standard CTC bowel preparation was sodium phosphate (phospho-soda), which was used in about 90% of our screening cases and was well tolerated in generally healthy adults without known or suspected renal or cardiac insufficiency. Although we had originally used two 45-mL doses of sodium phosphate spaced 3 hours apart during the DoD screening trial without complication (in more than 1300 asymptomatic adults), this represented "off-label" use according to U.S. Food and Drug Administration (FDA) guidelines. We subsequently showed that a single 45-mL dose of sodium phosphate was equally effective as the double-dose regimen,[5] which brought our preparation into compliance. If further purgation was needed, patients were instructed to take a bottle of magnesium citrate (included in the standard kit) in lieu of a second dose of sodium phosphate. We did not encounter any serious adverse effects among all the patients who took either the single-dose or double-dose sodium phosphate preparation. From a practical standpoint, most patients found it easier to swiftly drink the sodium phosphate undiluted, followed immediately by a clear-liquid chaser, such as a carbonated beverage. Alternatively, the solution can be diluted into an 8-ounce glass of clear juice or soda.

Because of concerns over rare instances of acute phosphate nephropathy, particularly in elderly patients with hypertension treated with angiotensin-converting enzyme (ACE) inhibitors, we generally avoided sodium phosphate in this group.[9] For nearly all patients in whom sodium phosphate was best avoided, magnesium citrate represented an acceptable substitute, given in liquid form in a 296-mL bottle. Because we find it somewhat less potent than sodium phosphate, we use a second bottle that is taken during step 2 along with the 2% barium (see www.virtuoctc.com). In 2008 following a formal retrospective study showing equivalence between the sodium phosphate and magnesium citrate preps (with more optimal fluid density with the latter approach),[7] we decided to switch to the magnesium citrate regimen as the standard CTC bowel preparation for our program. This has greatly streamlined patient scheduling because the need to screen for renal or cardiac insufficiency, or other contraindications for sodium phosphate, evaporated.

For patients who are severely compromised or tenuous and who cannot tolerate even moderate fluid or electrolyte shifts, we resort to polyethylene glycol (PEG), which is given as a 4-L solution. Although the safety profile of PEG is most favorable for such patients, this preparation is associated with the poorest compliance because of its taste and very large volume. Fortunately, this prep is only rarely necessary for CTC in our experience, accounting for less than 1% of cases. We generally have patients begin drinking the PEG solution around noon the day before CTC to allow more time for the oral contrast agents later on, with the goal of about one 8-ounce glass of PEG every 10 to 15 minutes until finished.

Regardless of which laxative is used, the dual oral contrast regimen is held constant, consisting of 2% barium followed by diatrizoate (see www.virtuoctc.com). We believe that the complementary actions of these two contrast agents, in conjunction with catharsis, provide for the optimal CTC preparation.[1] As with the sodium phosphate, the total volume of each oral contrast agent has been halved from the original trial and reduced to a single dose, without any discernible detriment to the fidelity of the prep. It should be noted that patients are instructed to drink 4 to 8 cups of clear liquid prior to moving on to steps 2 and 3 of the prep to maintain proper hydration. The basic rationale behind the specific order of the three prep components is that the laxative provides catharsis for the bulk removal of fecal material, the barium tags any residual solid stool that remains, and the diatrizoate serves the dual purpose of uniform fluid tagging and secondary catharsis.[1] To administer the barium prior to the primary catharsis would require a much greater volume because it would tag the entire stool bulk, nearly all of which will then be eliminated by the laxative. We strongly prefer the dilute 2% "CT grade" barium products over the 40% w/v high-density barium, which is unnecessarily dense and has led to difficulty at same-day OC with clogging of the endoscopic ports and channels. In our experience, the 2% barium has never caused a significant problem in nearly 2000 same-day colonoscopy studies performed following CTC.[1]

We have long suspected that the ionic water-soluble iodinated contrast containing diatrizoate is the true secret to success of this prep. Not only does the diatrizoate uniformly opacify the residual luminal fluid, but it also provides for a mild secondary catharsis and has a somewhat "slippery" consistency that seems to greatly decrease the amount of adherent solid debris. The last feature is key because adherent stool can be a major source of false-positive results and often precludes the preferred primary 3D polyp detection approach. Our limited experience with nonionic iodinated contrast agents (e.g., iohexol) suggests that the increase in adherent residual stool may override the benefit of its more palatable taste.

The use of oral contrast tagging improves the accuracy of CTC in several ways: it increases specificity by both tagging residual stool (barium effect) and decreasing the amount of adherent stool (diatrizoate effect), and it increases sensitivity by allowing for polyp detection in opacified fluid (diatrizoate effect). One potential pitfall that has actually become a useful interpretive asset for us is the tendency for true soft tissue polyps to demonstrate a thin surface coating of adherent contrast.[10] This contrast etching is generally seen only with true polyps and not with the surrounding colonic wall and therefore serves as a beacon for detection (see Chapter 20). Given the improved performance characteristics seen with the use of oral contrast tagging, we believe that it should be considered as standard CTC technique and should be used whenever possible. With regard to computer-aided detection (CAD), most algorithms until recently have been developed and tested without contrast tagging in mind. To be successful mov-

ing forward, CAD systems will need to address this issue and demonstrate acceptable performance for tagged cases.[11,12]

The issue of minimal or noncathartic bowel preparation for routine asymptomatic screening warrants consideration. To begin with, it must be made clear that the term "prepless" is a misnomer for minimal prep or noncathartic CTC approaches and should be avoided. In fact, some noncathartic approaches are perhaps more onerous than our low-volume cathartic standard prep because they often entail complicated and prolonged oral contrast regimens and dietary modifications, which may stretch out for 2 or 3 days. The main theoretical advantage to noncathartic CTC is the avoidance of laxatives, which would presumably result in increased patient compliance. However, there are a number of additional reasons why we believe that CTC without catharsis is not a "holy grail" or a singular solution.[13] First, primary 3D polyp detection may not be feasible with this approach because of the greater degree of residual solid stool. As discussed later in the interpretation section, limiting polyp detection to primary 2D is clearly a suboptimal approach for screening. Second, patients will not be able to undergo same-day optical colonoscopy if significant lesions are found. This "one-stop shop" service provided by our CTC program is highly valued by our patients and has been endorsed by the American Gastroenterological Association as the preferred method. The need for additional full preparation for subsequent colonoscopy on a separate day would negatively affect participation. The penalty for a false-positive call at noncathartic CTC is amplified because it involves an additional bowel preparation for an unnecessary invasive colonoscopy that likely could have been avoided with the standard cathartic CTC approach. Third, accuracy in a screening population will be lower because both false negatives (polyps obscured by stool) and false positives (stool masquerading as polyps) would almost certainly increase in a low-prevalence setting. Last, the low-volume cathartic preparations that we offer have been very well tolerated and are much less of a compliance barrier compared with the large-volume PEG prep used by our gastroenterologists. In the end, we feel that noncathartic CTC is worthy of further investigation and appears to be useful in certain symptomatic cohorts (see later). However, for screening purposes, this approach first needs to be validated in a sufficiently large trial because nearly any CTC technique appears promising when tested in small cohorts with high prevalence of disease. Aforementioned caveats aside, validation of noncathartic CTC for screening would be a useful alternative for those unwilling to take laxatives.

Beyond the screening setting, there are certain diagnostic scenarios that require a different approach to bowel preparation. In our experience with same-day CTC following incomplete OC, the lack of contrast tagging has resulted in false positives that likely could have been avoided if tagging were present. Beyond immediate scanning without additional preparation, other options to consider following incomplete OC include salvage oral contrast prior to same-day CTC, IV contrast in lieu of oral contrast, and scheduling CTC on a separate day to allow for standard preparation with oral contrast. Factors related to the OC examination that will influence our protocol decision include the fidelity of the prep, the presumed level of the colon reached, and whether or not a deep biopsy was performed. When same-day CTC is preferred, our current approach is to provide one 30-mL oral dose of diatrizoate and perform CTC about 2 hours later. Because patients have been sedated for OC, they may require additional recovery time before taking the oral contrast to reduce the risk of aspiration. Another diagnostic scenario where alterations should be considered is the symptomatic elderly and/or frail patient for whom the clinical question centers more on cancer detection than polyp detection. When combined with IV contrast (to help evaluate for both colorectal and extracolonic malignancy), a less aggressive bowel preparation may consist of only oral contrast without the use of cathartics. This approach is generally safer and more convenient, and these patients are often not candidates for same-day OC in any case.

There are some additional considerations prior to the actual CTC examination that are not strictly prep related but are still worth noting. We ask that patients taking Coumadin (warfarin) or Plavix (clopidogrel) continue these medications unless their referring physician specifically instructs them otherwise. The relatively low prevalence of large polyps or masses that would necessitate invasive colonoscopy generally does not warrant provision for same-day polypectomy in these patients. For patients with diabetes, we ask that they discuss with their doctor medication management and frequency of blood sugar testing prior to CTC. We also ask that patients who are otherwise eligible for same-day colonoscopy stop all nonsteroidal anti-inflammatory drug (NSAID) medications 5 days before their CTC examination. Although these medications will not affect the CTC study, it could have an impact on subsequent colonoscopy. Unlike anticoagulation therapy, short-term stoppage of NSAIDS is generally safe and does not require physician oversight. All of these considerations are included in the printed instructions found within the patient's prep kit (see www.virtuoctc.com).

Colonic Distention

Adequate distention of the colon, like proper bowel cleansing, is a critical component of technical success at CTC. It is important to understand that adequate or optimal distention is distinct from maximal distention because patient comfort and safety must be taken into account if CTC is to be widely embraced. Our distention protocol (described later) has continued to evolve and improve, resulting in inadequate segmental distention in less than 1% of patients. In general, gaseous distention for CTC can be achieved with either room air or CO_2, and the rate and degree of insufflation can be automated or manually controlled by either the patient or medical staff (technologist or physician). Rigid, large-caliber retention balloon catheters designed for the barium enema are seldom necessary for CTC screening. For the vast majority of screening patients, smaller and more flexible rectal catheters are preferred for reasons of patient comfort and safety. In our experience, the smaller caliber catheters with small, low-pressure retention cuffs specifically designed for CTC work very well. When a large rigid balloon catheter is deemed necessary because of laxity, appropriate caution should be taken.

It has become clear to us that automated CO_2 delivery represents the single best distention technique, with manual room air insufflation reserved only for certain extenuating circumstances, such as in an individual who is morbidly obese in whom the low pressure CO_2 cannot overcome the extrinsic pressure on the colon. Nearly all reported perforations at CTC have involved the use of manual staff-controlled room air insufflation in symptomatic patients, whereas the risk of perforation with automated or patient-controlled distention methods likely approaches zero for asymptomatic screening.[14] With regard to both study quality (i.e., degree of distention) and postprocedural discomfort, we have shown that automated CO_2 is superior to the manual room air technique.[15] The continuous low-pressure delivery provided with automated CO_2 reduces spasm and discomfort and provides better distention in segments with advanced diverticular disease. The much more rapid resorption of CO_2 through the colon wall (up to 150 times faster than room air) accounts for the improved comfort immediately following the procedure. Finally, one additional factor that has yet to receive much attention but is nonetheless important is staff preference. We have polled our CT technologists and found that they unanimously prefer the automated CO_2 technique over staff- or patient-controlled room air insufflation.[15] Significant time and effort may be required to coach individual patients to adequately self-insufflate with room air, whereas automated CO_2 requires relatively little explanation, and determination of an adequate endpoint is more straightforward. From the radiologist's perspective, the decreased operator dependence with automated CO_2 compared with manual staff-controlled insufflation results in more consistent distention and less variability from technologist to technologist.

The relative advantages of manual room air over automated CO_2 include its ubiquitous nature, low cost, and ability to distend the colon in patients who are morbidly obese when the low-pressure CO_2 cannot. In a very low-volume CTC practice, the increased costs associated with automated CO_2 (i.e., the machine itself and the customized tip and tubing assembly) could arguably offset the incremental gains in colonic distention and postprocedural discomfort. In addition, patient-controlled room air insufflation may result in less transient discomfort from rectal spasm during active distention compared with staff-controlled manual distention. Manual decompression of room air by the technologist prior to catheter withdrawal can also help alleviate postprocedure discomfort. Ultimately, the decision of which distention technique to use should be individualized to best suit a given patient or CTC program. However, going forward we firmly believe that automated CO_2 should be considered the front-line method for distention for any CTC program with adequate patient volumes.

There are several reasons why we believe that spasmolytics (especially those available in the United States) are generally unnecessary for CTC screening.[15] First, previous studies evaluating the effect of spasmolytics on colonic distention at CTC have found mixed but largely negative results, likely resulting in part from relaxation of the ileocecal valve. Second, needle administration of a drug adds invasiveness and patient discomfort, creates an opportunity for additional side effects, increases examination duration, and increases overall costs. Third, with our current distention protocol, nondiagnostic segmental distention is so uncommon that the need for spasmolytics is limited from the start. Last, even if some net benefit exists for using buscopan (hyoscine-N-butyl-bromide) compared with glucagon, this agent is not available for such use in the United States.

From our observational experiences and input from the CT technologists we have refined our protocol for colonic distention. To maintain efficiency, we have trained our CT technologists to independently obtain the entire CTC examination, including placement of the rectal catheter, quality assurance, and obtaining a decubitus series, as needed. The radiologist is only consulted for difficult or unusual situations, which allows more time for actual image interpretation. Before commencing with the examination, the patient is encouraged to use the restroom. The technologist inquires about the fidelity of the prep from the patient's perspective, but, assuming the patient generally followed the prep, we rarely halt the examination based on this subjective assessment. In fact, even when patients have eaten a solid breakfast during the day of bowel preparation, the CTC examination has generally been diagnostic.

Following rectal catheter placement, the patient remains in the left lateral decubitus for the initial 1.0 to 1.5 L of CO_2 delivered by the automated device. To reduce the transient discomfort related to rectal spasm, we have found it useful to initially set the equilibrium pressure at 17 to 20 mm Hg compared with maximum pressure of 25 mm Hg. The patient is then placed in the right lateral decubitus until about 3.0 to 3.5 L have been delivered in total, followed by supine positioning until a steady-state equilibrium has been reached, at which time scanning begins. The positional changes may help prevent underdistention related to CO_2 blockage from a fluid channel or bowel kink. Reversing the order of the decubitus positioning (right before left) is an acceptable variation to the protocol.

Transient pressure spikes of more than 30 or 40 mm Hg may be related to spasm, patient movement, or fluid block. Filling pressures are often less than 20 mm Hg, whereas equilibrium pressure while scanning is generally in the 20- to 25- mm Hg range. The volume of CO_2 "dispensed" can vary widely not only from differences in actual colonic volume, but also from variable degrees of reflux through the ileocecal valve, loss around the catheter, and continuous colonic resorption. Therefore, the total volume reading for CO_2 delivery has relatively little meaning and can range from 3 L to more than 10 L. It is imperative to perform MDCT acquisition at equilibrium with active replacement of CO_2. Some versions of the current CO_2 device in use will stop delivery when 4 L is reached and for every 2 L thereafter. CT technologists must be aware of this pitfall and know to press the reset button immediately prior to scanning if one of these levels has been reached. We perform the supine and prone scans at end expiration to raise the diaphragm and allow more room for the splenic flexure and transverse colon.

The CT scout image provides a general indication of overall colonic distention (Fig. 29-4). However, contrary to standard teaching, we have found that the CT scout image is unreliable for adequately assessing distention of the sigmoid and descending colon.[16] As a result, we have trained the CT technologists to recognize inadequate distention of the left colon by cine review of the 2D transverse images at the console while the patient remains on the scanner gantry. This step helps to ensure adequate distention of the left colon without the need for calling the patient back. If focal collapse persists at the *same point* on *both* supine *and* prone scans, a third set of images is obtained, generally in the right lateral decubitus position. This maneuver is necessary in a minority of cases but typically results in an overall diagnostic examination. In less than 1% of patients, nondiagnostic segmental evaluation will persist despite all of the these efforts. In such cases, we may offer the patient same-day unsedated flexible sigmoidoscopy in an attempt to complete their screening examination. Alternatively, a short interval for followup screening may be recommended. As noted previously, manual room air insufflation may help maintain adequate distention when CO_2 has failed in some individuals who are morbidly obese. One rare but important pitfall that has led to perforation with manual distention is inguinal herniation of the sigmoid colon.[17]

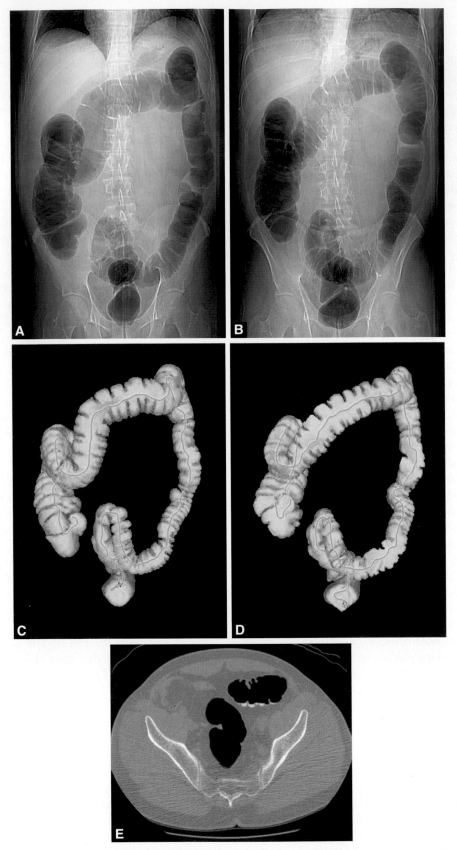

Figure 29-4   CT scout images for CTC. CT scout or "topogram" images are obtained in the supine **(A)** and prone **(B)** positions after a state of equilibrium has been reached with the automated carbon dioxide system. In a straightforward case like this without small bowel reflux, colonic tortuosity, or sigmoid diverticular disease, the scout views can provide a good assessment of overall distention, leading to an excellent CTC study **(C-E)**. In most cases, however, the CT technologist or radiologist should review the 2D reconstructions at the console to ensure adequate distention of the left colon **(E)**.

MDCT Scanning

Compared with CT coronary angiography and other temporally demanding protocols, CTC is a very forgiving examination with regard to scanner requirements. CTC is a noncontrast examination, the gas-filled large intestine is a relatively static structure, and the target lesion is sufficiently large (i.e., polyps >5 mm). As such, neither submillimeter collimation nor 64-channel scanners are necessary and may actually represent somewhat inefficient use of this more advanced technology. Just because one possesses the ability to image with ever-increasing spatial resolution does not mean that it always confers a net benefit. On the contrary, the increased dose required for submillimeter collimation likely outweighs any theoretical benefit for relevant polyp detection. State-of-the-art CTC requires only an 8-channel or 16-channel MDCT scanner. In fact, most CTC studies from the DoD multicenter screening trial were actually performed on 4-channel MDCT scanners, using a 4×2.5 mm detector configuration and 1-mm reconstruction interval.[1] Because the performance results were no different from the 8-channel scanners using an 8×1.25 mm detector configuration, this remains a viable and validated approach for detecting clinically relevant colorectal lesions.

Our current CTC scanning protocol remains relatively straightforward (see www.virtuoctc.com). Regardless of continuing advances in CTC technique and interpretation, the established practice of obtaining both supine and prone scans will likely always remain in place, given the invaluable complementary data provided and the ability to secondarily confirm suspected lesions that are detected on a single view. As discussed previously, the CT scout view provides a general indication of the overall quality of distention, but online review of the 2D transverse images can prevent nondiagnostic distention, particularly for the sigmoid colon.

Typical 16-channel MDCT scanning factors include a 0.5-second rotation time, 1.25-mm collimation, 1.375:1 pitch, 1.0-mm reconstruction interval, and 120 kV_p. Given the nature of the soft–tissue-air interface for polyp detection at CTC, it is widely recognized that the radiation dose can be significantly lowered from the usual diagnostic levels. To optimize the delivered dose, we now use a tube-current modulation system (Smart mA, GE Medical Systems) that modulates current in both the xy-plane and the z-direction. We have developed two protocols that have yielded significant dose reductions yet uniformly diagnostic examinations. For a typical low-dose series, as might be used in the supine position, we set the noise index at 50, the kV_p at 120, and the mA range at 30 to 300. For an ultra–low-dose series, as might be used in the prone position, we set the noise index at 70 and the kV_p at 140, and we keep the mA range at 30 to 150. This protocol results in a total effective dose that is typically less than 5 mSv. For MDCT scanners that are not equipped with a tube-current modulation system, one can generally use a technique in the range of 35 to 75 mAs, except for individualized increases in patients who are morbidly obese. Although further dose reduction is a desirable goal for evaluation of asymptomatic adults, we would also emphasize that the very small theoretical risk of low-dose radiation exposure is clearly outweighed by the actual risk of not being screened for colorectal cancer.[18,19]

With our current scanning parameters, each series can be kept at fewer than 500 images, with typically fewer than 1000 images for the total study. These source images are then sent to the CTC workstation for advanced modeling and interpretation and to PACS for storage. In addition to the thin-section source data, we automatically perform a second reconstruction of the supine dataset into a separate series of 5-mm-thick images at 3-mm intervals.[20] This additional series facilitates the review of extracolonic structures by providing fewer images (usually <100) with less image noise. This approach also allows for easier PACS retrieval when further evaluation of an extracolonic finding is needed because the source data are stored separately.

Because of the high diagnostic accuracy of CTC screening when oral contrast tagging and 3D polyp detection are used, we believe that the use of IV contrast is not indicated for asymptomatic screening. Without a clear benefit over our noncontrast protocol, the disadvantages of introducing IV contrast for CTC screening, which include increased time, costs, invasiveness, and risks, do not warrant its routine use at this time. Of course, we do us an IV contrast CTC protocol in certain diagnostic settings, most notably following incomplete colonoscopy from an occlusive carcinoma. IV contrast may also be used in some other cases following incomplete OC, occasionally for suspected submucosal lesions, and in certain frail or elderly symptomatic patients. In brief, the IV contrast protocol entails an initial low-dose noncontrast prone scan, followed by a postcontrast supine scan with standard diagnostic CT technique.

CTC INTERPRETATION

Although we have used and tested a wide variety of different CTC workstations from various manufacturers for research purposes over the years (e.g., from Philips, Vital Images, and GE), the only system that we have ever used at UW for direct patient care purposes is the Viatronix V3D system (Fig. 29-5; see also instruction videos on DVD). As a result of the Department of Defense screening trial, the Viatronix V3D system was the first to be clinically validated for colorectal screening and also the first to receive FDA approval for the specific purpose of screening. To us, it was clear that the most obvious advantage of the Viatronix V3D system over the other

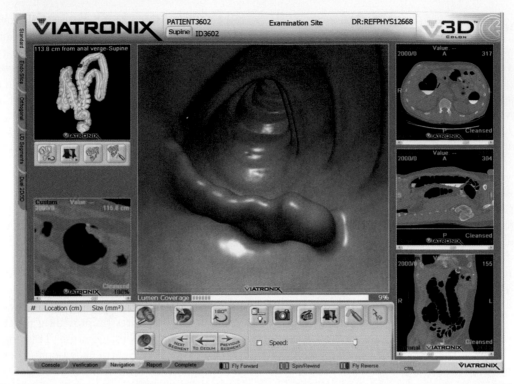

Figure 29-5 **Diagnostic interface of the Viatronix V3D Colon software system.** Screen capture of the CTC system shows the various 2D and 3D views present on the standard display. This system allows for time-efficient primary 3D evaluation and rapid 2D correlation and a host of diagnostic tools that facilitate the interpretation. A number of other windows and displays are available, but this standard window serves as our workhorse. (*See associated instructional video on DVD.*)

CTC systems was the ability to perform a more effective and time-efficient primary 3D polyp search, in addition to a number of other diagnostic advantages. In recent years, it has been gratifying to see that the 3D capabilities of several other CTC systems have greatly improved. Although not quite to the level of the Viatronix V3D, several can probably now be considered capable of effective primary 3D evaluation. The description of our clinical interpretive approach that follows applies specifically to the Viatronix V3D system. The 3D endoluminal fly-through and the various diagnostic tools are better demonstrated by the video clips in the associated DVD.

Refinements in our interpretation strategy and continued software improvements have resulted in faster and more accurate CTC interpretation. The supine and prone source CT images are sent to the V3D system, which then segments out the gas-filled intestine and generates a useful automated centerline for navigation (Fig. 29-6). The postprocessing required to create this model occurs in the background, while concurrent reading of already-processed studies transpires. With our biphasic 3D/2D interpretive approach, the radiologist has the option to commence with either primary 3D or primary 2D evaluation (Fig. 29-7). However, beyond a cursory 2D survey to primarily assess the quality of colonic preparation and distention, and to identify obvious masses, most polyp detection actually occurs on the 3D

endoluminal evaluation. The increased conspicuity of polyps on the 3D display renders nearly all relevant polyps to be readily identifiable, leaving the more tedious 2D search as largely a formality in most cases (see Chapter 17). However, in the minority of cases in which a significant amount of adherent residual stool or luminal fluid is present, or there is partial luminal collapse, primary 2D evaluation can serve a vital and often primary role. Of course, once a focal lesion is suspected, the 2D view is essential for internal characterization.

The 3D endoluminal fly-through is predominately a hands-free journey along the automated centerline, interspersed with manual mouse-driven navigation for selected regions and suspected abnormalities. A major drawback with the 3D endoluminal display on some CTC systems is the lack of unrestricted manual navigation. Primary 3D endoluminal review initially entailed bidirectional fly-through of the supine and prone models using a 90-degree field-of-view (FOV) angle, consisting of four total fly-throughs. More recently, we have found that widening the FOV angle to 120 degrees allows for one-way fly-through of each series (rectum to cecum on supine and cecum to rectum on prone) without sacrificing polyp detection.[21] For cases with suboptimal distention, however, bidirectional fly-through at 120 degrees may be prudent to adequately cover the mucosa. Regardless of the FOV angle or whether one-way or two-way

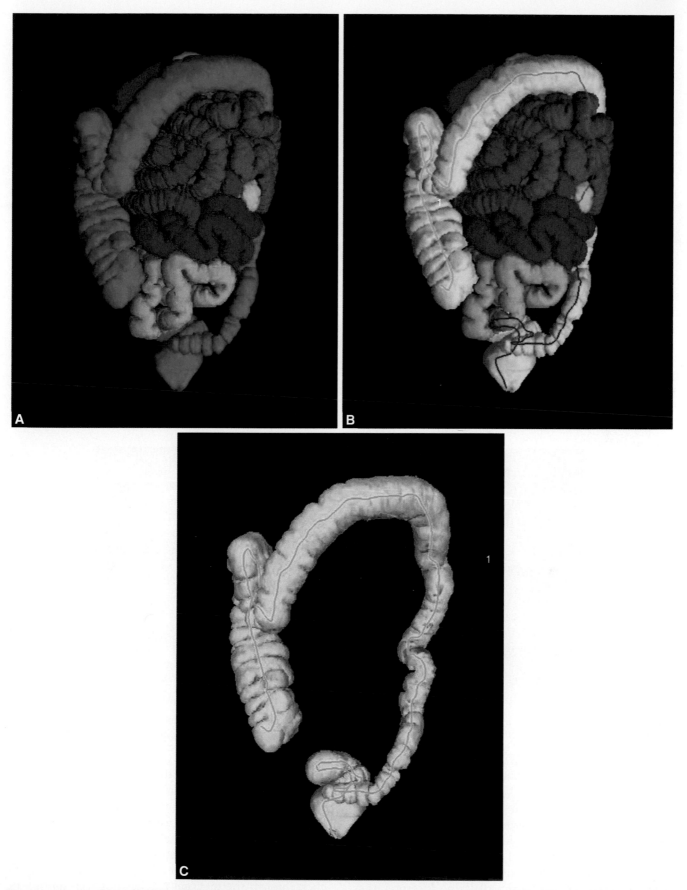

Figure 29-6   Segmentation of the large intestine. The CTC system we use extracts all gas-filled structures **(A)** and provides an automated centerline for each separate color-coded structure. The user simply selects the structures that represent the colon **(B),** which then disregards the rest, leaving behind the colon with an automated centerline for interpretation **(C).**

Illustration continued on following page

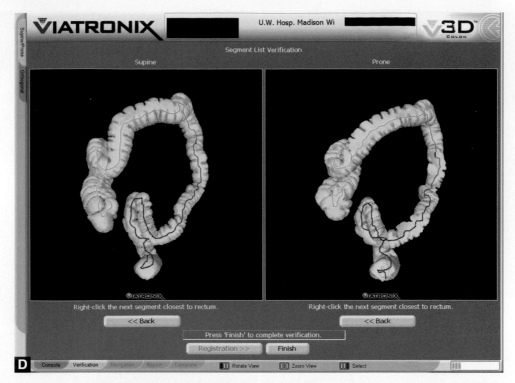

Figure 29-6 (Continued) **Segmentation of the large intestine.** The actual interactive interface **(D)** simultaneously displays both the supine and prone models, which can be rotated in any plane.

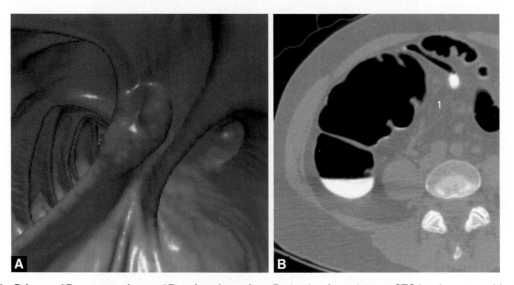

Figure 29-7 Primary 3D versus primary 2D polyp detection. Evaluation for polyps at CTC involves a combination of 3D and 2D displays. The 3D endoluminal view **(A)** increases the conspicuity of polyps among the normal folds. This image shows a normal ilieocecal valve and appendiceal orifice. For 2D evaluation **(B)**, a polyp window setting is used, which consists of a relatively wide width of 2000 HU centered at 0 HU. The use of oral contrast tagging increases accuracy for polyp assessment. For a variety of reasons (discussed in detail in Chapter 17), we favor the 3D display for initial polyp detection and the 2D view for confirmation.

navigation is used, the system continually tracks and updates the fraction of endoluminal surface covered (see Chapter 19). The automated marking of visualized areas not only increases reader confidence, but also avoids the need to start over if interrupted during interpretation. On average, 77% of the luminal surface is seen with uni-

directional flight and 94% for bidirectional flight with a 90-degree FOV.[22] Using the preferred 120-degree FOV, unidirectional coverage increases to about 90%. At this point, a missed region tool allows the reader to rapidly click through the mucosal patches not seen during the initial navigation, which generally increases coverage to

98% to 99% yet consumes only 10 to 20 seconds of interpretation time. The typical flight time from rectum to cecum (or vice versa) along the centerline is on the order of 1 minute for a normal case, with additional time needed to interrogate potential abnormalities. For most screening CTC cases, the entire study can be read in less than 10 minutes, but difficult or frankly positive cases will take longer.

Rapid interrogation of potential lesions detected on 3D can be accomplished by the usual 2D MPR (multiplanar reconstruction) correlation or with 3D translucency rendering, which provides information on the internal density of a lesion.[23] Translucency rendering is best demonstrated by the real-time video clips in the accompanying DVD. When used properly, the translucency rendering tool can decrease interpretation time by reducing the need for 2D confirmation of false positives, particularly tagged stool. The Viatronix V3D system has always allowed for electronic cleansing of the opacified residual luminal fluid and stool,[24] but we must clarify that, unlike the DoD screening trial, we have always kept this function disabled at UW.[1,25] In our experience, the disadvantages of digital fluid subtraction currently outweigh the benefits. The primary potential advantage of electronic fluid cleansing is to increase the degree of actual mucosal coverage per view (supine or prone). However, the subtraction artifacts that are often present at air-fluid-fold interfaces and also created by solid or semisolid material suspended in the fluid represent major diagnostic pitfalls.[24] These artifacts can greatly complicate and prolong the 3D evaluation and were likely a common source of false positives in our screening trial. The improvements to our prep have since resulted in relatively little residual fluid. Coupled with the complementary positional fluid shifts between the supine and prone series, the fluid level rarely overlaps between the two views in our experience.[26] Therefore, combined supine-prone 3D endoluminal evaluation of the gas-filled colon without electronic fluid subtraction reliably covers the entire mucosal surface. Furthermore, polyps are virtually never submerged on both views in our practice because even when a rare fluid overlap is present within a segment, it tends to be minimal (≤1 cm) and extremely unlikely to completely obscure a significant polyp. In addition, the 2D component of the biphasic interpretation ensures complete evaluation in the unusual cases where focal fluid overlap exists. The absence of subtraction artifacts allows for increased 3D endoluminal flight speed, which has doubled since the time of our screening trial, greatly reducing interpretation times.

When a suspicious lesion measuring 5 to 6 mm or greater is detected on 3D (or 2D) and confirmed to be composed of soft tissue on 2D, an electronic bookmark is placed. Of suspected polyps that are indeed real, the vast majority can also be identified on the alternative supine or prone view, which greatly increases overall diagnostic confidence. Our positive predictive value or concordance rate with OC for CTC-detected lesions is greater than 90%,[27] and it is even higher when the diagnostic confidence of the reader is greatest. Accurate linear measurement of polyps is not as straightforward as it may seem. Because the 2D measurement, which should always be optimized among the MPR views, tends to underestimate polyp size and the 3D view can overestimate size in some cases, we have found it useful to take both measurements into account before arriving at a final value.[28] In the future, polyp volume assessment may play a more prominent role because it is a better indicator of actual soft tissue mass present and more sensitive for detecting interval change.[29]

One factor related to CTC interpretation that should not be overlooked or undervalued is the reading environment. At both the National Naval Medical Center and the University of Wisconsin, we fought hard for and were fortunate enough to carve out a sequestered space for reading the CTC examinations. A logical location for a typical large group practice is the "3D lab" where other advanced visualization interpretations are performed. The real key is to be separated from the high-volume traffic of the typical body CT reading room, where the constant interruptions common to our daily practice might prove even more troubling with CTC interpretation. Assuming one is lucky enough to find a relatively isolated space, another feature that has become an ingrained component of our CTC interpretation experience is the luxury of listening to music while "flying." If at all possible in your practice, we highly recommend procuring musical accompaniment.

REPORTING OF RESULTS

The diagnostic algorithm for CTC screening is fairly simple. A screening CTC study is considered positive when any lesion ≥6 mm is detected. It must be emphasized that the polyps of greatest clinical significance will measure ≥10 mm in size. We offer same-day optical colonoscopy to all eligible patients with a positive CTC study, which avoids the need for additional preparation.[3,13,30] However because it is likely that the inherent neoplastic risk of one or two small polyps (6-9 mm) detected at CTC are outweighed by the procedural risks and costs associated with colonoscopic polypectomy, we also offer the option of noninvasive CTC surveillance for this C-RADS 2 category.[31-33] Although we agree with the 3-year surveillance interval recommended by C-RADS,[4] we were initially restricted to a 1- to 2-year followup regimen by our Institutional Review Board. We work closely with our gastroenterology colleagues, particularly with regard to same-day polypectomies. This "one-stop shop" capability ensures complete screening with a single bowel preparation, which greatly enhances patient satisfaction and compliance. We provide the colonoscopist with digital images, including the polyp location on the 3D map, 3D endoluminal projections, and 2D MPR images of the polyp(s). Special note is made of polyps located on the backside of folds, which are more easily missed at OC.[34]

The CTC dictation lends itself well to structured reporting in the form of a template. Our dictation shell includes subheadings for study indication, examination technique, colorectal findings, extracolonic findings, and final impression (Fig. 29-8). Although we use the C-RADS classification for our internal database and recordkeeping, we do not explicitly include this system in the dictated report to clinicians because we feel it unnecessarily complicates the communication. Instead, we simply describe the relevant colorectal and extracolonic findings and make our recommendations. For each relevant colorectal lesion detected at CTC, we report the linear size, segmental location, polyp morphology (pedunculated, sessile, or flat), and diagnostic confidence score for each polyp. For quantifying diagnostic confidence that a polyp is real, we have always used a three-point scale: a score of 3 indicates the highest confidence, 1 indicates the lowest confidence,

and 2 is intermediate. This diagnostic confidence score correlates well with the likelihood of finding a corresponding lesion at CTC and can provide useful information to the gastroenterologist and for program quality assurance.[27,35]

The CTC study is negative if no polyps are identified or if only potential diminutive lesions (≤5 mm) are seen. In these cases, which represent nearly 90% of our screening population, we recommend repeat colorectal screening in approximately 5 years, in concert with the recent American Cancer Society screening guidelines.[36] There are a number of reasons why no comment should be made of possible isolated diminutive lesions. First and foremost, they are simply not clinically relevant, yet their mention may raise undue anxiety in patients and referring physicians.[2,33,37] Furthermore, most diminutive "lesions" detected at CTC cannot be found at subsequent colonoscopy, representing either CTC false positives or colonoscopic false negatives. To avoid any confusion or false pretenses, we include the following disclaimer in all CTC reports: "Note: CT colonography is not intended for the detection of diminutives polyps (≤5 mm), the presence or absence of which will not change the clinical management of the patient" (Fig. 29-8). To date, we have not had a single complaint from our referring physicians regarding this statement. Reporting of extracolonic findings is discussed in detail in Chapters 27 and 28.

After routine screening CTC, individuals generally return to their regular activities, whether that happens to be work, home, or play. They generally have nothing to eat until we contact them within 1 to 2 hours with the polyp results. Given the relatively low positivity rate for asymptomatic screening, we do not have individuals waiting on site for results at our facility. If same-day colonoscopy is needed, arrangements can then be made after ensuring the patient is a suitable candidate and has a safe ride home. Of note, we generally do not communicate the extracolonic findings directly to patients because we feel that this exchange is better handled by the referring physician, who has presumably built a rapport with his or her patients.

Quality assurance is a critical component of any successful screening program, and we therefore take this seriously (see Chapter 28). We closely track our overall positive rate, nondiagnostic rate, OC referral rate, and concordance rate for cases that go on to OC.[27] We feel "concordance rate" is a more appropriate term than "positive predictive value" because we are finding that a significant proportion of discordant cases are ultimately found to be OC false negatives and not CTC false positives. We also make every attempt to follow up on potentially important extracolonic findings to ensure appropriate workup. We track our complication rate, but, at the time of this writing, we have yet to encounter any significant complications at CTC.

UW Screening CT Colonography Dictation Template

INDICATION: Routine colorectal cancer screening. [Revise if other indication]

TECHNIQUE: The patient underwent UW virtual colonoscopy bowel preparation the day before the exam, consisting of oral [magnesium citrate/PEG], 2% barium, and diatrizoate. Following automated carbon dioxide insufflation per rectum, low-dose supine and prone CT images were obtained without IV contrast. Images were sent to the Viatronix V3D workstation for combined 2D-3D evaluation of the colorectum for polyps.

FINDINGS:

COLON: [Comment on quality of prep and distention. Describe size, morphology, and location of any large (≥10 mm) or small (6-9 mm) polyps]

Note: CT colonography is not intended for the detection of diminutive colonic polyps (i.e., tiny polyps ≤5 mm), the presence or absence of which will not change management of the patient.

EXTRACOLONIC: [Note any relevant findings and specify in the impression whether additional work-up should be considered]

Note: Extracolonic evaluation is limited by the low-dose CT technique and the lack of IV contrast.

IMPRESSION: [Include relevant findings and follow-up recommendations]

Figure 29-8 **Dictation template for screening CTC at UW.** This shell includes the basic components of our CTC dictation. The black font provides the basic structure, technique, and caveats standard to most dictations, whereas the blue font provides guidance for mutable components particular to each case.

REFERENCES

1. Pickhardt PJ. Screening CT colonography: How I do it. *Am J Roentgenol.* 2007;189(2):290-298.

2. Pickhardt PJ, Choi JR, Hwang I, et al. Computed tomographic virtual colonoscopy to screen for colorectal neoplasia in asymptomatic adults. *N Engl J Med.* 2003;349(23):2191-2200.

3. Kim DH, Pickhardt PJ, Taylor AJ, et al. CT colonography versus colonoscopy for the detection of advanced neoplasia. *N Engl J Med.* 2007;357(14):1403-1412.

4. Zalis ME, Barish MA, Choi JR, et al. CT colonography reporting and data system: A consensus proposal. *Radiology.* 2005;236(1):3-9.

5. Kim DH, Pickhardt PJ, Hinshaw JL, Taylor AJ, Mukherjee R, Pfau PR. Prospective blinded trial comparing 45-mL and 90-mL doses of oral sodium phosphate for bowel preparation before computed tomographic colonography. *J Comp Assist Tomog.* 2007;31(1):53-58.

6. Van Uitert RL, Summers RM, White JM, Deshpande KK, Choi JR, Pickhardt PJ. Temporal and multiinstitutional quality assessment of CT colonography. *Am J Roentgenol.* 2008;191(5):1503-1508.

7. Agriantonios D, Kim DH, Pickhardt PJ, Hinshaw JL. Bowel preparation for CT colonography: a comparison of sodium phosphate and magnesium citrate. Chicago: RSNA Scientific Assembly; 2008.

8. Pickhardt PJ, Taylor AJ, Johnson GL, et al. Building a CT colonography program: Necessary ingredients for reimbursement and clinical success. *Radiology.* 2005;235(1):17-20.

9. Markowitz GS, Stokes MB, Radhakrishnan J, D'Agati VD. Acute phosphate nephropathy following oral sodium phosphate bowel purgative: An underrecognized cause of chronic renal failure. *J Am Soc Nephrol.* 2005;16(11):3389-3396.

10. O'Connor SD, Summers RM, Choi JR, Pickhardt PJ. Oral contrast adherence to polyps on CT colonography. *J Comp Assist Tomog.* 2006;30(1):51-57.

11. Summers RM, Franaszek M, Miller MT, Pickhardt PJ, Choi JR, Schindler WR. Computer-aided detection of polyps on oral contrast-enhanced CT colonography. *Am J Roentgenol.* 2005;184(1):105-108.

12. Summers RM, Yao JH, Pickhardt PJ, et al. Computed tomographic virtual colonoscopy computer-aided polyp detection in a screening population. *Gastroenterology.* 2005;129(6):1832-1844.

13. Pickhardt PJ. Colonic preparation for computed tomographic colonography: Understanding the relative advantages and disadvantages of a noncathartic approach. *Mayo Clin Proc.* 2007;82(6):659-661.

14. Pickhardt PJ. Incidence of colonic perforation at CT colonography: Review of existing data and implications for screening of asymptomatic adults. *Radiology.* 2006;239(2):313-316.

15. Shinners TJ, Pickhardt PJ, Taylor AJ, Jones DA, Olsen CH. Patient-controlled room air insufflation versus automated carbon dioxide delivery for CT colonography. *Am J Roentgenol.* 2006;186(6):1491-1496.

16. Choi M, Taylor AJ, VonBerge JL, Bartels CM, Pickhardt PJ. Can the CT scout reliably assess for adequate colonic distention at CT colonography? *Am J Roentgenol.* 2005;184(4):21-22.

17. Sosna J, Blachar A, Amitai M, et al. Colonic perforation at CT colonography: Assessment of risk in a multicenter large cohort. *Radiology.* 2006;239(2):457-463.

18. Brenner DJ, Elliston CD. Estimated radiation risks potentially associated with full-body CT screening. *Radiology.* 2004;232(3):735-738.

19. Radiation risk in perspective. Position statement of the Health Physics Society. McLean, VA: Health Physics Society. Adopted January 1996, revised August 2004.

20. Pickhardt PJ, Hanson ME, Vanness DJ, et al. Unsuspected extracolonic findings at screening CT colonography: Clinical and economic impact. *Radiology.* 2008;249(1):151-159.

21. Pickhardt PJ, Schumacher C, Kim DH. Polyp detection at 3D endoluminal CT colonography: sensitivity of one-way fly-through at 120-degree field-of-view angle. *J Comp Assist Tomog.* 2009, in press.

22. Pickhardt PJ, Taylor AJ, Gopal DV. Surface visualization at 3D endoluminal CT colonography: Degree of coverage and implications for polyp detection. *Gastroenterology.* 2006;130(6):1582-1587.

23. Pickhardt PJ. Translucency rendering in 3D endoluminal CT colonography: A useful tool for increasing polyp specificity and decreasing interpretation time. *Am J Roentgenol.* 2004;183(2):429-436.

24. Pickhardt PJ, Choi JHR. Electronic cleansing and stool tagging in CT colonography: Advantages and pitfalls with primary three-dimensional evaluation. *Am J Roentgenol.* 2003;181(3):799-805.

25. Pickhardt PJ. Differential diagnosis of polypoid lesions seen at CT colonography (virtual colonoscopy)—Author's response. *Radiographics.* 2004;24(6):1558-1559.

26. Pickhardt P, Kim D, Taylor A, Husain S. Complementary shifting of luminal fluid between supine and prone positioning at CT colonography: Implications for 3D mucosal coverage. Boston: 8th International VC Symposium; 2007.

27. Wise SM, Pickhardt PJ, Kim DH. Positive predictive value for polyps detected at screening CT colonography. Maui, HI: Annual Meeting for the Society of Gastrointestinal Radiologists; 2009.

28. Pickhardt PJ, Lee AD, McFarland EG, Taylor AJ. Linear polyp measurement at CT colonography: In vitro and in vivo comparison of two-dimensional and three-dimensional displays. *Radiology.* 2005;236(3):872-878.

29. Pickhardt PJ, Lehman VT, Winter TC, Taylor AJ. Polyp volume versus linear size measurements at CT colonography: Implications for noninvasive surveillance of unresected colorectal lesions. *Am J Roentgenol.* 2006;186(6):1605-1610.

30. Pickhardt PJ, Taylor AJ, Kim DH, Reichelderfer M, Gopal DV, Pfau PR. Screening for colorectal neoplasia with CT colonography: Initial experience from the 1st year of coverage by third-party payers. *Radiology.* 2006;241(2):417-425.

31. Pickhardt PJ, Kim DH, Cash BD, Lee AD. The natural history of small polyps at CT colonography. Rancho Mirage, CA: Annual Meeting for the Society of Gastrointestinal Radiologists; 2008.

32. Pickhardt PJ, Hassan C, Laghi A, et al. Clinical management of small (6- to 9-mm) polyps detected at screening CT colonography: A cost-effectiveness analysis. *Am J Roentgenol.* 2008;191(5):1509-1516.

33. Pickhardt PJ, Hassan C, Laghi A, et al. Small and diminutive polyps detected at screening CT colonography: A decision analysis for referral to colonoscopy. *Am J Roentgenol.* 2008;190(1):136-144.

34. Pickhardt PJ, Nugent PA, Mysliwiec PA, Choi JR, Schindler WR. Location of adenomas missed by optical colonoscopy. *Ann Intern Med.* 2004;141(5):352-359.

35. Pickhardt PJ, Choi JR, Nugent PA, Schindler WR. The effect of diagnostic confidence on the probability of optical colonoscopic confirmation of potential polyps detected on CT colonography: Prospective assessment in 1,339 asymptomatic adults. *Am J Roentgenol.* 2004;183(6):1661-1665.

36. Levin B, Lieberman DA, McFarland B, et al. Screening and surveillance for the early detection of colorectal cancer and adenomatous polyps, 2008: A joint guideline from the American Cancer Society, the US Multi-Society Task Force on Colorectal Cancer, and the American College of Radiology. *CA Cancer J Clin.* 2008;58(3):130-160.

37. Bond JH. Clinical relevance of the small colorectal polyp. *Endoscopy.* 2001;33(5):454-457.

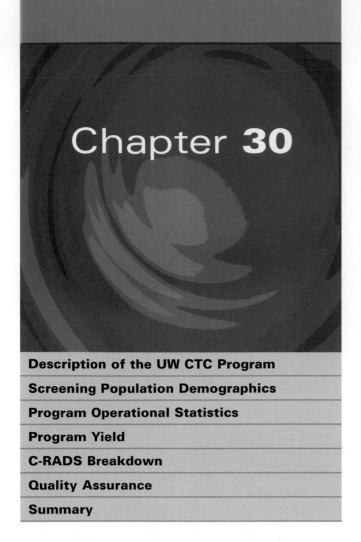

Chapter 30

Description of the UW CTC Program

Screening Population Demographics

Program Operational Statistics

Program Yield

C-RADS Breakdown

Quality Assurance

Summary

CTC Program Results at the University of Wisconsin

DAVID H. KIM, MD

PERRY J. PICKHARDT, MD

INTRODUCTION

Screening of asymptomatic, average-risk healthy individuals by CT colonography (CTC) holds great promise but is currently in fairly limited use in the United States. Except for a few notable exceptions, including the University of Wisconsin (UW) and the National Naval Medical Center, CTC screening is a low-volume endeavor for the majority of health care institutions around the country. The CTC program at UW represents the largest screening experience reimbursed by private third-party payers. This chapter examines the experience and results from an early interim analysis of the first 2000 to 3000 patients of this established CTC screening program. There are currently more than 6000 patients that have enrolled in the program, but even this is simply scratching the surface of potential volume.

DESCRIPTION OF THE UW CTC PROGRAM

The CT Colonography program at the University of Wisconsin has been in existence since April of 2004. The primary mission of the program is to screen average-risk adults of appropriate age by CTC to lower the future incidence of colorectal cancer (CRC). A much smaller

percentage of diagnostic CTC examinations are also performed for a variety of indications (see Chapter 9). The program draws mainly from the surrounding areas of Dane County, Wisconsin, although it also draws a small proportion of individuals from more distant regions because of its national reputation.

The UW CTC program is based within the Department of Radiology and runs in parallel with the gastroenterology-based UW optical colonoscopy (OC) program. Both are well-established clinical programs offered at the University of Wisconsin. Patients, in consultation with their physicians, simply choose one option or the other to undertake CRC screening. The CTC program uses an integrated model with therapeutic colonoscopy, where patients with nondiminutive polyps (≥ 6 mm) at CTC are offered the option of same-day removal at endoscopy. Such a practice model completely avoids the requirement for an additional bowel preparation.

CTC examinations are conducted in outpatient settings at UW regional clinics and on the main hospital campus. The CTC data from the different locations are networked to a central dedicated reading room in the main hospital. Currently, ten examinations slots are available among the various sites between 7:00 am and 10:00 am. The patients are allowed to leave the clinic or hospital immediately following the examination but are given the option to remain fasting until communication of results. The examinations are interpreted with conveyance of final results (in a formal report and verbally to the patient) within a 2-hour window. This allows for referral to colonoscopy for the small fraction of CTC patients who have an appropriately sized polyp. Therapeutic OC is typically performed in the late morning or early afternoon on the same day. The option of enrolling in an Institutional Review Board (IRB)-approved surveillance research protocol is available to patients with one or two small (6-9 mm) polyps (i.e., C-RADS [CT Colonography-Reporting and Data System] category C2). As an initial compromise, the followup interval was set at 2 years for patients with a 6- to 7-mm polyp, whereas for patients with an 8- to 9-mm polyp, the followup CTC was set at 1 year. We hope to expand these intervals as our longitudinal data emerge and demonstrate safety. The consensus C-RADS document reports that extended followup to 3 years is a valid consideration.[1]

The UW CTC program uses a team approach where each member has specific roles to maximize program results. The team is comprised of program nurse coordinators, administrative/data entry personnel, CTC technologists, and radiologists. An extensive database is maintained to allow coordination of clinical activities and research. Program responsibilities include maintenance of patient care lists to allow for scheduling of followup examinations at the appropriate time, resolution of discordant cases where a CTC abnormality is not seen at colonoscopy, and performance of appropriate quality metrics.

SCREENING POPULATION DEMOGRAPHICS

The majority of CTC cases in the UW program are screening in nature, and only a small percentage are diagnostic (<10%). The following population demographics (and program statistics described in following sections) concern only the screening group. The following statistics are based on interim analyses of the program (completed for groups ranging from 2195 to 3120 consecutive patients). These statistics have remained remarkably consistent within in a fairly narrow range since the inception of the program.[2]

The mean age of the CTC screening population seen at UW is 57 years old, with a standard deviation of 7 years. There is a female predominance (56% versus 44%). The vast majority of patients are asymptomatic, with only 2% of patients self-reporting symptomatology. Reported symptoms include changes in bowel habit, blood in stool, anemia, and abdomen pain that may have precipitated the examination. Only a minority (5%) report a positive family history. Consequently, the great majority of screened patients represent average-risk adults. The vast majority of patients are from the Dane county region referred from several primary care physician groups affiliated with the University of Wisconsin.

PROGRAM OPERATIONAL STATISTICS

A positive CTC examination is defined as one that has one or more polyps at least 6 mm in size. Examinations with possible diminutive-only polyps are considered negative. This is in compliance with recommendations outlined in C-RADS, which states that isolated diminutive polyps should not be reported at CTC.[1] The overall positive examination rate for screening at the UW CTC program is 13%. Consequently, the majority of screened patients (87%) are negative and are placed in the routine screening interval currently set at 5 years.[1,3] It is important to emphasize that the majority of patients who undergo CTC screening do not require a referral to colonoscopy. The screening evaluation is completed with a single CTC examination (Fig. 30-1).

Of the positive fraction (13%) potentially eligible for endoscopic referral, about 5% are C-RADS category C3 or C4, for which OC is recommended. The remaining 8% are C-RADS category C2, of which 3% chose immediate colonoscopy for polypectomy and 5% chose imaging surveillance through our IRB-approved research protocol. Therefore, 8% of the total CTC screening cohort undergo OC for polypectomy. Of this 8% fraction, which represents the OC referral rate, about 80% are able to undertake same-day colonoscopy. A small fraction of individuals proceed with colonoscopy at a later date either because of personal preference or an extenuating factor such as an anticoagulated state. In these cases, the patient requires a second bowel preparation prior to the therapeutic OC portion of the screening examination.

From a practical standpoint, this <10% eligible fraction for same-day optical colonoscopy translates into fewer than one referral to the gastrointestinal (GI) endoscopy service per day on average. Infrequently, there will be two referrals to GI in a single day but only very rarely will there be more than two. We highly encourage an integrated model of CTC/OC to allow a screening patient to obtain a complete workup within a single bowel preparation and visit. The alternative of multiple visits covering multiple days off from work is a less optimal situation, particularly because these individuals are often productive, functioning members of society.

The OC concordance rate for the program has remained remarkably constant at more than 90%,[4] despite various protocol changes and addition of CTC readers. We use this measure as a key quality metric of the program. It is a measure of whether a structural correlate exists at OC for a given lesion called at CTC. Structural correlates include not only true mucosal soft tissue polyps such as adenomas and hyperplastic polyps, but also vascular lesions such as venous blebs and deeper lesions such as submucosal masses. Pseudopolyps related to stool are not included as a true structural correlate. The concordance rate should be taken in the context of the OC referral rate. A high concordance rate associated with an OC referral rate in an appropriate range are measures of good program quality (see Chapter 28).

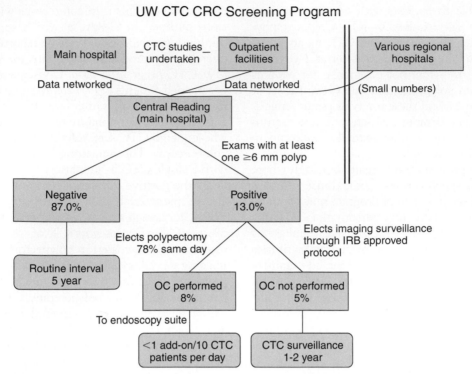

Figure 30-1 UW CTC program workflow. Flowchart demonstrates the overall organization and flow of the program. There are multiple sites where the examination can be conducted, with the data subsequently networked to a single reading area. An integrated model with OC is advocated in which those patients with a positive examination result can undergo therapeutic polypectomy on the same day.

PROGRAM YIELD

Colorectal Results

(Based on an interim program analysis on 3120 consecutive patients.[5])

The overall advanced neoplasia prevalence for the UW CTC screening population was 3.2% (n = 100) not including 158 individuals within a surveillance group. There were a total of 123 advanced neoplasms, including 14 invasive carcinomas. The average size of advanced neoplasms was 18.4 mm. The defining characteristic of advanced neoplasia was a large lesion size because 95% were at least 10 mm in size. Only 6 advanced adenomas in 5 patients were subcentimeter in size (not including the surveillance group). No subcentimeter cancers were present in this group (nor have we seen any subcentimeter cancers since). This yield of 123 advanced neoplasms was obtained through 561 total polypectomies. In comparison, primary OC screening in 3163 patients yielded 121 advanced neoplasms but required 2434 total polypectomies (resulting in 7 perforations).

Regardless of size, the majority of advanced adenomas were tubular adenomas. A significant fraction (34%) were tubulovillous histology, whereas only a small minority (3%) were purely villous. High-grade dysplasia was seen in 6.5%, all in the large category. Advanced adenomas were seen throughout the colon, with 40% proximal to the splenic flexure. Sessile and pedunculated morphol-

ogy accounted for the majority of advanced lesions (79%), with flat lesions accounting for a small minority. Serrated adenomas were infrequent at 3% of advanced neoplasia. Serrated adenomas were large, with an average size of 26 mm. Only one serrated adenoma contained high-grade dysplasia. Carpet lesions were seen in approximately 1 in every 500 patients or 0.2%, typically presenting as lesions larger than 50 mm. Carpet lesions were predominantly seen in either the rectum or cecum, correlating well with a prior barium enema era series.[6] They usually contained a significant villous component, some had high-grade dysplasia, and a small minority were malignant.

The overall prevalence for invasive carcinoma in our screening cohort has been about 0.2% to 0.3%, corresponding to approximately 1 unsuspected CRC for every 400 to 500 CTC screening examinations. The average size of CRC was 34 mm, presenting as large masses.

By this interim analysis, there were 158 patients in the CTC surveillance group harboring 193 polyps. Fifty-four patients with 70 polyps had returned for interval followup. Of this group, 67 polyps (96%) remained stable or regressed, and 3 increased in size. None had crossed the 10-mm threshold. Colonoscopic removal of the enlarging polyps revealed 3 tubular adenomas. No advanced adenomas were present within this group, nor were there cases of high-grade dysplasia or carcinoma in these preliminary results. Since this analysis, a substantial amount of surveillance data has accrued and is the primary topic of future investigations by our research group.

Extracolonic Results

(Based on an interim program analysis on 2195 consecutive patients.)[7]

The issue of extracolonic findings is a double-edged sword with both potential benefits and negative consequences (see Chapter 27). On the positive side, CTC can detect significant diagnoses such as unsuspected extracolonic cancers or aortic aneurysms to benefit the individual. On the negative side, it can unleash an imaging cascade for an ultimately benign finding, which can increase costs and anxiety and expose the person to potential complications. It is imperative that CTC programs handle this issue judiciously and consistently. The application of C-RADS will be a key to maintain quality and consistency between readers for the specific program.

In terms of the UW experience, the vast majority of CTC examinations (>90%) are negative for extracolonic findings or detect a finding of no consequence. It is important to realize that a CTC reader must feel comfortable in diagnosing benign lesions on this low-dose, noncontrast examination. If a radiologist is uncomfortable calling a benign cyst because of the limited technique, this would lead to unacceptable rates for correlative imaging. In the UW experience, we suggest further evaluation in less than 10% of patients (8.6% for the subgroup of 2195 consecutive screening patients). This has led to approximately 6% of patients who were ultimately worked up, with about 2.5% ultimately receiving a relevant new diagnoses, including a handful of extracolonic cancers (n = 9 for the 2195 group) and vascular aneurysms (n = 12). A large fraction of relevant diagnoses that ultimately were determined to be benign were related to adnexal cystic masses in females. The mean cost per patient for nonsurgical procedures has been calculated at an additional $31.02.

C-RADS BREAKDOWN

C-Category Percentages in C-RADS

The C-RADS C-category breakdown has remained stable over the experience of our program (Fig. 30-2). These percentages are helpful to calculate at regular intervals to confirm that there are not radical changes in percentages that may be a reflection of changing quality. Our C0 rate is less than 1%, which corresponds to nondiagnostic cases. The vast majority of examinations are in the C1 category (approximately 87%) and thus are negative. These patients are placed in the routine screening interval, which is currently set at 5 years. About 13% of cases are positive, ranging from C-RADS category C2 to C4. Of the

C2 category (7% to 8%), fewer than half (3%) choose polypectomy, whereas the majority elect imaging surveillance. Ultimately, approximately 8% undergo polypectomy, with 5% from the C3 and C4 categories.

E-Category Percentages in C-RADS

In a similar fashion, the C-RADS E-category breakdown has also been fairly stable throughout our program's existence (Fig. 30-3). As with the C categories, it is important to calculate these percentages at regular intervals to ensure that they remain in appropriate ranges. Particularly, it is important to assess for increasing E3 percentages, which may indicate a shift in interpretation where an individual is overcalling. In terms of extracolonic evaluation, the majority of examinations do not require additional workup because they reside in either the E1 or E2 category (90% combined). About 10% hold either E3 or E4 status, possibly requiring additional evaluation. The majority are E3 examinations (nearly 8%). As stated previously, about 2% to 3% are ultimately found to have a clinically relevant finding.

QUALITY ASSURANCE

The nondiagnostic rate encompassed by the C0 category for the UW program started out at about 1% and has continued to drop. The vast majority of completed examinations are thus interpretable. There are two main reasons for a nondiagnostic CTC examination: (1) because of a poor bowel prep in which there is too much untagged stool or (2) because of a persistently collapsed segment despite various maneuvers and additional series. In the case of

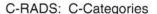

C-RADS: C-Categories

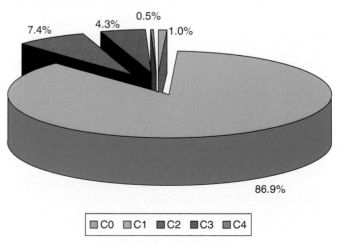

Figure 30-2 C-RADS C categories. Pie diagram demonstrates the percentage breakdown of the various C categories of C-RADS for the early UW CTC experience. These numbers have remained remarkably stable ever since.

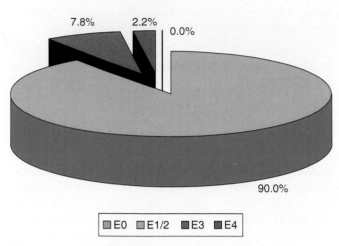

C-RADS: E-Categories

7.8%   2.2%   0.0%

90.0%

■ E0   ■ E1/2   ■ E3   ■ E4

Figure 30-3   C-RADS E categories. Pie diagram demonstrates the percentage breakdown of the various E categories of C-RADS for the early UW experience. As with the colonic breakdown, these numbers have remained remarkably stable.

poor bowel preparation, it is important to remember that even a large amount of *tagged* stool can still result in a diagnostic examination. It requires a predominantly two-dimensional (2D) approach (a 3D approach is precluded in this situation) with likely decreased sensitivities but can still be undertaken, as opposed to the untagged situation, in which adherent stool more easily mimics a soft tissue lesion. For the situation of a collapsed segment, it is important to remember that the vast majority of the colon has been evaluated. Often, it is only a short segment of sigmoid colon that cannot be adequately assessed and may need to be cleared by sigmoidoscopy. One of the key factors that has allowed us to maintain such a low nondiagnostic rate has been related to our programmatic approach to CTC. Our program coordinator is proactive in discussing with patients how to undertake the bowel preparation

and spends a considerable amount of time answering various questions. Similarly, our CTC technologists take great pride in problem solving to ensure that distention is adequate, particularly concerning the sigmoid colon.

Other quality metrics include the discordant case rate. These represent cases where a polyp called at CTC is not seen at OC. It is important to realize that these do not necessarily represent CTC false positives. It is just as likely that the finding represents an OC false negative. It is important to review these cases, and we regularly hold a discordant case conference to discuss management (e.g., does the patient require a repeat CTC, or is the consensus that it truly represents a CTC false positive?). The rate of discordant cases at UW is about 1% of all cases. Excluding about 20% of the cases currently in the process of discordant status resolution, CTC was ultimately correct (i.e., OC false negative) in approximately 30% of the cases, whereas OC was presumed to be correct for nearly 50% of the discordant cases.

The complication rate is extremely low for CTC. To date, no significant complications (e.g., perforations) have been encountered in our program's entire existence.

SUMMARY

It is hoped that the UW CTC program can serve as a prototype for developing CTC screening programs throughout the United States. An integrated model with therapeutic colonoscopy is favored to allow the small fraction of patients with significant positive results to complete their screening evaluation within a single visit. A team approach is needed to undertake the requirements of an effective screening program. The program is responsible for patients in followup, and various quality metrics should be applied at regular intervals. It is our hope that a network of similarly constructed CTC screening programs throughout the country will likely have a major impact on the prevalence of this wholly preventable cancer.

REFERENCES

1. Zalis ME, Barish MA, Choi JR, et al. CT colonography reporting and data system: A consensus proposal. *Radiology.* 2005;236(1):3-9.
2. Pickhardt PJ, Taylor AJ, Kim DH, Reichelderfer M, Gopal DV, Pfau PR. Screening for colorectal neoplasia with CT colonography: Initial experience from the 1st year of coverage by third-party payers. *Radiology.* 2006;241(2):417-425.
3. Levin B, Lieberman DA, McFarland B, et al. Screening and surveillance for the early detection of colorectal cancer and adenomatous polyps, 2008: A joint guideline from the American Cancer Society, the US Multi-Society Task Force on Colorectal Cancer, and the American College of Radiology. *CA Cancer J Clin.* 2008;58(3):130-160.
4. Wise SM, Pickhardt PJ, Kim DH. Positive predictive value for polyps detected at screening CT colonography. Maui, HI: Annual meeting for the Society of Gastrointestinal Radiologists; 2009.
5. Kim DH, Pickhardt PJ, Taylor AJ, et al. CT colonography versus colonoscopy for the detection of advanced neoplasia. *N Engl J Med.* 2007;357(14):1403-1412.
6. Rubesin SE, Saul SH, Laufer I, Levine MS. Carpet lesions of the colon. *Radiographics.* 1985;5(4):537-552.
7. Pickhardt PJ, Hanson ME, Vanness DJ, et al. Unsuspected extracolonic findings at screening CT colonography: Clinical and economic impact. *Radiology.* 2008;249(1):151-159.

Index